# Ovarian Endocrinology

# Ovarian Endocrinology

EDITED BY STEPHEN G. HILLIER

SENIOR LECTURER AND DIRECTOR
REPRODUCTIVE ENDOCRINOLOGY LABORATORY
DEPARTMENT OF OBSTETRICS
AND GYNAECOLOGY
UNIVERSITY OF EDINBURGH
CENTRE FOR REPRODUCTIVE BIOLOGY

OXFORD
BLACKWELL SCIENTIFIC PUBLICATIONS
LONDON EDINBURGH BOSTON
MELBOURNE PARIS BERLIN VIENNA

© 1991 by
Blackwell Scientific Publications
Editorial Offices:
Osney Mead, Oxford OX2 0EL
25 John Street, London WC1N 2BL
23 Ainslie Place, Edinburgh EH3 6AJ
3 Cambridge Center, Cambridge,
  Massachusetts 02142, USA
54 University Street, Carlton
  Victoria 3053, Australia

Other Editorial Offices:
Arnette SA
2, rue Casimir-Delavigne
75006 Paris
France

Blackwell Wissenschaft
Meinekestrasse 4
D-1000 Berlin 15
Germany

Blackwell MZV
Feldgasse 13
A-1238 Wien
Austria

First published 1991

Set by Setrite Typesetters, Hong Kong
Printed and bound in Great Britain by
Hartnolls Ltd, Bodmin, Cornwall

DISTRIBUTORS

Marston Book Services Ltd
PO Box 87
Oxford OX2 0DT
(*Orders*: Tel: 0865 791155
          Fax: 0865 791927
          Telex: 837515)

USA
Mosby-Year Book, Inc.
11830 Westline Industrial Drive
St Louis, Missouri 63141
(*Orders*: Tel: (800) 633−6699)

Canada
Mosby-Year Book Inc.
5240 Finch Avenue East
Scarborough, Ontario
(*Orders*: Tel: (416) 298−1588)

Australia
Blackwell Scientific Publications
(Australia) Pty Ltd
54 University Street
Carlton, Victoria 3053
(*Orders*: Tel: (03) 347−0300)

British Library
Cataloguing in Publication Data

Ovarian endocrinology.
 1. Medicine. Endocrinology
 I. Hillier, Stephen G.
 616.4

ISBN 0−632−02732−0

# Contents

# List of Contributors

R.F. ATEN PhD, *Reproductive Biology Section, Departments of Obstetrics and Gynecology, and Pharmacology, Yale University School of Medicine, New Haven, Connecticut, USA*

D.T. BAIRD DSc, FRCP(Ed), FRCOG, FRSE, *Department of Obstetrics and Gynaecology, University of Edinburgh Centre for Reproductive Biology, 37 Chalmers Street, Edinburgh EH3 9EW, UK*

H.R. BEHRMAN PhD, *Reproductive Biology Section, Departments of Obstetrics and Gynecology, and Pharmacology, Yale University School of Medicine, New Haven, Connecticut, USA*

M. BRÄNNSTRÖM MD, PhD, *Departments of Physiology, and Obstetrics and Gynaecology, University of Göteburg, Sweden*

B.R. CARR MD, *Department of Obstetrics and Gynecology, University of Texas Southwestern Medical Center at Dallas, 5323 Harry Hines Boulevard, Dallas, Texas 75235, USA*

K.J. DOODY MD, *Department of Obstetrics and Gynecology, University of Texas Southwestern Medical Center at Dallas, 5323 Harry Hines Boulevard, Dallas, Texas 75235, USA*

J.J. EPPIG PhD, *The Jackson Laboratory, Bar Harbor, Maine 04609, USA*

S. FRANKS MD, FRCP, *Department of Obstetrics and Gynaecology, St. Mary's Hospital Medical School, London W2 1PG, UK*

D.L. HEALY PhD, FRACOG, *Infertility Medical Centre, 62 Erin Street, Richmond, Victoria 3121, Australia*

S.G. HILLIER PhD, MRCPath, *Reproductive Endocrinology Laboratory, Department of Obstetrics and Gynaecology, University of Edinburgh Centre for Reproductive Biology, 37 Chalmers Street, Edinburgh EH3 9EW, UK*

P.O. JANSON MD, PhD, *Departments of Physiology, and Obstetrics and Gynaecology, University of Göteburg, Sweden*

W.L. MILLER MD, PhD, *Department of Pediatrics, University of California, San Francisco, California, 94143, USA*

**J.R. PEPPERELL** PhD, *Reproductive Biology Section, Departments of Obstetrics and Gynecology, and Pharmacology, Yale University School of Medicine, New Haven, Connecticut, USA*

**D.W. POLSON** MD, MRCOG, *Department of Obstetrics and Gynaecology, Withington Hospital, Nell Lane, West Didsbury, Manchester M20 8LR, UK*

**J.F. STRAUSS** III, MD, PhD, *Department of Obstetrics and Gynecology, University of Pennsylvania, School of Medicine, Philadelphia, Pennsylvania 19104, USA*

**A.J. ZELEZNIK** PhD, *Departments of Physiology and Obstetrics and Gynecology, University of Pittsburgh School of Medicine, Magee-Womens Hospital, Pittsburgh, Pennsylvania 15213, USA*

# Preface

Current impetus to research ovarian endocrinology can be traced back to two seminally important developments in reproductive medicine which occurred during the late 1970s. First, gene sequencing and cloning using recombinant DNA techniques. Significantly, the first human gene to be synthesized and cloned was a hormone: insulin. During the 1980s, myriad protein hormones, steroidogenic enzymes, 'growth factors' and receptors have been cloned and their molecular structures elucidated. Of particular relevance to reproductive endocrinology, the molecular approach has spawned fundamental insights on the structures of gonadotrophins and their receptors, steroidogenic enzymes and steroid receptors as well as providing new experimental tools with which to study mechanisms of hormone production and action at the cellular level. Armed with such tools, the mysteries of the ovarian 'black box' are beginning to be unravelled and it is now realistic to approach an understanding of the ovarian cycle—follicular growth/atresia, ovulation and luteinization—from the perspective of developmental biology, asking 'What are the factors which control the proliferation, differentiation and death of follicular somatic cells?' and 'How do these cells regulate oocyte development (and vice versa)?' Second, 'test-tube babies': although the first live baby arising out of *in vitro* fertilization (IVF) and embryo transfer involved a single oocyte collected during a spontaneous ovarian cycle, it immediately became apparent that transfer to the uterus of multiple embryos is necessary to maximize the chances of treatment success. The subsequent 'test-tube baby' explosion (estimated at over 20 000 live births world-wide by 1989) was fuelled by the use of ovarian stimulation therapy with exogenous gonadotrophins to override patients' spontaneous ovarian function and facilitate recovery of multiple oocytes for IVF and embryo transfer. Thus, the success of most contemporary forms of assisted reproduction (IVF, gamete-intrafallopian transfer [GIFT], ovulation induction, etc.) relies upon an ability, safely and predictably, to achieve controlled ovarian stimulation. This requirement has focused the attention of clinicians and scientists on the fundamentals of gonadotrophin action, encouraging a re-evaluation of the therapeutic strategies available for manipulating ovarian function: not only to bring about multiple follicular development in IVF/GIFT patients but also to treat more effectively women with ovulatory disorders in whom the aim is to stimulate maturation and ovulation of a single follicle so that conception might occur *in vivo*.

The molecular biology and 'test-tube baby' explosions have now come together to create a further development in reproductive medicine which will have its impact during the coming decade. The gonadotrophins follicle-stimulating hormone (FSH) and luteinizing hormone (LH) were first isolated in more or less pure forms over half a century ago. Purified pituitary gonadotrophins were used by Fevold and Greep *et al.* in their classic experiments which demonstrated unequivocally the need for both FSH and LH to stimulate ovarian follicular development and oestrogen secretion in hypophysectomized rats. Human pituitary gonadotrophins of equivalent purity have never been widely available for clinical use, but within the next few years pharmaceutical grades of human recombinant FSH and LH are both likely to become so. Taking account of recent advances in our understanding of gonadotrophin action at the cellular level, it should be possible to use these pure human gonadotrophins to devise improved strategies for stimulating ovarian function in infertile women.

It was with these thoughts in mind that I set out to structure a book from the perspectives of a select group of internationally renowned scientists and clinicians who are themselves generating, teaching and applying contemporary knowledge of ovarian endocrinology. My editorial role was greatly aided by the helpful co-operation of the contributors and the able assistance of my secretary Mrs Carol Irvine and Ms Karen Anthony of Book Production at Blackwell Scientific Publications. During preparation of the book, work in my own research laboratory was generously supported by the Wellcome Trust. As with any book of its sort, this one will be out of date by the time it is published. But the chapters it contains are authoritative if not exhaustive reviews which document current state-of-the-art and hint at directions in which research and clinical practice are likely to move during the decade ahead.

SGH
*Edinburgh, August, 1990*

# 1 The Ovarian Cycle

D.T. BAIRD

## Introduction

Hidden within the abdominal cavity protected from insults of the environment and trauma, the ovaries contain the genetic material which is passed on to future generations. These organs are unique amongst the glands of internal secretion in that their primary function is to produce gametes and all their endocrine activities subserve this function. The ovarian cycle is designed to ensure that mature female gametes (oocytes) are produced in good condition in the appropriate number at ovulation so that they are available for fertilization by sperm. Thus, in most species sexual behaviour is regulated by the cyclical secretion of ovarian hormones, which ensure that mating occurs at the appropriate time when eggs are ovulated. Human beings are an exception to this rule, which is one of the reasons for their relatively low fecundability. While the development of internal fertilization and viviparity in mammals is much less wasteful than external reproduction as utilized by birds and fish, it has imposed severe constraints. There is a finite number of offspring which can be carried through pregnancy and successfully reared after birth, and the number of eggs ovulated in each species must match accurately the optimal number of young. In every species the number of oocytes present in the ovaries greatly exceeds the number ovulated and hence a rigorous system of selection operates throughout the ovarian cycle.

Because the survival of the species depends on successful reproduction, the selection pressures to ensure the efficient working of this system are severe. The ovary secretes hormones which stimulate target

1   THE OVARIAN CYCLE

organs in the uterus, tubes and breasts as well as in the pituitary and certain parts of the brain. The correct functioning of the ovaries depends on a complex feedback mechanism involving the hypothalamus and anterior pituitary which ensures that development of egg-bearing follicles proceeds in an orderly manner. While the basic neuroendocrine mechanisms are similar in all mammals, each species has adapted the way in which the system is used to meet its specific requirements. For example, many species which inhabit areas of the Earth far from the Equator and, hence, are exposed to the stresses of cold and shortage of food during the winter, have evolved a system where the pattern of reproductive activity is influenced considerably by day length (Lincoln & Short, 1980). This seasonal change in reproductive activity is mediated by recognition of the change in day length via the retina and pineal gland. A similar photoperiod mechanism also exists in those animals which, like human beings, show little seasonal change in reproductive activity but it does not totally dominate the intrinsic rhythm.

The ovarian cycle is a means of restoring potential fertility after a sterile mating. In most mammals this is an infrequent occurrence but in present Western society with widespread use of contraception, repeated ovarian cycles and menstrual cycles are the norm. Morbidity associated with painful, heavy menses is extremely common and it has been suggested that the high incidence of cancer of the breast, endometrium and ovary may be due in part to cyclical stimulation of the target organs by oestrogen during repeated ovarian cycles (Doll, 1975).

The aim of this chapter is to provide an overview of the endocrine control of the ovarian cycle in women. Mention will be made of other primates where experimental evidence is available.

## Folliculogenesis

The ovaries are paired organs situated in the abdominal cavity and in women weigh c. 8 g each. Primordial follicles derived from gut mesentery are laid down in fetal life and persist scattered throughout the adult ovary mainly in the cortex (Baker, 1982). By a mechanism which is poorly understood a given number of oocytes is recruited each day for development — the process known as folliculogenesis. The initial stages of folliculogenesis are not dependent on gonadotrophins because they continue following hypophysectomy. However, by the time an antrum is formed (in women at a follicular diameter of c. 0.2 mm diameter) both follicle-stimulating hormone (FSH) and luteinizing hormone (LH) are required although the relative amounts probably vary depending on the stage of development.

The whole process of folliculogenesis in man takes approximately 6 months and occurs continually throughout life until the stock of oocytes is exhausted (Gougeon, 1982). The majority of follicles never ovulate and undergo atresia with the theca layers being restored to stroma (Peters & McNatty, 1980). The final 14 days of follicular development occur during the first half of the menstrual cycle and is totally dependent on the endocrine interaction of the ovary with the hypothalamo−pituitary unit.

Current evidence suggests that the follicle which will eventually ovulate is between 2 and 4 mm diameter at the beginning of each cycle (Baird, 1985). In women small antral follicles (≤5 mm diameter) have relatively low aromatase activity and, hence, the environment of small follicles is largely androgenic Fig. 1.1. Androgens have been shown to exert modulatory effects on granulosa cell function and in immature follicles they augment the ability of FSH to stimulate the production of cyclic adenosine monophosphate (cAMP) (Hillier, 1985). Any granulosa cell function which is mediated via an increase in intracellular cAMP is therefore susceptible to augmentation by androgens. One such function is the aromatization of androgens to oestrogen which is catalysed by the steroidogenic enzyme cytochrome P450aro (aromatase). The intercycle rise in the concentration of FSH stimulates aromatase activity in the granulosa cells of the small antral follicle which is then able to convert androstenedione and testosterone to oestradiol (Fig. 1.1). Thus the crucial factor in selecting or 'activating' the chosen follicle is the rise in FSH concentration. Further details of the cellular basis of FSH action on the ovary are given in Chapter 3.

The rise in the concentration of FSH as measured by radioimmunoassay is variable between individual women and appears modest (Fig. 1.2). Recent measurements of the bioactive FSH in serum have demonstrated a much more impressive rise in the concentration of FSH after luteal regression with a corresponding steep decline in the follicular phase of the cycle (Jia *et al.*, 1986; Reddi *et al.*, 1990) (Fig. 1.3). In the sera of women there are a large number of forms of FSH which

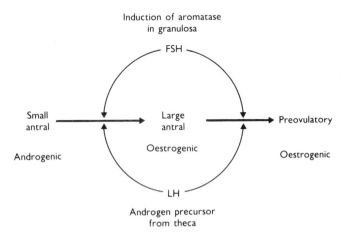

**Fig. 1.1.** Schematic representation of the development of a small antral follicle (<5 mm) to a large preovulatory follicle (20−25 mm). Both FSH and LH play a role in increasing the capacity to produce oestradiol.

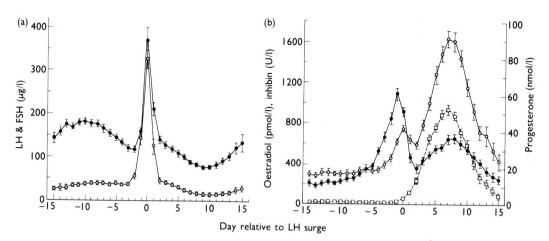

**Fig. 1.2.** Serum levels of gonadotrophins, ovarian steroids and inhibin during the menstrual cycle. (a) LH (○) and FSH (●); (b) inhibin (○), oestradiol (●) and progesterone (□). Results (mean±SEM) of assays on 33 normal women are normalized around the day of the LH surge (day 0). Reproduced with permission from McLachlan *et al.* (1990).

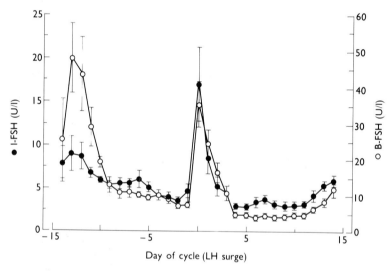

**Fig. 1.3.** Plasma immunoactive and bioactive FSH levels throughout the menstrual cycle (*n*=5). Immunoactive FSH (●) was determined by conventional radio-immunoassay, bioactive FSH (○) was determined by a modification of the rat granulosa cell bioassay initially described by Jia *et al.* (1986); both assays were standardized against the second International Reference Preparation (78/549). Results (mean±SEM) of assays on five normal volunteers are given relative to the day of the mid-cycle LH surge (day 0). Data reproduced with permission from Reddi *et al.* (1990).

differ in their change and, hence, biological activity (Wide, 1982). It may be that this change in the ratio of bio- to immunoactivity reflects differences in the forms of FSH.

Both theca and granulosa cells are involved in the synthesis of oestradiol by the antral follicle. Androstenedione and testosterone are produced by the theca interna cells under the stimulation of LH. These androgens are used as precursors for the synthesis of oestradiol by the granulosa cells. Most available evidence now suggests that the granulosa cells are the major (perhaps sole) source of oestrogen synthesis in the follicle (Dorrington & Armstrong, 1979). Although it was shown originally that preparations of theca cells were capable of synthesizing oestradiol *in vitro*, it was not possible to exclude some contamination with granulosa cells (Ryan & Petro, 1966). It has been calculated that over 99% of aromatase activity resides in the granulosa cells (Hillier *et al.*, 1981) and immunocytochemical techniques have since confirmed that aromatase is confined to the granulosa cell layers (Sasano *et al.*, 1989).

However, the amount of oestradiol secreted by the follicle is determined by both FSH and LH. FSH stimulates the aromatase activity of the granulosa cells antral follicles while LH stimulates the production of androgen precursors by the thecal layer. In this way the granulosa cells of small antral follicles are activated so that they can fully utilize the increased amount of androgen produced by the theca in response to the rise in LH, which also occurs following regression of the corpus luteum.

## Selection of the preovulatory follicle

The mechanism by which small follicles are selected for preovulatory development is not fully understood. In women there are up to 20 small antral follicles (2−5 mm diameter) distributed between the two ovaries at the time of luteal regression (McNatty, 1982; Baird, 1988). From this pool a single follicle is selected for further development while the remainder undergo regression. It may be that although these follicles are of similar size they are all at slightly different stages of development and that only one is at the optimal stage to benefit from the gonadotrophic environment which exists following regression of the corpus luteum, that is a high level of FSH and LH. In species like rats and pigs, it must be assumed that the development of several follicles is nearly synchronous so that multiple ovulation can occur (Fig. 1.4).

FSH plays a crucial role in this selection process. Large healthy antral follicles in women all contain detectable amounts of FSH while those with undetectable levels have much lower levels of oestrogen (McNatty & Baird, 1978). It has been suggested that local paracrine factors may play a role in selecting the dominant follicle (Goodman & Hodgen, 1983; Tonetta & DiZerega, 1989). While locally produced steroidal and non-steroidal factors probably modulate the responsiveness of the ovarian cells to gonadotrophins (see Chapter 3), it seems likely that the overriding mechanism involves classical blood-borne hormones. The fact that suppression of the development of secondary follicles

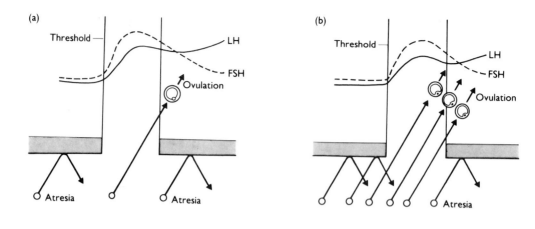

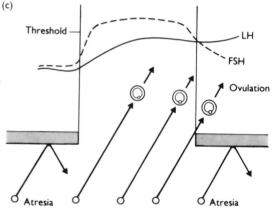

**Fig. 1.4.** Model for selection of the dominant follicle in the early follicular phase of the cycle. Only those small follicles which are at the optimal stage of development to benefit from the intercycle rise in FSH pass through the 'gate' and on to ovulation. Multiple ovulation can be produced by widening the gate or providing a greater number of synchronous follicles. (a) Single ovulation; (b) multiple ovulation — more follicles; (c) multiple ovulation — wider gate. Reproduced with permission from Baird (1987).

occurs in both ovaries equally, is incompatible with the suggestion that progesterone or any other factor diffusing locally from the corpus luteum suppresses or stimulates the selection of the dominant follicle (Baird, 1988).

Once selected, the chosen follicle ensures that development of further follicles is suppressed. Current evidence suggests that this dominance is effected by the suppression of FSH secretion due to the rise in levels of oestradiol secreted by the dominant follicle (Baird, 1987). Following enucleation of the dominant follicle, a period equivalent to the length of a normal follicular phase (12–14 days) elapses before ovulation occurs, indicating that a new small antral follicle requires to be recruited (Nilsson et al., 1982; Tonetta & DiZerega, 1989). If the level of oestrogen is raised prematurely in the early follicular phase (Vaitukaitis et al., 1971; Van Look et al., 1977a; Zeleznik, 1981) the concentration of FSH falls and development of the dominant follicle ceases, an effect which can be reversed by simultaneous administration of the antioestrogen clomiphene citrate. In rhesus monkeys a similar delay in follicular recruitment is seen when the concentration of FSH is suppressed by the administration of porcine follicular fluid containing large amounts of inhibin (Channing *et al.*, 1982). Although these experiments demonstrate that inhibin can suppress FSH, the fall in FSH during the follicular phase of the cycle occurs without any change in the secretion of inhibin and is more likely to be due to the rising levels of oestradiol (see Fig. 1.2).

As the follicle which will eventually ovulate approaches a diameter of about 10 mm, it begins to secrete increasing amounts of oestradiol. The concentration of oestradiol in venous blood draining the ovary containing the dominant follicle is 20-fold higher than that draining the contralateral side indicating that over 95% of the oestradiol produced in the follicular phase of the cycle is secreted by the preovulatory follicle (Baird & Fraser, 1975). Thus, by the mid-follicular phase the selected dominant follicle has a monopoly of the endocrine signals from the ovary and is able to dictate to the hypothalamo—pituitary unit the secretion of gonadotrophins which are optimal for its further development. In the sections which follow we shall consider the way in which these feedback mechanisms operate.

## Control of gonadotrophin secretion

Ovarian cyclicity is controlled by a feedback system involving the hypothalamus, anterior pituitary and the ovaries (Harris & Naftolin, 1970; Knobil, 1980) (Fig. 1.5) FSH and LH are secreted by the same cell in the anterior pituitary in response to stimulation by gonadotrophin-releasing hormone (GnRH) which interacts with specific receptors on the surface of the gonadotroph.

### Feedback functions of steroids and inhibin

Ovarian steroids feedback at the level of both the hypothalamus and anterior pituitary to regulate the secretion of gonadotrophins. The main ovarian steroids are oestradiol and progesterone, specific receptors for which are located in the hypothalamus and anterior pituitary. In recent years it has become apparent that the ovary secretes a protein hormone, inhibin, which inhibits the secretion of FSH selectively by interacting at the level of the anterior pituitary (de Jong, 1987; Burger *et al.*, 1987).

Inhibin is a glycoprotein composed of two subunits α and β linked together by disulphide bonds (Burger *et al.*, 1987). Two separate genes encode for each subunit both of which are derived from much larger precursors. Following cloning of the genes for inhibin the amino acid sequences of the protein were deduced and it was found that the smallest active molecule is *c.* 32 kDa (Mason *et al.*, 1985). The mechanism by which inhibin suppresses FSH is not clearly understood although it is known to inhibit the synthesis of FSH as well as its release.

Inhibin has been measured in human plasma using both bioassay

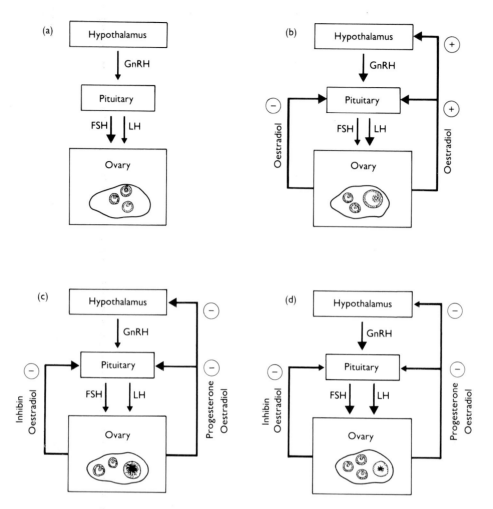

**Fig. 1.5.** Diagrammatic representation of the status of the hypothalamo−pituitary−
ovarian axis at progressive stages of the human ovarian cycle. (a) Early follicular phase:
at the beginning of the cycle both ovaries contain multiple immature follicles (<5 mm
diameter) therefore secretion of oestradiol is minimal. Pituitary secretion of LH and FSH
is raised (FSH greater than LH) due to withdrawal of the combined negative feedback
action of progesterone, oestradiol and inhibin produced by the previous corpus luteum.
The raised level of FSH stimulates the development of medium-sized follicles (≥5 mm)
and 'activates' oestrogen biosynthesis. (b) Late follicular phase: the preovulatory follicle
once selected (see Fig. 1.4) secretes oestradiol which exerts positive feedback control
over pituitary LH release and negative control over FSH. (c) Early luteal phase: after the
ovulation-inducing gonadotrophin surge, progesterone and oestradiol secreted by the
corpus luteum negatively regulate pituitary LH secretion. The corpus luteum also
secretes inhibin which acts jointly with oestradiol to suppress pituitary FSH release and
thereby suppress the growth of medium-sized antral follicles. (d) Late luteal phase: if
pregnancy is not initiated, the corpus luteum begins to undergo functional and structural
regression. As the combined negative feedback actions of luteal steroids and inhibin are
withdrawn, gonadotrophin levels adequate to sustain the growth of medium-sized antral
follicles are restored.

and immunoassay (Tsonis *et al.*, 1986; McLachlan *et al.*, 1987a, b). The concentration of inhibin is higher in ovarian venous than in peripheral blood indicating that it is secreted by the ovary (Illingworth *et al.*, 1989). Following oophorectomy the concentration falls to very low levels although the rate of fall is very slow due to an extremely long half-life (almost 24 h). Thus in adult women the ovary is the major (if not sole) source of inhibin which circulates in the blood stream although it is possible that it is produced by other organs in the body where it acts locally.

The concentration of inhibin in blood shows characteristic fluctuations throughout the cycle (McLachlan *et al.*, 1987a; 1990; Tsonis, McNeilly & Baird, 1987; Reddi *et al.*, 1990) (Fig. 1.2). During the follicular phase of the cycle the concentration remains fairly constant until within 2 or 3 days of ovulation. There is a peak coincidental to the preovulatory LH surge, followed by a dip and a marked rise in concentration during the luteal phase. The origin of this luteal phase rise is the corpus luteum, as indicated by the fact that the concentration is several-fold higher in ovarian venous plasma draining the ovary containing the corpus luteum than the contralateral side (Illingworth *et al.*, 1989).

The structure(s) responsible for the secretion of inhibin by the ovary in the follicular phase is not entirely clear. In non-human primates, mRNAs encoding the $\alpha$ and $\beta$ subunits of inhibin are expressed in the granulosa cells of antral follicles (Schwall *et al.*, 1990) which secrete inhibin when cultured *in vitro* (Hillier *et al.*, 1989). It is likely that the granulosa cells of most large human antral follicles can produce inhibin *in vivo* because its concentration in follicular fluid is extremely high (Baird *et al.*, 1988) and gonadotrophin-responsive production of inhibin by human granulosa cells has been demonstrated *in vitro* (Tsonis, Hillier & Baird, 1987; Hillier *et al.*, 1990). However, the concentration of inhibin in ovarian venous plasma draining the ovary containing the dominant follicle is similar to that draining the contralateral ovary; this suggests that several antral follicles in addition to the dominant follicle contribute equally to the ovarian secretion (Illingworth *et al.*, 1989). This conclusion would be compatible with the observation that the concentration of inhibin (unlike that of oestradiol) remains unchanged throughout the early and mid-follicular phase of the cycle. Thus the fall in secretion of FSH which occurs at this time of the follicular phase of the cycle and which is responsible for the selection of the ovulatory follicle cannot be due to inhibin but is a consequence of the increasing secretion of oestradiol (Fig. 1.5).

## LH and follicular endocrine function

What is the role of LH? In the early follicular phase of the cycle the concentration of LH rises as the suppressive effect of progesterone is removed following regression of the corpus luteum. The number of LH pulses increases from one every 4−6 h during the luteal phase to approximately one per hour during the mid-follicular phase. Each pulse of LH stimulates the secretion of androstenedione and testosterone by the theca layers of the follicle which are then converted into oestradiol by the granulosa cells. Thus the rise in the concentration of oestradiol throughout the follicular phase of the cycle reflects both the increased stimulation of the ovary by LH and the enhanced ability of the granulosa cells to convert androgen precursors into oestradiol (see Chapter 3).

### FSH and follicular endocrine function

In spite of the fall in the concentration of FSH which occurs in the follicular phase of the cycle, growth of the dominant follicle continues unabated. The mechanism by which the dominant follicle can survive in levels of FSH which are below the 'threshold' necessary to recruit further follicles is not fully understood, but implies that in some way it is more sensitive to FSH than other less favoured follicles (see Fig. 1.4). Recent evidence in hypogonadotrophic rhesus monkeys and women has confirmed that follicular development continues even if the dose of FSH falls below the threshold value (Zeleznik & Kubik, 1986; Glasier et al., 1988). It may be that the high intrafollicular levels of oestradiol enhance the responsiveness of granulosa cells to the action of FSH, as discussed further in Chapter 3.

Although the concentration of FSH falls in the mid- and late-follicular phase of the cycle, the dominant follicle requires a minimal level of FSH and LH throughout. Follicular development ceases in hypogonadotrophic women immediately following withdrawal of ex-ogenous gonadotrophins or pulsatile GnRH therapy (Brown et al., 1969; Polson et al., 1986) or in monkeys and women after the administration of antagonists of GnRH (Kenigsberg & Hodgen, 1986; Mais et al., 1986).

## Ovulation

Ovulation occurs as a result of a massive discharge of LH from the anterior pituitary (Yen et al., 1975). This preovulatory discharge of LH is due to the stimulation of the hypothalamo−pituitary unit by oestrogen. The exact mechanism of the positive feedback effects of oestradiol is not totally understood but probably involves action at both the hypo-thalamus and anterior pituitary (Fig. 1.5). Oestrogen sensitizes the gonadotrophs to the effects of GnRH so that throughout the follicular phase of the cycle there is progressively more LH released following injection of GnRH (Yen et al., 1972; Ross & Vande Wiele, 1974). In monkeys rendered hypogonadotrophic by destruction of the arcuate nucleus, cyclical ovarian function and ovulation can be restored by administration of GnRH pulses every hour (Wildt *et al.*, 1981) (see also Chapter 6). Because an LH surge occurs in these animals it has been claimed that the sensitization of the anterior pituitary is sufficient to account for the positive feedback effect of oestradiol and the LH surge (Knobil, 1980). Indeed, recent data has demonstrated a cessation of electrical activity associated with multi-unit recording from electrodes in the hypothalamus at the onset of the LH surge (Kesner *et al.*, 1987). In the rat and the sheep there is in addition an increase in the amount of GnRH secreted into the hypothalamic—hypophyseal portal vessels although the situation in the primate is not yet clear (Fink, 1979; Clarke & Cummins, 1982). At the onset of the LH surge and throughout its course well defined frequent pulses of LH can be identified in both women and rhesus monkeys (Marut *et al.*, 1981; Djahanbakhch *et al.*, 1984b). Presumably these reflect episodes of secretion of GnRH so it is likely that the LH surge is due to repeated discharge of GnRH acting on a pituitary, which is exquisitely sensitive to GnRH.

There is still doubt as to whether progesterone plays any role in the initiation of the LH surge in women. Prior to ovulation there is a rise in the concentration of progesterone which starts at about the onset of the LH surge (Johannson & Wide, 1969; Yussman & Taymor, 1970; Thorneycroft *et al.*, 1974; Testart *et al.*, 1982; Hoff *et al.*, 1983; Djahanbakhch *et al.*, 1984a). Progesterone facilitates the ability of oestrogen to provoke a discharge of LH and in the rat the timing of the LH surge on the afternoon of pro-oestrus, and is synchronized by the secretion of progesterone by the adrenal (Fink, 1979). In women some studies have reported a rise in the secretion of progesterone prior to the onset of the LH surge but in others the concentration only rises once the levels of LH have started to rise. As indicated above there is a progressive rise in the frequency of LH pulses in the late follicular phase and it may be difficult to decide precisely when the LH surge commences.

In a recent study in which blood samples were collected at 2-hourly intervals in the periovulatory period, the concentration of progesterone rose in parallel with that of LH at the onset of the surge (Hoff *et al.*, 1983). In order to investigate whether this preovulatory rise of progesterone was a cause or a consequence of the LH surge, the characteristics of LH and FSH release provoked by infusion of oestradiol alone or in combination with progesterone was examined in women in the mid-follicular phase of the cycle and in postmenopausal women receiving oestrogen replacement (Liu & Yen, 1983). While both regimes induced an LH surge, its magnitude and duration was significantly increased to a value which was similar to that found in the spontaneous cycle only when physiological amounts of progesterone were infused in addition to oestradiol. The results of this experiment strongly suggest that progesterone secreted by the ovary in response to LH enhances the positive feedback effects of oestradiol in the normal cycle.

11  THE OVARIAN CYCLE

The LH surge provokes a series of changes in the structure and function of the follicle which eventually result in ovulation and formation of the corpus luteum. About 12 h after the onset of the surge there is a progressive fall in the concentration of oestradiol in peripheral blood and in follicular fluid (Hoff *et al.*, 1983; Djahanbakhch *et al.*, 1984b; Van Look *et al.*, 1984). This fall in oestradiol secretion is not due to loss of ability of the granulosa cells to convert androgens to oestrogens because aromatase activity is maintained in cells aspirated from follicles on the point of ovulation (Hillier *et al.*, 1984). Rather it is more likely to be due to lack of precursor as indicated by the temporary decline in the concentration of androstenedione in follicular fluid and peripheral venous plasma after the LH surge. It is likely that LH receptors of the theca are desensitized by the high levels of LH (see Chapter 3).

The granulosa cells of the preovulatory follicle also contain LH receptors and respond to the LH surge by undergoing morphological changes known as luteinization. These cells start to produce progesterone and will form the granulosa—lutein cells of the corpus luteum. LH is also responsible for the physical changes in the follicle wall which result in ovulation (Espey, 1978). The collagen ground substance in the theca and surface epithelium begins to weaken due to the action of collagenase enzymes. In spite of a large increase in follicular fluid there is no increase in intrafollicular pressure due to the increased distensibility of the follicular wall. The mechanisms underlying the disintegration of collagen ground substance are complex and involve release of prostaglandins, plasminogen activator which converts plasminogen (a transudate from plasma into follicular fluid) into plasmin. The mechanism of follicular rupture is discussed in more detail in Chapter 5.

Coincidental to the LH surge there is a release of FSH. Its function is unknown but is responsible for the increase in mitotic activity in granulosa cells of small antral follicles in the early luteal phase of the cycle.

## The luteal phase

About 36 h after the onset of the LH surge, the follicular wall ruptures with extrusion of the egg and the corpus luteum is formed (Baird *et al.*, 1975). The basement membrane between the theca and granulosa layers is broken down and blood vessels which prior to ovulation have been confined to the theca layer, invade the luteinized granulosa cells. The corpus luteum is an extremely well vascularized endocrine gland with one of the highest blood flows per unit mass of any gland in the body. The invasion of blood capillaries is due to release of angiogenic factors including probably basic fibroblast growth factor (FGF) by the fibroblastic and blood cells, which together with the granulosa and luteal cells make up the corpus luteum (Findlay, 1986) (see Chapter 7).

The primate corpus luteum unlike those of many other species secretes oestradiol in addition to progesterone (Savard *et al.*, 1965; Baird, 1978; Rothchild, 1981). It is very likely that the granulosa—lutein cells are the origin of the oestradiol because the enzyme cytochrome P450aro has been localized by immunocytochemistry to these cells (Sasano *et al.*, 1989). We have recently shown that inhibin is present in these same cells as well as in the granulosa cells of the preovulatory follicle (Smith *et al.*, 1990b). Thus it appears that in primates the granulosa cells in the corpus luteum retain the ability to synthesize products which in other species are confined to the highly differentiated granulosa cells of the antral follicles.

The secretion of progesterone by the corpus luteum increases progressively until by day 10 after ovulation it has reached a maximum of *c.* 25 mg/day. The concentration of progesterone in luteal tissue and its capacity to produce progesterone when incubated *in vitro* is maximal in the early luteal phase (Swanston *et al.*, 1977; Richardson, 1986). Cholesterol in association with low-density lipoprotein (LDL) is the major blood-borne precursor used for the synthesis of progesterone (see Chapter 2), and it may be that the early corpus luteum has not yet acquired the full network of capillaries necessary to transport this steroidogenic precursor to the site of progesterone synthesis (Carr *et al.*, 1982).

The concentration of oestradiol and inhibin in peripheral plasma rise in the luteal phase in parallel with that of progesterone (McLachlan *et al.*, 1987b; 1990; Reddi *et al.*, 1990). In at least two species of subhuman primate (stump tail macaque and marmoset monkey) the corpus luteum also secretes inhibin and oestradiol although the luteal phase rise in the concentration of the latter is somewhat lower than that in women (Fraser *et al.*, 1989; Smith *et al.*, 1990a).

The secretion of the luteal hormones is under the control of LH. LH but not FSH increases the production of progesterone, oestradiol and inhibin when added to luteal slices or dispersed luteal cells incubated *in vitro* (Savard *et al.*, 1965; Tsonis *et al.*, 1987a). This is hardly surprising because high-affinity receptors for LH but not FSH or prolactin are present on luteal cells throughout the luteal phase (McNeilly *et al.*, 1980; Rajaniemi *et al.*, 1981; Bramley *et al.*, 1987). *In vivo*, each pulse of LH is followed by an increase in the concentration of progesterone and oestradiol (Backström *et al.*, 1982; Filicori *et al.*, 1984). In the late luteal phase when the frequency of LH pulses has dropped to one or two/24 h, the concentration of progesterone may fall to low levels between pulses. Injection of human chorionic gonadotrophin (hCG) is followed by an increase in the concentration of progesterone and if its administration is continued the luteal phase can be prolonged for several days (Hanson *et al.*, 1971).

These observations suggesting that the corpus luteum is dependent on LH, have received strong support from experiments in the monkeys and women in which potent antagonists of GnRH have been administered at different stages of the luteal phase (Mais *et al.*, 1986; Fraser *et al.*, 1989; McLachlan *et al.*, 1989). At all stages of the cycle there is a prompt cessation of LH pulses after the administration of the antagonist followed immediately by a decline in the concentration of progesterone, oestradiol and inhibin. Subsequent luteal activity appears to depend on the duration of action and dose of the antagonist. Repeated doses of a potent antagonist results in prolonged suppression of progesterone secretion, luteal regression and premature menstruation. Small doses of shorter duration are followed by temporary suppression of progesterone secretion and subsequent partial or complete recovery of luteal function (Fraser *et al.*, 1987).

In summary, all the available evidence suggests that the human corpus luteum is dependent throughout its life span on continuous support by pituitary LH. It is possible that other luteotrophic factors such as prolactin may be involved in maintaining the morphological integrity of the corpus luteum although normal luteal function, as judged by the concentration of progesterone in peripheral plasma, still occurs when the secretion of prolactin is inhibited by administration of the dopamine agonist, bromocriptine (Schultz *et al.*, 1976).

The hormones produced by the corpus luteum have profound effects in the secretion of gonadotrophins by the anterior pituitary (Fig. 1.5). During the luteal phase over 90% of the ovarian hormones is secreted by the corpus luteum and, hence, the secretory products of this structure dominate the feedback signals (Baird & Fraser, 1975). Progesterone inhibits the activity of the so-called 'pulse-generator', the synchronized network of hypothalamic neurones which synthesize and discharge GnRH (Knobil, 1980). As the frequency of LH pulses falls in response to rising levels of progesterone there is a rise in the amplitude of each pulse. This change in the pattern of LH during the luteal phase is almost certainly due to progesterone because it can be mimicked by the administration of progesterone during the follicular phase (Soules *et al.*, 1984) and is temporarily reversed by the antigestagen mifepristone (RU 486) (Critchley & Baird, 1986). If the corpus luteum is enucleated there is a rise in the concentration of LH and an increase in the frequency of LH pulses.

Oestradiol also contributes to the control of LH during the luteal phase (Fig. 1.5). Administration of oestradiol in large amounts suppresses the concentration of LH further and results in premature regression of the corpus luteum. Following administration of antioestrogens such as clomiphene or tamoxifen there is an increase in the frequency but not in the amplitude of LH pulses suggesting that oestradiol enhances the suppressive effect of progesterone during the luteal phase. In the presence of progesterone, oestradiol is unable to induce an LH surge by positive feedback presumably because the frequency of GnRH pulses is insufficient to prime the anterior pituitary. Thus, during the luteal phase under the combined effects of oestradiol and progesterone the concentration of LH is suppressed to the lowest level observed throughout the cycle.

While progesterone has a profound effect on the secretion of LH, it has little influence on the concentration of FSH the secretion of which is controlled by oestradiol and inhibin, although their relative importance has not yet been determined (Fig. 1.5). Passive immunization of rhesus monkeys with antiserum to oestradiol results in a rise in the secretion of FSH and development of large antral follicles (Zeleznik *et al.*, 1987). Similar experiments investigating the role of inhibin have not yet been reported in primates although in sheep both oestradiol and inhibin play a role in regulating the secretion of FSH in the luteal phase (Mann *et al.*, 1989).

As the corpus luteum is the source of oestradiol and inhibin during the luteal phase and their secretion is controlled by LH not FSH, there is no negative feedback loop operative to control the secretion of FSH the secretion of which falls below the threshold necessary to sustain the growth of medium sized antral follicles. Thus during the luteal phase of the menstrual cycle all antral follicles $\geq 5$ mm diameter are atretic and make an insignificant contribution to the secretion of ovarian hormones (McNatty *et al.*, 1983). During this stage of the cycle follicular development is suppressed and only recommences when the concentration of FSH and LH rise during regression of the corpus luteum (Baird *et al.*, 1984).

## Luteal regression

About 10–12 days after its formation the levels of progesterone start to decline indicating the regression of the corpus luteum (Fig. 1.2). There is a parallel fall in the concentration of oestradiol and inhibin suggesting that a common mechanism is operating to suppress the secretory capacity of luteal cells. There is no significant decline in the secretion of LH observed at this time. Rather the frequency of LH pulses increases, although the corpus luteum is apparently unable to respond by a rise in the secretion of progesterone. These findings indicate that luteal regression cannot be explained solely on the basis of withdrawal of luteotrophic support. In many species, for example sheep, pig, guinea pig, luteal regression is due to the release of prostaglandin $F_{2\alpha}$ from the uterus following priming with oestradiol and progesterone (Horton & Poyser, 1976). Prostaglandin $F_{2\alpha}$ reaches the ovary by a local countercurrent mechanism between the utero-ovarian vein and the ovarian artery (McCracken *et al.*, 1971; Baird, 1977). On reaching the ovary prostaglandin $F_{2\alpha}$ stimulates the secretion of oxytocin from the corpus luteum which acts on the uterus to provoke further release of prostaglandin $F_{2\alpha}$ (Flint & Sheldrick, 1982). Thus a positive feedback loop is created which ensures the demise of the corpus luteum. The mechanism by which prostaglandin $F_{2\alpha}$ prevents the stimulation of the synthesis of progesterone is not fully understood and is discussed in detail in Chapter 7.

In primates it is unlikely that prostaglandin $F_{2\alpha}$ of uterine origin is essential for luteal regression because normal ovarian cycles occur in women with congenital absence of the uterus or following hysterectomy (Neill et al., 1969; Beling et al., 1970; Fraser et al., 1973). It is more likely that some local self-destruct mechanism ensures that the corpus luteum becomes unresponsive to LH (Baird, 1985). LH receptors are present in high concentrations in corpora lutea in the mid- and late luteal phase but decline strikingly in corpora albicantia (McNeilly et al., 1980). However, there are great difficulties in obtaining corpora lutea timed precisely in relation to the onset of luteal regression and, hence, we still do not know whether the loss of LH receptors is a cause or consequence of luteal regression.

The corpus luteum produces a number of substances which are potential inhibitors of the synthesis of progesterone. Oestradiol inhibits the conversion of pregnenolone to progesterone by luteal cells of monkeys and women incubated in vitro (Williams et al., 1979). In women there is a progressive increase in the ratio of oestradiol to progesterone as the corpus luteum ages (Swanston et al., 1977; Fujita et al., 1981) and in the rhesus monkey there is a striking increase in the ability of luteal cells to convert androgens to oestradiol which may account for the high levels of oestradiol present in the corpus luteum of this species at luteal regression (Stouffer et al., 1980). Conflicting effects of oxytocin on progesterone production by human luteal cells have been reported. One study showed suppression by high concentrations of oxytocin (Tan et al., 1982), while another carefully conducted study using dispersed luteal cells discerned no effect on basal or hCG-stimulated progesterone production even at very high concentrations of the peptide (Richardson, 1986). There is also controversy as to whether the human corpus luteum produces oxytocin but even the reported values are below those which have been shown to have any effect on progesterone production (Wathes et al., 1982; Khan-Dawood & Dawood, 1983; Auletta & Flint, 1988; Auletta et al., 1988; Wathes, 1989).

A more likely candidate for a local luteolytic agent is prostaglandin $F_{2\alpha}$. The concentration of prostaglandin $F_{2\alpha}$, which probably reflects the biosynthetic potential of the luteal cells in response to the trauma of collection, is maximal in corpora albicantia (Schutt et al., 1976; Swanston et al., 1977; Patwardhan & Lanthier, 1985). However, the concentration of prostaglandin $F_{2\alpha}$ is also high in the recently formed corpus luteum, falling to low levels in the mid-luteal phase. These seemingly anomalous findings do not negate any role for prostaglandin $F_{2\alpha}$ if it is postulated that the corpus luteum becomes increasingly sensitive to luteolytic agents as it progresses into the late luteal phase when the level of luteotrophic support is minimal. Thus the maintenance of the corpus luteum is dependent on a balance between LH on the one hand and on the other hand, a range of potentially luteolytic factors including oestrogen, prostaglandin $F_{2\alpha}$ and possibly oxytocin. Further details of the cell-to-cell interactions which involve actions of LH and locally produced luteolysins in luteal regression are provided in Chapter 7.

**Luteal rescue**

If pregnancy is to become successfully established the maintenance of the corpus luteum and continued secretion of progesterone is essential. Around the start of implantation, about 7 days after ovulation, the embryo secretes hCG which stimulates increased secretion of progesterone by the corpus luteum. By day 8 of the luteal phase of the pregnant cycle, the concentration of progesterone is already higher than in the non-pregnant cycle (Lenton & Woodward, 1988). Although the rescue of the corpus luteum is undoubtedly due to hCG the mechanism is not fully understood. The amounts of hCG secreted by the trophoblast increase exponentially and very rapidly reach levels which might be expected to downregulate the synthesis of LH receptors. However, receptors for LH are apparently maintained at luteal phase levels in the corpus luteum at early pregnancy although not unexpectedly *c.* 90% are occupied by hCG (Bramley *et al.*, 1987). The lifespan of the corpus luteum in the non-pregnant cycle can only be maintained by exogenous hCG in amounts far in excess of those required to occupy sufficient receptors to stimulate maximally the production of progesterone. It is possible, therefore, that at levels present during early pregnancy not only does it act as a surrogate for LH in stimulating the secretion of progesterone, but also has a more generalized luteotrophic role by antagonizing the processes involved in luteal regression.

# Determination of cycle length

An unusual feature of the ovarian cycle of primates including man compared with many other mammals is the long 14-day follicular phase (Baird, 1988). The length of the follicular phase is determined by the time taken for a small antral follicle to reach maturity when it secretes sufficient oestrogen to provoke a preovulatory LH surge. In primates this process takes at least 14 days because the largest healthy antral follicle at the time of luteal regression is only 2−4 mm containing *c.* 1 million granulosa cells. In contrast, in species like sheep and cattle with short follicular phases (3−7 days) the development of large antral follicles continues throughout the luteal phase and ovulation is only prevented by the inhibitory action of progesterone. When the levels of progesterone fall at luteal regression, the secretion of LH and oestradiol rises and ovulation occurs within a few days.

It has been previously suggested that the long follicular phase in women is related to the fact that the corpus luteum secretes oestradiol and inhibin in addition to progesterone (Baird et al., 1975; Baird, 1988). Both hormones are potent inhibitors of the secretion of FSH, levels of which during the luteal phase fall below that necessary to 'activate' small antral follicles (Fig. 1.5). In contrast the corpus luteum of the sheep does not secrete either oestradiol or inhibin which arise from the antral follicles throughout the cycle. Thus a negative feedback loop between follicles in the ovary and the hypothalamo–pituitary unit continues to function and follicular development occurs continually throughout the luteal phase.

The teleological reason for the lengthening of the follicular phase in primates is unknown. The retention of the ability to secrete oestradiol and inhibin by the granulosa–lutein cells may have evolved in menstruating primates in order to allow sufficient time for repair and proliferation of the endometrium before ovulation.

The length of the luteal phase appears to be more constant. In all mammals a period of priming with progesterone is necessary before the uterine environment is favourable for the development and implantation of the embryo. Short and/or inadequate luteal phases are usually associated with infertility (Jones, 1973).

Thus the length of the ovarian cycle is dependent on the time taken to develop a mature follicle and the intrinsic lifespan of the corpus luteum. The length of the cycle is normal in hypogonadotrophic women in whom ovarian activity is stimulated by exogenous GnRH given in pulses at a fixed frequency every 90 min throughout the cycle (Leyendecker & Wildt, 1983; Jacobs et al., 1985). Thus the 'zeitbeger' of the ovarian cycle is in the ovary not in some cyclical centre in the brain.

## Perimenopausal ovary

Throughout life there is a progressive loss of the fixed stock of oocytes in the ovaries and by c. 50 years of age the depletion is such that very few oocytes remain and ovarian cyclicity ceases (Baker, 1982). The menopause is the last menstrual period and is characterized by ovarian failure with raised levels of gonadotrophins.

During the last few years leading up to the menopause there is a marked increase in the variability in the length of the menstrual cycle which reflects the alteration in ovarian function (Treloar et al., 1967; Sherman et al., 1979). Overall the length of the menstrual cycle shortens significantly throughout reproductive life from a mean of 28 to 26 days.

The few detailed studies of the endocrine changes in cycles during this menopausal transition have shown a wide range in pattern (Sherman & Korenmann, 1975; Van Look et al., 1977b; Metcalf et al., 1982). In some women normal cycles continue until the last menstrual period. In others a short follicular phase is associated with an elevation of FSH levels in the early and mid-follicular phase of the cycle which are suppressed to normal during the luteal phase. The concentration of LH, oestradiol and progesterone are all within the normal range. Recent data has confirmed a long held suspicion that the monotrophic elevation in the concentration of FSH is due to a reduced secretion of inhibin. (E.A. Lenton & A.J. Woodward, unpublished data). As the number of oocytes in the ovaries is depleted, there are presumably few antral follicles which are the source of inhibin in the follicular phase. The levels of oestradiol are normal because over 90% is secreted by the dominant follicle. In the luteal phase the secretion of FSH is suppressed because at this stage of the cycle virtually all the inhibin and oestradiol is secreted by the corpus luteum.

The prolonged menstrual cycles found in the perimenopausal years are associated with periods of temporary ovarian failure when the levels of oestradiol remain persistently low (Baird, 1988). There is a progressive rise in the concentration of FSH until eventually raised levels of oestradiol indicate a developing follicle. It is presumed that the population of follicles has fallen below that necessary to ensure the presence in the ovary of at least one suitable small antral follicle each month. Follicular development during these cycles may be abnormal with anovulation or short luteal phases.

## Menopausal ovary

Following the menopause the ovary is not totally devoid of endocrine activity, although there are few or no antral follicles. The stromal tissue stains positive for $3\beta$-hydroxysteroid dehydrogenase, indicating the ability to synthesize progesterone. When stromal homogenates from postmenopausal ovaries are incubated in vitro the main steroid product is androstenedione and testosterone. These androgens are present in higher concentrations in ovarian venous plasma than in peripheral plasma indicating that they are secreted in vivo (Judd et al., 1974). However, although the ovarian secretion of testosterone contributes to c. 25–50% of the total production rate, the secretion of androstenedione is trivial compared with that of the adrenals (Siiteri & MacDonald, 1973). The bulk of oestrogens in postmenopausal women is not secreted by ovary or adrenal but is derived by conversion in peripheral tissues such as that from androstenedione.

# Conclusion and summary

The ovary is in a continuous state of flux. Even during periods of apparent quiescence recruitment of primordial follicles into the pool of growing antral follicles occurs throughout reproductive life until the stock of oocytes is exhausted at the menopause. Once recruited the follicles continue to grow and differentiate until they are lost through atresia. During the final selection and growth of the preovulatory follicle, the endocrine environment is hostile to all but the chosen follicle ensuring that a single egg is ovulated. The length of the cycle is determined by the corpus luteum and the selected follicle which appear to have a fixed lifespan. Both structures require gonadotrophins but their lifespan is not dictated by a central clock; rather the hormones they secrete feed back to establish the gonadotrophic pattern of the ovarian cycle.

# References

Auletta, F.J. & Flint, F. (1988) Mechanisms controlling corpus luteum function in sheep, cows, non human primates and women especially in relation to the time of luteolysis. *Endocr. Rev.*, **9**, 88–105.

Auletta, F.J., Jones, D.S.C. & Flint, A.P.F. (1988) Does the human corpus luteum synthesize neurohypophysial hormones? *J. Endocrinol.*, **116**, 163–5.

Backström, C.T., McNeilly, A.S., Leask, R. & Baird, D.T. (1982) Pulsatile secretion of LH, FSH, prolactin, oestradiol and progesterone during the human menstrual cycle. *Clin. Endocrinol., (Oxf.)*, **7**, 29–42.

Baird, D.T. (1977) Local utero–ovarian relationships. In Crighton, D.B., Foxcroft, G.R., Haynes, N.B. & Lamming, G.E. (eds) *Control of Ovulation*, pp. 217–233. Butterworths, London.

Baird, D.T. (1978) Synthesis and secretion of steroid hormones by the ovary *in vivo*. In Zuckerman, S. & Weir, B.J. (eds) *The Ovary*, 2nd edn, Vol 3, pp. 305–57. Academic Press, London.

Baird, D.T. (1983) Factors regulating the growth of the preovulatory follicle in the sheep and the human. *J. Reprod. Fertil.*, **69**, 343–52.

Baird, D.T. (1985) Control of luteolysis. In Jeffcoate, S.L. (ed.) *The Luteal Phase*, pp. 25–42. Wiley, Chichester.

Baird, D.T. (1987) A model for follicular selection and ovulation: Lesson from superovulation. *J. Steroid Biochem.*, **27**, 15–23.

Baird, D.T. (1988) The primate ovary: critique and perspectives. In Stouffer, R.L. (ed.) *The Primate Ovary*, pp. 249–59. Plenum Press, New York.

Baird, D.T., Backström, T., McNeilly, A.S., Smith S.K. & Wathen, C.G. (1984) Effect of enucleation of the corpus luteum at different stages of the luteal phase of the human menstrual cycle on subsequent follicular development. *J. Reprod. Fertil.*, **70**, 615–24.

Baird, D.T., Baker, T.G., McNatty, K.P. & Neal, P. (1975) Relationship between the secretion of the corpus luteum and the length of the follicular phase of the ovarian cycle. *J. Reprod. Fertil.*, **45**, 611–19.

Baird, D.T. & Fraser, I.S. (1975) Concentration of oestrone and oestradiol in follicular fluid and ovarian venous blood of women. *Clin. Endocrinol. (Oxf.)*, **4**, 259–66.

Baird, D.T., Tsonis, C.G., Messinis, I.E., Templeton, A.A. & McNeilly, A.S. (1988) Inhibin levels in gonadotropin-treated cycles. *Ann. N.Y. Acad. Sci.* **541**, 153–61.

Baker, T.G. (1982) Oogenesis and ovulation. In Austin, C.R. & Short, R.V. (eds) *Reproduction in Mammals*, 2nd edn, pp. 17–45. Cambridge University Press, Cambridge.

Beling, C.G., Marcus, L. & Markham, M. (1970) Functional activity of the corpus luteum following hysterectomy. *J. Clin. Endocrinol. Metab.* **30**, 30–9.

Bramley, T.A., Stirling, D., Swanston, I.A., Menzies, G.S., McNeilly, A.S. & Baird, D.T. (1987) Specific binding sites for gonadotrophin-releasing hormone LH/chorionic gonadotrophin, low-density lipoprotein, prolactin and FSH in homogenates of human corpus luteum. II: Concentrations throughout the luteal phase of the menstrual cycle and early pregnancy. *J. Endocrinol.* **113**, 317–27.

Brown, J.B., Evans, J.H., Adey, F.D., Taft, H.P. & Townsend, L. (1969). Factors involved in induction of fertile ovulation with human gonadotrophins. *Br. J. Obstet. Gynaecol.*, **76**, 289–307.

Burger, H.G., DeKretser, D.M., Findlay, J.K. & Igarashi, M. (eds) (1987) *Inhibin — Non-Steroidal*

*Regulation of Follicle Stimulating Hormone Secretion*, (Serono Symposia, Vol 42). Raven Press, New York.

Carr, B.R., MacDonald, P.C. & Simpson, E.R. (1982) The role of lipoproteins in the regulation of progesterone secretion by the human corpus luteum. *Fertil. Steril.*, **38**, 303–11.

Channing, C.P., Anderson, L.D., Hoover, D.J., Kolena, J., Osteen, K.G., Pomerantz, S.H. & Tanabe, K. (1982) The role of non-steroidal regulators in control of oocyte and follicular maturation. *Recent Prog. Horm. Res.*, **38**, 331–400.

Clarke, I.J. & Cummins, J.T. (1982) The temporal relationships between gonadotropin releasing hormone (GnRH) and luteinizing hormone (LH) secretion in ovariectomised ewes. *Endocrinology*, **111**, 1737–9.

Critchley, H.O.D. & Baird, D.T. (1986) Antigestogen RU 486 increases LH secretion in the luteal phase of the cycle. *J. Endocrinol.*, Suppl. **108** (Abstr. 95).

de Jong, F.H. (1987) Inhibin — Its nature, site of production and function. *Oxf. Rev. Reprod. Biol.*, **9**, 1–53.

Djahanbakhch, O., Warner, P., McNeilly, A.S. & Baird, D.T. (1984a) Pulsatile release of LH and oestradiol during the periovulatory period in women. *Clin. Endocrinol. (Oxf.)*, **20**, 579–89.

Djahanbakhch, O., Warner, P., McNeilly, A.S., Swanston, I.A. & Baird, D.T. (1984b) Changes in prolactin in relation to those of FSH, oestradiol, androstenedione and progesterone around the preovulatory surge of LH in women. *Clin. Endocrinol. (Oxf.)*, **20**, 463–72.

Doll, R. (1975) The epidemiology of cancers of the breast and reproductive system. *Scot. Med. J.*, **20**, 305–15.

Dorrington, J.H. & Armstrong, D.T. (1979) Effects of FSH on gonadal functions. *Recent Prog. Horm. Res.*, **35**, 301–42.

Espey, L.L. (1978) A comprehensive model of ovulation. In Jones, R.E. (ed) *The Vertebrate Ovary*, pp. 503–32. Plenum Press, New York.

Filicori, M., Butler, J.P. & Crowley, W.F. (1984) Neuroendocrine regulation of the corpus luteum in the human. *J. Clin. Invest.*, **73**, 1638–47.

Findlay, J.K. (1986) Angiogenesis in reproductive tissues. *J. Endocrinol.*, **111**, 357–66.

Fink, G. (1979) Neuroendocrine control of gonadotrophin secretion. *Br. Med. Bull.*, **35**, 155–60.

Flint, A.P.F. & Sheldrick, G.L. (1982) Ovarian secretion of oxytocin is stimulated by prostaglandin. *Nature*, **297**, 587–8.

Fraser, I.S., Baird, D.T., Hobson, B.M., Michie, E.A. & Hunter, W. (1973) Cyclical ovarian function in women with congenital absence of the uterus and vagina. *J. Clin. Endocrinol. Metab.*, **36**, 634–7.

Fraser, H.M., Neston, J.J. & Vickery, B.H. (1987) Suppression of luteal function by a luteinizing hormone-releasing hormone antagonist during the early luteal phase in the stumptailed macaque

monkey and the effects of subsequent administration of human chorionic gonadotropin. *Endocrinology*, **121**, 612–18.

Fraser, H.M., Robertson, D.M. & DeKretser, D.M. (1989) Immunoactive inhibin concentrations in serum throughout the menstrual cycle of the macaque: suppression of inhibin during the luteal phase after treatment with an LHRH antagonist. *J. Endocrinol.*, **121**, R9–R12.

Fujita, Y., Mori, T., Suzuki, A., Nihnobu, K. & Nishimura, T. (1981) Functional and structural relationships in steroidogenesis *in vitro* by human corpus lutea during development and regression. *J. Clin. Endocrinol. Metab.*, **53**, 744–51.

Glasier, A.F., Baird, D.T. & Hillier, S.G. (1988) FSH and the control of follicular growth. *J. Steroid. Biochem.*, **32**, 167–70.

Goodman, A.L. & Hodgen, D. (1983) The ovarian triad of the primate menstrual cycle. *Recent Prog. Horm. Res.*, **39**, 1–67.

Gougeon, A. (1982) Rate of follicular growth in the human ovary. In Rolland, R., van Hall, E.V., Hillier, S.G. McNatty, K.P. & Schoemaker, J. (eds) *Follicular Maturation and Ovulation*, pp. 155–63. Excerpta Medica, Amsterdam.

Hanson, F.W., Powell, J.E. & Stevens, V.C. (1971) Effects of hCG and human pituary LH on steroid secretion and functional life of the human corpus luteum. *J. Clin. Endocrinol. Metab.*, **32**, 211–15.

Harris, G.W. & Naftolin, F. (1970) The hypothalamus and control of ovulation. *Br. Med. Bull.*, **26**, 3–9.

Hillier, S.G. (1985) Sex steroid metabolism and follicular development in the ovary. *Oxf. Rev. Reprod. Biol.*, **7**, 168–222.

Hillier, S.G., Reichert, L.E. Jr. & van Hall, E.V. (1981) Control of preovulatory follicular estrogen biosynthesis in the human ovary. *J. Clin. Endocrinol. Metab.*, **51**, 847–56.

Hillier, S.G., Wickings, E.J., Afnan, M., Margara, R.A. & Winston, R.M.L. (1984) Granulosa cell steroidogenesis before *in vitro* fertilization. *Biol. Reprod.*, **31**, 679–86.

Hillier, S.G., Wickings, E.J., McNeilly, A.S., Reichert, L.E. Jr., Illingworth, P. & Baird, D.T. (1990) Hormone-dependent production of inhibin by cultured human granulosa cells. *J. Endocrinol.*, Suppl. **124** (Abstr. 69).

Hillier, S.G., Wickings, E.J., Saunders, P.T.K., Shimisaki, S., Reichert, L.E. Jr. & McNeilly, A.S. (1989) Hormonal control of inhibin production by primate granulosa cells. *J. Endocrinol.*, **123**, 65–73.

Hoff, J.F., Quigley, M.E. & Yen, S.S.C. (1983) Hormonal dynamics at mid-cycle: a re-evaluation. *J. Clin. Endocrinol. Metab.*, **57**, 792–6.

Horton, E.W. & Poyser, N.L. (1976) Uterine luteolytic hormone: a physiological role for prostaglandin $F_{2\alpha}$. *Physiol. Rev.*, **56**, 913–19.

Illingworth, P.J., Reddi, K., Smith, K. & Baird, D.T. (1989) Ovarian vein concentrations of inhibin during the human menstrual cycle. *J. Endocrinol.,* Suppl. **123** (Abstr. 62).

Jacobs, H.S., Abdulwahid, N., Adams, J., Armar, N.A., Brook, C.G.D., Chambers, G.R., Craft, I. *et al.* (1985) Endocrine control of follicular growth in humans. In Rolland, R., Heineman, M.J., Hillier, S.G. & Vemer, H. (eds) *Gamete Quality and Fertility Regulation,* pp. 257–70. Excerpta Medica, Amsterdam.

Jia, X.C., Kessel, B., Yen, S.S.C., Tucker, E.M. & Hsueh, A.J.W. (1986) Serum bioactive follicle stimulating hormone during the human menstrual cycle and in hyper and hypogonadotropic states: application of a sensitive granulosa cell aromatase bioassay (GAB). *J. Clin. Endocrinol. Metab.,* **62**, 1243–1249.

Johansson, E.D.B. & Wide, L. (1969) Periovulatory levels of plasma progesterone and luteinizing hormone in women. *Acta Endocrinol. Copenh.,* **62**, 82–8.

Jones, G.S. (1973) Luteal phase defect. In Denamur, R. & Netter, A. (eds) *Le Corps Jaune,* pp. 401–19. Masson, Paris.

Judd, H.L., Judd, G.E., Lucas, W.E. & Yen, S.S.C. (1974) Endocrine function of the post menopausal ovary: concentration of androgens and estrogens in ovarian and peripheral vein blood. *J. Clin. Endocrinol. Metab.,* **39**, 1020–4.

Kenigsberg, D. & Hodgen, G.D. (1986) Ovulation inhibition by administration of weekly gonadotropin-releasing hormone antagonist. *J. Clin. Endocrinol. Metab.,* **62**, 734–41.

Kesner, J.S., Wilson, R.C., Kaufman, J-M., Hotchkiss, J., Chen, Y., Yamamoto, H., Pardo, R.R. & Knobil, E. (1987) Unexpected responses of the hypothalamic gonadotropin-releasing hormone 'pulse generator' to physiological estradiol inputs in the absence of the ovary. *Proc. Natl. Acad. Sci. USA,* **84**, 8745–9.

Khan-Dawood, F.S. & Dawood, M.Y. (1983) Human ovaries contain immunoreactive oxytocin. *J. Clin. Endocrinol. Metab.,* **57**, 1129–32.

Knobil, E. (1980) The neuroendocrine control of the menstrual cycle. *Recent Prog. Horm. Res.,* **36**, 53–88.

Lenton, E.A. & Woodward, A.J. (1988) The endocrinology of conception cycles and implantation in women. *J. Reprod. Fertil.,* Suppl. **36**, 1–15.

Leyendecker, G. & Wildt, L. (1983) Induction of ovulation with chronic intermittent (pulsatile) administration of GnRH in women with hypothalamic amenorrhoea. *J. Reprod. Fertil.,* **69**, 397–409.

Lincoln, G.A. & Short R.V. (1980) Seasonal breeding: nature's contraceptive. *Recent Prog. Horm. Res.,* **36**, 1–52.

Liu, J.H. & Yen, S.S.C. (1983) Induction of the midcycle gonadotropin surge by ovarian steroids in women: a critical evaluation. *J. Clin. Endocrinol. Metab.,* **57**, 797–802.

McCracken, J.A., Baird, D.T. & Goding J.R. (1971) Factors affecting the secretion of steroids from the transplanted ovary in the sheep. *Recent Prog. Horm.*

Res., **27**, 537–82.

McLachlan, R.I., Cohen, N.L., Dahl, K.D., Bremner, W.L. & Soules, M.R. (1990) Serum inhibin levels during the periovulatory interval in normal women: relationship with sex steroid and gonadotrophin levels. *Clin. Endocrinol. (Oxf.),* **32**, 39–48.

McLachlan, R.I., Cohen, N.L., Vale, W.W., Rivier, J.E., Burger, H.G., Bremner, W.J. & Soules, M.R. (1989) The importance of luteinizing hormone in the control of inhibin and progesterone secretion by the human corpus luteum. *J. Clin. Endocrinol. Metab.,* **68**, 1078–85.

McLachlan, R.I., Robertson, D.M., Healy, D.L., Burger, H.G. & DeKretser, D.M. (1987a) Circulating immunoreactive inhibin levels during the normal menstrual cycle. *J. Clin. Endocrinol. Metab.,* **65**, 954–61.

McLachlan, R., Robertson, D.M., Healy, D.L., Findlay, J.K., DeKretser, D.M. & Burger, H.G. (1987b) The radioimmunoassay of human serum inhibin. In Burger, H.G., DeKretser, D.M., Findlay, J.K. & Igarashi, M. (eds) (1987) *Inhibin — Non-Steroidal Regulation of Follicle Stimulating Hormone Secretion,* Serono Symposia, Vol 42, pp. 105–18. Raven Press, New York.

McNatty, K.P. (1982) Ovarian follicular development from the onset of luteal regression in human and sheep. In Rolland, R., van Hall, E.V., Hillier, S.G., McNatty, K.P. & Schoemaker. J. (eds) *Follicular Maturation and Ovulation,* pp. 1–18. Excerpta Medica, Amsterdam.

McNatty, K.P. & Baird, D.T. (1978) Relationship between follicle-stimulating hormone, androstenedione and oestradiol in human follicular fluid. *J. Endocrinol.,* **76**, 527–31.

McNatty, K.P., Hillier, S.G., van den Boogard, A.M.J., Trimbos-Kemper, T.C.M., Reichert, L.E. Jr. & van Hall, E.V. (1983) Follicular development during the luteal phase of the human menstrual cycle. *J. Clin. Endocrinol. Metab.,* **56**, 1022–31.

McNeilly, A.S., Kerin, J., Swanston, I.A., Bramley, T.A. & Baird, D.T. (1980) Changes in the binding of human chorionic gonadotrophin/luteinizing hormone, follicle stimulating hormone and prolactin to human corpora lutea during the menstrual cycle and pregnancy. *J. Endocrinol.,* **87**, 315–25.

Mais, V., Kazer, R.R., Cetel, N.S., Rivier, J., Vale, W.W. & Yen, S.S.C. (1986) The dependency of folliculogenesis and corpus luteum function on pulsatile gonadotropin secretion in cycling women using a gonadotropin-releasing hormone antagonist as a pulse. *J. Clin. Endocrinol. Metab.,* **62**, 1250–5.

Mann, G.E., Campbell, B.K., McNeilly, A.S. & Baird, D.T. (1989) Passively immunizing ewes against inhibin during the luteal phase of the oestrous cycle raises the plasma concentration of FSH. *J. Endocrinol.,* **123**, 383–91.

Marut, E.L., Williams, R.F., Cowan, B.D., Lynch, A., Lerner, S.P. & Hodgen, G.D. (1981) Pulsatile pituitary gonadotropin secretion during the maturation of the dominant follicle in monkeys: estrogen positive feedback enhances the biological activity of LH. *Endocrinology*, **109**, 2270–2.

Mason, A.J., Hayflick, J.S., Ling, N., Esch, K., Ueno, N., Ying, S.Y., Guillemin, *et al.* (1985) Complementary DNA sequences of ovarian follicular fluid inhibin show precursor structure and homology with transforming growth factor-β. *Nature*, **318**, 659–63.

Metcalf, M.G., Donald, R.A. & Livesey, J.H. (1982) Pituitary–ovarian function before, during and after the menopause: a longitudinal study. *Clin. Endocrinol. (Oxf.)*, **17**, 489–94.

Neill, J.D., Johansson, E.D.B. & Knobil, E. (1969) Failure of hysterectomy to influence the normal pattern of cyclic progesterone secretion in the rhesus monkey. *Endocrinology*, **84**, 464–5.

Nilsson, L., Wikland, M. & Hamberger, L. (1982) Recruitment of an ovulatory follicle in the human following follicle-ectomy and lute-ectomy. *Fertil. Steril.*, **37**, 30–4.

Patwardhan, V.V. & Lanthier, A. (1985) Luteal phase variations in endogenous concentrations of prostaglandins PGE and PGF and in the capacity of their *in vitro* formation in the human corpus luteum. *Prostaglandins*, **30**, 91–8.

Peters, H. & McNatty, K.P. (1980) *The Ovary*. Granada Publishing, London.

Polson, D.W., Sagle, M., Mason, H.D., Adams, J., Jacobs, H.S. & Franks, S. (1986) Ovulation and normal luteal function during LHRH treatment of women with hyperprolactinaemic amenorrhoea. *Clin. Endocrinol. (Oxf.)*, **24**, 531–7.

Rajaniemi, H.J., Ronnberg, L., Kauppila, A., Ylostalo, P., Jalkanen, M., Saastamoinen, J., Selander, J. *et al.* (1981) Luteinizing hormone receptors in human ovarian follicles and corpora lutea during the menstrual cycle and pregnancy. *J. Clin. Endocrinol. Metab.*, **108**, 307–13.

Reddi, K., Wickings, E.J., McNeilly, A.S., Baird, D.T. & Hillier, S.G. (1990) Circulating bioactive follicle stimulating hormone and immunoreactive inhibin during the normal human menstrual cycle. *Clin. Endocrinol. (Oxf.)*, **33**, 547–557.

Richardson, M.C. (1986) Hormonal control of ovarian luteal cells. *Oxf. Rev. Reprod. Biol.*, **8**, 321–78.

Ross, G.T. & Vande Wiele, R.L. (1974) The Ovaries. In Williams, R.H. (ed) *Textbook of Endocrinology*, 5th edn, Chapter 7. W.B. Saunders, London.

Rothchild, I. (1981) The regulation of the mammalian corpus luteum. *Recent Prog. Horm. Res.*, **37**, 183–298.

Ryan, K.J. & Petro, Z. (1966) Steroid biosynthesis by human ovarian granulosa and theca cells. *J. Clin. Endocrinol. Metab.*, **26**, 146–52.

Sasano, H., Okamoto, M., Mason, J.I., Simpson, E.R., Mendelson, C.R., Sasano, N. & Silverberg, S.G. (1989) Immunolocalization of aromatase, 17-α hydroxylase, and side-chain-cleavage cytochromes P-450 in the human ovary. *J. Reprod. Fertil.*, **85**, 163–9.

Savard, K., Marsh, J.M. & Rice, B.F. (1965) Gonadotrophins and ovarian steroidogenesis. *Recent Prog. Horm. Res.*, **21**, 285–356.

Schultz, K.D., Geiger, W., Del Pozo, E., Lose, K.H., Kunzig, H.J. & Lancranjan, I. (1976) An influence of prolactin-inhibitor Bromocriptin (CB154) on human luteal function *in vivo*. *Arch. Gynakol.*, **221**, 93–7.

Schutt, D.A., Clarke, A.H., Fraser, I.S., Goh, P., McMahon, G.R., Saunders, D.M. & Shearman, R.P. (1976) Changes in concentration of prostaglandin F and steroids in human corpora lutea in relation to growth of the corpus luteum and luteolysis. *J. Endocrinol*, **71**, 453–4.

Schwall, R.H., Mason, A.J., Wilcox, J.N., Bassett, S.G. & Zeleznik, A.J. (1990) Cellular localization of inhibin/activin subunit expression in the primate ovary. *Mol. Endocrinol.*, **4**, 75–9.

Sherman, B.M. & Korenmann, S.G. (1975) Hormonal characteristics of the human menstrual cycle throughout reproductive life. *J. Clin. Invest.*, **55**, 699–706.

Sherman, B.M., Wallace, R.B. & Treloar, A.E. (1979) The menopausal transition: endocrinological and epidemiological considerations. *J. Biosocial Sci.*, Suppl. **6**, 19–35.

Siiteri, P.K. & MacDonald, P.C. (1973) Role of extraglandular estrogen in human endocrinology. In Field, J. (ed) *Handbook of Physiology*, Vol II, pp. 615–29. Williams & Wilkins, Baltimore.

Smith, K.B., Lunn, S.F. & Fraser, H.M. (1990a) Inhibin secretion in the common marmoset monkey. *J. Endocrinol.*, **126**, 489–495.

Smith, K.B., Millar, M.R., McNeilly, A.S. Fraser, H.M. & Baird, D.T. (1990b) Immunocytochemical localisation of inhibin in the human corpus luteum. *J. Reprod. Fertil.* Abstract Series No. 5 (Abstr. 64).

Soules, M.R., Steiner, R.A., Clifton, D.K., Cohen, N.L., Askel, S. & Bremner, W.J. (1984) Progesterone modulation of pulsatile LH secretion in normal women. *J. Clin. Endocrinol. Metab.*, **58**, 378–83.

Stouffer, R.L., Bennett, L.A. & Hodgen, G.D. (1984) Estrogen production by luteal cells isolated from rhesus monkeys during the menstrual cycle: correlation with spontaneous luteolysis. *Endocrinology*, **106**, 519–25.

Swanston, I.A., McNatty, K.P. & Baird, D.T. (1977) Concentration of prostaglandin $F_{2\alpha}$ and steroids in the human corpus luteum. *J. Endocrinol*, **73**, 115–22.

Tan, G.J.S., Tweedale, R. & Biggs, J.S.G. (1982) Oxytocin may play a role in the control of the human corpus luteum. *J. Endocrinol.*, **95**, 65–70.

Testart, J., Frydman, R., Nahoul, K., Grenier, J., Feinstein, M.C., Roger, M. & Scholler, R. (1982) Steroids and gonadotropins during the late preovulatory phase of the menstrual cycle. Time relationships between plasma hormone levels and luteinizing hormone surge onset. *J. Steroid Biochem.*, **17**, 675–82.

Thorneycroft, I.H., Sribyatta, B., Tom, W.K., Nakamura, R.M. & Mishell, D.R. Jr. (1974) Measurements of serum LH, FSH, progesterone, 17αhydroxyprogesterone and estradiol-17β levels at 4 hour intervals during the periovulatory phase of the menstrual cycle. *J. Clin. Endocrinol. Metab.*, **39**, 754–8.

Tonetta, S.A. & DiZerega, G.S. (1989) Intragonadal regulation of follicular maturation. *Endocrinol. Rev.*, **10**, 205–29.

Treloar, A.E., Boynton, R.E., Behn, B.G. & Brown, B.W. (1967) Variation of the human menstrual cycle through reproductive life. *Int. J. Fertil.*, **12**, 77–126.

Tsonis, C.G., McNeilly, A.S. & Baird, D.T. (1986) Measurement of exogenous and endogenous inhibin in sheep serum using a new and extremely sensitive bioassay for inhibin based on inhibition of ovine pituitary FSH secretion *in vitro. J. Endocrinol.*, **110**, 341–52.

Tsonis, C.G., Hillier, S.G. & Baird, D.T. (1987) Production of inhibin bioactivity by human granulosa-lutein cells: stimulation by FSH and testosterone *in vitro. J. Endocrinol.*, **112**, R11–14.

Tsonis, C.G., McNeilly, A.S. & Baird, D.T. (1987) Production and secretion of ovarian inhibin. In Burger, H.G., DeKretser, D.M., Findlay, J.K. & Igarashi, M. (eds) *Inhibin — Non-Steroidal Regulation of Follicle Stimulating Hormone Secretion*, Serono Symposia, Vol 42, pp. 203–19. Raven Press, New York.

Van Look, P.F.A., Hunter, W.M., Corker, C.S. & Baird, D.T. (1977a) Failure of positive feedback in normal men and subjects with testicular feminization. *Clin. Endocrinol. (Oxf.)*, **7**, 353–366.

Van Look, P.F.A., Lothian, H., Hunter, W.M., Michie, E.A. & Baird, D.T. (1977b) Hypothalamic–pituitary ovarian function in perimenopausal women. *Clin. Endocrinol. (Oxf.)*, **7**, 13–21.

Van Look, P.F.A., Templeton, A.A., Swanston, I.A., Angell, R.R., Aitken, J., Hendry, R. & Baird, D.T. (1984) The effect of hCG on steroid levels in human Graafian follicles. *Proceedings of the 3rd Joint Meeting of British Endocrine Societies* (Abstr. 160).

Vaitukaitis, J.L., Bermudez, J.A., Cargille, M., Lipsett, M.B. & Ross, G.T. (1971) New evidence for an anti-estrogenic action of clomiphene citrate in women. *J. Clin. Endocrinol. Metab.*, **32**, 503–8.

Wathes, D.C. (1989) Oxytocin and vaspression in the gonads. *Oxf. Rev. Reprod. Biol.*, **11**, 226–82.

Wathes, D.C., Swann, R.W., Pickering, B.J., Porter, G., Hull, M.G.R. & Drife, J.O. (1982) Neurohypophyseal hormones in the human ovary. *Lancet*, **ii**, 410–12.

Wide, L. (1982) Male and female forms of human follicle stimulating hormone in serum. *J. Clin. Endocrinol. Metab.*, **55**, 682–8.

Wildt, L., Hausler, A., Hutchison, J.S., Marshall, G. & Knobil, E. (1981) Estradiol as a gonadotropin releasing hormone in the rhesus monkey. *Endocrinology*, **108**, 2011–13.

Williams, M.T., Roth, M.S., Marsh, J.M. & Lemaire, W.J. (1979) Inhibition of human chorionic gonadotropin-induced progesterone synthesising estradiol in isolated human luteal cells. *J. Clin. Endocrinol. Metab.*, **48**, 437–40.

Yen, S.S.C., Lasley, B.L., Wang, C.F., LeBlanc, H. & Siler, T.I.M. (1975) The operating characteristics of the hypothalamic–pituitary system during the menstrual cycle and observations on biological action of somatostatin. *Recent Prog. Horm. Res.*, **31**, 331–63.

Yen, S.S.C., van den Berg, G., Rebar, R. & Ehara, Y. (1972) Variation of pituitary responsiveness to synthetic LRF during different phases of the menstrual cycle. *J. Clin. Endocrinol. Metab.*, **35**, 931–4.

Yussman, M.A. & Taymor, M.L. (1970) Serum levels of follicle stimulating and luteinizing hormone and plasma progesterone related to ovulation by corpus luteum biopsy. *J. Clin. Endocrinol. Metab.*, **30**, 396–9.

Zeleznik, A.J. (1981) Premature elevation of systemic estradiol reduces serum levels of follicle-stimulating hormone and lengthens the follicular phase of the menstrual cycle in rhesus monkeys. *Endocrinology*, **109**, 352–5.

Zeleznik, A.J., Hutchison, J.S. & Schuler, H.M. (1987) Passive immunization with antioestradiol antibodies during the luteal phase of the menstrual cycle potentiates the perimenstrual rise in serum gonadotrophin concentrations and stimulates follicular growth in cymomologous monkeys (*Macaca fascicularis*). *J. Reprod Fertil.*, **80**, 403–10.

Zeleznik, A.J. & Kubik, C.J. (1986) Ovarian responses in macaques to pulsatile infusion of follicle-stimulating hormone (FSH) and luteinizing hormone: increased sensitivity of the maturing follicle to FSH. *Endocrinology*, **119**, 2025–32.

# 2 Molecular Basis of Ovarian Steroid Synthesis

J.F. STRAUSS III & W.L. MILLER

## Introduction

The principal ovarian hormones are steroids, oestradiol and progesterone, secreted by the preovulatory follicle and corpus luteum. Major pathways of steroid hormone synthesis in the ovaries are illustrated in Fig. 2.1. Primary components of the ovarian steroidogenic machinery include: (1) proteins that participate in the acquisition of cholesterol, including lipoprotein receptors and enzymes involved in *de novo* cholesterol synthesis; (2) mixed-function oxidases that catalyse the cleavage of carbon side-chains from the sterol nucleus (cytochrome P450scc and cytochrome P450c17), introduce hydroxyl groups (cytochrome P450c17) and aromatize the A ring (cytochrome P450aro); (3) the oxido-reductases (or hydroxysteroid dehydrogenases) that

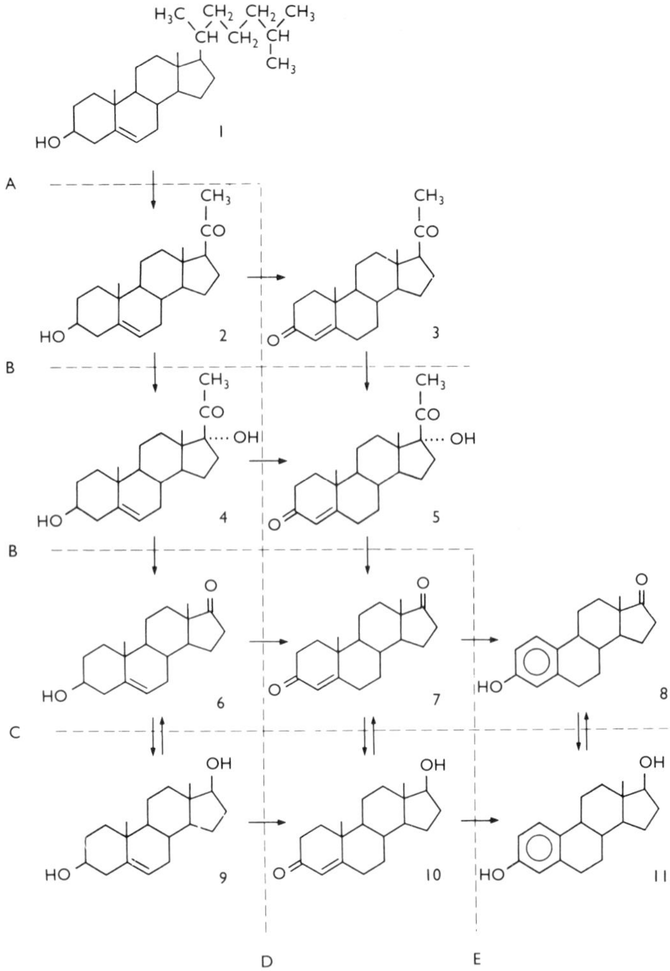

**Fig. 2.1.** Pathways of ovarian steroid hormone synthesis. Enzymes: (A) cholesterol side-chain cleavage (P450scc); (B) 3β-Hydroxysteroid dehydrogenase/$\Delta^{5\text{-}4}$ isomerase; (C) 17-hydroxylase/C-17,20-lyase (P450c17); (D) 17β-hydroxysteroid dehydrogenase; (E) aromatase (P450aro). Steroids: (1) cholesterol; (2) pregnenolone; (3) 17-hydroxypregnenolone; (4) progesterone; (5) 17-hydroxyprogesterone; (6) dehydroepiandrosterone; (7) androstenedione; (8) oestrone; (9) androstenediol; (10) testosterone; (11) oestradiol.

catalyse in some cases, reversibly, the oxidation or reduction of oxy functions at C-3, C-17 and C-20 (e.g. 3β-hydroxysteroid dehydrogenase, 17β-hydroxysteroid dehydrogenase and 20α-hydroxysteroid dehydrogenase); (4) reductases, that irreversibly reduce the $\Delta^4$ olefinic bond of the A ring of $\Delta^4$-3 keto steroids (e.g. 5α-reductase).

In this chapter we will review the molecular basis of ovarian steroidogenesis, emphasizing the structure and function of the proteins and their genes involved in hormone synthesis, the mechanisms that underlie the control of their expression, and genetic defects that impair the steroid-secretory functions of the ovaries.

# Acquisition of cholesterol by steroidogenic cells

## *De novo* cholesterol synthesis

Steroidogenic cells in the ovaries readily synthesize cholesterol from acetyl coenzyme A and rates of sterol synthesis are enhanced in response to trophic stimulation, or when ovarian cells are deprived of an exogenous source of cholesterol (i.e. lipoproteins) (Strauss *et al.*, 1981; Nestler *et al.*, 1989). 3-Hydroxy-3-methylgluratyl coenzyme A reductase (HMG-CoA reductase), the rate-determining enzyme in *de novo* cholesterol synthesis, generally parallels steroidogenic activity. This enzyme exists in phosphorylated (inactive) and non-phosphorylated (active) forms, and most of the enzyme in ovarian tissue is phosphorylated. The strongest correlation between steroidogenesis and HMG-CoA reductase is with total enzyme activity (i.e. phosphorylated plus non-phosphorylated enzyme). The importance of HMG-CoA reductase phosphorylation/dephosphorylation to the control of *de novo* sterol synthesis in steroidogenic glands is uncertain.

In the rat and rabbit ovary there is a striking increase in HMG-CoA activity during the luteinization of follicles initiated by treatment with exogenous gonadotrophin. In the rat, the increase in enzyme activity is transient (Schuler *et al.*, 1981; Hedin *et al.*, 1987) whereas it is more sustained in the rabbit (Kovanen *et al.*, 1978). This periovulatory peak of HMG-CoA reductase activity may reflect the need of developing luteal cells to supplement their cholesterol requirements or to generate other mevalonate-derived products including dolichol, ubiquinone and isopentenyl RNA.

## Uptake and metabolism of lipoproteins by ovarian cells

Ovarian cells take up cholesterol from circulating lipoproteins by receptor-mediated and non-receptor-mediated mechanisms. The pathways and the specific lipoprotein classes favoured depend upon the species and cell type in question.

### *Low-density lipoproteins (LDL)*

These are taken up primarily by a receptor-mediated mechanism; less than 10% of LDLs are accumulated by a receptor-independent process (Gwynne & Strauss, 1982; Nestler *et al.*, 1989). Human granulosa–lutein cells express numerous LDL receptors recognizing apolipoproteins B and E on their surfaces (Fig. 2.2). These receptors are located on microvilli and are later concentrated in 'coated pits' which usually reside at the base of the microvilli. The 'pits' have a coating of clathrin on their cytoplasmic face which can undergo a transition from a hexagonal to a pentagonal array, which provides the driving force for

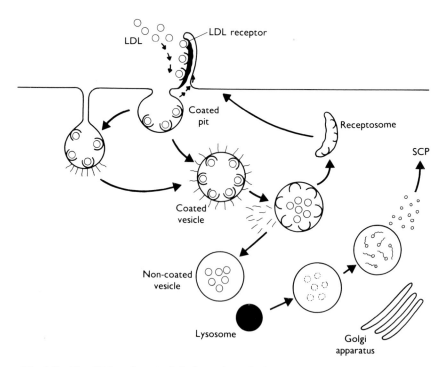

**Fig. 2.2.** The 'LDL pathway' of cholesterol uptake by steroidogenic cells. LDL binds to receptors that are internalized in coated vesicles. LDL is separated from its receptor, which is recycled back to the plasma membrane. LDL then travels in non-coated vesicles to the vicinity of the Golgi apparatus where lysosomal hydrolases are introduced. Acid proteinases degrade LDL apolipoproteins to amino acids and acid lipase frees cholesterol from esters. Free cholesterol then diffuses out of lysosomes and may be transferred to organelles with the assistance of sterol-carrier proteins (SCP).

internalization of the 'pit'. The internalized lipoproteins are ultimately moved to the lysosomal apparatus after being separated from the receptors, which are recycled back in receptosomes to the plasma membrane. LDL protein is degraded and cholesteryl esters are hydrolysed by acid lipase in the lysosomal system.

### High-density lipoproteins (HDL)

HDL-bearing apolipoprotein E (apo E) may be metabolized by the LDL pathway because apo E associates with the LDL (B/E) receptor. Steroidogenic cells, including ovarian granulosa cells, synthesize and secrete apo E (Driscoll *et al.*, 1985; Wyne *et al.*, 1989). These cells may therefore be able to modify the apolipoprotein composition of HDL in their environment to direct the particles for uptake via the B/E receptor. Elaboration of apo E appears to be under hormonal regulation such that apo E synthesis is increased in parallel with cellular demands for cholesterol.

Apo E-free HDL also provides cholesterol to ovarian cells (Gwynne & Strauss, 1982). While this has been demonstrated convincingly for rodent species, there is evidence that apo E-free HDL can deliver cholesterol to bovine, porcine and human granulosa cells *in vitro*. The mechanics of cholesterol delivery from apo E-free HDL remain to be elucidated, but it is evident that the process is completely different from the 'LDL pathway'.

A high-affinity binding site for HDL has been demonstrated in rat ovarian tissue. The characteristics of HDL-binding to this high-affinity site are quite different from the binding of LDL to its receptor in that binding is highly temperature dependent, relatively insensitive to proteases, does not require calcium, and is not inhibited by polyanions. Unlike LDLs, HDLs do not seem to associate preferentially with clathrin-coated areas of the plasma membrane. A putative HDL-binding protein with a molecular weight of *c.* 80 kDa has been detected by ligand blotting in ovarian membranes (Ghosh & Menon, 1986). In marked contrast, radiation inactivation and target analysis suggest the molecular mass of the HDL-binding site on human fibroblast membranes to be 16 kDa (Mendel *et al.*, 1988). These discrepancies could be explained by the different methodologies employed as well as differences in the size of the HDL-binding site in steroidogenic tissues and fibroblasts.

It has been suggested that apo A-I is the apolipoprotein that interacts with the HDL-binding site (Monaco *et al.*, 1987), but other data indicate that apo A-II and the apo Cs are recognized (Hwang & Menon, 1985; Schreiber *et al.*, 1985). The broad specificity of the HDL-binding site, which may be due primarily to hydrophobic interactions, distinguishes it from the LDL receptor. However, specific binding to either intact cells or plasma membranes is inhibited by modifying the tyrosyl residues of HDL particles with tetranitromethane (Nestler *et al.*, 1985b). Nevertheless, tetranitromethane-modified HDL particles exhibit substantial 'non-specific' or 'low-affinity' binding and stimulate steroidogenesis by rat granulosa cells as well as native HDL. This suggests that any interaction of HDL with the cell surface may be sufficient for the transfer of sterol.

In contrast to the 'LDL pathway', the amount of HDL sterol accumulated by steroidogenic cells exceeds the amount of apolipoprotein taken up, and relatively little apolipoprotein degradation occurs (Gwynne & Strauss 1982; Nestler *et al.*, 1989). In addition, ultrastructural studies of the uptake of HDL by rat ovarian cells reveal that a relatively small amount of HDL apolipoprotein is internalized. These observations suggest that the delivery of HDL sterol involves a non-endocytotically mediated net flux of cholesterol from HDL into cells. Moreover, HDL-delivered free cholesterol is utilized for hormone synthesis in preference to esterified sterol (Nestler *et al.*, 1985a; Parinaud *et al.*, 1987). This suggests that independent mechanisms are involved in the uptake of the free and esterified sterol moieties of HDL.

Mechanisms underlying the uptake of free cholesterol and sterol ester from HDL remain to be elucidated. Some studies suggest that membrane phospholipids regulate binding of HDL and facilitate the transfer of sterols from HDL into cells. Alternatively, hepatic lipase could play a role by hydrolysing HDL phospholipids. This would increase the sterol:phospholipid molar ratio of the HDL particles, thereby enhancing the transfer of free cholesterol to cells. Indeed, treatment of HDL with phospholipase $A_2$ increases its ability to stimulate progesterone synthesis by human granulosa cells (Parinaud et al., 1987). Hepatic lipase could also participate in this aspect of HDL metabolism by serving as a transfer protein, or by generating lysophospholipids which could form micelles with sterol esters, allowing them to permeate the cell membrane. Ovarian tissues, particularly corpora lutea, contain substantial hepatic lipase activity which appears to originate in the liver and be taken up from the circulation and bound to the surface of endothelial cells in the ovary (Hixenbaugh et al., 1989). After delivery of sterols, HDL particles may dissociate from the cell surface and return to the circulation, accounting for the disproportionate accumulation of HDL sterols relative to apolipoproteins.

Current evidence indicates that HDL-delivered cholesteryl esters are not metabolized in ovarian cells by lysosomal hydrolases. Lysosomotrophic agents such as chloroquine do not inhibit the conversion of HDL-delivered radiolabelled sterol esters into steroids, and it is likely that other sterol esterases, like the cytosolic neutral sterol esterase, hydrolyse these esters to release free cholesterol (Nestler, et al., 1985b).

Alternative routes of HDL metabolism include internalization and lysosomal degradation and retroendocytosis. Secretion of apo E by the cells would convert apo E-free HDL into particles capable of being processed through the LDL pathway. HDL uptake via the transferrin receptor may also occur as a result of transferrin binding to HDL. This 'piggy-backing' could lead to retroendocytosis, which is the normal cycle for transferrin bound to its receptor. Thus, the 'HDL pathway' encompasses several potential steps: (1) binding and delivery/dissociation of sterol; (2) absorptive endocytosis and degradation; and (3) retroendocytosis.

## Use of cholesterol synthesized *de novo* v. lipoprotein-associated cholesterol

Most steroidogenic cells rely on combined uptake of lipoproteins and *de novo* cholesterol biosynthesis to generate precursors for steroidogenesis. Lipoprotein-associated cholesterol is the predominant source of precursor for cells which produce large quantities of hormone, such as those of the corpus luteum (Brown et al., 1979; Gwynne & Strauss, 1982; Nestler et al., 1989). Radiotracer studies in humans reveal that plasma cholesterol is almost fully equilibrated with the steroidogenic pool of sterol (Bolte et al., 1974). Imaging of steroidogenic tissues with radiocholesterol analogues (using [131]I- or [75]Se-labelled selenomethyl derivatives) is possible because of the voracious appetite of steroidogenic glands for plasma cholesterol (Gross *et al.*, 1984). Moreover, inhibitors of HMG-CoA reductase (e.g. mevinolin) do not have a major impact on circulating steroid hormone levels in man (Illingworth & Corbin, 1985; Farnsworth *et al.*, 1987). These findings are consistent with the notion that human steroidogenic cells utilize circulating cholesterol as a major substrate for hormone synthesis.

'Book-keeping' of cholesterol dynamics in human organs cannot be readily accomplished, but estimates of the contributions of various sources of cholesterol to steroidogenesis have been obtained in laboratory animals with techniques that quantify sterol synthesis *de novo*, receptor and non-receptor mediated lipoprotein uptake (Koelz *et al.*, 1982; Spady & Dietschy, 1983, 1985; Spady *et al.*, 1987). These studies demonstrate that in non-human primates and rats, active steroidogenic glands accumulate the majority of their cholesterol from lipoproteins. In other species like the hamster and guinea pig, cholesterol synthesized *de novo* makes a more significant contribution.

Studies *in vitro* with human ovarian tissues have shown enhanced secretion of hormones when cells or explants are cultured in the presence of lipoproteins (Tureck & Strauss, 1982; Carr *et al.*, 1982; Soto *et al.*, 1984). Ovarian cells cultured in serum-free or lipoprotein-deficient medium undertake markedly increased secretion of steroids when lipoproteins are introduced to the medium. Furthermore, in the presence of an adequate supply of lipoprotein-carried cholesterol, inhibition of HMG-CoA reductase does not suppress steroidogenesis (Goldstein & Brown, 1990).

## Fluctuations in plasma lipoprotein concentrations and compartmentalization in steroidogenic tissues

Lipoprotein profiles are influenced by steroidal hormones including oestrogens and androgens and synthetic progestational agents. Changes in plasma lipoprotein content and composition occur during the menstrual cycle and during the reproductive cycles of animals, but these cyclic changes are not sufficient to alter the function of steroidogenic glands which derive precursor cholesterol from circulating lipoproteins (Lussier-Cacan *et al.*, 1977; Jones *et al.*, 1988).

The ability of certain ovarian cells to synthesize steroid hormones appears to be affected by their access to lipoproteins. A partial blood—follicle barrier excludes high molecular weight substances including LDL from the follicular antrum. Thus, LDL cannot reach the granulosa cells in the preovulatory follicle until after the mid-cycle surge of LH which initiates breakdown of the follicular wall and vascularization of the developing corpus luteum (Carr *et al.*, 1982). Moreover, follicular fluid is rich in glycosaminoglycans which prevent LDL from association with LDL receptors (Bellin *et al.*, 1987). Therefore, utilization of LDL-cholesterol for steroidogenesis is constrained in the follicular micro-environment, which may in turn restrain steroid hormone synthesis until after ovulation has occurred (see Chapter 6).

### Regulation of *de novo* cholesterol synthesis, and uptake and metabolism of lipoproteins

Stimulation of steroidogenesis by gonadotrophins usually results in an associated increase in sterol synthesis and uptake of lipoprotein-carried cholesterol. The increase in *de novo* cholesterol synthesis is due mainly to an increase in HMG-CoA reductase activity which results from increased accumulation of the enzyme protein (Schuler *et al.*, 1981; Azhar *et al.*, 1984; Rodgers *et al.*, 1987a; Hedin *et al.*, 1987). The increase in enzyme protein is a consequence of increased enzyme synthesis, due at least in part to a rise in mRNA encoding the enzyme (Golos & Strauss, 1988). This response is quite rapid, and increases in HMG-CoA reductase enzyme are seen within hours of applying trophic stimulation. Since HMG-CoA reductase protein turns over rapidly, trophic hormones might also affect enzyme stability, an aspect of regulation which has yet to be explored in ovarian cells.

Transcription of the gene encoding HMG-CoA reductase is driven by positive promoter elements which have been defined in the 5' flanking DNA sequence. Although the *trans* factors that bind to these *cis* elements have not yet been identified, they appear to be different from the factors that bind to the positive promoter of the LDL receptor gene. The positive promoter is suppressed by negative feedback of a cholesterol precursor or metabolite (Saucier *et al.*, 1985; Osborne *et al.*, 1988; Takagi *et al.*, 1989). There is evidence that an oxysterol or a hydroxylanosterol, is the effector molecule. Preliminary data reveal the presence of a cytochrome P450 which generates 26-hydroxycholesterol in many tissues, particularly steroidogenic glands. This enzyme is inhibited by progestins and the antifungal agent, ketoconazole, but not by aminoglutethimide. Indeed, addition of aminoglutethimide to isolated steroidogenic mitochondria promotes increased C-26 hydroxylation of cholesterol, presumably because substrate is diverted from P450scc and pregnenolone and progesterone, inhibitors of the 26-hydroxylase, are therefore not made (J.F. Strauss III, R. Fischer & J.M. Trzaskos, unpublished observations). The oxysterols may act to control gene transcription after binding to an oxysterol 'receptor'. This receptor is believed to function in a manner similar to steroid hormone receptors, in this situation blocking the action of the factor(s) which binds to the positive promoter (Fig. 2.3). Chemical cross-linking studies as well as ligand-binding studies with radiolabelled oxysterols have demonstrated an oxysterol-binding protein monomer with a molecular

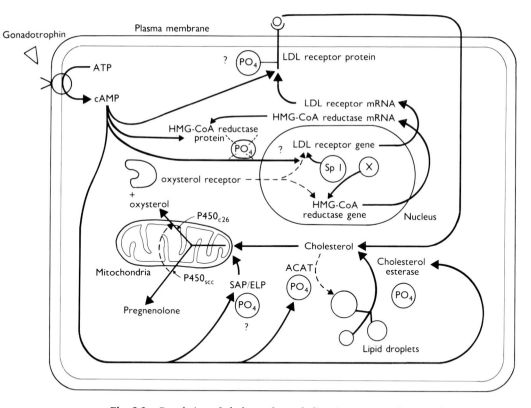

**Fig. 2.3.** Regulation of cholesterol metabolism in ovarian cells. Stimulation of the ovarian cell by gonadotrophin increases production of cAMP. cAMP exerts multiple actions to promote steroidogenesis and increase synthesis and uptake of cholesterol; it may promote dephosphorylation of HMG-CoA reductase, thereby acutely activating existing enzyme; it may also cause the LDL receptor to be phosphorylated in its cytoplasmic tail which might enhance receptor recycling; promotes phosphorylation of cholesterol esterase (causing its activation) and acyl CoA:cholesterol acyl transferase (ACAT), (causing its inhibition). This shifts cholesterol out of the esterified storage pool and makes it available for hormone synthesis. cAMP may increase the levels of steroidogenesis-activator peptide (SAP) and or endozepine-like peptide (ELP), perhaps promoting their phosphorylation. This would increase access of cholesterol to mitochondrial cytochrome P450scc. Sterol-carrier protein (SCP₂), not shown here, may also be phosphorylated such that its ability to move cholesterol to the mitochondria is increased. As a result of increased progestogen synthesis, mitochondrial 26-hydroxylase (P450c26) activity may be inhibited, reducing production of oxysterol which mediates negative feedback inhibition of HMG-CoA reductase and LDL receptor gene expression. This would result in diminished inhibition of the positive promoter, activated by Sp1 in the case of the LDL receptor gene, and another *trans* factor (x) in the case of HMG-CoA reductase. This in turn would lead to increased transcription of both genes and more HMG-CoA reductase and more LDL receptors. cAMP may also lessen the ability of the oxysterol to suppress LDL receptor gene expression, perhaps, by phosphorylation of the oxysterol receptor. Solid lines reflect stimulation of a reaction, dashed lines inhibition.

weight of *c.* 97 kDa in cell extracts, which is the putative oxysterol receptor (Taylor *et al.*, 1988).

The rapid increase in HMG-CoA reductase levels which precede increased steroidogenesis is due to diminished sterol negative feedback.

Inhibition of steroid hormone synthesis with aminoglutethimide almost completely blocks the rise in HMG-CoA reductase activity and enzyme protein levels (Schuler *et al.*, 1981). Inhibition of steroidogenesis in the presence of 25-hydroxycholesterol, which is a potent negative feedback regulator, prevents the rise in HMG-CoA reductase mRNA (Golos & Strauss, 1988). These findings are all consistent with the idea that stimulation of steroidogenesis depletes cells of a sterol negative feedback effector (e.g. due to inhibition of 26-hydroxycholesterol P450 by pregnenolone or progesterone) which causes increased synthesis of HMG-CoA reductase and probably other enzymes involved in cholesterol synthesis (Fig. 2.3).

LDL receptor levels correlate with the steroidogenic activity of ovarian cells. In the human corpus luteum, receptors are most abundant in the mid-luteal phase, when progesterone secretion is greatest, and least abundant in regressed corpora lutea (corpora albicanti) and stromal tissue (Ohashi *et al.*, 1982; Bramley *et al.*, 1987a,b). Stimulation of granulosa–lutein cells with gonadotrophins increases LDL receptors and consequently the ability of these cells to take up and metabolize LDL. The increase in LDL receptors is due to enhanced synthesis of receptor protein, which is driven by accumulation of the mRNA encoding the receptor, presumably as a result of increased transcription (Golos *et al.*, 1985, 1986; Golos & Strauss, 1987). Although trophic hormones acting via cyclic adenosine monophosphate (cAMP)-mediated postreceptor signalling (see Chapter 3) have well-documented stimulatory effects on LDL receptor levels, other trophic factors including insulin-like growth factor (IGF-I) promote granulosa cell LDL metabolism by mechanisms that may not involve cAMP (Veldhuis *et al.*, 1987; Veldhuis & Rogers, 1987).

Similar to regulation of HMG-CoA reductase, transcription of the LDL receptor gene is subject to negative feedback by a cholesterol precursor or metabolite (Takagi *et al.*, 1989). The LDL receptor gene has a positive promoter which appears to be responsive to the transcription factor, Sp1 (Sudhof *et al.*, 1987; Dawson *et al.*, 1988). The 5' flanking DNA regions of the LDL receptor and HMG-CoA reductase genes contain a related sequence (GTG G/C GGTG) which may be the *cis* elements which confer sterol negative feedback control of these genes. This octanucleotide sequence could be the core of the binding site for a sterol-dependent protein (e.g. receptor for the regulatory sterol) that suppresses the activity of the positive promoter.

When steroidogenesis in human granulosa–lutein cells is stimulated in the presence of aminoglutethimide, an inhibitor of cholesterol side-chain cleavage, or when cells are stimulated in the presence of 25-hydroxycholesterol and aminoglutethimide, expression of the LDL receptor gene is increased, but not to the same extent as it is in the absence of the inhibitor and hydroxysterol (Takagi & Strauss, 1989).

This contrasts with the control of HMG-CoA reductase where the stimulation of gene expression is almost completely blocked. Thus, there is differential regulation of the mRNAs encoding HMG-CoA reductase and LDL receptor in the face of sterol negative feedback which might allow steroidogenic cells to acquire lipoprotein-associated cholesterol even when cellular sterol pools are replete. It remains to be determined how the differential regulation of HMG-CoA reductase and LDL receptor gene expression is effected. cAMP might stimulate gene transcription or produce some modification in the negative feedback mechanism that normally controls the LDL receptor gene. Although cAMP increases LDL receptor synthesis and raises LDL receptor mRNA levels in cultured human granulosa cells, the 5' flanking DNA of the LDL receptor gene (up to 6.5 kb) does not appear to contain an enhancer element that is responsive to cAMP (Takagi & Strauss, 1989). It therefore seems likely that expression of the LDL receptor gene occurs in the face of sterol negative feedback because the feedback signal is in some way attenuated by cAMP (e.g. phosphorylation of an oxysterol binding protein which reduces its ability to suppress transcription of the LDL receptor gene).

Gonadotrophic stimulation enhances LDL metabolism as well as promoting uptake of LDL. The apparent rate of internalization and degradation of LDL is increased in gonadotrophin-stimulated cells (Golos et al., 1985). This has been documented by determining the ratio of cell-surface bound and internalized lipoprotein to degraded [$^{125}$I]-LDL. This ratio decreases in human and rat granulosa cells exposed to trophic hormones, indicating accelerated processing of LDL. Using colloidal gold labelled LDL particles to identify the structural basis of this postreceptor enhancement of LDL metabolism, it has been shown that both the rate of internalization as well as the movement of LDL particles to the lysosomal apparatus are augmented (J. Foster, J.F. Strauss III & L.G. Paavola, unpublished observations).

The cytoplasmic tail of the bovine adrenal LDL receptor can be phosphorylated (Kishimoto et al., 1987). However whether phosphorylation of receptor occurs in intact cells, if it is under hormonal control, and the potential significance of phosphorylation with regard to receptor function (i.e. its effect on internalization or recycling) are not yet known.

Ovarian accumulation of HDL is increased by gonadotrophins and trophic stimulation of cells in vitro increases the uptake of HDL-associated cholesterol and cholesteryl ethers (Gwynne & Strauss, 1982; Nestler et al., 1989). The mechanisms by which trophic agents increase the uptake of HDL-cholesterol are not yet known. Is synthesis of HDL binding sites required? Are the various pathways by which HDL can be metabolized by the cells altered co-ordinately? Do trophic hormone-induced alterations in cellular sterol balance affect the activity of the 'HDL pathway'? All of these questions remain to be answered.

# Cholesteryl ester dynamics in steroidogenic cells

A characteristic feature of steroidogenic ovarian cells is abundant cytoplasmic lipid droplets containing cholesteryl esters. Sterol esters in these droplets are synthesized by acyl coenzyme A: cholesterol acyltransferase (ACAT), located in the rough endoplasmic reticulum (Tavani *et al.*, 1982). The lipid droplets may bud off from the endoplasmic reticulum after accumulation of newly synthesized sterol esters.

Polyunsaturated fatty acids (e.g. linolenic acid, arachidonic acid, docosapentenoic acid and docosahexenonic acid) taken up from circulating lipoproteins or derived by elongation and desaturation within steroidogenic cells are esterified to cholesterol (Strauss *et al.*, 1977; O'Meara *et al.*, 1985). The accumulation of the long-chain polyunsaturated fatty acids in sterol esters may reflect ACAT preference for these fatty acyl coenzyme As (CoAs) and/or differential rates of mobilization of esters of long-chain polyunsaturates. The pattern of fatty acid esterification to sterols changes with the functional status of ovarian cells suggesting specific metabolic roles for these lipids, perhaps as precursors of prostanoids and/or lipoxygenase products (Tuckey *et al.*, 1984).

The lipid-droplet sterol esters are hydrolysed by a soluble sterol ester hydrolase. This enzyme, a protein with a molecular weight of 84 kDa, is activated by phosphorylation of serine residues by cAMP-dependent protein kinase (Trzeciak & Boyd, 1974; Colbran *et al.*, 1986). Steroidogenic cells also contain a neutral pH-optimum, particulate sterol ester hydrolase activity, which in some ovarian tissues is altered in response to trophic stimulation (see Strauss *et al.*, 1981). However, the role of this enzyme in the turnover of cellular sterol esters remains to be defined.

The sterol esters in ovarian cells are in a dynamic state, and the size and number of lipid droplets change as the pool expands or contracts (Claesson, 1954). The quantity of sterol ester stored is determined by the availability of cholesterol to the cell through synthesis *de novo* or accumulation of lipoprotein-associated cholesterol on the one hand, and the steroidogenic activity of the cell on the other (Strauss *et al.*, 1981). Lowering of circulating cholesterol levels in experimental animals in the presence of active steroidogenesis reduces ovarian cholesterol ester stores. Cells cultured in lipoprotein-poor medium also have minimal levels of sterol esters, but addition of lipoprotein results in sterol ester accumulation. Gonadotrophic stimulation diverts cholesterol away from the ACAT reaction and into the steroidogenic pool. Conversely, inhibition of steroid hormone synthesis increases the storage of sterol esters.

There appears to be a continuous cycle of ester synthesis and hydrolysis in ovarian cells (Flint & Armstrong, 1973). Factors controlling the synthetic arm of this cycle include the availability of cholesterol to ACAT (Tavani *et al.*, 1982) (the primary factor in the short-term regulation of sterol ester synthesis), the level of ACAT activity (determined by the amount of enzyme protein), and possibly the lipid milieu of the enzyme. In addition, the activity of ACAT may be inhibited by phosphorylation of the enzyme. Thus, phosphorylation of ACAT (inhibition) and the cytosolic cholesterol ester hydrolase (activation) would result in complimentary changes in the metabolism of cellular sterol esters increasing availability of free cholesterol (Suckling *et al.*, 1983). However, the impact of phosphorylation on flux through the ACAT reaction *in vivo* is as yet unknown. Steroidal products may also affect ACAT activity. Inhibition of ACAT by progesterone can readily be observed *in vitro*, and under certain circumstances progestins may also suppress the synthesis of sterol esters in intact cells (Simpson & Burkhart, 1980a,b).

A portion of the cholesterol synthesized *de novo* or entering cells from the circulation appears to be targeted for esterification, even under circumstances where the availability of exogenous cholesterol is limited (Veldhuis *et al.*, 1985). Thus, inhibition of ACAT with Sandoz compound 58−035 increases steroid synthesis by granulosa cells cultured in lipoprotein-poor medium, presumably because more cholesterol is available for hormone production. However, compound 58−035 does not affect steroidogenesis when cells are cultured in the presence of an adequate supply of lipoprotein-associated cholesterol.

The rate of cholesteryl ester hydrolysis is determined by the activity of the sterol ester hydrolase, which is set by the amount of enzyme protein and its phosphorylation state. Access of enzyme to the lipid-droplet substrate represents another possible locus of control. The cDNA for the hormone-sensitive lipase has recently been cloned, but to-date there are no published reports on the control of expression of this gene using the molecular probes (Holm *et al.*, 1988).

## Cytochrome P450s

The three mixed function oxidases involved in ovarian steroidogenesis are members of the cytochrome P450 family, so-called because they exhibit a characteristic shift in the Soret absorbance peak from 420 to 450 nm upon reduction in the presence of carbon monoxide (Hall, 1986). All P450 enzymes contain *c.* 500 amino acids and have a haem-binding region near the carboxy terminus. The steroid-binding sites of ovarian and other steroidogenic P450 enzymes have considerable similarity in primary structure (Picado-Leonard & Miller, 1988). Cytochrome P450 enzymes require oxygen and reducing equivalents derived from NADPH for catalytic activity. The electrons from NADPH are transferred to the cytochrome P450s by either a mitochondrial or microsomal electron-transport chain with an obligatory flavoprotein constituent.

## The cholesterol side-chain cleavage system (cytochrome P450scc)

Cholesterol side-chain cleavage, which yields pregnenolone and iso-capraldehyde, is the first committed step in steroid hormone synthesis (Fig. 2.1). This reaction takes place in the inner mitochondrial membrane and is the major rate-determining step in steroid hormone synthesis (Fig. 2.4). It is catalysed by cytochrome P450scc and its associated electron-transport system, consisting of a flavoprotein reductase (ferredoxin reductase or adrenodoxin reductase), and an iron sulphur protein shuttle (ferrodoxin or adrenodoxin), which carries electrons to cytochrome P450scc (Miller, 1988). The three components of the cholesterol side-chain cleavage system have been purified to homogeneity from bovine adrenals, and full length cDNAs for the bovine and human proteins have been cloned. The genes for human cytochrome P450scc, adrenodoxin reductase and adrenodoxin have also been cloned and sequenced.

### The cholesterol side-chain cleavage reaction

The cholesterol side-chain cleavage reaction entails three catalytic cycles: the first two lead to the introduction of hydroxyl groups at positions C-22 and C-20, and the third results in cleavage of the side-chain between these carbons. Each catalytic cycle requires one molecule of

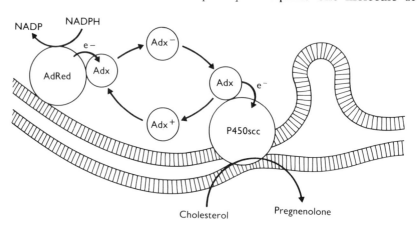

**Fig. 2.4.** Electron transport to mitochondrial cytochrome P450. Adrenodoxin (ferredoxin) reductase (AdRed), a flavoprotein loosely bound to the inner mitochondrial membrane, accepts electrons ($e^-$) from NADPH, converting it to NADP. These electrons are passed to adrenodoxin (ferredoxin) (Adx), an iron–sulphur protein freely diffusible in solution in the mitochondrial matrix. Electrons from charged adrenodoxin ($Adx^-$) are accepted by a cytochrome P450 such as P450scc shown here. The uncharged adrenodoxin ($Adx^+$) then returns to the adrenodoxin reductase for another pair of electrons. For P450scc, three pairs of electrons must be transported to the P450 to convert cholesterol to pregnenolone. It is likely that the inner and outer mitochondrial membranes become more closely opposed during active steroidogenesis, facilitating the flux of hydrophobic steroid molecules (from Miller, 1988).

NADPH and one molecule of oxygen, such that the overall stoichiometry is as follows (Hall, 1986):

cholesterol + 3 NADPH + 3 $H^+$ + 3 $O_2$ → pregnenolone + isocapraldehyde + 4 $H_2O$ + 3 $NADP^+$

The sterol substrate remains bound to a single active site on cytochrome P450scc due to the tight binding of the reaction intermediates. The $K_d$ for binding of cholesterol is $c$. 5000 nM, whereas the $K_d$'s for (22R) 22-hydroxycholesterol and (20R, 22R) 20,22-dihydroxycholesterol are 4.9 and 81 nM, respectively. Thus, once cholesterol is bound to the enzyme it is committed to complete the reaction sequence. The estimated $K_d$ for pregnenolone is 2900 nM, which permits the dissociation of the final reaction product from the enzyme (Lambeth, 1985; Hall, 1986).

Binding of cholesterol to the hydrophobic haem pocket of cytochrome P450scc is the slowest phase of the side-chain cleavage reaction. The lipid milieu of this integral membrane protein can influence the binding of cholesterol, as cardiolipin increases the affinity of purified cytochrome P450scc for sterol (Lambeth, 1985). Molecular models derived from the study of cholesterol analogues and purified enzyme indicate that C-22 of the cholesterol molecule lies within 0.4 Å of the enzyme's haem iron, and C-20 lies 1.54 Å further away (Heyl et al., 1986). The first hydroxylation in the reaction probably occurs at C-22 because of its closer proximity to the haem iron. The introduction of the 22R hydroxyl group may cause a relative shift of 1−2 Å in the position of the substrate to bring C-20 close to the haem iron, and permit the second hydroxylation reaction to occur. The process of cholesterol side-chain scission is not well understood, other than the requirements for NADPH and $O_2$. Cleavage of the 20,22-dihydroxycholesterol side-chain does not involve incorporation of oxygen into either pregnenolone or isocapraldehyde, and most authors believe that olefins and epoxides are not intermediates (Teicher et al., 1978).

The shuttling of reducing equivalents to cytochrome P450scc is accomplished by ferredoxin in a cycle of reduction and oxidation. Ferredoxin forms a 1:1 complex with ferrodoxin reductase, which catalyses reduction of the iron−sulphur protein. The reduced ferredoxin then dissociates and forms a 1:1 complex with cytochrome P450scc, is then oxidized and subsequently returns for recharging to ferredoxin reductase. Ferredoxin reductase has a greater affinity for oxidized ferredoxin than the reduced protein. The binding of cholesterol to cytochrome P450scc increases the enzyme's affinity for reduced ferredoxin by $c$. 20-fold. These differences in binding affinities promote flux of reducing equivalents to substrate-charged cytochrome P450scc (Lambeth et al., 1979, 1980; Hanukoglu et al., 1981; Lambeth & Pember, 1983). Supply of electrons to cytochrome P450scc does not seem to be a rate-determining factor in the cholesterol side-chain cleavage reaction.

## Structure of the cholesterol side-chain cleavage system: the proteins, mRNAs and their genes

Mature cytochrome P450scc is the 50 kDa protein product of a 2.0 kb mRNA which is encoded by a gene spanning some 20 kb, consisting of nine exons split by eight introns (Morohashi *et al.*, 1984, 1987; Chung *et al.*, 1986). Human beings have only one gene for cytochrome P450scc, located on chromosome 15 (Table 2.1). The enzyme is synthesized as a larger protein which is transported into the mitochondria and subsequently processed to the mature enzyme by a metal ion-requiring endoprotease (Matocha & Waterman, 1985).

Ferredoxin reductase (Table 2.1) exists in two forms, a protein of 41 kDa and another of 42 kDa (Suhara *et al.*, 1982). Both are products of a single gene which resides in man on chromosome 17 cen→ q25 (Hanukoglu *et al.*, 1987; Sagara *et al.*, 1987; Solish *et al.*, 1988). The two forms of the enzyme arise from alternate splicing of the mRNA precursor such that 18 additional nucleotides, encoding six amino acids, are inserted into the middle of one form of the mRNA. The alternatively spliced mRNA containing the six extra codons represents 10−20% of the total ferredoxin reductase mRNA (Solish *et al.*, 1988). The significance of cells having two ferredoxin reductases is not yet known but it appears that all steroidogenic tissues contain both forms of mRNA (S.B. Solish & W.L. Miller, unpublished results). Ferredoxin reductase and ferredoxin are synthesized as larger proteins containing leader sequences rich in basic amino acids, typical of proteins imported into mitochondria. These preproteins, like cytochrome P450scc, are processed to the mature forms by an endoprotease.

The iron−sulphur protein, ferredoxin, is generated from a large

**Table 2.1.** Characteristics of genes encoding steroidogenic enzymes

| Enzymes | No. genes | Exons | Size (kb) | Location | mRNA sizes (kb) | Mature protein size (kDa) |
|---|---|---|---|---|---|---|
| P450scc | 1 | 9 | >20 | 15 | 2 | 50 |
| Ferredoxin reductase | 1 | 12 | 6−12 | 17 cen→q25 | 2 | 41 |
| Ferredoxin | 1 | 5 | >30 | 11 q13→qter | 1.0, 1.4, 1.7 | 12.3 |
| Pseudogenes | 2 | — | c.2 | 20 cen→q13.1 | | |
| P450$_{c17}$ | 1 | 8 | 6.6 | 10 | 2 | 50 |
| P450aro | 1−?2 | 10 | >40 | 15 q21.1 | 2.4, 2.7, 3.0, 3.5 | 55 |
| 3β-hydroxysteroid dehydrogenase | 1 | 3 | 8 | 1p11→13 | 1.7 | 42 |
| 17β-hydroxysteroid dehydrogenase (oestrone → oestradiol) | 2 | ? | 5−6 | 17 cen→q25 | 1.4 | 35 |
| 20α-hydroxysteroid dehydrogenase | ? | ? | ? | ? | ? | 36 |
| 5α reductase | 1 | ? | ? | ? | 2.5 | 29 |

gene (or genes) which spans more than 20 kb (Table 2.1) located in man on chromosome 11q13→ qter (Morel et al., 1988). At least two processed ferredoxin pseudogenes are located on chromosome 20. The human gene has four exons, the first of which encodes a 60 amino acid signal-peptide and the other three exons code for the 124 amino acids of the mature polypeptide (Chang et al., 1988). The human ferredoxin gene appears to have a single promoter whereas the bovine gene appears to have two promoters which generate two mRNA species, differing in their 5′ ends with respect to which DNA sequences constitute the first exon. Only one of these two mRNAs appears to be translated. Multiple ferredoxin mRNAs are found, ranging between 1 and 1.75 kb in size, due to the presence of four polyadenylation sites in the 3′ untranslated region (Okamura et al., 1985, 1987; Picado-Leonard et al., 1988). This long 3′ untranslated region may be involved in regulating the half-life of the mRNA (S.T. Brentano & W.L. Miller, unpublished results).

Molar ratios of the three components of the cholesterol side-chain cleavage complex vary according to the steroidogenic tissue in question. In the bovine corpus luteum, the ferredoxin reductase:ferredoxin: cytochrome P450scc ratio is 1:2.5:3 (Hanukoglu & Hanukoglu, 1986). The expression of each protein is subject to differential regulation by gonadotrophins (see below).

## Intracellular transport of cholesterol and its access to cholesterol side-chain cleavage enzyme

The rate of formation of pregnenolone in steroidogenic cells is determined by: (1) the availability of cholesterol to the mitochondria (Toaff et al., 1979); (2) the access of cholesterol to the inner mitochondrial membranes (Nakamura et al., 1980; Privalle et al., 1987); (3) the quantities present of cholesterol side-chain cleavage enzyme and its flavoprotein and iron−sulphur protein co-factors; (4) the degree of enzyme activity expressed (Simpson et al., 1987b). Acute alterations in steroidogenesis generally result from changes in the availability of cholesterol to the enzyme and perhaps its expressed activity, whereas longer-term alterations involve all of these factors.

The cytoskeleton, controlled by gonadotrophins in ovarian cells, seems to play a central role in the intracellular movement of cholesterol (Hall, 1985; Amsterdam & Rotmensch, 1987). The steroidogenic response to gonadotrophic stimulation can be inhibited by agents that disrupt the cellular assembly of microfilaments and microtubules (see Strauss et al., 1981). Cytochalasins, which prevent polymerization of microfilaments, inhibit steroidogenesis and movement of cholesterol to the mitochondria. Introduction of antibodies to actin, or introduction of DNase (which also binds to actin and inhibits microfilament function) can also interfere with steroidogenesis and transport of cholesterol to mitochondria. The antimicrotubular agent vinblastine also inhibits intracellular transport of cholesterol.

Mechanisms by which the cytoskeleton facilitates movement of sterols are not understood. The cytoskeleton could simply maintain organelles in a favourable assemblage (e.g. lipid droplets in association with mitochondria). Alternatively, it might promote the distribution of proteins required for cholesterol movement to specific organelles (e.g. sterol carrier proteins). Paradoxically, under certain conditions cytoskeletal inhibitors increase basal steroidogenesis (Carnegie & Tsang, 1988). This facilitative effect may be due to disruption of cellular architecture, thereby increasing sterol access to the mitochondria. Disruption of the cytoskeleton might also increase cellular concentrations of cAMP (Saltarelli et al., 1984).

Carrier proteins may play a role in sterol transport. These include the basic 13 kDa polypeptide, sterol-carrier protein$_2$ (SCP$_2$), and fatty-acid binding protein (11.3 kDa), also called a sterol-carrier protein by some investigators (Conneely et al., 1984; Vahouny et al., 1987). Both of these proteins are found in steroidogenic tissues and are located in endoplasmic reticulum, mitochondria, peroxisomes and cytosol. Moreover, trophic hormones increase the synthesis of these proteins and affect their intracellular distribution (Van Noort et al., 1986, 1988; Trzeciak et al., 1987). SCP$_2$ facilitates the movement of cholesterol from lipid droplets to mitochondria in cell-free systems and also increases synthesis of pregnenolone when added to isolated mitochondria (Vahouny et al., 1987). Liposome-mediated transfer of SCP$_2$ antibodies to adrenal cells partially inhibits steroidogenesis (Chanderbhan et al., 1986).

SCP$_2$ probably facilitates the movement of sterol by removing cholesterol from membranes rather than by acting as a true carrier. This distinguishes SCP$_2$ action from that of fatty-acid binding protein, which complexes with its ligand. Fatty-acid binding protein is found in mitochondria and its distribution within the cell is also affected by trophic hormones (Conneely et al., 1984). Whether this protein is actually involved in sterol movement is unknown (Vahouny et al., 1987). However, since steroidogenic mitochondria oxide fatty acids as a major means of generating ATP, it is possible that both SCP$_2$ and a fatty-acid binding protein function in concert to promote formation of pregnenolone (Flint & Denton, 1970).

Other short-lived peptides also appear to be involved in the distribution of cholesterol from outer to inner mitochondrial membranes. Indeed, the factor that promotes intramitochondrial sterol movement seems to be a key effector of the acute steroidogenic responses to stimulation with gonadotrophin. This was first suggested by acute inhibition of steroid synthesis in rats treated with cycloheximide, an inhibitor of protein synthesis, but not with inhibitors of DNA or RNA synthesis (see Strauss et al., 1981). Cycloheximide causes a rapid, reversible reduction in formation of pregnenolone without affecting levels of cytochrome P450scc in mitochondria (Simpson *et al.*, 1978; Toaff *et al.*, 1979). Although steroidogenic activities of intact mitochondria isolated from tissues or cells exposed to cycloheximide are diminished, if the organelles are disrupted by sonication they display normal abilities to synthesize pregnenolone. Intact mitochondria of cycloheximide-treated tissues accumulate sterol in the outer membrane, but this sterol cannot effectively enter the inner membrane steroidogenic pool (Privalle *et al.*, 1987). Disruption of the mitochondrial architecture makes this sterol available to the enzyme system. Furthermore, when mitochondria from tissues or cells that have been exposed to cycloheximide are incubated with hydroxysterols (which can readily move between membranes) they synthesize as much steroid as do control organelles (Toaff *et al.*, 1979). These findings suggest that a protein or polypeptide with a short half-life, but whose mRNA is relatively long lived, plays a role in distributing cholesterol between the outer and inner mito-chondrial membranes.

Several candidates have been proposed as the so-called 'labile protein' or 'cycloheximide-sensitive factor' involved in mitochondrial cholesterol distribution. Farese and co-workers (Farese, 1987) suggested that the factor might be a polyphosphoinositide, synthesized by en-zymes with short half-lives. Large concentrations of exogenous poly-phosphorylated polar lipids can stimulate mitochondrial pregnenolone synthesis, and there are reports of increased synthesis of polyphos-phoinositides by ovarian cells in response to trophic hormones. How-ever, the effects of phospholipids *in vitro* may reflect artefactual alter-ations in mitochondrial membranes. Moreover, there are conflicting reports regarding the stimulation of polar lipid synthesis in steroidogenic cells by trophic hormones (Tanaka & Strauss, 1982). Thus, it seems unlikely that polyphosphoinositides function as key physiological regu-lators of cholesterol side-chain cleavage.

A more likely candidate for the 'labile protein' was recently de-scribed by Pedersen and Brownie (Pedersen & Brownie, 1983, 1987; Pedersen, 1987). This is a polypeptide of 2.2 kDa that can be isolated from steroidogenically active tissues including rat adrenal, ovary and a testicular tumour. The level of this polypeptide is low in tissues treated jointly with trophic hormones and cycloheximide, and non-steroidogenic tissues contain negligible quantities as compared with steroidogenic glands. This polypeptide, named steroidogenesis-activator peptide (SAP), dose-dependently stimulated pregnenolone synthesis by intact mitochondria up to four-to-five fold. SAP has been purified to homogeneity from a rat testicular tumour and its amino acid sequence has been determined. Interestingly, the primary sequence is almost completely identical to that of the carboxy terminus of the minor (78 kDa) heat-shock protein, glucose-regulated protein (Ting & Lee, 1988), suggesting that SAP is derived from the larger protein (Gregoire &

Pedersen, 1989). The significance of this relationship and the way in which cycloheximide could act to block the generation of SAP remain to be determined.

Another candidate for the 'labile protein' is a peptide recently isolated from bovine adrenal (Yanagibashi *et al.*, 1988). This peptide: (1) stimulates the conversion of exogenously added cholesterol to pregnenolone in isolated bovine adrenal mitochondria; (2) increases the concentration of cholesterol in inner and outer mitochondrial membranes; (3) increases the transport of cholesterol from the outer to the inner mitochondrial membranes; (4) increases the binding of cholesterol to cytochrome P450scc. Isolation and sequencing of this peptide has shown it to contain 84 amino acids with a molecular weight of 9.7 kDa. Except for two absent carboxy-terminal amino acids, its sequence is identical to that of bovine endozepine, a factor that inhibits binding of diazepam to gamma-aminobutyric acid (GABA) receptors in bovine brain (Besman *et al.*, 1989). These intriguing findings raise a number of interesting possibilities including the existence of GABA receptor-like molecules on mitochondria which receive and transduce the endozepine-like polypeptide signal.

The exact mechanism(s) of action of the 'labile factor' still remains to be defined. One possible way in which it could promote steroidogenesis is by altering contacts between inner and outer mitochondrial membranes permitting sterol to move by membrane flow (Stevens *et al.*, 1985). Alternatively, a mitochondrial cholesterol translocator may exist that is regulated by the factor (Lambeth *et al.*, 1987).

### Control of cholesterol side-chain cleavage enzyme levels

Immunocytochemical localization of cytochrome P450scc in human, bovine and rat ovarian tissue reveals an interesting pattern of enzyme distribution (Goldring *et al.*, 1986; Rodgers *et al.*, 1986a,b,c; Zlotkin *et al.*, 1986; Goldschmidt *et al.*, 1989; Sasano *et al.*, 1989). Cytochrome P450scc is detectable in the theca interna and in the granulosa cell layer of preovulatory follicles. Interestingly, granulosa cells in the cumulus oophorus do not contain detectable cytochrome P450scc until after ovulation, whereas the enzyme is present in mural granulosa cells throughout late preovulatory development. In luteal tissue, the enzyme is found in granulosa–lutein and theca–lutein cells. The relative abundance of cytochrome P450scc mRNA during follicular development parallels changes in cellular levels of the enzyme protein (Figs 2.5 and 2.6). In the rat, cytochrome P450scc mRNA levels are low in granulosa and thecal cells of small antral follicles. However, mRNA levels in these cells increase during preovulatory follicular development (stimulated by FSH: see Chapter 3) to reach a maximum during the process of luteinization (Goldring *et al.*, 1986; McMasters *et al.*, 1987; Goldschmit *et al.*, 1989). Abundant levels of mRNA and enzyme protein are main-

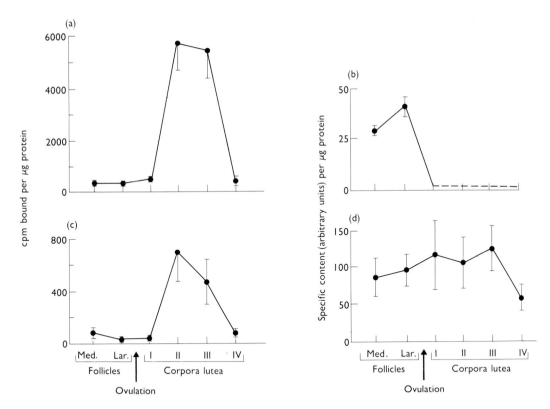

**Fig. 2.5.** Contents of (a) cytochrome P450scc, (b) cytochrome P450c17, (c) adrenodoxin (ferredoxin), and (d) NADPH-cytochrome P450 reductase in follicles and corpora lutea at progressive stages of the bovine ovarian cycle, determined by Western blotting. Follicles are classified as 'medium' (10 mm average diameter), or 'large' (16 mm average diameter); corpora lutea are designated I, II, III and IV, corresponding to the early, early–mid, mid–late, and late luteal phases of the oestrous cycle. (Modified from Waterman *et al.*, 1986.)

tained in luteal tissue throughout pregnancy, even though there is a marked decline in serum progesterone levels before parturition occurs. A generally similar pattern of change in levels of cytochrome P450scc protein and mRNA has been found in the follicles and corpora lutea of cows and pigs (Funkenstein *et al.*, 1983; Rodgers *et al.*, 1987; Tuckey *et al.*, 1988).

In the human fetal ovary, little cytochrome P450scc mRNA can be discerned even though adrenodoxin mRNA is present (Voutilainen & Miller, 1986; Voutilainen *et al.*, 1988). The relative lack of cytochrome P450scc mRNA in fetal ovaries is consistent with the idea that they are steroidogenically quiescent. The presence of adrenodoxin mRNAs in the relative absence of expression of the cytochrome P450scc gene is consistent with adrenodoxin's role as a generic electron transfer factor for all forms of mitochondrial P450, and not only with those involved in steroidogenesis.

Thus, the level of cholesterol side-chain cleavage enzyme protein

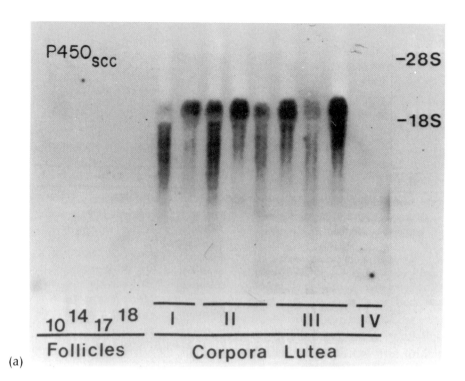

(a)

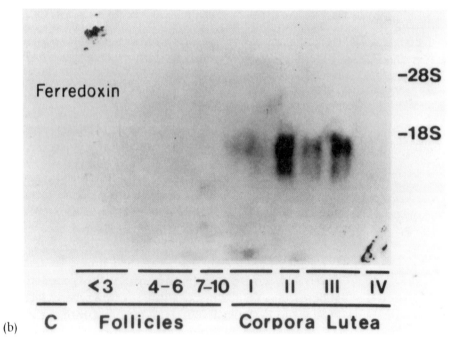

(b)

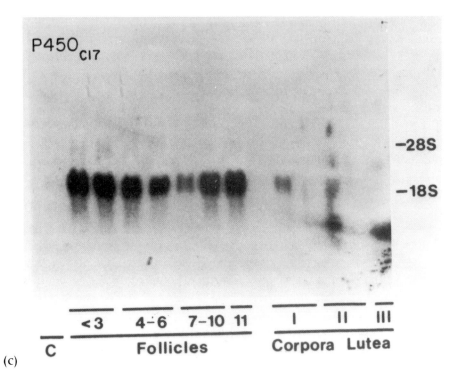

(c)

**Fig. 2.6.** Relative levels of cytochrome P450scc (a), cytochrome P450c17 (b), and NADPH-cytochrome P450 reductase (c) mRNAs in follicles and corpora lutea at progressive stages of development throughout the bovine ovarian cycle. Total RNA was size-fractionated by agarose-gel electrophoresis and analysed by Northern blotting (20 μg total RNA/track for the P450scc blot; 5 μg poly $(A)^+$/track for the two other blots). Individual follicles (10, 14, 17 and 18 mm diameter) were used for the P450scc blot; ovarian cortex (c) and individual (11 mm) or pooled (<3 mm, 4−6 mm and 7−10 mm) follicles for the two other blots. Corpora lutea are designated I, II, III and IV, corresponding to the early, early−mid, mid−late, and late luteal phases of the oestrous cycle. (Modified from Rodgers *et al.*, 1987b.)

generally reflects follicular and luteal steroidogenic capacity (Fig. 2.5). Gonadotrophins or cAMP analogues act via cAMP-dependent protein kinase (see Chapter 3) to increase the synthesis of cytochrome P450scc, ferredoxin and ferredoxin reductase, in association with increased accumulation of the mRNAs which encode them (Tuckey & Stevenson, 1986; Waterman *et al.*, 1986; Goldring *et al.*, 1987; Simpson *et al.*, 1987b; Trzeciak *et al.*, 1986).

Levels of mRNA for cytochrome P450scc and ferredoxin in steroidogenic tissues parallel those of their encoded proteins (Voutilainen *et al.*, 1986, 1988; Golos *et al.*, 1987; Miller, 1988; Picado-Leonard *et al.*, 1988; Solish *et al.*, 1988; Ringler *et al.*, 1989). These mRNAs appear to rise primarily as a result of increased gene transcription. This is demonstrated by the fact that inhibitors of RNA synthesis block trophic hormone-induced increases in the mRNAs, and more directly by analysing transcription using nuclear run-off assays (John *et al.*, 1986).

Hormonal induction of expression using 5′ flanking (promoter) DNA from the P450scc and adrenodoxin genes has also been demonstrated in gene transfer systems (Chung *et al.*, 1989; Inoue *et al.*, 1988; C.C.D. Moore & W.L. Miller, unpublished results). However, the effects of trophic agents on mRNA stability have not been rigorously investigated and it is possible that steady-state mRNA levels are also subject to post-transcriptional control. Although upregulation of synthesis of the cholesterol side-chain cleavage system is viewed as a 'long-term' response, increases in gene transcription and mRNA levels occur within hours, so even this response is relatively rapid. Stimulatory effects of gonadotrophins and cAMP analogues on levels of cytochrome P450scc protein and mRNA in pig and rat granulosa cells are enhanced by a local regulatory action of oestrogen (Toaff *et al.*, 1983; Richards *et al.*, 1987) (see Chapter 3). In rat, upregulation of P450scc gene expression during preovulatory follicular development is followed by what appears to be constitutive expression of the gene in corpora lutea (Richards *et al.*, 1987). This may also be the case in primates where short-term deprivation of luteotrophic support does not impair progesterone production (see Chapter 6). The factors that account for sustained, gonadotrophin-independent expression of the cytochrome P450scc gene in luteal tissues have yet to be elucidated.

Using a fusion gene construct introduced into Y-1 mouse adrenal cells the 5.4 kb long 5′ flanking DNA of the human cytochrome P450scc gene has been shown to contain a *cis* element that confers responsiveness to cAMP (Inoue *et al.*, 1988). This portion of the 5′ flanking DNA of the gene also contains elements conferring tissue-specificity of gene expression. The exact sequences required for cAMP responsiveness and tissue-specificity are not yet known but preliminary data indicate that only a few hundred bases of the 5.4 kb DNA are involved (C.C.D. Moore & W.L. Miller, unpublished observations). The 5′-flanking region of the ferredoxin gene contains canonical promoters including a TATA box and two GC boxes (Chang *et al.*, 1988) and the first 333 bases of upstream 5′ flanking DNA are sufficient to drive expression of the gene (Chung *et al.*, 1989). Further upstream there are sequences highly homologous to glucocorticoid and oestrogen response elements, but it is not yet known if this gene is regulated by these steroids.

Synthesis of a short-lived protein(s) seems to be required in some circumstances for enhanced transcription of the cytochrome P450scc and adrenodoxin genes to occur, as the stimulatory effects of trophic hormones or cAMP analogues are blocked by the presence of the protein synthesis inhibitor, cycloheximide (Simpson *et al.*, 1987b). The putative protein(s) whose synthesis is blocked has sometimes been termed steroid hydroxylase inducing protein (SHIP). Whether there is a SHIP and if so, whether single or multiple related factors control individual genes remains to be determined. Furthermore, not in all cell types does inhibition of protein synthesis block the accumulation of these mRNAs in response to stimulation by trophic hormones (Golos *et al.*, 1987; Picado-Leonard *et al.*, 1988). Thus if SHIPs exist in these systems they are either already induced or have long half-lives, rendering the effects of trophic hormones on steroidogenic enzyme mRNAs insensitive to inhibition of protein synthesis.

Factors other than trophic pituitary hormones, hCG and cAMP can modulate expression of the cytochrome P450scc gene. Insulin-like growth factors (IGFs) increase cytochrome P450scc and ferredoxin synthesis by porcine granulosa cells (Veldhuis *et al.*, 1986; Veldhuis & Rogers, 1987); and mRNAs for IGFs and steroidogenic enzymes are co-ordinately controlled in human tissues (Voutilainen & Miller, 1987, 1988). The mechanisms by which IGFs regulate synthesis of the components of the cholesterol side-chain cleavage system are not yet understood.

The synthesis of cytochrome P450scc in bovine granulosa cells is increased by the presence of LDL. This finding is interesting in light of the general ability of substrate to induce P450 enzyme activity (Funkenstein *et al.*, 1984). The cytochrome P450scc gene might contain positive control elements that are activated by cholesterol or a cholesterol metabolite.

The cholesterol side-chain cleavage system can be expressed in non-steroidogenic cells (e.g. COS-1 cells) by introducing constructs containing full-length cDNAs for cytochrome P450scc and ferredoxin under the control of a suitable promoter (Zuber *et al.*, 1988). The enzyme system can therefore be synthesized, processed and introduced into the mitochondria of cells that do not normally make steroid hormones. Although cells transfected with these constructs synthesize pregnenolone, steroidogenic activity is not enhanced by cAMP analogues. Thus, the ability to mobilize cholesterol and to transfer it to the side-chain cleavage system in a cAMP-responsive fashion is unique to steroidogenic cells.

### Control of cholesterol side-chain cleavage enzymic activity

The expressed activity of the cholesterol side-chain cleavage system may be influenced by the phosphorylation of its components, including cytochrome P450scc (which can be phosphorylated by calcium dependent protein kinase) and ferredoxin (which is phosphorylated by cAMP-dependent protein kinase) (Vilgrain *et al.*, 1984; Monnier *et al.*, 1987). Although the importance of the phosphorylation state of these proteins to the control of steroidogenesis remains obscure (are they phosphorylated in intact cells?), this form of covalent modification of extant proteins might either enhance or diminish their catalytic activities. Indeed, phosphorylation of ferredoxin promotes its functional activity in reconstituted systems (Monnier *et al.*, 1987).

## 17-Hydroxylase/C-17,20-lyase (cytochrome P450c17)

Pregnenolone and progesterone, both $C_{21}$ steroids, can be hydroxylated at C-17 as well as converted into $C_{19}$ androgens [dehydroepiandrosterone (DHA) and androstenedione, respectively] by a single microsomal enzyme, cytochrome P450c17 (Nakajin & Hall, 1981a,b; Nakajin *et al.*, 1981). Molecular cloning has established that human cytochrome P450c17 is encoded by a single gene residing on chromosome 10, yielding a mRNA of c. 2 kb (Matteson *et al.*, 1986b; Chung *et al.*, 1987). The intron−exon structure of this gene is unique, but there are clear similarities between its structure and that of cytochrome P450c21, another member of the same gene superfamily. There are also structural similarities between the cytochrome P450 proteins encoded by these two genes. Similarities in their intron/exon structures, hydropathy profiles, and the structures of their haem-binding and steroid-binding sites indicate the P450c17 and P450c21 proteins to be more similar than their 28% amino acid sequence homology would suggest (Picado-Leonard & Miller, 1987). The human genome appears to contain two other gene sequences related to that of cytochrome P450c17 (Matteson *et al.*, 1986b). The nature and location of these sequences are not yet known.

Convincing evidence that cytochrome P450c17 carries out 17-hydroxylation as well as removal of the 17,20 side-chain on ring D of the steroid nucleus was derived from studies with the purified protein (Nakajin *et al.*, 1981), and confirmed by studies in which non-steroidogenic cells were transformed with a bovine cytochrome P450c17 expression vector and found to express both 17-hydroxylase and 17,20-lyase activities (Zuber *et al.*, 1986). Several factors may determine whether the substrate undergoes 17-hydroxylation or scission of the 17,20 bond including the nature and concentration of the substrate and the flux of reducing equivalents. $\Delta^5$ substrates are favoured for 17,20 bond-cleavage while 17-hydroxylation predominates at low substrate concentrations (Nakajin *et al.*, 1984; Zuber *et al.*, 1986). Cytochrome P450c17 receives two electrons from NADPH (Fig. 2.7). The first is transferred rapidly by P450 reductase, and the second is transferred more slowly from either P450 reductase or cytochrome $b_5$ (Jefcoate *et al.*, 1986). Increasing the ratio of P450 reductase or cytochrome $b_5$ to P450c17 *in vitro* increases the relative ratio of 17,20 lyase activity to 17-hydroxylase activity (Onoda & Hall, 1982; Yanagibashi & Hall, 1986).

In the human ovarian follicle, expression of the cytochrome P450c17 gene appears to be restricted to thecal cells, consistent with these cells being major intrafollicular sites of androgen synthesis (see Chapter 3). This has been demonstrated by Northern blot analysis of RNA extracted from isolated cells as well as immunocytochemical staining of ovarian sections with a specific antibody (Voutilainen *et al.*, 1986; Sasano *et al.*,

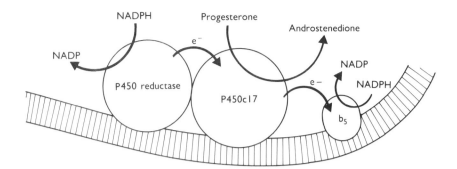

**Fig. 2.7.** Electron transport to microsomal cytochrome P450. P450 reductase, a flavoprotein distinct from adrenodoxin reductase, accepts electron pairs from NADPH, thus converting it to NADP. These electrons are then passed directly to a cytochrome P450, such as P450c17 shown here. Transfer of the second electron from P450 reductase is slow; hence, this second electron may alternatively be provided by cytochrome $b_5$ (from Miller, 1988).

1989). Studies on bovine ovarian tissue also reveal expression of cytochrome P450c17 in thecal cells but not granulosa cells (Rodgers *et al.*, 1986a,b,c, 1987b). These findings support the notion that tissue-specific regulation of this gene occurs in the ovaries and also, indirectly, support the 'two-cell, two gonadotrophin' mechanism of oestrogen synthesis whereby thecal cells are believed to provide the androgen substrate aromatized by granulosa cells in the preovulatory follicle (see Chapter 3). The molecular basis for the restriction of cytochrome P450c17 gene expression to specific steroidogenic cells is not yet known. However, its elucidation is likely to provide considerable new insight into the control of tissue-specific steroidogenesis in the ovaries and other steroidogenic tissues.

LH, acting via cAMP-mediated postreceptor signalling, increases cytochrome P450c17 levels in thecal cells by promoting synthesis of the enzyme protein, attendant upon increased production of P450c17 mRNA (Richards *et al.*, 1987). ACTH stimulates P450c17 levels in a similar manner in the adrenal (DiBlasio *et al.*, 1987). Interestingly, in mature Graafian follicles, the ovulation-inducing surge of LH causes a reduction in the level and activity of thecal cytochrome P450c17 (Hedin *et al.*, 1987; Rodgers *et al.*, 1986a,b,c, 1987b) (Figs. 2.5 and 2.6), effectively terminating preovulatory follicular oestrogen synthesis. The mechanisms by which LH causes this response remains unknown (see Chapter 3).

The 5' flanking nucleotide sequence of the human cytochrome P450c17 gene has several unique structural features, including (1) four nearly identical copies of a 50-55-base sequence resembling the nucleotide sequence of steroid-hormone response elements, and (2) a sequence that is related to the consensus sequences of cAMP and phorbol-ester response elements (Picado-Leonard & Miller, 1987). However, when fragments of DNA from these putative regulatory regions of the gene are fused to a reporter gene and transferred into different host cells (mouse cells: adrenal Y-1, Leydig MA-10 or L; human cells: HeLa or JEG-3 choriocarcinoma) they do not influence transcription of the reporter gene. Instead, cAMP-inducibility and tissue-specificity of expression appear to be conferred by only 107 base-pairs of 5' flanking DNA. Furthermore, a region suppressible by dexamethasone lies between 230 and 770 bases upstream, outside the sequence with glucocorticoid response element-like repeats (Picado-Leonard et al., 1989). These observations vividly demonstrate that the function of DNA segments cannot be determined solely by inspection of their nucleotide sequences. In testicular Leydig cells, cytochrome P450c17 is subject to rapid inhibition by oestrogens. This response involves the oestradiol receptor, consistent with direct steroidal control of the expression of this gene (Nozu et al., 1981a; Nozu et al., 1981b).

## Aromatase (cytochrome P450aro)

Aromatase is the granulosa cell enzyme crucial to preovulatory follicular oestrogen synthesis (see Chapter 3). This cytochrome P450 catalyses two sequential hydroxylations of the angular C-19 methyl group of the steroid nucleus, resulting in its elimination, and a third hydroxylation of the $2\beta$-hydroxyl group which results in subsequent aromatization of the steroid A-ring (Miller, 1988; Mendelson et al., 1988a). The reaction sequence occurs at a single active site on the enzyme and requires three electron pairs donated from three molecules of NADPH via the action of NADPH flavoprotein cytochrome P450 reductase and three molecules of oxygen (Thompson & Siiteri, 1974a,b) (Fig. 2.7).

The 55 kDa aromatase protein has been purified from human placenta and a full length cDNA for the enzyme has been cloned (Mendelson et al., 1985; Chen et al., 1988; Evans et al., 1986; Nakajin et al., 1986; Simpson et al., 1987a; Corbin et al., 1988). Cytochrome P450aro cDNAs hybridize in Northern blots with mRNAs of 2.4, 2.7, 3.0 and 3.5 kb. Interestingly, aromatase mRNA profiles suggest a degree of tissue-specificity among steroidogenic tissues with adipose tissue expressing transcripts 3.0 and 3.5 kb long, and placenta transcripts of 2.4, 2.7 and 3.0 kb long. Multiple sizes of P450aro mRNA (1.9, 2.6 and 3.3 kb) are also found in the rat ovary (Hickey et al., 1988). Southern blot analyses of human DNA under stringent hybridization conditions (Chen et al., 1988) suggests the existence of two or more aromatase genes, while others (Corbin et al., 1988) find evidence for only one gene located on chromosome 15 (the chromosome which also bears cytochrome P450scc and a dioxin-induced cytochrome P450). One aromatase gene that has been partially characterized is at least 40 kb long, consisting of 10 exons (E.R. Simpson, personal communication).

A variety of hormones have been reported to stimulate accumulation of cytochrome P450aro mRNA in ovarian and extragonadal tissues including gonadotrophins (FSH) [Follicle-stimulating hormone], IGF-I, cAMP analogues, phorbol esters (which may enhance stimulatory actions of cAMP) and glucocorticoids (Steinkampf *et al.*, 1987, 1988). Epidermal growth factor (EGF) antagonizes the stimulatory effects of some of these agents (Mendelson *et al.*, 1988a, b), consistent with its suspected role as a local modulator of follicular endocrine function (see Chapter 3).

Gonadotrophins also stimulate NADPH cytochrome P450 reductase. In granulosa cells, synthesis and specific activity of the flavoprotein are both increased by treatment with FSH or analogues of cAMP (Durham *et al.*, 1985). Thus gonadotrophins stimulate oestrogen synthesis by increasing the cellular production of electron transport proteins as well as P450scc, P450c17 and P450aro enzyme proteins.

In the human ovary, cytochrome P450aro is detectable by immunocytochemical analysis in the granulosa cells of maturing antral follicles (Sasano *et al.*, 1989), consistent with the high level of aromatase enzyme activity expressed by granulosa cells in oestrogen-secretory preovulatory follicles (Hillier *et al.*, 1981). In the corpus luteum P450aro is located in granulosa−lutein cells. The enzyme protein is not detectable in any other ovarian cell type. In rat ovaries, P450aro mRNA is low in small antral follicles and increases during FSH-stimulated preovulatory development to a peak after administration of an ovulation-inducing dose of human chorionic gonadotrophin (hCG) (Hickey *et al.*, 1988). Enzyme and mRNA levels during pregnancy in the rat display a unique pattern of change, being low early on, rising in mid- and late pregnancy but declining at parturition. Under these circumstances, alterations in enzyme and mRNA levels are not always concordant with changes in follicular and luteal oestradiol synthesis, indicating that regulation of aromatization involves transcriptional and post-transcriptional control.

## Hydroxysteroid dehydrogenases

The hydroxysteroid dehydrogenases or oxido-reductases catalyse the interconversion of steroidal alcohols and carbonyls in a positional and stereospecific manner. However, they frequently display a range of substrate specificities (e.g. the ability to oxidize and/or reduce 17β- and 20α-oxy functions). These enzymes are located in the microsomes and in the cytosol and utilize NAD(H) or NADP(H) as co-factors. They carry out ordered sequential reactions, the first step of which is binding of the pyridine nucleotide co-factor. The monomeric forms of these enzymes have molecular weights of *c.* 35 kDa. The existing literature on hydroxysteroid dehydrogenases is replete with assertions of iso-enzymes having different subcellular localizations, steroidal substrate specificities and co-factor requirements. These claims will either be substantiated or refuted as specific enzymes are purified to homogeneity and analysed by molecular cloning. Whereas cytochrome P450 steroidogenic enzymes catalyse reactions that are rate-determining, the oxido-reductases do not usually play key regulatory roles in steroid hormone synthesis.

## 3β-Hydroxysteroid dehydrogenase/$\Delta^5$-$\Delta^4$ isomerase

3β-Hydroxysteroid dehydrogenase/$\Delta^5$-$\Delta^4$ isomerase is a microsomal enzyme that utilizes $NAD^+$ as a co-factor (Miller, 1988). It converts pregnenolone into progesterone, 17-hydroxypregnenolone into 17-hydroxyprogesterone, and dehydroepiandrosterone into androstenedione (Fig. 2.1). Inhibitors of 3β-hydroxysteroid dehydrogenase/ $\Delta^5$-$\Delta^4$ isomerase (e.g. epostane) effectively block progesterone synthesis and interrupt pregnancy (Bigerson et al., 1986).

A variety of biochemical studies suggest the existence of multiple 3β-hydroxysteroid dehydrogenase/$\Delta^5$-$\Delta^4$ isomerase enzymes with differing specificities for $C_{19}$ and $C_{21}$ steroids (e.g. Gibb & Hagerman, 1976). Clinical identification of patients with presumptive 3β-hydroxysteroid dehydrogenase deficiency of adrenal but not of gonadal tissues also support the existence of isozymes (Pang et al., 1983; Cravioto et al., 1986). However, tissue- or substrate-specific isozymes have not yet been isolated.

Very recently, some success has been achieved in purifying 3β-hydroxysteroid dehydrogenase. The rat testis and bovine adrenal enzyme appears to be a single protein of c. 46 kDa which possesses both dehydrogenase and isomerase activities (Ishii-Ohba et al., 1986a,b). The N-terminal amino acid sequence of the human placental enzyme has been determined and a full-length cDNA cloned (Luu-The et al., 1989b). The predominant 3β-hydroxysteroid dehydrogenase mRNA is 1.7 kb in length, derived from a gene which lies on chromosome 1 in human beings.

3β-Hydroxysteroid dehydrogenase/$\Delta^5$-$\Delta^4$ isomerase activity in the human corpus luteum has been localized to the perimitochondrial endoplasmic reticulum by electron microscope cytochemistry (Laffargue et al., 1972). The enzyme is therefore positioned to act upon pregnenolone produced by the mitochondrial cholesterol side-chain cleavage system. Because ovarian cells have a large capacity to generate progesterone when presented with exogenous pregnenolone, 3β-hydroxysteroid dehydrogenase/$\Delta^5$-$\Delta^4$ isomerase is not thought to be a rate-determining enzyme in steroidogenesis. Even though the enzyme is apparently present in excess, its levels in ovarian cells change during the life-cycle of the follicle and corpus luteum. Moreover, enzyme activity is upregulated both in vivo and in vitro by gonadotrophins (Hsueh et al., 1984). For example, 8-bromo cAMP increases 3β-hydroxysteroid dehydrogenase/$\Delta^5$-$\Delta^4$ isomerase mRNA levels in human granulosa cells in vitro (Y. Tremblay, B. Marcotte, J.F. Strauss III & F. Labrie, unpublished observations).

## 17β-Hydroxysteroid dehydrogenase

Reversible interconversion of oestrone and oestradiol, and andro-stenedione and testosterone is catalysed by 17β-hydroxysteroid dehydrogenase, also termed 17-ketosteroid reductase. Studies using extracts from a variety of tissues indicate that these enzymes utilize both NADH and NADPH as co-factors, are loosely bound to microsomal membranes and have a monomeric molecular weight of *c.* 35 kDa (Engel & Groman, 1974). The placental enzyme exists as a 68 kDa homodimer with one NADPH binding site per monomer. 17β-Hydroxysteroid dehydrogenase activity from human ovarian extracts is recovered primarily in the cytosolic fraction. This enzyme is far more efficient in coverting oestrone to oestradiol than androstenedione to testosterone (Pittaway *et al.*, 1977).

17β-Hydroxysteroid dehydrogenase cDNA clones have been isolated from placental libraries (Peltoketo *et al.*, 1988; Luu-The *et al.*, 1989a). One of these cDNAs was used to show that the human genome has two 'placental-type' 17β-hydroxysteroid dehydrogenase genes esti-mated to be 5−6 kb in size, located on chromosome 17cen→q25 (Tremblay *et al.*, 1989). The gene(s) is expressed in luteinized granulosa cells and placenta, and both of these tissues contain a prominent 1.4 kb mRNA which hybridizes with this cDNA. This mRNA species was not detected in adrenal tissue or RNA extracted from a Leydig cell tumour. These observations suggest that the enzyme responsible for converting androstenedione to testosterone might be substantially different from that which catalyses the interconversion of oestrone and oestradiol (Bogovich & Payne, 1980; Barbieri *et al.*, 1988). Levels of 17β-hydroxysteroid dehydrogenase mRNA are regulated by cAMP.

## 20α-Hydroxysteroid dehydrogenase

20α-Hydroxysteroid dehydrogenase is a NADP(H)-dependent enzyme which catalyses the reversible oxidation and reduction of the C-20 oxy function of $C_{21}$ steroids. This enzyme is located in microsomes and the cytosol. The enzyme has an estimated molecular weight of 36 kDa (Pongsawasdi & Anderson, 1984; Pineda *et al.*, 1985). A single enzyme catalyses oxidation and reduction of the C-17 and C-20 oxy functions of steroids in the placenta. This may also be true for the ovarian enzyme since the placental-type 17β-hydroxysteroid dehydrogenase gene is expressed in luteinized granulosa cells (Tremblay *et al.*, 1989).

In the ovary, 20α-hydroxysteroid dehydrogenase is believed to function primarily as a catabolic enzyme, converting progesterone into a biologically inert steroid, 20α-hydroxyprogesterone. The enzyme has been studied in rat, mouse, rabbit and human ovarian tissues. The most extensive work has been carried out in the rat where it has been shown that 20α-hydroxysteroid dehydrogenase increases in regressing rat luteal tissue (Rodway & Kuhn, 1975). The activity of this enzyme in the rat ovary is suppressed by prolactin (Pupkin et al., 1966; Hashimoto & Wiest, 1969; Lamprecht et al., 1969; Lahav et al., 1977) but increased by luteinizing hormone (LH) in vivo and in vitro. (Hsueh et al., 1984). Its appearance in rat corpora lutea was induced by treatment in vivo with prostaglandin $F_{2\alpha}$ (Strauss & Stambaugh, 1974), presumably because of the antigonadotrophic action of this prostanoid (see Chapter 7). No information is available on the regulation of this enzyme in human ovaries.

## Steroid reductases

The reductases are microsomal proteins that catalyse the reduction of the $\Delta^4$-olefinic bonds of the steroid A-ring producing either 5α- or 5β-reduced steroids utilizing NADPH as a co-factor. The action of 5α-reductase on $C_{19}$ steroids produces biologically active 5α-reduced androgens, whereas 5α-reduction of $C_{21}$ steroids yields compounds with no known functions in the ovary or female reproductive tract (Zmigrod et al., 1972).

### 5α-Reductase

5α-Reductase is present in the ovaries, liver, kidneys, skin and brain. This enzyme has diverse functions in that it generates a potent androgen by converting testosterone into 5α-dihydrotestosterone, and participates in the catabolism of steroids including androgens, progestins and corticosteroids. The enzyme is localized in various subcellular fractions including the nuclear membranes, the endoplasmic reticulum, mitochondria and cytosol. This broad pattern of distribution could be related in part to the enzyme's function in different tissues. Recently it was shown that solubilized 5α-reductase is a 29 kDa protein encoded by a 2.5 kb mRNA derived from a single gene (Farkash et al., 1988; Andersson et al., 1989).

   5α-Reductase activity has been well studied in the rodent ovary (Eckstein & Lerner, 1977; Eckstein & Nimrod, 1977). The enzyme activity is high in prepubertal ovarian tissue (stromal cells), and these glands produce copious amounts of 5α-reduced androgens, mainly androsterone (Erickson et al., 1985). This enzyme is also present in ovarian tissues of other species, including women, but it has not been well characterized in terms of its cellular distribution (Wise & Fields, 1978).

   FSH suppresses 5α-reductase in the rat follicle (Payne et al., 1989). This inhibitory effect may be augmented by the action of steroid hormones. Progesterone and testosterone are competitive substrates for 5α-reductase whereas oestradiol is a non-competitive inhibitor, with concentrations of 1 μM of this steroid exerting a significant inhibitory effect (Eckstein & Nimrod, 1977). Since follicular-fluid oestradiol concentrations reach up to 10 μM in the preovulatory follicle, it is possible that follicular 5α-reductase activity is modulated by oestrogen. Conversely, 5α-reduced androgens are competitive inhibitors of granulosa cell aromatase which have the potential to act reciprocally and modulate the synthesis of oestrogens (Hillier et al., 1980).

## Co-ordinated expression of genes encoding steroidogenic enzymes: some unresolved issues

Gonadotrophins generally increase the activities of steroidogenic enzymes in ovarian cells (a notable exception to this being the periovulatory suppression of thecal cytochrome P450c17 by LH, as discussed above). Although various postreceptor signalling systems influence ovarian steroid synthesis (see Chapter 3), gonadotrophins appear to act primarily via adenylyl cyclase signalling to regulate the transcription of genes encoding steroidogenic enzymes and related proteins. Intracellular cAMP action increases the abundance of the mRNAs encoding all three components of the cholesterol side-chain cleavage system, including P450scc which carries out the rate-determining reaction in steroid synthesis. The cyclic nucleotide also mediates positive regulation by LH of cytochrome P450c17 and NADPH cytochrome P450 reductase mRNAs (in thecal cells), and positive regulation by FSH of P450aro and 17β-hydroxysteroid dehydrogenase mRNAs (in granulosa cells), thereby establishing the ovarian capacity for oestrogen synthesis.

Based on studies of inhibitors of protein synthesis which block the effects of cAMP analogues on transcription of steroid hydroxylase genes, the actions of cAMP may require the intermediacy of an inducing protein (SHIP) (see above). The nature of this protein(s) and the gene(s) which encodes it remain to be explored. Even though cAMP promotes the accumulation of the various mRNAs encoding steroidogenic enzymes in specific ovarian cell types, kinetics of the mRNA responses differ: perhaps as a result of differential sensitivity to cAMP, to a protein-inducer, or to the integrated action of other modulatory factors on mRNA synthesis and/or degradation (e.g. locally produced steroids, IGFs, EGF, etc.) acting by as of yet unknown mechanisms. How can FSH, acting via intracellular cAMP, raise the level of P450aro mRNA in granulosa cells without causing an equivalent increase in P450scc mRNA? Why does thecal P450c17 rise during follicular growth in response to gonadotrophic stimulation and then decline following the ovulation-inducing LH surge, and how does the same LH surge simultaneously stimulate marked accumulation of P450scc mRNA in luteinizing follicular cells? Given these perplexing observations, it seems reasonable to entertain ideas of cellular compartmentalization or dosage effects such that genomic responses are related to the concentration of cAMP produced and/or the temporal pattern of cAMP accumulation.

It is evident that cAMP must activate a protein kinase, which in turn, presumably phosphorylates proteins which control gene transcription (i.e. *trans* acting factors). These factors could act directly on cAMP response elements (CRE), such as those identified in the 5' flanking DNA regions of certain genes (e.g. chorionic gonadotrophin and somatostatin genes). A DNA-binding protein which binds to the TGACGTCA sequence has recently been identified and its cDNA cloned (Hoeffler *et al.*, 1988). The cDNA for the 34 kDa protein hybridizes with mRNAs of 7 and 3 kb in human steroidogenic tissues (L.-C. Kao, C.E. McKnight & J.F. Strauss III, unpublished observations). This protein, which is known to be phosphorylated by protein kinases, is presumably one potential regulator of transcriptional activity in the cAMP cascade. The consensus sequence of the *cis* element required for responsiveness to protein kinase C (TGACTCA) is similar to the CRE nucleotide sequence and a *trans* factor (*Jun*) which mediates the action of protein kinase C can bind to this *cis* element. It is therefore possible to envision synergistic as well as competitive interactions between these intracellular signalling pathways. However, classical or related CRE sequences and AP-2 response elements (CCCCAGGC) which may also confer cAMP regulation on genes, are found only in some steroidogenic enzyme genes. Moreover, inspection of the 5' flanking DNA of the steroidogenic enzyme genes which have been sequenced reveals no strikingly common motifs other than canonical promoters. Other genes may be under direct transcriptional control by cAMP and the products of these genes might then modulate transcription of steroidogenic enzyme genes.

The regulation of cholesterol synthesis *de novo* and LDL receptors occurs primarily through modulation due to cholesterol negative feedback with some reinforcing action of cAMP on the expression of the LDL receptor gene (Takagi & Strauss, 1989). The control of cholesterol acquisition at the genomic level therefore appears to be coupled to the cellular utilization of sterol for steroid synthesis.

## Genetic defects in ovarian steroid synthesis

Several well-characterized genetic disorders affect steroidogenesis in the ovaries and adrenals (for review see Miller & Levine, 1987). The most well studied at the molecular level are the more common abnormalities in cortisol biosynthesis (21-hydroxylase and 11β-hydroxylase deficiencies), but molecular analyses have also been undertaken of several mutant genes which more directly affect steroid synthesis in the ovaries, including cytochrome P450scc and cytochrome P450c17. Southern blot analyses of genomic DNA from affected individuals suggests that most of the defects are due to point mutations. Notably, there are no known deficiencies in aromatase and it is likely that a defect in cytochrome P450aro prevented the expression of its enzymic activity would be lethal. This is somewhat puzzling in view of the survival of subjects with cytochrome P450c17 deficiency who are deficient in the ability to produce androgens and oestrogens.

While numerous studies of gene polymorphisms for 21-hydroxylase have been reported (Miller & Morel, 1989), restriction fragment length polymorphism (RFLP) analyses of other genes encoding steroidogenic enzymes have not been described. Thus, the extent of polymorphisms, their frequency in various populations, and the association of specific RFLPs with various states of ovarian dysfunction (e.g. polycystic ovarian disease, luteal phase defects) are unknown.

## Abnormalities in LDL and LDL receptors

Subjects with hypobetalipoproteinaemia have virtually no circulating LDL and both luteal and placental progesterone production are well below normal (Illingworth *et al.*, 1982; Parker *et al.*, 1986) (See Fig. 9.11). Deficiencies in adrenal steroidogenesis are also discernible in subjects with familial homozygous hypercholesterolaemia who have abnormal expression of LDL receptors due to a variety of mutations in the structural gene (Illingworth *et al.*, 1983; Boizel *et al.*, 1986). The fact that maximal steroidogenesis is compromised when circulating LDL levels are low, or if cells have a defect in their ability to take up LDL, is evidence that LDL-associated cholesterol is an important substrate for steroidogenesis in man. However, since hormone production does still continue in these circumstances, human steroidogenic cells must be able to accommodate, either by accumulating cholesterol in association with other lipoproteins or by synthesizing cholesterol *de novo*.

## Cholesterol side-chain cleavage (P450scc) deficiency

Deficiency in cholesterol side-chain cleavage activity (also known as congenital lipoid adrenal hyperplasia) is a rare lethal defect that prevents the synthesis of all steroid hormones. Of the 32 patients reported in the literature, only 11 have survived (Hauffa *et al.*, 1985). Cytochrome P450scc protein is not found in adrenal (Koizumi *et al.*, 1977) or testicular mitochondria (Hauffa *et al.*, 1985). Southern blot analysis of DNA from three unrelated affected subjects revealed no gross deletions in the single cytochrome P450scc gene (Matteson *et al.*, 1986a). Hence, this disorder may be caused by point mutations which affect gene transcription or result in an inactive gene product. Although disorders of the genes encoding ferredoxin reductase and ferredoxin would also disrupt cholesterol side-chain cleavage activity, it is quite unlikely that defects in these genes cause congenital lipoid adrenal hyperplasia. Ferredoxin reductase and ferredoxin appear to be generic co-factors for all mitochondrial forms of cytochrome P450 and are widely distributed in non-steroidogenic tissues (Picado-Leonard et al., 1988; Solish et al. 1988). Abnormalities of either of these components of the cholesterol side-chain cleavage system would therefore disrupt other vital enzyme systems, including renal vitamin D 1α-hydroxylase and hepatic 26-hydroxylase. The hypothetical syndrome resulting from defective ferredoxin reductase or ferredoxin should include congenital lipoidal adrenal hyperplasia, vitamin D-resistant rickets, and cholestatic jaundice. Such a syndrome has not been reported. By contrast, disorders of factors involved in the transport of cholesterol to the mitochondria or in the binding of cholesterol to P450scc cannot be ruled out. It will be of interest to examine the potential roles of SAP, endozepine, and $SCP_2$ in this disorder.

### 3β-Hydroxysteroid dehydrogenase deficiency

Deficiencies in 3β-hydroxysteroid dehydrogenase occur as severe and attenuated forms (Bongiovanni, 1981, 1984). The severe form is rare and often fatal. It is characterized by abnormal adrenal and gonadal steroidogenesis with accumulation of large circulating concentrations of $\Delta^5$-steroids. The attenuated form of the enzyme deficiency is more common and generally presents during or after puberty (Pang et al., 1983). In females, the partial deficit in adrenal steroidogenesis leads to increased concentrations of $\Delta^5$-steroids, including pregnenolone and dehydroepiandosterone sulphate. Adrenal stimulation with ACTH results in an increased ratio of 17-hydroxypregnenolone to 17-hydroxy-progesterone. Ovarian function may be normal in affected individuals (Medina et al., 1986), but can be impaired in some subjects, either as a result of abnormal ovarian steroidogenesis or as a result of accumulation of adrenal androgens (Zachmann et al., 1979). The molecular basis of the various forms of this enzyme deficiency and apparent selective involvement of certain steroidogenic glands is unknown.

### 17-Hydroxylase/C-17,20-lyase (P450c17) deficiency

Although it is clear that a single protein, P450c17, mediates both 17-hydroxylase activity and 17,20-lyase activity (see above), separate deficiency states have been reported for each enzyme activity. Deficient 17,20-lyase activity in the presence of 17-hydroxylase activity is rare (Zachmann et al., 1972; Goebelsmann et al., 1976), suggesting a point mutation in P450c17 that permits pregnenolone or progesterone to be bound and undergo 17-hydroxylation but which prohibits receipt of a second pair of electrons to mediate 17,20-lyase activity. This is similar to the situation in simple virilizing congenital adrenal hyperplasia, where a mutated P450c21 enzyme can 21-hydroxylate deoxycorticosterone but not 17α-hydroxyprogesterone (Miller & Levine, 1987; Miller & Morel, 1989).

Deficient P450c17 activity impairs the formation of sex steroids, so that XX females with this disorder are phenotypically normal, except for the absence of pubic and axillary hair elicited by adrenal androgens. Females have sexual infantilism, primary amenorrhoea, minimal or undetectable sex steroids, persistently elevated gonadotrophins, and may have significant hypertension due to adrenal oversecretion of deoxycorticosterone (Miller & Levine, 1987). The testes of genetic XY males with this disorder produce little or no sex steroids, consequently these individuals have either a completely female phenotype or a degree of pseudohermaphroditism. Since both XX and XY individuals with P450c17 deficiency have a female phenotype, the condition may be generally diagnosed only when the subject, having been raised as female, is referred for sexual infantilism and primary amenorrhoea.

Southern blot analysis of genomic DNA from patients with 17-hydroxylase deficiency has not revealed large alterations in the gene (Bradshaw et al., 1987). A mutant P450c17 gene from a Japanese subject had a single point mutation resulting in a stop codon (TGA) at amino acid 17 in exon 1, preventing translation of the mRNA (Yanese et al., 1988). Other patients have detectable P450c17 mRNA and protein in their gonadal tissue but lack significant enzyme activity, indicating the presence of a point mutation which impairs catalytic function (Winter et al., 1989). A mutant gene with a four-base duplication in exon 8, which encodes the carboxy terminus of the enzyme, has also been described. This shifts the mRNA reading frame, changing the carboxy-terminal amino acid sequence and resulting in a protein devoid of enzymic activity (Kagimoto et al., 1988).

A recent case-report described a woman with 17-hydroxylase deficiency who underwent treatment for infertility by *in vitro* fertilization (Rabinovici et al., 1989). Follicular development occurred in response to ovarian stimulation with human menopausal gonadotrophins despite undetectable levels of oestradiol and extremely low androgen concentrations in peripheral blood and follicular fluid. Although she did not become pregnant, mature oocytes were collected which fertilized and underwent pre-implantation embryonic development *in vitro*. These observations challenge the existing notion that oestrogen has an important local role in follicular maturation.

## 17β-Hydroxysteroid dehydrogenase deficiency

17β-Hydroxysteroid dehydrogenase deficiency is a known cause of familial male pseudohermaphroditism (Saez et al., 1971; Goebelsmann et al., 1973; Ulloa-Aguirre et al., 1985). As noted earlier, the enzyme converting oestrone to oestradiol may be distinct from the enzyme that interconverts androstenedione and testosterone. There is only one report of a young woman with presumed ovarian 17β-hydroxysteroid dehydrogenase deficiency (Pang *et al.*, 1987). This female and her younger sisters had symptoms of androgen (androstenedione) excess of ovarian origin, including hirsutism and polycystic ovarian disease. Peripheral conversion of androstenedione to testosterone was normal. Conclusive documentation of deficient 17β-hydroxysteroid dehydrogenase activity in ovarian tissue was not provided, although the pattern of steroids in blood in response to provocative testing was consistent with reduced levels of this enzyme. The relatively normal sexual development of the patient would be consistent with her intact ability to undertake peripheral conversion of 17-ketosteroids to 17-hydroxy compounds.

### 5α-Reductase deficiency

Well recognized as a cause of ambiguous genitalia in males, symptoms of 5α-reductase deficiency in women have not been well characterized. A fertile female homozygous for 5α-reductase deficiency was reported by Imperato-McGinley *et al.* (1974). This would suggest that 5α-reduced steroids are not critically important to ovarian function. However, existing data do not rule out the possibility that subtle alterations in ovarian activity occur in association with this condition.

## Molecular diagnosis of ovarian dysfunction: the future?

At present, cDNA probes for several steroidogenic enzymes including 5α-reductase and 3β-hydroxysteroid dehydrogenase have just been cloned and sequenced. The availability of these probes, particularly the 3β-hydroxysteroid dehydrogenase cDNA and genomic clones will help identify the molecular basis of disorders of ovarian and adrenal steroidogenesis which are currently ill-defined (e.g. late-onset cryptic 3β-hydroxysteroid dehydrogenase defect). Knowledge of the ways in which gonadotrophins and growth factors interact to regulate steroidogenic enzyme gene expression may also provide insight into underlying causes of various forms of ovarian dysfunction. Given the pace of recent discoveries, it should be possible to broach many of the outstanding questions in ovarian steroidogenesis during the coming decade.

## Acknowledgements

We thank Dr John E. Shively for sharing his data before publication and Ms Deborrah Coffin for her assistance in the preparation of this manuscript. Supported by NIH Grant HD06274 and a grant from the Mellon Foundation to Jerome F Strauss III, and by NIH grant DK37922 and grant 6-396 from the March of Dimes to Walter L. Miller.

# References

Amsterdam, A. & Rotmensch, S. (1987) Structure-function relationships during granulosa cell differentiation. *Endocr. Rev.*, **8**, 309−37.

Andersson, S., Bishop, R.W. & Russel, D.W. (1989) Expression, cloning and regulation of steroid 5α-reductase, an enzyme essential to male sexual differentiation. *J. Biol. Chem.*, **264**, 16249−55.

Azhar, S., Chen, Y.D.I. & Reaven, G.M. (1984) Gonadotropin modulation of 3-hydroxy-3-methylglutaryl coenzyme A reductase activity in desensitized, luteinized rat ovary. *Biochemistry*, **23**, 4533−8.

Barbieri, R.L., Rein, M.S., Hornstein, M.D. & Ryan, K.D. (1988) Rat leydig cell and granulosa cells 17-ketosteroid reductase: subcellular localization and substrate specificity. *Am. J. Obstet. Gynecol.*, **159**, 1564−9.

Bellin, M.E., Veldhuis, J.D. & Ax, R.L. (1987) Follicular fluid glycosaminoglycans inhibit degradation of low-density lipoproteins and progesterone production by porcine granulosa cells. *Biol. Reprod.*, **37**, 1179−84.

Besman, M.J., Yanagibashi, K., Lee, T.D., Kawamura, M., Hall, P.F. & Shively, J.E. (1989) Identification of des-endozepine as an effector of ACTH-dependent adrenal steroidogenesis: Stimulation of cholesterol delivery is mediated by the peripheral benzodiazepine receptor. *Proc. Natl. Acad. Sci. USA* (in press).

Bigerson, L, Odlind, V. & Johansson, E.D.B. (1986) Effects of epostane on progesterone synthesis in early human pregnancy. *Contraception*, **33**, 401−10.

Bogovich, K. & Payne, A.H. (1980) Purification of rat testicular microsomal 17-ketosteroid reductase. Evidence that 17-ketosteroid reductase and 17β-hydrogenase are distinct enzymes. *J. Biol. Chem.*, **255**, 5552−9.

Boizel, R., DePeretti, E., Cathiard, A.M., Halimi, S., Bost, M., Berthezene, F. & Saez, J.M. (1986) Pattern of plasma levels of cortisol, dehydroepiandrosterone and pregnenolone sulfate in normal subjects and in patients with homozygous familial hypercholesterolemia during ACTH infusion. *Clin. Endocrinol. (Oxf.)*, **25**, 363−71.

Bolte, E., Coudert, S. & Lefebvre, Y. (1974) Steroid production from plasma cholesterol II. In vivo conversion of plasma cholesterol to ovarian progesterone and adrenal C19 and C21 steroids in humans. *J. Clin. Endocrinol. Metab.*, **38**, 394−400.

Bongiovanni, A.M. (1981) Acquired adrenal hyperplasia: with special reference to 3β-hydroxysteroid dehydrogenase. *Fertil. Steril.*, **35**, 599−608.

Bongiovanni, A.M. (1984) Congenital adrenal hyperplasia due to 3β-hydroxysteroid dehydrogenase deficiency. In New, M.I. & Levine, L.S. (eds) *Adrenal Diseases in Childhood, Pediatric and Adolescent Endocrinology*, Vol. 13, pp. 72−82. Karger. Basel.

Bradshaw, K.D., Waterman, M.R., Couch, R.T., Simpson, E.R. & Zuber, M.X. (1987) Characterization of complementary deoxyribonucleic acid for human adrenocortical 17α-hydroxylase. A probe for analysis of 17α-hydrolase deficiency. *Mol. Endocrinol.*, **1**, 348−54.

Bramely, T.A., Stirling, D., Swanston, I.A., Menzies, G.S. & Baird, D.T. (1987a) Specific binding sites for LH/chorionic gonadotropin, low density lipoprotein, prolactin, and FSH in homogenates of human corpus luteum. I: Validation of methods. *J. Endocrinol.*, **113**, 305−15.

Bramely, T.A., Stirling, D., Swanston, I.A., Menzies, G.S., McNeilly, A.S. & Baird, D.T. (1987b) Specific binding sites for gonadotropin-releasing hormone, LH/chorionic gonadotropin, low-density lipoprotein, prolactin and FSH in homogenates of human corpus luteum II. Concentrations throughout the luteal phase of the menstrual cyclic and early pregnancy. *J. Endocrinol.*, **113**, 317−27.

Brown, M.S., Kovanen, P.T. & Goldstein, J.L. (1979) Receptor-mediated uptake of lipoprotein-cholesterol and its utilization for steroid synthesis in the adrenal cortex. *Recent Prog. Horm. Res.*, **35**, 215−49.

Carnegie, J.A. & Tsang, B.K. (1988) The cytoskeleton and rat granulosa cell steroidogenesis: possible involvement of microtubules and microfilaments. *Biol. Reprod.*, **38**, 100−8.

Carr, B.R., MacDonald, P.C. & Simpson, E.R. (1982) The role of lipoproteins in the regulation of progesterone secretion by the human corpus luteum. *Fertil. Steril.*, **38**, 303−11.

Chanderbhan, R.F., Kharroubi, A.T., Noland, B.J., Scallen, T.J. & Vahouny, G.V. (1986) Sterol carrier protein2: further evidence for its role in adrenal steroidogenesis. *Endocr. Res.*, **12**, 351−70.

Chang, C.-V., Wu, D.-A., Lai, C.C., Miller, W.L. & Chung, B.C. (1988) Cloning and structure of the human adrenodoxin gene. *DNA*, **7**, 609−15.

Chen, S., Besman, M.J., Sparkes, R.S., Zollman, S., Klisak, I., Mohandas, T., Hall, P.F. & Shively, J.E. (1988) Human aromatase: cDNA cloning, Southern blot analyses, and assignment of the gene to chromosome 15. *DNA*, **7**, 27−38.

Chung, B.C., Lai, C.C., Lin, C.H. & Chang, C.Y. (1989) Analysis of the human adrenodoxin promoter: evidence for its activity. *Biochem. Biophys. Res. Commun.*, **159**, 343−8.

Chung, B.C., Matteson, K.H., Voutilainen, R., Mohandas, T.K. & Miller, W.L. (1986) Human cholesterol side-chain cleavage enzyme P450scc: cDNA cloning, assignment of the gene to chromosome 15, and expression in the placenta. *Proc. Natl. Acad. Sci. USA*, **83**, 8962−6.

Chung, B.C., Picado-Leonard, J., Haniu, M., Bienkowski, M., Hall, P.F., Shively, J.E. & Miller, W.L. (1987) Cytochrome P450c17 (steroid 17α hydroxylase/17,20 lyase): Cloning of human adrenal and testis cDNAs indicates the same gene is expressed in both tissues. *Proc. Natl. Acad. Sci. USA*, **84**, 407−11.

Claesson, L. (1954) The intracellular localization of esterified cholesterol in the living interstitial gland cell of the rabbit ovary. *Acta Physiol. Scand.*, **31**, 53−78.

Colbran, R.J., Garton, A.J., Cordle, S.R. & Yeaman, S.J. (1986) Regulation of cholesterol ester hydrolase by cyclic AMP-dependent protein kinase *FEBS Lett.* **201**, 257−61.

Conneely, O.M., Headon, D.R., Olson, C.D., Ungar, F. & Dempsey, M.E. (1984) Intramitochondrial movement of adrenal sterol carrier protein with cholesterol in response to corticotropin. *Proc. Natl. Acad. Sci. USA*, **81**, 2970−4.

Corbin, C.J., Graham-Lorence, S., McPhaul, M., Mason, J.I., Mendelson, C.R. & Simpson, E.R. (1988) Isolation of a full-length cDNA insert encoding human aromatase system cytochrome P-450 and its expression in nonsteroidogenic cells. *Proc. Natl. Acad. Sci. USA*, **85**, 8949−52.

Cravioto, M.D.C., Ulloa-Aquirre, A., Bermudez, J.A., Herrera, J., Lisker, R., Mendez, J.P., & Perez-Palacios, G. (1986) A new inhibited variant of 3β-hydroxysteroid dehydrogenase-isomerase deficiency syndrome evidence for the existence of two isoenzymes. *J. Clin. Endocrinol. Metab.*, **62**, 360−7.

Dawson, R.A., Hofmann, S.L., Van der Westhuyzen, D.R., Sudhof, T.C., Brown, M.J. & Goldstein, J.L. (1988) Sterol-dependent repression of low-density lipoprotein receptor promoter mediated by 16-base pair sequence adjacent to binding for transcription factor Sp 1. *J. Biol. Chem.*, **263**, 3372−9.

DiBlasio, A.M., Voutilainen, R., Jaffe, R.B. & Miller, W.L. (1987) Hormonal regulation of mRNA for P450scc (cholesterol side-chain cleavage enzyme) and P450c17 (17α-hydroxylase/17,20 lyase) in cultured human fetal adrenal cells. *J. Clin. Endocrinol. Metab.*, **65**, 170−5.

Driscoll, D.M., Schreiber, J.M., Schmit, V.M. & Getz, G.S. (1985) Regulation of apolipoprotein E synthesis in rat ovarian granulosa cells. *J. Biol. Chem.*, **260**, 9031−8.

Durham, C.R., Zhu, H., Masters, B.S.S., Simpson, E.R. & Mendelson, C.R. (1985) Regulation of aromatase activity of rat granulosa cells: induction of synthesis of NADPH-cytochrome P-450 reductase by FSH and dibutyryl cyclic AMP. *Mol. Cell. Endocrinol.*, **40**, 211−19.

Eckstein, B. & Lerner, N. (1977) Changes in ovarian 5α steroid reductase and 20α-hydroxysteroid dehydrogenase activity produced by induction of first ovulation with gonadotropin. *Biochim. Biophys. Acta*, **489**, 143−9.

Eckstein, B. & Nimrod, A. (1977) Properties of microsomal $\Delta^4$-3-ketosteroid 5α-reductase in immature rat ovary. Inhibition by estradiol 17β. *Biochim. Biophys. Acta*, **499**, 1−9.

Engel, L.L. & Groman, E.V. (1974) Human placental 17β-estradiol dehydrogenase: characterization and structural studies. *Recent Prog. Horm. Res.*, **30**, 139−69.

Erickson, G.F., Magoffin, D.A., Dyer, C.A. & Hoteditz, C. (1985) The ovarian androgen producing cells: A review of structure function relationships. *Endocr. Rev.*, **6**, 371−99.

Evans, C.T., Ledesma, D.B., Schultz, T.Z., Simpson, E.R. & Mendelson, C.R. (1986) Isolation and characterization of a complementary DNA specific for human aromatase system P-450 mRNA. *Proc. Natl. Acad. Sci. USA*, **83**, 6387−91.

Farese, R.V. (1987) An update on the role of phospholipid metabolism in the action of steroidogenic agents. *J. Steroid Biochem.*, **27**, 737−43.

Farkash, Y., Soreg, H. & Orly, J. (1988) Biosynthesis of catalytically active rat testosterone 5α-reductase in microinjected Xenopus oocytes: evidence for tissue specific differences in translatable mRNA. *Proc. Natl. Acad. Sci. USA*, **85**, 5824−8.

Farnsworth, W.J., Hoeg, J.M., Maher, M., Brittain, E.H., Sherins, R.J. & Brewer, H.B. Jr. (1987) Testicular function in type II hyperlipoproteinemic patients treated with levastatin (mevinolin) or neomycin. *J. Clin. Endocrinol. Metab.*, **65**, 546−50.

Flint, A.P.F. & Armstrong, D.T. (1973) Activities of enzymes responsible for steroid biosynthesis and cholesterol ester metabolism in rabbit ovarian interstitial tissue and corpora lutea. *Biochem. J.*, **132**, 301−11.

Flint, A.P.F. & Denton, R.M. (1970) Metabolism of endogenous sterol ester by the superovulated rat ovary *in vivo*. *Biochem. J.*, **116**, 79−82.

Funkenstein, B., Waterman, M.R., Masters, B.S.S. & Simpson, E.R. (1983) Evidence for the presence of cholesterol side chain cleavage cytochrome P-450 and adrenodoxin in fresh granulosa cells. Effects of follicle-stimulating hormone and cyclic AMP on cholesterol side chain cleavage cytochrome P-450 synthesis and activity. *J. Biol. Chem.*, **258**, 10187−91.

Funkenstein, B., Waterman, M.R. & Simpson, E.R. (1984) Induction of cholesterol side-chain cleavage cytochrome P-450 and adrenodoxin by follicle stimulating hormone 8-bromo-cyclic AMP and low density lipoprotein in cultured bovine granulosa cells. *J. Biol. Chem.*, **259**, 8572−7.

Ghosh, K.K. & Menon, K.M.J. (1988) Identification of gonadotropin inducible high density lipoprotein receptors in the solubilized membranes from rat ovary. *Biochem. Biophys. Res. Commun.*, **134**, 1006−14.

Gibb, W. & Hagerman, D.D. (1976) The specificity of the 3β-hydroxysteroid dehydrogenase activity of bovine ovaries toward dehydroepiandrosterone and pregnenolone: evidence for multiple enzymes.

*Steroids*, **25**, 31−41.

Goebesmann, U., Horton, R., Mestman, J.H., Arce, J.J., Nagata, Y., Nakamura, R.M., Thorneycroft, I.H. & Mishell, D.R. Jr. (1973) Male pseudohermaphroditism due to testicular 17-hydroxysteroid dehydrogenase deficiency. *J. Clin. Endocrinol. Metab.*, **36**, 867−79.

Goebelsmann, U., Zachmann, M., Davajan, V., Israel, R., Mestman, J.H. & Mishell, D.R. (1976) Male pseudohermaphroditism consistent with 17,20 desmolase deficiency. *Gynecol. Obstet. Invest.*, **7**, 138−56.

Goldring, N.B., Durica, J.M., Lifka, J., Hedin, L., Ratoosh, S.L., Miller, W.L., Orley, J. & Richards, J.S. (1987) Cholesterol side-chain cleavage P450 (P450scc) mRNA: Evidence for hormonal regulation in rat ovarian follicles and constitutive expression in corpora lutea. *Endocrinology*, **120**, 1942−50.

Goldring, N.B., Fakash, Y., Goldschmidt, D. & Orley, J. (1986) Immunofluorescent probing of the mitochondrial cholesterol side-chain cleavage cytochrome P-450 expressed in differentiating granulosa cells in culture. *Endocrinology*, **119**, 2821−32.

Goldschmit, D., Kraicer, P. & Orley, J. (1989) Periovulatory expression of cholesterol side-chain cleavage cytochrome P-450 in cumulus cells. *Endocrinology*, **124**, 369−78.

Goldstein, J.L. & Brown, M.S. (1990) Regulation of the mevalonate pathway. *Nature*, **343**, 425−30.

Golos, T.G., August, A.M. & Strauss, J.F. III (1986) Expression of low density lipoprotein receptor in cultured human granulosa cells: regulation by human chorionic gonadotropin, cyclic AMP and sterol. *J. Lipid Res.*, **27**, 1089−96.

Golos, T.G., Miller, W.L. & Strauss, J.F. III (1987) Human chorionic gonadotropin and 8-bromo-cyclic adenosine monophosphate promote an acute increase in cytochrome P450scc and adrenodoxin messenger RNAs in cultured granulosa cells by a cycloheximide-insensitive mechanism. *J. Clin. Invest.*, **80**, 896−9.

Golos, T.G., Soto, E.A., Tureck, R.W. & Strauss, J.F. III (1985) Human chorionic gonadotropin and 8-bromo-adenosine 3′,5′-monophosphate stimulate [$^{125}$I] low density lipoprotein uptake and metabolism by luteinized human granulosa cells in culture. *J. Clin. Endocrinol. Metab.*, **61**, 633−8.

Golos, T.G. & Strauss, J.F. III (1987) Regulation of low density lipoprotein receptor gene expression in cultured human granulosa cells: Roles of human chorionic gonadotropin, 8-bromo-3′,5′-cyclic adenosine monophosphate and protein synthesis. *Mol. Endocrinol.*, **1**, 321−6.

Golos, T.G. & Strauss, J.F. III (1988) 8-bromoadenosine cyclic 3′,5′-phosphate rapidly increases 3-hydroxy-3-methyl-glutaryl coenzyme A reductase mRNA in human granulosa cells: Role of cellular sterol balance in controlling the response to tropic stimulation. *Biochemistry*, **27**, 3503−6.

Gregoire, J. & Pedersen, R.C. (1989) ACTH control of steroidogenesis activator polypeptide and glucose regulated protein-78 in rat adrenal cortex. *Proceedings of the 71st Annual Meeting of the Endocrine Society.* Seattle, WA. Abstr. 1442.

Gross, J.D., Shapiro, B., Thrall, J.H., Freitas, J.E. & Beierwaltes, W.H. (1984) The scintigraphic imaging of endocrine organs. *Endocr. Rev.*, **5**, 221−81.

Gwynne, J.T. & Strauss J.F. III (1982) The role of lipoproteins in steroidogenesis and cholesterol metabolism in steroidogenic glands. *Endocr. Rev.*, **3**, 295−329.

Hall, P.F. (1985) The role of the cytoskeleton in the supply of cholesterol for steroidogenesis. In Strauss, J.F. III & Menon, K.M.J. (eds) *Lipoprotein and Cholesterol Metabolism in Steroidogenic Tissues*, pp. 207−17. George F. Stickley Co., Philadelphia.

Hall, P.F. (1986) Cytochromes P-450 and the regulation of steroid synthesis. *Steroids*, **48**, 131−96.

Hanukoglu, I., Gutfinger, T., Haniu, M. & Shively, J.K. (1987) Isolation of a cDNA for adrenodoxin reductase (ferredoxin-NADP$^+$ reductase). Implications for mitochondrial cytochrome P-450 systems. *Eur. J. Biochem.*, **169**, 449−55.

Hanukoglu, I. & Hanukoglu, Z. (1986) Stoichiometry of mitochondrial cytochromes P-450, adrenodoxin and adrenodoxin reductase in adrenal cortex and corpus luteum. Implications for membrane organization and gene regulation. *Eur. J. Biochem.*, **157**, 27−31.

Hanukoglu, I., Spitsberg, V., Bumpus, J.A., Dus, K.M. & Jefcoate, C.R. (1981) Adrenal mitochondrial cytochrome P-450scc: cholesterol and adrenodoxin interactions at equilibrium and during turnover. *J. Biol. Chem.*, **256**, 4321−8.

Hashimoto, I. & Wiest, W.G. (1969) Luteotrophic and luteolytic mechanisms in rat corpora lutea. *Endocrinology*, **84**, 886−92.

Hauffa, B.P., Miller, W.L., Grumbach, M.M., Conte, F.A. & Kaplan, S.L. (1985) Congenital adrenal hyperplasia due to deficient cholesterol side-chain cleavage activity (22,22 desmolase) in a patient treated for 18 years. *Clin. Endocrinol. (Oxf.)*, **23**, 481−93.

Hedin, L., Rodgers, R.J., Simpson, E.R. & Richards, J.S. (1987) Changes in content of cytochrome P450$_{17\alpha}$, cytochrome P450scc and 3-hydroxy-3-methylglutaryl CoA reductase in developing rat ovarian follicles and corpora lutea: correlation with thecal steroidogenesis. *Biol. Reprod.*, **37**, 211−23.

Heyl, B.L., Tyrrell, D.J. & Lambeth, J.D. (1986) Cytochrome P-450scc-substrate interactions. Role of the 3β-and-side-chain hydroxyls in binding to oxidized and reduced forms of the enzyme. *J. Biol. Chem.*, **261**, 2743−9.

Hickey, G.J., Chen, S., Besman, M.J., Shiveley, J.E., Hall, P.F., Gaddey-Kurten, D. & Richards, J.S. (1988) Hormonal regulation, tissue distribution and content of aromatase cytochrome P450 messenger ribonucleic acid and enzyme in rat ovarian follicles and corpora lutea: relationship to estradiol biosynthesis. *Endocrinology*, **122**, 1426−36.

Hillier, S.G., Reichert, L.E.R. Jr. & van Hall, E.V. (1981) Control of preovulatory follicular estrogen biosynthesis in the human ovary. *J. Clin. Endocrinol. Metab.*, **52**, 847−56.

Hillier, S.G., van den Boogaard, A.J.M., Reichert, L.E. Jr. & van Hall, E.V. (1980) Intraovarian sex steroid hormone interactions and the control of follicular maturation: aromatization of androgens by human granulosa cells *in vitro J. Clin. Endocrinol. Metab.*, **50**, 640−7.

Hixenbaugh, E.A., Sullivan, T.R. Jr., Strauss, J.F. III, Laposata, E.A., Komaromy, M. & Paavola, L.G. (1989) Hepatic lipase in the rat ovary. Ovaries cannot synthesize hepatic lipase but accumulate it from the circulation. *J. Biol. Chem.*, **264**, 4222−30.

Hoeffler, J.P., Mayer, T.E., Yun Y., Jameson, J.L. & Habener, J.F. (1988) Cyclic AMP-responsive DNA-binding protein: structure based on a cloned placental cDNA. *Science*, **242**, 1430−3.

Holm, C., Kirchgessner, T.G., Svenson, K.L., Fredrickson, G., Nilsson, A., Miller, C.G., Shively, J.E. et al. (1988) Hormone-sensitive lipase: sequences, expression, and chromosomal localization to 19 cent-q13.3. *Science*, **241**, 1503−6.

Hsueh, A.J.W., Adashi, E.Y., Jones, P.B. & Welsh, T.H. Jr. (1984) Hormonal regulation of the differentiation of cultured ovarian granulosa cells. *Endocr. Rev.* **5**, 76−126.

Hwang, J. & Menon, K.M.J. (1985) Binding of apolipoprotein A-I and A-II after recombination with phospholipid resides to the high density lipoprotein receptor of luteinized rat ovary. *J. Biol. Chem.*, **260**, 5660−8.

Illingworth, D.R. & Corbin, D. (1985) The influence of mevinolin on the adrenal cortical response to corticotropin in heterozygous familial hypercholesterolemia. *Proc. Natl. Acad. Sci. USA*, **82**, 6291−4.

Illingworth, D.R., Corbin, D.K., Kemp, E.D. & Keenan, E.J. (1982) Hormone changes during the menstrual cycle in abetalipoproteinemia-reduced luteal phase progesterone in a patient with hypobetalipoproteinemia. *Proc. Natl. Acad. Sci. USA*, **78**, 6685−9.

Illingworth, D.R., Lees, A.M. & Lees, R.S. (1983) Adrenal cortical function in homozygous familial hypercholesterolemia. *Metabolism*, **30**, 1045−52.

Imperato-McGinley, J., Guerreo, L., Gautier, T. & Peterson, R.E. (1974) Steroid 5α reductase deficiency in man: an inherited form of male pseudohermaphroditism. *Science*, **186**, 1213−15.

Inoue, H., Higashi, Y., Morohashi, K. & Fujii-Kuriyama, Y. (1988) The 5′ flanking region of the human P-450(scc) gene shows responsiveness to cAMP-dependent regulation in a transient gene-expression system of Y-1 adrenal tumor cells. *Eur. J. Biochem.*, **171**, 435−40.

Ishii-Ohba, H., Juano, H. & Tamaoki, B. (1986a) Purification and properties of testicular 3β-hydroxy-5-ene steroid dehydrogenase and 5-ene-4-ene isomerase. *J. Steroid Biochem.*, **25**, 555−60.

Ishii-Ohba, H., Saiki, N., Inano, H. & Tamaoki, B. (1986b) Purification and characterization of rat adrenal 3β-hydroxysteroid dehydrogenase with steroid 5-ene-4-ene-isomerase. *J. Steroid Biochem.*, **24**, 753−60.

Jefcoate, C.R., McNamara, B.C. & DiBartolomeis, M.S. (1986) Control of steroid synthesis in adrenal fasciculata cells. *Endocr. Res.*, **12**, 315−50.

John, M.E., John, M.C., Boggaram, V., Simpson, E.R. & Waterman, M.R. (1986) Transcriptional regulation of steroid hydroxylase genes by corticotropin. *Proc. Natl. Acad. Sci. USA*, **83**, 4715−19.

Jones, D.Y., Judd, J.T., Taylor, P.R., Campbell, W.S. & Nair, P.P. (1988) Menstrual cycle effects on plasma lipids. *Metabolism*, **37**, 1−2.

Kagimoto, M., Winter, J.S.D., Kagimoto, K., Simpson, E.R. & Waterman, M.R. (1988) Structural characterization of normal and mutant human 17α-hydroxylase genes molecular bases of the example of combined 17α-hydroxylase/17,20-lyase deficiency. *Mol. Encocrinol.*, **2**, 567−70.

Kishimoto, A., Brown, M.S., Slaughter, C.A. & Goldstein, J.L. (1987) Phosphorylation of serine 833 in cytoplasmic domain of low density lipoprotein receptor by a high molecular weight enzyme resembling casein kinase III. *J. Biol. Chem.*, **262**, 1344−51.

Koelz, H.R., Sherrill, B.C., Turley, S.D. & Dietschy, J.M. (1982) Correlation of low and high density lipoprotein binding *in vivo* with rates of lipoprotein degradation in the rat: a comparison of lipoproteins of rat and human origin. *J. Biol. Chem.*, **257**, 8061−72.

Koizumi, S., Kyoyo, S., Miyawaki, T., Kidani, H., Funabashi, T., Nakashima, H., Nakauma, Y., et al. (1977) Cholesterol side-chain cleavage enzyme activity and cytochrome P450 content in adrenal mitochondria of a patient with congenital lipoid adrenal hyperplasia (Prader disease). *Clin. Chim. Acta*, **77**, 301−6.

Kovanen, P.T., Goldstein, J.L. & Brown, M.S. (1978) High levels of 3-hydroxy-3-methylglutaryl coenzyme A reductase activity and cholesterol synthesis in the ovary of the pregnant rabbit. *J. Biol. Chem.*, **253**, 5126−32.

Laffargue, P., Chamlian, A. & Adechy-Senkoel, L. (1972) Localization probable en microscopie electronique de la 3β-hydroxysteroide dehydrogenase, de la glucose-6-phosphate dehydrogenase et de la NADH diaphorase dans le corps jaune ovarien de la femme. *J. Microsc.*, **13**, 325−37.

Lahav, M., Lamprecht, S.A., Amsterdam, A. & Lindner, H.R. (1977) Suppression of 20α-hydroxysteroid dehydrogenase activity in cultured rat luteal cells by prolactin. *Mol. Cell. Endocrinol.*, **6**,

293−302.

Lambeth, J.D. (1985) Cholesterol side chain cleavage in adrenal cortex: comparison of the purified phospholipid vesicle-reconstituted system with isolated rat mitochondria. In Strauss, J.F. III & Menon, K.M.J. (eds) *Lipoprotein and Cholesterol Metabolism in Steroidogenic Tissues*, pp. 237−41. George F. Stickley Co., Philadelphia.

Lambeth, J.D. & Pember, S.D. (1983) Cytochrome P-450scc-adrenodoxin complex: Reduction properties of the substrate-associated cytochrome and relation of the reduction states of heme and iron-sulfur centers to association of the proteins. *J. Biol. Chem.*, **258**, 5596−602.

Lambeth, J.D., Seybert, D. & Kamin, H. (1979) Ionic effects on adrenal steroidogenic electron transport: The role of adrenodoxin as an electron shuttle. *J. Biol. Chem.*, **254**, 7255−64.

Lambeth, J.D., Seybert, D.W. & Kamin, H. (1980) Phospholipid vesicle-reconstituted cytochrome P-450scc; mutually facilitated binding of cholesterol and adrenodoxin. *J. Biol. Chem.*, **255**, 138−43.

Lambeth, J.D., Xu, X.X. & Glover, M. (1987) Cholesterol sulfate inhibits adrenal mitochondrial cholesterol side chain cleavage at a site distinct from cytochrome P-450scc. Evidence for an intramitochondrial cholesterol translocator. *J. Biol. Chem.*, **262**, 9181−6.

Lamprecht, S.A., Lindner, H.R. & Strauss, J.F. III (1969) Induction of 20α-hydroxysteroid dehydrogenase in rat corpora lutea by pharmacological blockade of prolactin secretion. *Biochim. Biophys. Acta*, **187**, 133−43.

Lussier-Cacan, S., Bolte', Z., Bidallier, M., Huang, Y.S. & Davignon, J. (1977) Cyclic fluctuations of plasma cholesterol in the female miniature swine and its relationship to progesterone secretion. *Proc. Soc. Exp. Biol. Med.*, **154**, 471−4.

Luu-The, V., Labrie, C., Zhao, H.F., Couët, J., Lachance, Y., Simard, J., Leblanc, G. *et al.* (1989) Characterization of cDNAs for human 17β-dehydrogenase and assignment of the gene to chromosome 17: evidence of two mRNA species with distinct 5'-termini in human placenta. *Mol. Endocrinol.*, **3**, 1301−9.

Luu-The, V., Lachance, Y., Labrie, C., Leblanc, G., Thomas, J.L., Strickler, R.C. & Labrie, F. (1989) Full length cDNA sequence of human 3β-hydroxy-5-ene steroid dehydrogenase. *Mol. Endocrinol.*, **3**, 1310−12.

McMasters, K.M., Dickson, L.A., Shamy, R.V., Robischo, K., MacDonald, G.J. & Moyle, W.R. (1987) Rat cholesterol side-chain cleavage enzyme (P-450cc). Use of a cDNA probe to study the hormonal regulation of P-450scc messenger RNA levels in ovarian granulosa cells. *Gene*, **57**, 1−9.

Matocha, M.F. & Waterman, M.R. (1985) Synthesis and processing of mitochondrial steroid hydroxylases. *In vivo* maturation of the precursor of cyto-chrome P-450scc cytochrome P-450$_{11\beta}$ and adrenodoxin. *J. Biol. Chem.*, **260**, 12259−65.

Matteson, K.J., Chung, B., Urdea, M.S. & Miller, W.L. (1986a) Study of cholesterol side-chain cleavage (20,22 desmolase) deficiency causing congenital lipoid adrenal hyperplasia using bovine-sequence P450scc oligodeoxyibonucleotide probes. *Endocrinology*, **118**, 1296−305.

Matteson, K.J., Picado-Leonard, J., Chung, B., Mohandas, T.K. & Miller, W.L. (1986b) Assignment of the gene for adrenal P450$_{c17}$ (17α-hydroxylase/17,20 lyase) to human chromosome 10. *J. Clin. Endocrinol. Metab.*, **63**, 789−91.

Medina, M., Herrera, J., Flores, M., Martin, O., Bermudez, J.A. & Zarate, A. (1986) Normal ovarian function in a mild form of late-onset 3β-hydroxysteroid dehydrogenase deficiency. *Fertil. Steril.*, **46**, 1021−5.

Mendel, C.M., Junitake, S.T., Kane, J.P. & Kempner, E.S. (1988) Radiation inactivation of binding sites for high density lipoproteins in human fibroblast membranes. *J. Biol. Chem.*, **263**, 1314−19.

Mendelson, C.R., Corbin, C.J., Means, G.D., Marthis, J.M., Graham-Lorence, S., Merrill, J.C. & Simpson, E.R. (1988a) The aromatase cychrome P-450 gene and its regulation. In Imura, H. *et al.* (eds) *Progress in Endocrinology*, pp. 483−90. Elsevier Science Publishers, Netherlands.

Mendelson, C.R., Merrill, J.C., Steinkampf, M.P. & Simpson, C.R. (1988b) Regulation of the synthesis of aromatase cytochrome P-450 in human adipose, stromal and ovarian granulosa cells. *Steroids*, **50**, 51−9.

Mendelson, C.R., Wright, E.E., Evans, C.T., Porter, J.C. & Simpson, E.R. (1985) Preparation and characterization of polyclonal and monoclonal antibodies against human aromatase cytochrome P-450 (P-450arom) and their use in its purification. *Arch. Biochem. Biophys.*, **243**, 480−91.

Miller, W.L. (1988) Molecular biology of steroid hormone synthesis. *Endocr. Rev.*, **9**, 295−318.

Miller, W.L. & Levine, L.S. (1987) Molecular and clinical advances in congenital adrenal hyperplasia. *J. Pediatr.*, **111**, 1−17.

Miller, W.L. & Morel, V. (1989) Molecular genetics of 21-hydroxylase deficiency. *Annu. Rev. Genet.*, **23**, 371−93.

Monaco, L., Bond, H.M., Howell, K.E. & Cortese, R. (1987) A recombinant apo A-1-protein hybrid reproduces the binding parameters of HDL to its receptor. *EMBO J.*, **6**, 3253−60.

Monnier, N., Defaye, G. & Chambaz, E.M. (1987) Phosphorylation of bovine and adrenodoxin. Structural study and enzymatic activity. *Eur. J. Biochem.*, **169**, 147−53.

Morel, Y., Picado-Leonard, J., Wu, D.A., Chang, C.Y., Mohandas, T.K., Chung, B. & Miller, W.L. (1988) Assignment of the functional gene for adrenodoxin to chromosome 11q13→qter and of adrenodoxin pseudogenes to chromosome 20 cen →q13.1. *Am. J. Hum. Genet.*, **43**, 52−9.

Morohashi, K., Fujii-Kuriyama, Y., Okada, Y., Sogawa, K., Hirose, T., Inayama, S. & Omera, T. (1984) Molecular cloning and nucleotide sequence of cDNA for mRNA of mitochondrial cytochrome P-450(scc) of bovine adrenal cortex. *Proc. Natl. Acad. Sci. USA*, **81**, 4647−51.

Morohashi, K., Sogawa, K., Omura, T. & Fujii-Kuriyama, Y. (1987) Gene structure of human cytochrome P-450(scc), cholesterol desmolase. *J. Biochem.*, **101**, 879−87.

Nakajin, S. & Hall, P.F. (1981a) Microsomal cytochrome P-450 from neonatal pig testis. Purification and properties of a $C_{21}$ steroid side-chain cleavage system (17α-hydroxylase-$C_{17,21}$-lyase). *J. Biol. Chem.*, **256**, 3871−6.

Nakajin, S. & Hall, P.F. (1981b) Testicular microsomal cytochrome P450 for $C_{21}$ steroid side-chain cleavage. *J. Biol. Chem.*, **256**, 6134−9.

Nakajin, S., Shinoda, M. & Hall, P.F. (1986) Purification to homogeneity of aromatase from human placenta. *Biochem. Biophys. Res. Commun.*, **134**, 704−10.

Nakajin, S., Shinoda, M., Maniu, M., Shively, J.E. & Hall, P.F. (1984) $C_{21}$ steroid side-chain cleavage enzyme from porcine adrenal microsomes. Purification and characterization of the 17α-hydroxylase/$C_{17,20}$ lyase cytochrome P450. *J. Biol. Chem.*, **259**, 3971−6.

Nakajin, S., Shively, J.E., Yuan, P. & Hall, P.F. (1981) Microsomal cytochrome P-450 from neonatal pig testis: two enzymatic activities (17α-hydroxylase and $C_{17,20}$ lyase) associated with one protein. *Biochemistry*, **20**, 4037−42.

Nakamura, M., Watanuki, M., Tilley, B.E. & Hall, P.F. (1980) Effect of adrenocorticotrophin on intracellular cholesterol transport. *J. Endocrinol.*, **84**, 179−88.

Nestler, J.E., Bamberger, J., Rothblat, G.H. & Strauss J.F. III (1985a) Metabolism of high density lipoproteins reconstituted with [$^3$H] cholesteryl ester and [$^{14}$C] cholesterol in the rat, with special reference to the ovary. *Endocrinology*, **117**, 502−10.

Nestler, J.E., Chacko, G.K. & Strauss J.F. III (1985b) Stimulation of rat ovarian cell steroidogenesis by high density lipoproteins modified with tetranitromethane. *J. Biol. Chem.*, **260**, 7316−21.

Nestler, J.E., Takagi, K. & Strauss, J.F. III (1989) Lipoprotein and cholesterol metabolism in cells that synthesize steroid hormones. In Esfahani, M. & Swaney, J. (eds) *Advances in Cholesterol Research*. Telford Press (in press).

Nozu, K., Dutau, M.L. & Catt, K.J. (1981) Estradiol receptor-mediated regulation of steroidogenesis in gonadotropin-desensitized Leydig cells. *J. Biol. Chem.*, **256**, 1915−22.

Nozu, K., Matsurra, S., Catt, K.J. & Dufau, M.L. (1981) Modulation of Leydig cell androgen biosynthesis and cytochrome P-450 levels during estrogen treatment and human chorionic gonadotropin-induced densitization. *J. Biol. Chem.*, **256**, 10012−17.

Ohashi, M., Carr, B.R. & Simpson, E.R. (1982) Lipoprotein binding sites in human corpus luteum membrane fractions. *Endocrinology*, **110**, 1477−82.

Okamura, T., John, M.E., Zuber, M.X., Simpson, E.R. & Waterman, M.R. (1985) Molecular cloning and amino acid sequence of the precursor form of bovine adrenodoxin: Evidence for a previously unidentified COOH-terminal peptide. *Proc. Natl. Acad. Sci. USA*, **82**, 5705−9.

Okamura, T., Kagimoto, M., Simpson, E.R. & Waterman, M.R. (1987) Multiple species of bovine adrenodoxin mRNA. Occurrence of two different mitochondrial precursor sequences associated with the same mature sequence. *J. Biol. Chem.*, **262**, 10335−8.

O'Meara, M.L., Tuckey, R.C. & Stevenson, P.M. (1985) A comparison of the lipid classes and essential fatty acid content of rat plasma lipoproteins and ovary. *Int. J. Biochem.*, **17**, 1027−30.

Onoda, M. & Hall, P.F. (1982) Cytochrome $b_5$ stimulates purified testicular microsomal P-450 (C21 side-chain cleavage). *Biochem. Biophys. Res. Commun.*, **108**, 454−60.

Osborne, T.F., Gil, G., Goldstein, J.L. & Brown, M.S. (1988) Operator constitutive mutation of 3-hydroxy-3-methylglutaryl coenzyme A reductase promoter abolishes protein binding to sterol regulatory element. *J. Biol. Chem.*, **263**, 3380−7.

Pang, S., Levine, L.S., Stoner, E., Opitz, J.M., Pollack, M.S., Dupont, B. & New, M.I. (1983) Non salt-losing congenital adrenal hyperplasia due to 3β-hydroxysteroid dehydrogenase deficiency with normal glomerulosa function. *J. Clin. Endocrinol. Metab.*, **56**, 808−18.

Pang, S., Softness, B., Sweeney, W.J. III & New, M.I. (1987) Hirsutism, polycystic ovarian disease, and ovarian 17-ketosteroid reductase deficiency. *N. Engl. J. Med.*, **316**, 1295−301.

Parinaud J., Perret, B., Ribbes, H., Chap, H., Pontonnier, G. & Douste-Blasy, L. (1987) High density lipoprotein and low density lipoprotein utilization by human granulosa cells for progesterone synthesis in serum-free culture: respective contributions of free and esterified cholesterol. *J. Clin. Endocrinol Metab.*, **64**, 409−17.

Parker, C.R., Illingworth, D.R., Bissonnette, J. & Carr, B.R. (1986) Endocrine changes during pregnancy in a patient with homozygous familial hypobetalipoproteinemia. *N. Engl. J. Med.*, **314**, 557−60.

Payne, D.W., Resnick, C.E. & Adashi, E. (1989) Inhibition of steroid 5α-reduction by FSH in immature rat granulosa cell cultures; possible role of 5α-reductase as a pubertal switch. *36th Annual Meeting of the Society for Gynecologic Investigation*, San Diego, CA. Abstr. 252.

Pedersen, R.C. (1987) Steroidogenesis activator polypeptide (SAP) in the rat ovary and testes. *J. Steroid Biochem.*, **27**, 731−5.

Pedersen, R.C. & Brownie, A.C. (1983) Cholesterol side-chain cleavage in the rat adrenal cortex: Isolation of a cycloheximide-sensitive activator peptide. *Proc. Natl. Acad. Sci. USA*, **80**, 1882−6.

Pedersen, R.C. & Brownie, A.C. (1987) Sequence of steroidogenesis activator polypeptide (SAP) isolated from a rat Leydig cell tumor. *Science*, **236**, 188−90.

Peltoketo, H., Isomaa, V., Maentausta, O. & Vihko, R. (1988) Complete amino acid sequence of human placental 17β-hydroxysteroid dehydrogenase deducted from cDNA. *FEBS Lett.*, **239**, 73−7.

Picado-Leonard, J., Mellon, S.H., Brentano, S.T. & Miller, W.L. (1989) Tissue-specific and cAMP-responsive elements in the P450c17 gene. *Pediatr. Res.*, **24**, 90A (Abstr. 524).

Picado-Leonard, J. & Miller, W.L. (1987) Cloning and sequence of the human gene for P450$_{c17}$ (steroid 17α-hydroxylase/17,20 lyase): similarity to the gene for P450$_{c21}$. *DNA*, 6, 439−48.

Picado-Leonard, J. & Miller, W.L. (1988) Homologous sequences in steroidogenic enzymes, steroid receptors, and a steroid binding protein suggest a consensus steroid binding sequence. *Mol. Endocrinol.*, **2**, 1145−50.

Picado-Leonard, J., Voutilainen, R., Kao, L.-C., Chung, B.C., Strauss, J.F. III & Miller, W.L. (1988) Human adrenodoxin: cloning of three cDNAs and cycloheximide enhancement in JEG-3 cells. *J. Biol. Chem.*, **2633**, 3240−3244 (corrected, p. 11016).

Pineda, J.A., Salinas, M.E. & Warren, J.C. (1985) Purification and characterization of 20α-hydroxysteroid dehydrogenase from bull testis. *J. Steroid Biochem.*, **23**, 1001−6.

Pittaway, D.E., Anderson, R.N. and Givens, J.R. (1977) Characterization of human ovarian estradiol-17β oxidoreductase activity. *Acta Endocrinol. Copenh.*, **85**, 624−35.

Pongsawasdi, P. & Anderson, B.M. (1984) Kinetic studies of rat ovarian 20α-hydroxysteroid dehydrogenase. *Biochim. Biophys. Acta*, **799**, 51−8.

Privalle, C.T., McNamara, B.C., Dherwal, M.S. & Jefcoate, C.R. (1987) ACTH control of cholesterol side-chain cleavage at adrenal mitochondrial cytochrome P-450scc. Regulation of intramitochondrial cholesterol transfer. *Mol. Cell. Endocrinol.*, **53**, 87−101.

Pupkin, M., Bratt, H., Weisz, J., Lloyd, C.H. & Balogh, K. Jr. (1966) Dehydrogenases in the rat ovary. I. A histochemical study of $\Delta^5$-3β- and 20α-hydroxysteroid dehydrogenase and enzymes of carbohydrate oxidation during the estrous cycle. *Endocrinology*, **79**, 316−22.

Rabinovici, H.J., Blankenstein, J., Goldman, B., Rudak, E., Dor, E., Pariente, C., Geier, A. *et al.* (1989) In vitro fertilization and primary embryonic cleavage are possible in 17α-hydroxylase deficiency despite extremely low intrafollicular 17β-estradiol. *J. Clin.*

*Endocrinol. Metab.*, **68**, 693−7.

Richards, J.S., Johnson, T., Hedin, L., Lifka, J., Ratoosh, S., Durica, J.M. & Goldring, W.B. (1987) Ovarian follicular development from physiology to molecular biology. *Recent Prog. Horm. Res.*, **43**, 231−70.

Ringler, G.E., Kao, L-C., Miller, W.L. & Strauss, J.F. III (1989) Effects of 8-bromo-cAMP on expression of endocrine functions by cultured human trophoblast cells. Regulation of specific mRNAs. *Mol. Cell Endrocrinol.*, **61**, 13−21.

Rodgers, R.J., Mason, J.I. Waterman, M.R. & Simpson, E.R. (1987a) Regulation of synthesis of 3-hydroxy-3-methylglutaryl coenzyme A reductase in the bovine ovary *in vivo* and *in vitro*. *Mol. Endocrinol.*, **1**, 172−80.

Rodgers, R.J., Rodgers, H.F., Hall, P.F., Waterman, M.R. & Simpson, E.R. (1986a) Immunolocalization of cholesterol side-chain-cleavage cytochrome P-450 and 17α-hydroxylase cytochrome P-450 in bovine ovarian follicles. *J. Reprod. Fertil.*, **78**, 627−38.

Rodgers, R.J., Rodgers, H.F., Waterman, M.R. & Simpson, E.R. (1986b) Immunolocalization of cholesterol side-chain-cleavage cytochrome P-450 and ultrastructural studies of bovine corpora lutea. *J. Reprod. Fertil.* **78**, 639−52.

Rodgers, R.J., Waterman, M.R. & Simpson, E.R. (1986c) Cytochromes P-450$_{scc}$, P-450$_{17\alpha}$, adrenodoxin and reduced nicotinamide adenine dinucleotide phosphate-cytochrome P-450 reductase in bovine follicles and corpora lutea. Changes in specific contents during the ovarian cycle. *Endocrinology*, **118**, 1366−74.

Rodgers, R.J., Waterman, M.R. & Simpson, E.R. (1987b) Levels of messenger ribonucleic acid encoding cholesterol side-chain cleavage cytochrome P-450, 17α-hydroxylase cytochrome P-450, adrenodoxin and low density lipoprotein receptor in bovine follicles and corpora lutea throughout the ovarian cycle. *Mol. Endocrinol.*, **1**, 274−9.

Rodway, R.G. & Kuhn, N.J. (1975) Hormonal control of luteal 20α hydroxysteroid dehydrogenase and $\Delta^5$-3β-hydroxysteroid dehydrogenase during luteolysis in the pregnant rat. *Biochem. J.*, **152**, 433−43.

Saez, M.N., De Peretti, E., Morera, A.M., Davis, M. & Bertrand, J. (1971) Familial male pseudohermaphroditism with gynecomastia due to a testicular 17-ketoreductase defect. I. Studies *in vivo*. *J. Clin. Endocrinol. Metab.*, **32**, 604−10.

Sagara, Y., Takata, Y., Miyata, T., Hara, T. & Horiuchi, T. (1987) Cloning and sequence analysis of adrenodoxin reductase cDNA from bovine adrenal cortex. *J. Biochem.*, **102**, 1333−6.

Saltarelli, D., de la Ilosa-Hermier, P., Tertrin-Clary, C. & Hermier, C. (1984) Effects of antimicrotubular agents on cAMP production and in steroidogenic responses of isolated rat Leydig cells. *Biol. Cell.*, **52**, 259−66.

Sasano, H., Okamoto, M., Mason, J.I., Simpson, E.R., Mendelson, C.R., Sasano, W. & Silverberg, S.G. (1989) Immunolocalization of aromatase, 17α-hydroxylase and side-chain cleavage cytochrome, P-450 in the human ovary. *J. Reprod. Fertil.*, **85**, 163–9.

Saucier, J.E., Kandutsch, A.A., Taylor, F.R., Spencer, J.A., Phirwa, S. & Goyen, A.K. (1985) Identification of regulatory oxysterols, 24(s), 25-epoxycholesterol and 25-hydroxycholesterol in cultured fibroblasts. *J. Biol. Chem.*, **260**, 14571–9.

Schreiber, J.R., Edelstein, C. & Scanu, A.M. (1985) Effect of high-density lipoproteins with varying ratios of apolipoprotein A-1 to apolipoprotein A-II on steroidogenesis by cultured rat ovary granulosa cells. *Biochim. Biophys. Acta*, **835**, 169–75.

Schuler, L.A., Toaff, M.E. & Strauss, J.F. III (1981) Regulation of ovarian cholesterol metabolism: control of 3-hydroxy-3-methylglutaryl coenzyme A reductase and acyl coenzyme A: cholesterol acyl transferase. *Endocrinology*, **108**, 1476–82.

Simpson, E.R. & Burkhart, M.F. (1980a) Acyl coA: cholesterol acyl transferase activity in human placental microsomes: inhibition by progesterone. *Arch. Biochem. Biophys.*, **200**, 79–85.

Simpson, E.R. & Burkhart, M.F. (1980b) Regulation of cholesterol metabolism by human choriocarcinoma cells in culture: effect of lipoproteins and progesterone in cholesteryl ester synthesis. *Arch. Biochem. Biophys.*, **200**, 86–92.

Simpson, E.R., Evans, C.T., Corbin, C.J., Powell, F.E., Ledesma, D.B. & Mendelson, C.R. (1987a) Sequence of cDNA inserts encoding aromatase cytochrome P-450 (P-450arom). *Mol. Cell. Endocrinol.*, **52**, 267–72.

Simpson, E.R., McCarthy, J.L. & Peterson, J.A. (1978) Evidence that the cycloheximide-sensitive site of adrenocorticotropic hormone action is in the mitochondrion: changes in pregnenolone formation, cholesterol content, and the electron paramagnetic resonance spectra of cytochrome P-450 *J. Biol. Chem.*, **253**, 3135–9.

Simpson, E.R., Mason, J.I., John, M.E., Zuber, M.X., Rodgers, R.J. & Waterman, M.R. (1987b) Regulation of the biosynthesis of steroidogenic enzymes. *J. Steroid Biochem.*, **27**, 801–5.

Solish, S.B., Picado-Leonard, J., Morel, Y., Kuhn, R.W., Mohandas, T.K., Hanukoglu, I. & Miller, W.L. (1988) Human adrenodoxin reductase: two mRNAs encoded by a single gene on chromosome 17 cen → q25 are expressed in steroidogenic tissues. *Proc. Natl. Acad. Sci. USA*, **85**, 7104–8.

Soto, E.A., Silavin, S.L., Tureck, R.W. & Strauss, J.F. III (1984) Stimulation of progesterone synthesis in luteinized human granulosa cells by human chorionic gonadotropin and 8-bromo-adenosine-3',5'-monophosphate: the effect of low density lipoprotein. *J. Clin. Endocrinol. Metab.*, **58**, 813–37.

Spady, D.K. & Dietschy, J.M. (1983) Sterol synthesis in vivo in 18 tissues of the squirrel monkey, guinea pig, rabbit, hamster, and rat. *J. Lipid Res.*, **24**, 303–15.

Spady, D.K. & Dietschy, J.M. (1985) Rates of cholesterol synthesis and low-density lipoprotein uptake in the adrenal glands of the rat, hamster and rabbit in vivo. *Biochim. Biophys. Acta*, **836**, 167–75.

Spady, D.K., Huettinger, M., Bilheimer, D.W. & Dietschy, J.M. (1987) Role of receptor-independent low density lipoprotein transport in the maintenance of tissue cholesterol balance in the normal and WHHL rabbit. *J. Lipid Res.*, **28**, 32–41.

Steinkampf, M.P., Mendelson, C.R. & Simpson, E.R. (1988) Effects of epidermal growth factor and insulin-like growth factor 1 on the levels of mRNA encoding aromatase cytochrome P-450 in human ovarian granulosa cells. *Mol. Cell. Endocrinol.*, **59**, 93–9.

Steinkampf, M.P., Simpson, E.R. & Mendelson, C.R. (1987) Regulation by follicle stimulating hormone of the synthesis of aromatase cytochrome P450 in human granulosa cells. *Mol. Endocrinol.*, **1**, 465–70.

Stevens, V.L., Tribble, D.L. & Lambeth, J.D. (1985) Regulation of mitochondrial compartment volumes in rat adrenal cortex by ether stress. *Arch. Biochem. Biophys.*, **242**, 324–7.

Strauss, J.F. III, Schuler, L.A., Rosenblum, M.F. & Tanaka, T. (1981) Cholesterol metabolism by ovarian tissue. *Adv. Lipid Res.*, **18**, 99–157.

Strauss, J.F. III, Seifter, E., Lien, E.L., Goodman, D.B.P. & Stambaugh, R.L. (1977) Lipid metabolism in regressing rat corpora lutea of pregnancy. *J. Lipid. Res.*, **18**, 246–58.

Suckling, K.E., Tocher, D.R., Smelhe, C.G. & Boyd, G.S. (1983) *In vitro* regulation of bovine adrenal cortical acyl-CoA: cholesterol acyltransferase and comparison with rat liver enzyme. *Biochim. Biophys. Acta*, **753**, 422–9.

Sudhof, T.C., Van der Westhuyzen, D.R., Goldstein, J.L., Brown, M.S. & Russell, D.W. (1987) Three direct repeats and a TATA-like sequence are required for regulated expression of the human low density lipoprotein receptor gene. *J. Biol. Chem.*, **262**, 10773–9.

Suhara, K., Nakayama, K., Takikawa, O. & Katagiri, M. (1982) Two forms of adrenodoxin reductase from mitochondria of bovine adrenal cortex. *Eur. J. Biochem.*, **125**, 659–64.

Takagi, K., Alvarez, J.G., Favata, M.F., Trzaskos, J.M. & Strauss, J.F. III (1989) Control of LDL receptor gene promoter activity. Ketoconazole inhibits serum-lipoprotein but not oxysterol suppression of gene transcription. *J. Biol. Chem.*, **264**, 12352–7.

Takagi, K. and Strauss, J.F. III (1989) Control of low density lipoprotein gene expression in steroidogenic cells. *Can. J. Physiol. Pharmacol.*, **67**, 968–73.

Tanaka, T. & Strauss, J.F. III (1982) Stimulation of luteal mitochondrial cholesterol side-chain cleavage by cardiolipin. *Endocrinology*, **110**, 1592–8.

Tavani, D.M., Tanaka, T., Strauss, J.F. III & Billheimer, J.T. (1982) Regulation of acyl coenzyme A: cholesterol acyltransferase in the luteinized rat ovary: observations with an improved enzymatic assay. *Endocrinology*, **111**, 974–800.

Taylor, F.R., Kandutsch, A.A., Anzalone, C., Phirwa, S. & Spencer, T. (1988) Photo-affinity labelling of the oxysterol receptor. *J. Biol. Chem.*, **263**, 2264–9.

Teicher, B.A., Koizumi, N., Koreeda, M. & Talalay, P. (1978) Biosynthesis of pregnenolone form cholesterol by mitochondrial enzymes of bovine adrenal cortex. The question of the participation of the 20(22) olefins and 20,22-epoxides of cholesterol. *Eur. J. Biochem.*, **91**, 11–19.

Thompson, E.A. Jr. & Siiteri, P.K. (1974a) Utilization of oxygen and reduced nicotinamide adenine dinucleotide phosphate by human placental microsomes during aromatization of androstenedione. *J. Biol. Chem.*, **249**, 5364–72.

Thompson, E.A. Jr. & Siiteri, P.K. (1974b) The involvement of human placental microsomal cytochrome P450 in aromatization. *J. Biol. Chem.*, **249**, 5373–8.

Ting, J. & Lee, A.S. (1988) Human gene encoding the 78000 dalton glucose-regulated protein and its pseudogene: Structure, conservation, and regulation. *DNA*, **7**, 275–86.

Toaff, M.E., Strauss, J.F. III, Flickinger, G.L. & Shattil, S.J. (1979) Relationship of cholesterol supply to luteal mitochondrial steroid synthesis. *J. Biol. Chem.*, **254**, 3977–82.

Toaff, M.E., Strauss, J.F. III & Hammond, J.M. (1983) Regulation of cytochrome P-450scc in immature procine granulosa cells by FSH and estradiol. *Endocrinology*, **112**, 1156–8.

Tremblay, Y., Ringler, G.E., Morel, Y., Mohandas, T.K., Labrie, F., Strauss J.F. III & Miller, W.L. (1989) Regulation of the gene for estrogenic 17-ketosteroid reductase lying on chromosome 17 cen-q25. *J. Biol. Chem.*, **264**, 20458–62.

Trzeciak, W.H. & Boyd, G.S. (1974) Activation of cholesteryl esterase in bovine adrenal cortex. *Eur. J. Biochem.*, **46**, 201–7.

Trzeciak, W.H., Simpson, E.R., Scallen, T.J., Vahouny, G.V. & Waterman, M.R. (1987) Studies on the synthesis of sterol carrier protein₂ in rat adrenocortical cells in monolayer culture. Regulation by ACTH and dibutyryl cyclic 3',5'-AMP. *J. Biol. Chem.*, **262**, 3713–17.

Trzeciak, W.H., Waterman, M.R. & Simpson, E.R. (1986) Synthesis of the cholesterol side-chain cleavage enzymes in cultured rat ovarian granulosa cells. Induction by follicle stimulating hormone and dibutyryl adenosine 3',5'-monophosphate. *Endocrinology*, **119**, 323–30.

Tuckey, R.C., Kostadinovic, Z. & Stevenson, P.M. (1988) Ferredoxin and cytochrome P-450scc concentrations in granulosa cells of porcine ovaries during follicular cell growth and luteinization. *J. Steroid Biochem.*, **31**, 201–5.

Tuckey, R.C., Lee, G., Costa, N.D. & Stevenson, P.M. (1984) The composition and distribution of lipid granules in the rat ovary. *Mol. Cell. Endocrinol.*, **38**, 187–95.

Tuckey, R.C. & Stevenson, P.M. (1986) Ferredoxin reductase levels in the ovaries of pigs and super-ovulated rats during follicular cell growth and luteinization. *Eur. J. Biochem.*, **161**, 629–33.

Tureck, R.W. & Strauss, J.F. III (1982) Progesterone synthesis by luteinized human granulosa cells in culture: the role of *de novo* sterol synthesis and lipoprotein-carried sterol. *J. Clin. Endocrinol. Metab.*, **54**, 367–73.

Ulloa-Aquirre, A., Bassol, S., Poo, Mendez, J.P., Mutchinick, D., Robles, L. & Perez-Palacios, G. (1985) Endocrine and biochemical studies in a 46XY phenotypically male infant with 17 ketosteroid reductase deficiency. *J. Clin. Endocrinol. Metab.*, **60**, 634–3.

Vahouny, G.V., Chanderbhan, R.F., Kharroubi, A., Noland, B.J., Pastuszyn, A. & Scallen, T.J. (1987) Sterol carrier and lipid transfer proteins. *Adv. Lipid Res.*, **22**, 83–113.

Van Noort, M., Rommerts, F.F.G., Van Amerongen, A. & Wirtz, K.W.A. (1986) Localization and hormonal regulation of the non-specific lipid transfer protein (sterol carrier protein₂) in rat testis. *J. Endocrinol.*, **109**, R13–16.

Van Noort, M., Rommerts, F.F.G., Van Amerongen, A. & Wirtz, K.W.A. (1988) Regulation of sterol carrier protein 2(SCP2) levels in the soluble fraction of rat Leydig cells, kinetics and the possible role of calcium influx. *Mol. Cell. Endocrinol.*, **56**, 133–40.

Veldhuis, J.D., Nestler, J.E. & Strauss, J.F. III (1987) The insulin-like growth factor, somatomedin C, stimulates low density lipoprotein metabolism by swine granulosa cells. *Endocrinology*, **121**, 340–6.

Veldhuis, J.D. & Rodgers, R.J. (1987) Mechanisms subserving the steroidogenic synergism between follicle-stimulating hormone and insulin-like growth factor I (somatomedin C). Alterations in cellular sterol metabolism in swine granulosa cells. *J. Biol. Chem.*, **262**, 7658–64.

Veldhuis, J.D., Rodgers, R.J., Dee, A. & Simpson, E.R. (1986) The insulin-like growth factor, somatomedin C, induces synthesis of cholesterol side-chain cleavage cytochrome P-450 and adrenodoxin in ovarian cells. *J. Biol. Chem.*, **261**, 2499–502.

Veldhuis, J.D., Strauss, J.F. III, Silavin, S.L. & Kolp, L.A. (1985) The role of cholesterol esterification in ovarian steroidogenesis: studies in cultured swine granulosa cells using a novel inhibitor of acyl coenzyme A: cholesterol acyltransferase. *Endocrinology*, **116**, 25–30.

Vilgrain, I., Defaye, I. & Chambaz, E.M. (1984) Adrenocortical cytochrome P-450 responsible for cholesterol side chain cleavage (P-450scc) is phosphorylated by the calcium-activated phospholipid-sensitive protein kinase (protein kinase C). *Biochem. Biophys. Res. Commun.*, **125**, 554−61.

Voutilainen, R. & Miller, W.L. (1986) Developmental expression of genes for the steroidogenic enzymes P450scc (20,22 desmolase), P450c17 (17α hydroxylase/17/20 lyase) and P450c21 (21-hydroxylase) in the human fetus. *J. Clin. Endocrinol. Metab.*, **63**, 1145−50.

Voutilainen, R. & Miller, W.L. (1987) Coordinate trophic hormone regulation of mRNAs for insulin-like growth factor II and the cholesterol side-chain cleavage enzyme, P450scc in human steroidogenic tissues. *Proc. Natl. Acad. Sci. USA*, **84**, 1590−4.

Voutilainen, R. & Miller, W.L. (1988) Developmental and hormonal regulation of mRNAs for insulin-like growth factor II and steroidogenic enzymes in human fetal adrenal and gonads. *DNA*, **7**, 9−15.

Voutilainen, R., Picado-Leonard, J., DiBlasio, A.M. & Miller, W.L. (1988) Hormonal and developmental regulation of adrenodoxin messenger ribonucleic acid in steroidogenic tissues. *J. Clin. Endocrinol. Metab.*, **66**, 383−8.

Voutilainen, R., Tapananinen, J., Chung, B., Matteson, K.J. & Miller, W.L. (1986). Hormonal regulation of P450scc (20,22 desmolase) and P450c17 (17α-hydroxylase/17,20 lyase) in cultured human granulosa cells. *J. Clin. Endocrinol. Metab.*, **63**, 202−7.

Waterman, M.R., Mason, J.I., Zuber, M.X., John, M.E., Rodgers, R.J. & Simpson, E.R. (1986) Control of gene expression of adrenal steroid hydroxylases and related enzymes. *Endocr. Res.*, **12**, 393−408.

Winter, J.S.D., Couch, R.M., Miller, J., Perry, Y.S., Ferreira, P., Bayadala, L. & Shackleton, C.H.C. (1989) Combined 17-hydroxyiase and 17,20-desmolase deficiencies evidence for synthesis of a defective cytochrome P450$_{17}$. *J. Clin. Endocrinol. Metab.*, **68**, 309−16.

Wise, T.H. & Fields, M.J. (1978) Analysis for the 5α-steroid reductase in the bovine ovary with ($^{14}$C)-progesterone and ($^{14}$C) testosterone. *J. Steroid Biochem.*, **9**, 1207−15.

Wyne, K.L., Schreiber, J.R., Larsen, A.L. & Getz, G.S. (1989) Regulation of apoliproprotein E biosyntheses by cAMP and phorbol esters in rat ovarian granulosa cells. *J. Biol. Chem.*, **264**, 981−9.

Yanagibashi, K. & Hall, P.F. (1986) Role of electron transport in the regulation of the lyase activity of C21 side-chain cleavage P450 from porcine adrenal and testicular microsomes. *J. Biol. Chem.*, **261**, 8429−33.

Yanagibashi, K., Ohno, Y., Kawamura, M. & Hall, P.F. (1988) The regulation of intracellular transport of cholesterol in bovine adrenal cells: purification of a novel protein. *Endocrinology*, **123**, 2075−82.

Yanase, T., Kagimoto, M., Matsui, N., Simpson, E.R. & Waterman, M.R. (1988) Combined 17α-hydroxylase/17,20-lyase deficiency due to a stop codon in the N-terminal region of 17α-hydroxylase cytochrome P-450. *Mol. Cell. Endocrinol.*, **59**, 249−53.

Zachmann, M., Forest, M.G. & De Peretti, E. (1979) 3β-hydroxysteroid dehydrogenase deficiency: follow-up study in a girl with pubertal bone age. *Horm. Res.*, **11**, 292−302.

Zachmann, M., Vollmin, J.A., Hamilton, W. & Prader, A. (1972) Steroid 17,20-desmolase deficiency: a new cause of male pseudohermaphroditism. *Clin. Endocrinol. (Oxf.)*, **1**, 369−85.

Zlotkin, T., Farkash, Y. & Orly, J. (1986) Cell-specific expression of immunoreactive cholesterol side chain cleavage cytochrome P-450 during follicular development in the rat ovary. *Endocrinology*, **119**, 2809−20.

Zmigrod, A., Lindner, H.R. & Lamprecht, S.A. (1972) Reductive pathways of progesterone metabolism in the rat ovary. *Acta Endocrinol. Copenh.* **67**, 141−52.

Zuber, M.X., Mason, J.I., Simpson, E.R. & Waterman, M.R. (1988) Simultaneous transfection of COS-1 cells with mitochondrial and microsomal steroid hydroxylases: Incorporation of a steroidogenic pathway into non-steroidogenic cells. *Proc. Natl. Acad. Sci. USA*, **85**, 699−703.

Zuber, M.X., Simpson, E.R. & Waterman, M.R. (1986) Expression of bovine 17α-hydroxylase cytochrome P450 cDNA in non-steroidogenic (COS-1) cells. *Science*, **234**, 1258−61.

# 3 Cellular Basis of Follicular Endocrine Function

S.G. HILLIER

## Introduction

During the follicular phase of the human menstrual cycle, the follicle destined to ovulate increases in size from a diameter of 2–5 mm to over 20 mm and becomes the major ovarian source of secreted oestrogen. This oestrogen-secretory stage in its development encompasses a programmed sequence of cell growth and differentiation in the follicle wall which terminates with ovulation and transformation of the follicle into a corpus luteum. The entire sequence of events depends upon primary (endocrine) stimulation of the ovaries by the gonadotrophins follicle-stimulating hormone (FSH) and luteinizing hormone (LH), underpinned by local (paracrine and autocrine) levels of control emanating from within the follicle itself.

The aim of this chapter is to survey current concepts of gonadotrophin-regulated preovulatory follicular development and endocrine function, emphasizing the intrafollicular regulatory mechanisms underlying synthesis and secretion of oestrogen by the ovaries. Knowledge of this subject has increased substantially during the past decade and several comprehensive reviews of the relevant literature are available (Hillier *et al.*, 1980a, 1981, 1985; Richards 1980;

Richards *et al.*, 1987; Dorrington *et al.*, 1983; Hsueh *et al.*, 1984, 1989; Adashi *et al.*, 1985; Gore-Langton & Armstrong, 1988; Tonetta & DiZerega, 1989).

## Gonadotrophins and preovulatory follicular development

Normal preovulatory follicular development and oestrogen secretion depend upon appropriate stimulation of the ovaries by adequate amounts of both FSH and LH. Relative requirements for stimulation by each gonadotrophin at progressive stages of follicular development are illustrated schematically in Fig. 3.1.

Multiple antral follicles capable of entering preovulatory stages of development are usually present in the ovaries at the beginning of a normal menstrual cycle. Such 'incipient' preovulatory follicles are between 2 and 5 mm in diameter, comprising a fluid-filled antral cavity surrounded by inner granulosa (in which the cumulus-enclosed secondary oocyte is embedded) and outer thecal cell layers separated by a lamina basalis. Tonic stimulation of the ovaries by both FSH and

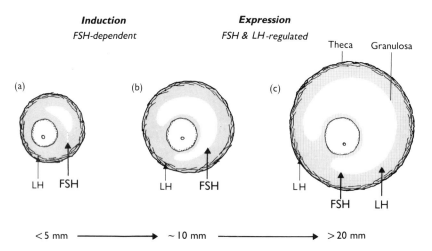

**Fig. 3.1.** Development-related requirements for follicular stimulation by gonadotrophins. FSH receptors are located on granulosa cells and LH receptors on thecal cells throughout antral follicular development. (a) Incipient preovulatory follicles (~5 mm diameter) present at the beginning of a menstrual cycle continue to develop in response to the intercycle FSH rise. (b) By the midfollicular phase a single 'dominant' follicle is 'selected' (see text), being the largest (≥10 mm diameter) healthy follicle in either ovary. Due to the inductive action of FSH, granulosa cells in this follicle will have proliferated and acquired LH receptors and steroidogenic enzymes including P450aro (aromatase) crucial to oestrogen synthesis. (c) During the mid-late follicular phase, preovulatory follicular growth and expression of endocrine function (oestrogen secretion) depend on joint stimulation by FSH and LH and the follicle becomes increasingly responsive to each gonadotrophin. Ovulation is induced by the mid-cycle LH surge which is released when follicular diameter is ≥20 mm and oestrogen secretion rate is maximal.

LH is required for follicles to achieve this stage of development whereas selectively increased stimulation by FSH in the face of tonic stimulation by LH is required for preovulatory growth and oestrogen secretion to begin (Fig. 3.1). During the second half of the follicular phase, oestrogen synthesis in the preovulatory follicle becomes directly responsive to LH as well as FSH.

## Function of FSH

Increased secretion of FSH by the pituitary gland constitutes the primary signal for preovulatory follicular development to begin (Hsueh et al., 1989). This occurs in response to withdrawal of steroid/inhibin-mediated ovarian feedback inhibition of pituitary FSH release as the corpus luteum of the previous cycle regresses (see Chapter 1). It requires 10–12 days of sustained stimulation by FSH for an c. 5-mm diameter follicle to attain a full preovulatory diameter of ≥20 mm. During this period, the granulosa cell content of such a follicle doubles five or six times to reach over 50 million (McNatty, 1981). FSH stimulates granulosa cell proliferation directly and induces LH-responsive mechanisms in these cells which subserve the steroid-secretory functions of the preovulatory follicle and (after ovulation) the corpus luteum. Important FSH-induced developments in granulosa cell function during this period include increased secretion of glycosaminoglycans which contribute to the formation of follicular fluid (Ax & Ryan, 1979; Yanagashita et al., 1981); increased synthesis of steroids (progesterone and oestradiol) reflected in the rising follicular fluid steroid level (McNatty, 1981), induction of LH receptors functionally coupled to steroidogenesis (Channing & Tsafriri, 1977), and overall increased responsiveness to FSH and LH (Richards, 1980; Hsueh et al., 1984; Hillier, 1985).

Granulosa cells are the only ovarian cells which possess measurable FSH receptors and binding of FSH to its receptor on the cell surface activates adenylyl cyclase-mediated postreceptor signalling (see below), leading to increased expression of diverse mRNAs encoding proteins crucial to granulosa cell proliferation and differentiation (Richards et al., 1987). Known FSH-responsive genes are listed in Table 3.1. They include the LH receptor itself (Segaloff et al. 1990) and some major steroidogenic enzymes, notably aromatase (P450aro), the cytochrome P450 crucial to oestrogen synthesis (Mendelson et al., 1988); proteases such as tissue plasminogen activator; regulatory peptides such as inhibin subunits and follistatin; and a 'heat-shock' protein. Other genes expected to be under direct FSH control include the LH receptor (McFarland et al., 1989) and insulin-like growth factors (IGFs) which are implicated in the autocrine control of granulosa cell development (Oliver et al., 1989) (see later).

**Table 3.1.** FSH-inducible genes in ovarian granulosa cells

| mRNA | Reference |
|---|---|
| P450scc | Richards *et al.*, 1987 |
| P450aro | Steinkampf *et al.*, 1987; Hickey *et al.*, 1988 |
| RIIβ subunit of type II cAMP-dependent protein kinase | Hedin *et al.*, 1987 |
| Tissue plasminogen activator | O'Connell *et al.*, 1987; Ohlsson *et al.*, 1988 |
| Renin | Kim *et al.*, 1987 |
| Apoliprotein E | Wyne *et al.*, 1989 |
| Prostaglandin endoperoxide synthase | Richards *et al.*, 1987 |
| Inhibin α-subunit | Woodruff *et al.*, 1987 |
| Inhibin $β_A$-and $β_B$-subunits | Turner *et al.*, 1989 |
| Pro-opiomelanocortin | Young *et al.*, 1989 |
| Heat-shock protein (hsp90) | Ben-Ze'ev & Amsterdam, 1989 |
| Follistatin | Shimasaki *et al.*, 1989 |
| LH receptor | Segaloff *et al.*, 1990 |

## Function of LH

The steroid-secretory function of the preovulatory follicle, like that of the corpus luteum, is critically dependent on LH. Increased follicular oestrogen secretion occurs during the second half of the follicular phase when the frequency of pulsatile LH discharge by the pituitary increases and FSH secretion declines. At mid-cycle, oestrogen secretion is suppressed by the mid-cycle LH surge which simultaneously initiates follicle rupture, corpus luteum formation and onset of luteal pro-gesterone secretion (Yen, 1986). After ovulation, tonic stimulation by LH transiently sustains the steroid-secretory function of the corpus luteum (Filicori *et al.*, 1984). If pregnancy occurs, the functional lifespan of the corpus luteum is extended by the direct action of trophoblastic human chorionic gonadotrophin (hCG) (see below).

Granulosa cells develop LH receptors in response to stimulation by FSH (see above), both gonadotrophins can thereby act directly to stimulate granulosa cell steroidogenesis in the preovulatory follicle (Channing & Tsafriri, 1977). LH receptors are also located on thecal/interstitial cells and steroidogenesis (androgen synthesis) in these cells is under direct LH control throughout the menstrual cycle (Erickson *et al.*, 1985). LH acts via its receptor in the plasma membrane of granulosa−lutein cells and thecal/interstitial cells to stimulate steroid synthesis mediated by adenylyl cyclase signalling (Marsh, 1976; Golos *et al.*, 1987; Magoffin, 1989). Intracellular signalling via inositol lipid hydrolysis also contributes to the actions of LH and hCG on steroido-genesis in luteinized granulosa cells (Davis *et al.*, 1984; Leung & Wang, 1989) (see below).

## Postreceptor signalling and gonadotrophin action

Receptor-activated increases in adenylyl cyclase activity and intracellular production of cyclic adenosine monophosphate (cAMP) mediate the effects of FSH (on immature granulosa cells) and LH (on thecal cells and mature granulosa cells) (Richards *et al.*, 1987). Other factors trans-mit information into these cells via receptor-activated tyrosine kinase or phosphoinositide (PI) hydrolysis, thereby modulating cellular responsiveness to gonadotrophins (Fig. 3.2.).

### Adenylyl cyclase

The pivotal role of intracellular cAMP in mediating gonadotrophin action on gonadal cells has been recognized for many years (Marsh,

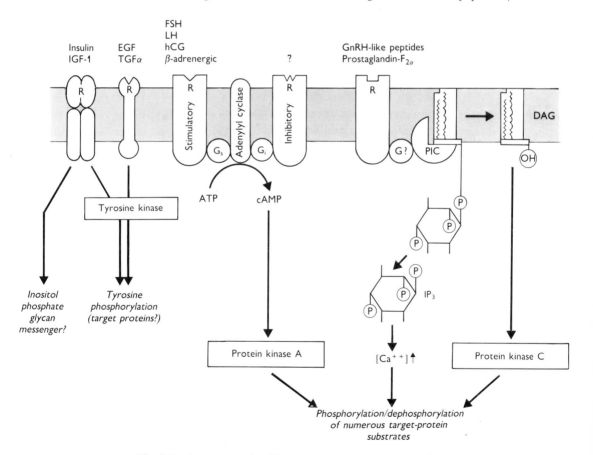

**Fig. 3.2.** Postreceptor signalling pathways in ovarian follicular cells (based on Michell, 1989).

77 FOLLICULAR ENDOCRINE FUNCTION

1976). Binding of gonadotrophins to their receptors on the cell surface activates adenylyl cyclase to increase the formation of cAMP which stimulates the activity of cAMP-dependent protein kinase (protein kinase A). Protein kinase A exists as a tetrameric complex comprising two regulatory subunits (which bind cAMP) and two catalytic subunits with phosphotransferase activity (Beebe et al., 1989). Binding of cAMP to the regulatory subunits of protein kinase A depresses the phospho-transferase activity of its catalytic subunits, permitting phosphorylation of protein substrates which either stimulate steroidogenesis acutely or exert longer-term inductive effects by increasing rates of transcription of cAMP-regulated genes (Kurten & Richards, 1989). The nature of the proteins phosphorylated by protein kinase A and the mechanism(s) by which transcription is increased are not yet understood (Roesler et al., 1988)

Hormonal activation of cAMP formation involves the sequential action of three proteins: (1) the receptor; (2) a guanine nucleotide coupling protein (G protein) termed $G_s$ and comprising three subunits $\alpha_s$, $\beta$ and $\gamma$; and (3) adenylyl cyclase (Johnson & Dhanasekaran, 1989). Receptors which regulate adenylyl cyclase activity are transmembrane glycoproteins with the hormone-binding site on the outer membrane surface and a signalling domain at the cytoplasmic face of the membrane. Binding of gonadotrophin to its receptor triggers a conformational change and opens up the nucleotide binding site of $G_s$. In its unactivated form the $G_s$ nucleotide binding-site binds guanosine diphosphate (GDP). However, once activated by hormone binding the $G_s$ nucleotide binding-site releases GDP and binds instead to guanosine triphosphate (GTP), the most abundant guanine nucleotide present in cells. Once GTP binds, the $\alpha$-subunit of $G_s$ is released into the surrounding membrane to activate adenylyl cyclase. Since the free $\alpha$-subunit of $G_s$ has intrinsic GTPase activity, it rapidly converts bound GTP to GDP, thereby halting the activation of additional adenylyl cyclase and allowing the GDP-liganded $\alpha$-subunit to reassociate into an inactive $\alpha_s$, $\beta$, $\gamma$ trimer. Agents which inhibit rather than stimulate adenylate cyclase do so by activating receptors that interact with $G_i$, a second and more abundant trimeric G protein. In such cases, activated $G_i$ counteracts the stimulatory effects of $G_s$ on adenylyl cyclase and inhibits steroidogenesis (Michell, 1989).

The molecular structure of the FSH receptor appears to be similar to those of the receptors for LH/hCG and thyroid-stimulating hormone (TSH) (Ascoli & Segaloff, 1989; Segaloff et al., 1990). The structure of the LH/hCG receptor, predicted from its complementary DNA sequence (McFarland et al., 1989), consists of a large (341-amino acid) extracellular domain connected to a 26-residue signal peptide via a 333-residue region containing seven transmembrane sequences (Fig. 3.3.). The presence of seven transmembrane domains is a common feature of G protein-associated receptors (e.g. $\beta_2$ adrenergic agonists,

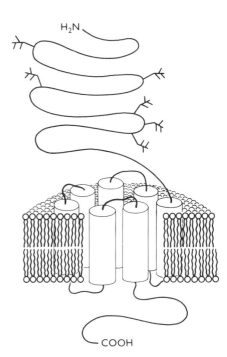

**Fig. 3.3.** Postulated model for the LH/hCG receptor in the plasma membrane. Above the membrane bilayer is the extracellular space; below is cytoplasmic. Reproduced with permission from McFarland *et al.* (1989).

serotonin and acetylcholine) (Johnson & Dhanasekaran, 1989). Each transmembrane domain is envisaged to represent one transit of the folded polypeptide through the plasma membrane and cytoplasmic loops linking the transmembrane domains are likely sites of productive interactions with G proteins. The large putative hormone-binding extra-cellular domain of the receptor for LH/hCG appears to set it apart from other members of the G protein coupled receptor family in which the hormone-binding site appears to be formed in part by the assemblage of extracellular loops linking the seven transmembrane domains (Mc-Farland *et al.*, 1989). Based upon sequence similarities and structural homologies shared by the α-subunits of their G proteins, all members of the G protein-coupled receptor family characterized to-date are thought to have evolved from a common ancestral receptor (Michell, 1989).

### Tyrosine kinases

Granulosa cells also possess other receptors which regulate intracellular tyrosine kinase activity. Receptors in this category include those for epidermal growth factor (EGF/TGFα) (Feng *et al.*, 1987) and insulin-like growth factor (IGF)-I (Adashi *et al.*, 1985; Gates *et al.*, 1987). The ligand-binding and tyrosine kinase domains of the EGF/TGFα receptor are on separate portions of a single polypeptide chain spanning the plasma membrane: the ligand-binding site is outside coupled to tyrosine kinase inside. The IGF-I receptor is similar to the insulin receptor in that it has ligand-binding sites on separate subunits of a multi-subunit receptor protein spanning the plasma membrane (Sibley *et al.*, 1988). However, for both types of receptor, binding of ligand to the extracellular binding site(s) activates intracellular tyrosine kinase, promoting the phosphorylation of tyrosine residues in protein involved in cell growth and/or differentiation (Michell, 1989).

Factors which stimulate postreceptor signalling involving tyrosine kinases promote cell proliferation and positively (insulin or IGF-I) or negatively (EGF/TGFα) regulate gonadotrophin-induced steroidogenesis (see later). They are therefore strongly implicated in the local regulation of cellular responsiveness to gonadotrophins in the pre-ovulatory follicle.

### Phosphoinositide (PI) metabolism

Endocrine and paracrine information affecting follicular development and steroid synthesis is also fed into ovarian cells via the products of increased inositol lipid hydrolysis in the plasma membrane (Leung & Wang, 1989). Receptors using this signalling system transmit information by G protein coupled activation of a phospholipase, phosphoinositidase C (PIC), which metabolizes PI to inositol triphosphate and 1,2-diacylglycerol (Berridge, 1987a). Inositol triphosphate formation triggers pulsed mobilization of $Ca^{2+}$ in the cytoplasm via rapid opening and closing of ATP-dependent calcium channels in the endoplasmic reticulum. Regulation of cytosolic $Ca^{2+}$ has long been known to be important to cell growth and function (Gilman, 1987). 1,2-diacylglycerol produced by PI metabolism activates calcium-dependent protein kinase(s) (protein kinase C) which is also intimately involved in the control of cell growth and differentiation (Nishizuka, 1988). The 'bifurcating signal pathway' based on inositol phosphate/$Ca^{2+}$ and 1,2-diacylglycerol/protein kinase C (Berridge, 1987a) is therefore of fundamental importance to widely divergent physiological processes, including the activation of gene transcription by growth factors (Berridge, 1987b; Whitman & Cantley, 1988).

LH stimulates PI metabolism in granulosa—lutein cells (Davis *et al.*, 1984; Leung & Wang, 1989), and ovarian follicles and corpora lutea are sites of protein kinase C activity (Noland & Dimino, 1986). Activation of protein kinase C in immature granulosa cells (Kasson *et al.*, 1985; Shinohara *et al.*, 1985) and thecal/interstitial cells (Hofeditz *et al.*, 1988) is associated with inhibition of gonadotrophin-stimulated steroidogenesis. On the other hand, luteal cells respond to activation of protein kinase C with acute increases in cAMP production and steroid synthesis (Davis *et al.*, 1989; Wheeler & Veldhuis, 1989). Thus granulosa cells show development-related responses to activation of protein kinase C. Many non-steroidal factors with putative intrafollicular regulatory functions activate PI signalling, including various protein growth factors, bombesin, vasopressin, gonadotrophin-releasing hormone (GnRH)-like peptide(s), angiotensin II and prostaglandin $F_{2\alpha}$ (Michell, 1989). Paracrine activation of protein kinase C is therefore likely to be of major importance to the modulation of gonadotrophin (cAMP)-stimulated cell growth and function in ovarian follicles (Berridge, 1987b).

## Histogenetic basis of ovarian steroidogenesis

Steroid synthesis and metabolism occurs under gonadotrophic control in three principal ovarian cell types: interstitial, thecal and granulosa. Stromal interstitial and thecal cells characteristically synthesize mainly $C_{19}$ steroid (androgens); granulosa cells synthesize $C_{21}$ steroids and aromatize androgens to oestrogens (see Chapter 2).

### Interstitial cells (stroma)

Secondary interstitial cells derived from the thecae of degenerated follicles are sites of $C_{19}$ steroid synthesis in the ovarian stroma (Erickson et al., 1985). Androgen is quantitatively the major class of steroid produced by these cells since they lack P450aro (Sasano et al., 1989). Androgen synthesis in stromal interstitial cells is under LH control mediated by LH receptors and intracellular cAMP, similar to androgen synthesis in the theca interna (see below). Stromal androgen synthesis beginning long before puberty onset, is sustained throughout the reproductive years and persists after the menopause. Postmenopausal ovaries contain relatively large amounts of secondary interstitial tissue with little or no steroidogenically active follicular/luteal tissue. Steroid-secretory cells, morphologically similar to testicular Leydig cells, are prominent in the hilar region of such ovaries. Androgen (mainly androstenedione) is therefore the major ovarian endocrine secretion after the menopause (Ross & Schreiber, 1986).

### Thecal cells

The theca interna regulated by LH is the principal cellular site of follicular androgen synthesis (Tsang et al., 1979). During the follicular phase of the human menstrual cycle, the ovary contributes c. 30% of the total blood androstenedione and the adrenal accounts for the rest. Towards mid-cycle, the ovarian contribution rises to c. 60% due to increased synthesis and secretion of the steroid by the LH-stimulated theca of the preovulatory follicle, reflecting its role as a precursor for oestradiol (Baird, 1977).

The rate-limiting conversion of $C_{21}$ substrates to $C_{19}$ androgen steroids is catalysed by P450c17 (see Chapter 2), a steroidogenic cytochrome P450 expressed in the ovary predominantly, if not exclusively, by thecal/interstitial cells and theca−lutein cells (Richards *et al.*, 1987; Sasano *et al.*, 1989). P450c17 exhibits both 17-hydroxylase and C-17,20-lyase activities and converts pregnenolone and progesterone to dehydroepiandrosterone (DHA) and androstenedione via the corresponding 17-hydroxylated $C_{21}$ intermediates (17-pregnenolone and 17-progesterone). Androstenedione and DHA are each present at high concentrations in human follicular fluid (Fowler *et al.*, 1977; McNatty, 1981; Dehennin *et al.*, 1987), indicating that both the $\Delta^4$ (progesterone to androstenedione) and $\Delta^5$ (pregnenolone to DHA) routes of androgen synthesis are operative in thecal cells (McAllister *et al.*, 1989).

$C_{21}$ precursors used in thecal androgen synthesis may be derived from adjacent granulosa cells (Short, 1962), or synthesized intracellularly from acetate or blood-borne LDL-cholesterol (Erickson *et al.*, 1985). Uptake of cholesterol, cholesterol side-chain cleavage activity (P450scc) and P450c17 are all positively regulated by LH via adenylyl cyclase signalling (Magoffin, 1989). The enzyme which converts DHA to androstenedione (3β-hydroxysteroid dehydrogenase/$\Delta^{5-4}$ isomerase) appears to be constitutively expressed in thecal cells (Erickson *et al.*, 1985). P450aro is absent or expressed at extremely low levels (Sasano *et al.*, 1989).

## Granulosa cells

During advanced preovulatory development stimulated by FSH, granulosa cells express P450aro (Steinkampf *et al.*, 1987; Hickey *et al.*, 1988; Sasano *et al.*, 1989) and become major if not exclusive sites of intrafollicular oestrogen synthesis (Hillier *et al.*, 1981) (Fig. 3.4). Granulosa cells do not express P450c17 and therefore are unable to synthesize androgens *de novo*. However, they do express 3β-hydroxysteroid dehydrogenase/$\Delta^{5-4}$ isomerase (Redhead *et al.*, 1983), 17-ketoreductase (Bjersing, 1967) and 5α-reductase (McNatty,

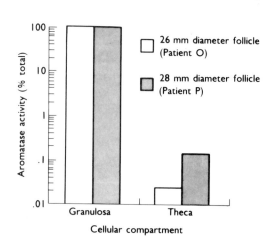

**Fig. 3.4.** Relative distribution of aromatase activity among theca and granulosa cells in the preovulatory follicle from each of two women (26 mm follicle from subject O; 28 mm follicle from subject P) dissected from ovaries removed during the late-follicular phase of spontaneous menstrual cycles. The values are means of three to six measurements on isolated cell suspensions, extrapolated on the basis of cell recoveries to give total aromatase activity (100%) (Hillier *et al.*, 1981).

1981) and can therefore metabolize DHA and androstenedione to bio-logically active androgens which serve local regulatory functions, including testosterone and 5α-dihydrotestosterone (Hillier, 1985) (see below). Granulosa cells are also sites of steroid conjugation (Lischinsky *et al.*, 1983) and high concentrations of DHA sulphate accumulate in follicular fluid (Dehennin *et al.*, 1987).

Progesterone synthesis is only a minor granulosa cell function before the onset of the LH surge. However, LH-responsive steroidogenic enzymes crucial to progesterone synthesis in the corpus luteum are induced by FSH during preovulatory granulosa cell development, notably P450scc (Funkenstein *et al.*, 1984; Richards *et al.*, 1987). Granulosa cells isolated from preovulatory follicles are therefore able to undertake high rates of progesterone synthesis in response to stimulation by LH or HCG *in vitro*. (Channing & Tsafriri, 1977; Hillier & Wickings, 1985).

## Preovulatory follicular oestrogen secretion

Gonadotrophins and steroidogenic precursors are borne into the pre-ovulatory follicle by the afferent vasculature of the theca interna; ef-ferent blood vessels convey oestradiol synthesized in the follicular wall into the ovarian venous effluent. Preovulatory follicular oestrogen syn-thesis is thereby subject to gonadotrophic and haemodynamic control.

### Gonadotrophic control

Oestrogen secretion by the preovulatory follicle depends on the co-ordinated steroidogenic potential of its thecal and granulosa cells (Falck,

**Fig. 3.5.** Contemporary 'two-cell, two-gonadotrophin' model of follicular oestradiol biosynthesis. Androstenedione ($C_{19}$) synthesis from cholesterol ($C_{27}$) via $C_{21}$ steroid intermediates occurs in the theca under LH control. Aromatase, the granulosa cell enzyme which converts androstenedione to oestradiol ($C_{18}$), is induced by FSH. FSH also induces LH receptors coupled to steroid synthesis in granulosa cells: aromatase is therefore under direct control by both FSH and LH in the preovulatory follicle. Androstenedione synthesized in thecal cells enters the efferent follicular vasculature to be secreted as the major follicular androgen and also traverses the lamina basalis, and enters adjacent granulosa cells where it is aromatized to oestradiol. Only the lamina basalis stands between mural granulosa cells and thecal blood vessels in many regions of the follicle wall. Oestradiol formed in granulosa cells is thereby discharged into the ovarian vein, accounting for the follicular-phase increase in ovarian oestradiol secretion. Modified from Armstrong and Dorrington (1979) and Hillier (1985).

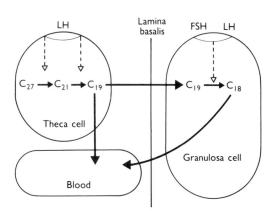

1959; Short, 1962; Bjersing, 1967; Ryan, 1979), controlled by FSH and LH (Armstrong & Dorrington, 1979). Principal tenets of the widely accepted 'two-cell, two gonadotrophin' model of oestrogen synthesis (Fig. 3.5.) are that (1) LH stimulates the synthesis of precursor androgen (androstenedione) in the theca interna, (2) thecal androgens traverse the extracellular space and enter adjacent granulosa cells, where (3) FSH stimulates the aromatization of precursor androgen into oestradiol. The scheme illustrated in Fig. 3.5 accommodates the ability of granulosa cell aromatase, following induction by FSH, to respond directly to stimulation by LH, as revealed by *in vitro* experiments using rat (Wang *et al.*, 1981) and human preovulatory granulosa cells (Hillier *et al.*, 1983) (see Fig. 3.6).

Since LH stimulates androgen formation (by thecal cells) and aromatization (in granulosa cells) it directly regulates oestrogen production at the theca−granulosa cell interface in the preovulatory follicle. Secreted oestradiol effects positive feedback control of pituitary LH release and thereby stimulates its own formation (Yen, 1986). This dynamic interaction leads to a gradual increase in the integrated circulating LH level and each pulse of LH delivered to the preovulatory follicle stimulates concurrent bursts of androstenedione and oestradiol discharge into the ovarian vein (Baird *et al.*, 1981). Rates of androgen synthesis in the theca appear to be closely tuned to rates of aromatization in the granulosa cell layer (Hillier *et al.*, 1981). A local feedback loop (granulosa on theca) may be operative, mediated by oestradiol, other follicular steroids and/or tissue-specific regulatory proteins (see below). This relationship breaks down at mid-cycle when the LH surge is triggered and follicular oestrogen secretion declines shortly before ovulation.

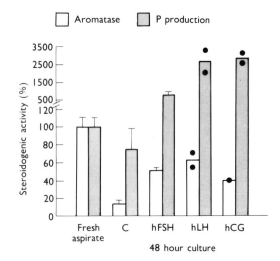

**Fig. 3.6.** Demonstration of FSH- and LH-responsive aromatase activity and progesterone synthesis in granulosa cells aspirated from a human preovulatory follicle. Extant steroidogenic activity (100%) measured in freshly isolated cells is compared with the activity measured after culturing for 48 h as a cell monolayer in the absence (C) or presence of gonadotrophin: hFSH (LER 8/116, 75 ng/ml) or hLH (LER 960, 30 ng/ml). Results are expressed as mean percentage activity (±SE or range of duplicates) relative to that of the freshly isolated cells. Note (1) the precipitate decline in aromatase activity in the absence of gonadotrophic stimulation; (2) the amelioration of this decline by FSH, LH, and hCG; and (3) the pronounced stimulatory effects of all three gonadotrophins on progesterone synthesis. Reproduced with permission from Hillier *et al.* (1983).

### Vascular control

The theca interna of the preovulatory follicle is highly vascularized and contains large numbers of steroidogenically active cells richly endowed with surface receptors for LH (Zeleznik *et al.*, 1981). It is therefore ideally equipped to take up blood-borne precursor cholesterol and respond to circulating LH with increased rates of androgen synthesis. The avascular granulosa cell layer is exposed to high concentrations of aromatizable androgen which reach it by diffusion from the theca interna. Cells in the outermost (mural) granulosa cell layer are thought to be particularly active sites of aromatization since they have higher levels of cytochrome P450 (Zoller & Weisz, 1978) and LH receptors than granulosa cells located distally to the lamina basalis (Amsterdam *et al.*, 1975). Moreover, mural granulosa cells are in close contact with thecal blood vessels, being separated only by the lamina basalis in many regions of the follicle wall. They can therefore respond immediately to changes in the circulating level of LH and discharge the oestrogen they produce more or less directly into the efferent blood system of the preovulatory follicle (Zeleznik *et al.*, 1981).

## Development-related cellular responses to gonadotrophins

Granulosa and thecal cells in ovarian follicles undergo development-related changes in responsiveness to FSH and LH which help explain the initiation, maintenance and termination of oestrogen secretion by the preovulatory follicle (Zeleznik *et al.*, 1977). As discussed later, there is increasing evidence that locally produced steroidal and non-steroidal factors as well as the gonadotrophins themselves control these developments.

### Responses of granulosa cells to FSH

FSH-responsive aromatase activity and progesterone synthesis in granulosa cells increase markedly during preovulatory follicular development in rat (Hillier *et al.*, 1978; Zeleznik *et al.*, 1977), human (Hillier *et al.*, 1981) and non-human primate ovaries (Harlow *et al.*, 1988) (see Fig. 3.7). This development is a direct cellular response to FSH, entailing amplification of cAMP-mediated intracellular signalling (Hillier *et al.*, 1980b; Richards, 1980). The underlying molecular mechanism remains to be fully clarified but is known to involve increased formation of the regulatory RIIβ subunit of type II protein kinase A (Hedin *et al.*, 1987) and attendant increases in the expression of several other cAMP-responsive genes, including the steroidogenic enzymes P450aro and P450scc (Richards *et al.*, 1987). Such an FSH-induced increase in granulosa cell sensitivity to FSH appears to be crucial to the mechanism

**Fig. 3.7.** Development-dependent increase in granulosa cell sensitivity to FSH. Granulosa cells were isolated from small (0.5–1.0 mm diameter) and large (≥2.0 mm; i.e. preovulatory) follicles in late follicular-phase marmoset (*Callithrix jacchus*) ovaries. The cells were cultured for 48 h at 37°C in the presence of increasing concentrations of FSH LER-8/116 (hFSH). Aromatase activity was determined at 48 h by measuring oestradiol production (by radioimmunoassay) during a further 3-h incubation of washed cell monolayers in the presence of 1.0 μM testosterone as an exogenous aromatase substrate. Data are mean ± SE from incubations in triplicate. Note the *c.* 10-fold increase in sensitivity to FSH shown by the granulosa cells obtained from large follicles. Redrawn from Harlow *et al.* (1988).

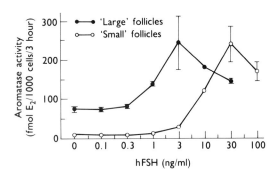

by which the preovulatory follicle can continue to grow and secrete oestrogen during the late follicular phase of the menstrual cycle when FSH levels are declining (Zeleznik & Hillier, 1984; Hillier *et al.*, 1988; Glasier *et al.*, 1989).

### Responses of granulosa cells to LH

Granulosa cells also acquire increased responsiveness to LH during advanced preovulatory follicular development (Zeleznik *et al.*, 1977; Hillier *et al.*, 1978), which is another important reason why the pre-ovulatory follicle is able to secrete oestrogen despite undergoing re-duced stimulation by FSH in the late follicular phase (Zeleznik & Hillier, 1984). The key to this crucial development is the induction by FSH of cell-surface LH receptors functionally coupled to the same cAMP-mediated signalling pathway(s) activated by FSH (Birnbaumer & Kirchik, 1983; Richards *et al.*, 1987).

### Selection of the dominant follicle

The inductive action of FSH on granulosa cell aromatase and the sub-sequent responsiveness of this enzyme system to stimulation by gon-adotrophins are central to the mechanism by which usually only one oestrogensecretory follicle develops, secretes oestrogen and ovulates in human menstrual cycles (Zeleznik & Hillier, 1984). When the plasma FSH level rises at the beginning of the follicular phase, multiple follicles with varying potentials for FSH-dependent development are present in the ovaries. These follicles require varying degrees of stimulation by FSH to in order to undergo preovulatory development and the follicle which eventually matures and ovulates is thought to be the one whose granulosa cells most rapidly acquire high levels of aromatase and LH receptor in response to the intercycle FSH rise: i.e. the one with the lowest FSH 'threshold' (Brown, 1978; Hillier, 1981). During the mid-follicular phase, oestradiol secretion by this follicle begins to increase and the steroid feeds back to negatively regulate pituitary FSH secretion. This causes a progressive reduction in the circulating FSH level and thereby limits the FSH-dependent development of other follicles with relatively high threshold FSH requirements. Thus only one follicle becomes fully mature, protected against the fall in circulating FSH by its relatively high responsiveness to both FSH and LH.

The mechanism which establishes the variable FSH threshold requirements of individual follicles at the beginning of each menstrual cycle is not understood. However, as discussed in the next section, there is increasing evidence that regulatory actions of locally produced steroidal and non-steroidal factors are involved.

### Termination of follicular oestrogen secretion

Several hours after the onset of the ovulation-inducing LH surge, ovarian oestrogen secretion and plasma oestradiol levels decline because androgen (aromatase precursor) synthesis in the theca interna of the preovulatory follicle (Hillier, 1985). The mechanism by which thecal androgen synthesis is suppressed is not understood but appears to entail thecal 'desensitization' to LH, brought about by the extreme increase in circulating levels of the gonadotrophin which characterize this stage of the menstrual cycle. The desensitization process seems to involve impaired coupling of the LH receptor to the guanine nucleotide-binding regulatory protein $G_s$ (Birnbaumer & Kirchik, 1983; Ekstrom & Hunzicker-Dunn, 1989) and thecal 17-hydroxylase/C-17,20 lyase activity is inhibited (Erickson et al., 1985; Richards et al., 1987). Once the LH surge subsides and follicular rupture has occurred, thecal androgen synthesis is reinitiated in the corpus luteum. The LH surge does not suppress granulosa cell aromatase activity in the preovulatory follicle and may even enhance it (Hillier & Wickings, 1985). Granulosa cell progesterone synthesis is also enhanced by the LH surge, in anticipation of the steroid-secretory function of the corpus luteum (see Chapter 6).

# Paracrine signalling and follicular endocrine function

Paracrine control is a generalized form of bioregulation whereby one cell-type in a tissue selectively influences the activity of an adjacent cell-type through the biosynthesis and release of chemical messengers which diffuse into the parenchyma and act specifically on neighbouring target cells (Franchimont, 1986). The term 'paracrine' was initially invoked to explain cell–cell interactions in the digestive tract mediated by locally produced gut peptides (Van Noorden & Polak, 1979). The particular relevance of paracrine control to the co-ordination of thecal and granulosa cell function in the ovarian follicle has become increasingly apparent hand-in-hand with the application of modern cell and molecular biology techniques to study the growth and differentiation of follicular cells *in vitro*. Selected aspects of this follicular paracrine system are assessed here.

## Steroidal regulation

The 'two-cell, two gonadotrophin' model of oestrogen synthesis in the preovulatory follicle (see above) provided the first satisfactory explanation of the cellular basis of oestrogen synthesis and laid the foundations for modern concepts of a follicular paracrine system (Armstrong & Dorrington, 1979). Oestrogens had long been recognized as intrafollicular 'organizers' which promote granulosa cell development and responsiveness to gonadotrophins *in vivo* (Gaarenstrom & de Jongh, 1946; Hisaw, 1947; Goldenberg *et al.*, 1973; Richards, 1980), and locally produced androgens were implicated in the control of follicular atresia (Louvet *et al.*, 1975). Towards the end of the 1970s, the increased use of primary granulosa cell culture systems to study androgen action *in vitro* revealed unexpected abilities of aromatizable and non-aromatizable androgens to act alone (Schomberg *et al.*, 1976; Lucky *et al.*, 1977) and synergistically with FSH (Armstrong & Dorrington, 1976; Nimrod & Lindner, 1976) to stimulate synthesis of progesterone and aromatase activity (Daniel & Armstrong, 1980; Hillier & de Zwart, 1981). With the demonstration that granulosa cells possess androgen receptors (Schreiber & Ross, 1976) which mediate androgenic augmentation FSH-induced granulosa cell differentiation (Hillier *et al.*, 1977; Hillier & de Zwart, 1981), it was suggested that LH-induced thecal androgens, besides serving as aromatase substrates, might function as 'intercellular (theca→granulosa) regulators which mediate certain follicular requirements for stimulation by LH' (Hillier *et al.*, 1982). Regulatory roles in the follicular paracrine system for androgens along with oestrogens, other steroids and diverse non-steroidal factors are now widely accepted (Gore-Langton & Armstrong, 1988; Tonetta & DiZerega, 1989) (see Fig. 3.8).

### Androgens

Androgens produced by thecal cells cross the lamina basalis, penetrate the granulosa cell layer and accumulate in follicular fluid (Tsang *et al.*, 1979; McNatty, 1981). Although there is experimental evidence for involvement of androgens in follicular atresia (see below), androgen levels in follicular fluid of atretic follicles do not differ markedly from those in healthy follicles of a comparable size (Brailly *et al.*, 1981;

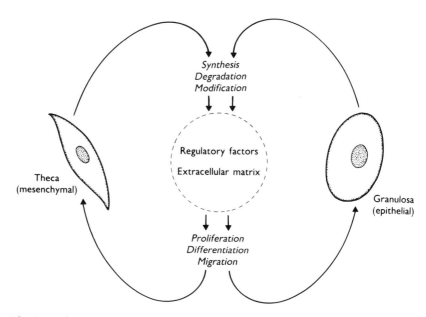

**Fig. 3.8.** The follicular paracrine system. The interaction between granulosa and thecal cells in the follicle wall can be likened to the classic form of epithelio–mesenchymal interaction which occurs during general tissue morphogenesis in the embryo. Each cell type responds selectively to endocrine stimulation by FSH (granulosa) and LH (theca) by producing soluble (steroidal and non-steroidal) regulatory factors and extracellular matrix which effect paracrine and autocrine control of cell proliferation, differentiation and migration in the maturing follicle.

Westergaard, 1986). Depending on stage of development (controlled by FSH), granulosa cells express enzymes which interconvert andro-stenedione and other steroids with potential regulatory functions in the follicle wall, including testosterone (via 17-ketoreductase: Bjersing, 1967), 5α-reduced androgens (via 5α-reductase: McNatty *et al.*, 1979), oestradiol (via aromatase: McNatty *et al.*, 1979) and catechol oestrogens (via oestrogen hydroxylase: Hammond *et al.*, 1986).

For several mammalian species, including a non-human primate (Harlow *et al.*, 1986), it has been shown that FSH-induced differen-tiation of cultured granulosa cells is modulated by the presence of androgens at concentrations found in follicular fluid (Hillier, 1985; Daniel & Armstrong, 1986; Hsueh, 1986). Receptor-mediated androgen action in granulosa cells leads to increased generation of extracellular cAMP and attendant amplification of cAMP-dependent biochemical processes initiated by FSH. Androgens active in this regard include testosterone and androstenedione as well as their non-aromatizable 5α-reduced congeners. The net effect is enhanced granulosa cell sensi-tivity to stimulation by FSH, suggesting a possible role for locally produced androgens in modulating follicular threshold requirements for stimulation by FSH (see above).

Experiments *in vivo* using oestrogen-pretreated, hypophysectomized immature rats have shown that the degree of concomitant stimulation with FSH is a major determinant of granulosa cell response to androgen. In the absence of FSH, treatment with LH/hCG to stimulate ovarian androgen production (Louvet *et al.*, 1975) or administration of exogenous androgen (Hillier & Ross, 1979) promotes follicular atresia. On the other hand, joint treatment with FSH and androgen promotes normal preovulatory follicular development and oestrogen secretion (Armstrong & Papkoff, 1976). Hyperstimulation with LH (? causes excessive follicular androgen production) inhibits preovulatory follicular steroid synthesis and stimulates atresia (Armstrong *et al.*, 1989; Opavsky & Armstrong, 1989). However, androgen action in granulosa cells at advanced stages of differentiation is difficult to assess since these cells more efficiently aromatize androgens to oestrogen which reduces the potential for direct effects of androgen (Harlow *et al.*, 1988). On the other hand, $5\alpha$-reduced androgen metabolites may be produced which are competitive aromatase inhibitors and hence have the potential to suppress oestrogen synthesis (Hillier *et al.*, 1980a; Shaw *et al.*, 1989).

### Oestrogens

Oestrogen is an intrafollicular autocrine regulator (i.e. having an action within the cell which produces it). Treatment of hypophysectomized immature female rats with exogenous oestrogen stimulates granulosa cell mitosis, raises gonadotrophin receptor levels and amplifies follicular responsiveness to exogenously administered gonadotrophin (Goldenberg *et al.*, 1973; Richards, 1980; Hsueh *et al.*, 1984). At the intracellular level, oestrogen augments FSH-induced expression of the regulatory subunit RII$\beta$ of type II cAMP-dependent protein kinase (Richards *et al.*, 1987) and the steroidogenic enzymes P450aro and P450scc (Richards *et al.*, 1987; Toaff *et al.*, 1983). Oestrogen also stimulates expression of inhibin $\alpha$- and $\beta_B$-subunit mRNAs (Turner *et al.*, 1989) and augments FSH-induced inhibin production by cultured rat granulosa cells (Bicsak *et al.*, 1988).

Regulatory actions of oestrogen in granulosa cells are thought to be mediated by binding of the steroid to receptor(s) which regulate rates of transcription from oestrogen responsive genes (Richards *et al.*, 1987). A protein with the physicochemical properties of an oestrogen receptor has been detected by ligand-binding assays in nuclei and cytosol from whole ovaries and granulosa cells (Saiduddin & Zassenhaus, 1977; Kudolo *et al.*, 1984a; Richards, 1985). However, at least one other oestrogen-binding species is present in rat granulosa cells which could also participate in oestrogen action (Kudolo *et al.*, 1984b). The finding that mouse ovaries express at least two mRNA species which cross-hybridize with RNA probes complementary to the steroid-binding domain of the mouse oestrogen receptor provides further evidence that steroid binding sites other than that of the 'classic' oestrogen receptor might mediate autocrine oestrogen action in the ovaries (Hillier *et al.*, 1989).

Whether oestrogens exert significant regulatory actions in human granulosa cells is less certain and the only relevant data have come from non-human primate models. In an immunocytochemical study of monkey ovaries, granulosa cells stained negatively for the oestrogen receptor whereas intense positive staining occurred in the ovarian surface epithelium (Hild-Petito *et al.*, 1988). Treatment of cultured marmoset granulosa with oestradiol augmented FSH-inducible inhibin production without enhancing steroidogenesis (Hillier *et al.*, 1989).

The raised follicular fluid oestrogen level in the preovulatory follicle is thought likely to contribute to the intrafollicular mechanism whereby a single preovulatory follicle is selected to ovulate in the human menstrual cycle. Although there is no direct evidence to support regulatory oestrogen action in human granulosa cells, granulosa cell aromatase activity (Hillier *et al.*, 1981) and follicular fluid oestradiol levels (Bomsel-Helmreich *et al.*, 1979; McNatty, 1981) increase during preovulatory follicular development and correlate positively with follicular 'health' (Hillier, 1985). Once selected (see above), the preovulatory follicle is presumed to be developmentally favoured through the activation of a local positive feedback loop in which the oestrogen it produces stimulates granulosa cell proliferation and augments responsiveness of these cells to gonadotrophins, thereby causing further increases in oestrogen formation, and so on (Hillier, 1981; McNatty, 1981; Hsueh *et al.*, 1984).

Granulosa cell oestrogen is also implicated as a paracrine regulator of thecal cell function (Leung & Armstrong, 1980; Hillier, 1985) and may be involved in the suppression of thecal androgen synthesis in response to the mid-cycle LH surge (Erickson *et al.*, 1985).

### Catechol oestrogens

Assessment of direct oestrogen action in isolated granulosa cell systems may be complicated by the fact that preovulatory granulosa cells have an increased capacity to metabolize oestradiol to catechol oestrogens (Hammond *et al.*, 1986). Catechol oestrogens have been identified in ovarian follicular fluids from various species, including man (Dehennin *et al.*, 1984) and 2-hydroxyoestradiol augments FSH-induced synthesis of progesterone and aromatization of androgens in cultured granulosa cells (Hudson & Hillier, 1985). Other evidence suggests that catechol oestrogens can inhibit granulosa cell proliferation (Spicer & Hammond, 1989). These findings therefore point to intrafollicular regulatory functions for catechol oestrogens.

## Non-steroidal regulation

Neither FSH nor oestrogen exert mitogenic effects on granulosa cells *in vitro* whereas they do so when administered *in vivo* (Hammond & English, 1987). This raises the question of whether locally produced 'growth factors' co-ordinate mitogenic and differentiative actions of gonadotrophins and sex steroids. Candidates for such a role include IGFs, EGF, TGFs, inhibins and activins, fibroblast growth factors (FGFs) and cytokines.

### IGFs

The IGFs (IGF-I and IGF-II) are a family of low molecular weight single-chain peptides which share considerable structural and functional homologies with proinsulin (Froesch *et al.*, 1985). IGF-I and IGF-II each cross-react with the insulin receptor and receptors for insulin and both factors are present on most cells (Rechler & Nissley, 1985), including thecal and granulosa cells in the human ovary (Poretsky *et al.*, 1985). Receptors for insulin and IGF-I also share structural and functional similarities, including intracellular signalling involving tyrosine kinases (Sibley *et al.*, 1988) (see above). Both IGFs exert endocrine effects on tissue growth throughout the body, being secreted by the liver under the control of growth hormone (GH) (Slack, 1989). IGFs are also synthesized and act locally in various tissues including muscle, bone and gonads (Adashi *et al.*, 1985).

There is increasing evidence that stimulatory effects of FSH on granulosa cell growth and differentiation are subject to positive paracrine/autocrine regulation by IGFs (Adashi *et al.*, 1989; Hammond *et al.*, 1988). Granulosa cells express IGF-I receptors which increase in number following treatment with FSH *in vitro* (Adashi *et al.*, 1986). Induction by FSH of granulosa cell steroidogenesis, expression of LH receptors, deposition of proteoglycans, and responsiveness to β-adrenergic agonists, are augmented by the presence of physiological concentrations of IGF-I or supraphysiological concentrations of insulin (Adashi *et al.*, 1985). The stimulatory effects of insulin on granulosa cells is explained by cross-reaction with granulosa cell IGF-I receptors. The stimulatory action of IGF-I on FSH-induced cytodifferentiation entails amplification of intracellular cAMP action, as opposed to a net increase in cAMP production (Adashi *et al.*, 1985). IGF-I also synergizes with oestradiol to promote granulosa cell steroidogenesis (Veldhuis *et al.*, 1986).

Granulosa cells are intrafollicular sites of IGF-I mRNA expression (Oliver *et al.*, 1989) and synthesis of IGF-I (Hammond *et al.*, 1985), regulated by gonadotrophins, oestradiol and GH (Jia *et al.*, 1986). Autocrine regulatory actions of IGF-I in isolated granulosa cells have been observed *in vitro*. Presence of a neutralizing monoclonal antibody to IGF-I in granulosa cell culture medium inhibited the stimulatory effects of FSH, oestradiol, growth hormone and charcoal-treated follicular fluid on progesterone production (Mondschein et al., 1989). Granulosa cells also synthesize a low molecular weight (34 kDa) IGF-binding protein which is likely to participate in the regulation of cellular growth responses to IGFs (Suikkari et al., 1989; Ui et al., 1989). Thus there is good experimental evidence to propose that IGF-I exerts autocrine control over granulosa cell growth and differentiation in the ovaries.

Although thecal cells are not sites of discernible IGF-I gene expression (Oliver et al., 1989), they possess IGF-I receptors (Poretsky et al., 1985; Cara & Rosenfield, 1988), and both basal and LH-stimulated synthesis of androgen in cultured thecal/interstitial cells can be enhanced by treatment with insulin or IGF-I (Barbieri et al., 1983, 1986; Hernandez et al., 1988; Cara & Rosenfield, 1988; Magoffin et al., 1990). IGF-I of granulosa cell origin therefore has the potential to exert paracrine control over the theca interna as well as exerting autocrine control within the granulosa cell layer. This is reminiscent of the situation in non-gonadal tissues in which IGFs promote cell differentiation, such as muscle and bone. In such tissues IGFs are also found in epithelia (where they appear to be concerned mainly with the maturation of the differentiated epithelial cell types) rather than in the underlying mesenchyme (Slack, 1989).

IGF-II has been identified in significant amounts in human follicular fluid (Ramasharma et al., 1986) and is produced in vitro by proliferating granulosa cell cultures obtained from human ovaries (Ramasharma & Li, 1987). Stimulation of steroid synthesis in such cells by treatment with FSH, hCG or dibutyryl cAMP co-ordinately induces expression of IGF-II mRNA, suggesting an autocrine/paracrine role for IGF-II in stimulating granulosa cell proliferation (Miller, 1988).

### EGF and TGFα

EGF and TGFα are closely related gene products with similar properties which bind to the same receptors (Massagué, 1983; Derynck, 1986). The active factors are polypeptides consisting of c. 50 amino acids which have been shown to modulate development of epidermis, breast, and gut; act as angiogenic factors and may mediate hypercalcaemia (Gill et al., 1987; Waterfield, 1989). Granulosa cells express hormonally-regulated receptors for EGF/TGFα (Feng et al., 1987). Treatment in vitro with EGF/TGFα promotes granulosa cell proliferation (Gospodarowicz & Bialecki, 1979) and interferes with the induction by FSH of functional cell differentiation (expression of LH receptors, aromatase activity and progesterone synthesis, inhibin synthesis) (Jones et al., 1982; Knecht & Catt, 1983; Franchimont et al., 1986; Steinkampf et al., 1988). Intrafollicular expression of TGFα has been localized to the theca interna (Kudlow et al., 1987). EGF/TGFα of thecal origin is therefore likely to be involved in the paracrine control of granulosa cell responsiveness to FSH, serving to enhance cell proliferation and inhibit steroidogenesis.

## *TGFβ*

TGFβs are 25 kDa homodimeric proteins usually expressed in regions of epithelio-mesenchymal interaction, notably during embryonic organogenesis (Slack, 1989). They are multi-functional regulators of cell growth, differentiation and function which either stimulate or inhibit cellular proliferation *in vitro* depending on the cells, growth conditions and presence of other growth factors (Roberts *et al.*, 1988).

Ovarian thecal (Skinner *et al.*, 1987; Bendell & Dorington, 1988) and granulosa cells (Kim & Schomberg, 1989) have been identified as sites of TGFβ synthesis, and steroid synthesis in both cell types is influenced by treatment with TGFβ *in vitro*. In rat granulosa cell cultures, treatment with TGFβ modulates stimulatory effects of FSH and inhibitory effects of EGF/TGFα on LH-receptor induction (Knecht *et al.*, 1986) as well as steroidogenesis (Adashi & Resnick, 1986; Feng *et al.*, 1986). TGFβ also promotes granulosa cell proliferation *in vitro* (Dorrington *et al.*, 1988). In rat thecal/interstitial cell cultures, TGFβ inhibits androgen synthesis and stimulates progesterone accumulation (Magoffin *et al.*, 1989). TGFβ is therefore a potential autocrine regulator of steroid synthesis in both cell types as well as a possible mediator of paracrine theca−granulosa cell interaction in the follicle wall.

The effect of TGFβ on granulosa cell growth and differentiation may depend upon the concomitant degree of exposure to FSH. In cultured rat granulosa cells, TGFβ was shown to augment cell responsiveness (cAMP production, LH-receptor induction and steroidogenesis) to low doses of FSH but attenuate responsiveness to high-dose FSH (Knecht *et al.*, 1987). This important finding suggests a mechanism whereby locally produced TGFβs might contribute to the establishment of interfollicular variations in FSH thresholds in the human menstrual cycle (see above).

One way in which TGFβs are known to affect tissue morphogenesis is by influencing the abundance and architecture of the extracellular matrix as well as the ability of cells to interact with it (Massagué, 1987). Various mesenchymal and epithelial cell types whose growth and differentiation are affected by TGFβs respond to these factors with elevated deposition of cell-adhesion proteins such as fibronectin, production of protease inhibitors and expression of integrin receptors (Roberts *et al.*, 1988). It is noteworthy that granulosa cell differentiation is associated with reduced deposition of fibronectin (Skinner *et al.*, 1985), and that extracellular matrix has been shown to influence granulosa cell responsiveness to gonadotrophins *in vitro* (Amsterdam *et al.*, 1989). Granulosa−theca interaction in the developing follicle may therefore be likened to classic forms of epithelio–mesenchymal tissue interaction involving TGFβs and other locally produced regulatory factors (Slack, 1989), as illustrated in Fig. 3.8.

### Inhibins and activins

Mature inhibin is a 32 kDa glycoprotein which has been isolated from ovarian follicular fluid as two distinct forms composed of a common α-subunit and one of two β-subunits $\beta_A$ and $\beta_B$ (Ling et al., 1985; Miyamoto et al., 1985; Rivier et al., 1985; Robertson et al., 1985; Vale et al., 1988; Ying, 1988). Treatment of pituitary cell cultures with inhibin suppresses FSH secretion whereas treatment with the homo-dimeric $\beta_A$, $\beta_A$ form of inhibin, termed activin (Vale et al., 1986) or FSH-releasing protein (FRP) (Ling et al., 1986), stimulates FSH release (Tsonis & Sharpe, 1986). These properties seem likely to reflect physio-logical functions of inhibin and activin in the human endocrine system, notably during the luteal phase of the menstrual cycle when inhibin is secreted in large amounts by the corpus luteum (see Chapters 1 and 6).

The three inhibin subunits are encoded by separate genes (Mason et al., 1985, 1986; Forage et al., 1986; Mayo et al., 1986; Esch et al., 1987) whose expression in granulosa cells is developmentally regulated and inducible by FSH (Woodruff et al., 1987, 1988; Turner et al., 1989). The α- and $\beta_B$-subunit mRNAs, but not $\beta_A$-subunit mRNA, are also inducible by treatment with oestradiol in vitro (Turner et al., 1989). Secretion of inhibin protein by rat (Erickson & Hsueh, 1978; Suzuki et al., 1987; Bicsak & Hsueh, 1988; Bicsak et al., 1988; Zhang et al., 1988), bovine (Henderson & Franchimont, 1983), human (Tsonis et al., 1987) and non-human primate granulosa cells (Hillier et al., 1989) is also regulated by gonadotrophins and sex steroids in vitro.

The human preovulatory follicle does not secrete important amounts of inhibin until the mid-cycle LH surge begins. However, inhibin and activin are both believed to serve local regulatory functions within developing ovarian follicles (de Jongh, 1988). Interest in the putative intragonadal function(s) of these factors is fuelled by the high degree of structural homology (30–40%) which exists between them and the members of a family of growth factors which are synthesized from precursors of high molecular weight and expressed during embryo-genesis and organogenesis across a wide range of animal phyla (Roberts et al., 1988; Vale et al., 1988). Members of this gene family include TGFβ, Mullerian duct inhibiting substance (MIS; causes Mullerian duct re-gression in males), decapentaplegic gene complex (DPPC; active during insect embryogenesis) and vg1 protein (a mesoderm-inducing factor in frog embryos). Moreover, bone marrow expresses inhibin $\beta_A$ mRNA and human leukaemic cells produce activin (Eto et al., 1987). Treatment with activin in vitro stimulated erythroid differentiation (haemoglobin accumulation) in human erythroleukaemic cell cultures and this effect was inhibited by co-treatment with inhibin (Yu *et al.*, 1987), further emphasizing the likelihood that inhibin-related subunits and dimeric proteins play roles in tissue growth and differentiation.

It remains to be determined just what are the regulatory functions of inhibin and activin, their precursors free or their subunits in ovarian follicles (Burger & Findlay, 1990). Inhibin was shown to augment LH-stimulated androstenedione in thecal cell cultures whereas activin was inhibitory (Hsueh *et al.*, 1987). In rat granulosa cell cultures, inhibin purified from porcine (Ying *et al.*, 1986), but not bovine (Hutchinson *et al.*, 1987) follicular fluid inhibited aromatase activity. Reasons for the discrepancy are uncertain but may reside in the specific forms of inhibin and experimental conditions used. Activin enhanced FSH-stimulated aromatase activity in rat granulosa cells but inhibited pro-gesterone production (Hutchison *et al.*, 1987). Activin also inhibited the growth of Chinese hamster ovary cells in culture. Treatment with inhibin alone had no significant effect on ovarian cell growth but it partially overcame the inhibitory effect of activin (Gonzalez-Manchon & Vale, 1989). It seems likely that future research will unravel important regulatory functions for this family of peptides in the ovary.

### FGFs

FGFs are 'heparin-binding growth factors' (Burgess & Maciag, 1989) which control the proliferation, differentiation and other activities of mesoderm and neurectoderm derived cells. Basic (b)FGF is relatively abundant in pituitary, brain, adrenals and ovaries, as opposed to acidic FGF which is restricted to brain and other neural tissues (Slack, 1989).

The corpus luteum is a rich source of bFGF and the factor is thought to play an important local role as an angiogenic factor during luteal development (Gospodarowicz & Ferrara, 1989). The factor is also implicated in the local control of granulosa cell proliferation and differ-entiation in the preovulatory follicle. Bovine granulosa cells express the bFGF gene and produce bioactive bFGF, furthermore, their pro-liferation in tissue culture is stimulated by the presence of bFGF (Neufeld *et al.*, 1987). bFGF is not a mitogen for cultured rat granulosa cells but it inhibits FSH-mediated induction of LH receptors, reversibly attenuates FSH induction of aromatase activity and stimulates progesterone syn-thesis in these cells (Baird & Hsueh, 1986). bFGF is therefore thought likely to exert autocrine regulatory influences over granulosa cell growth and differentiation. Because of its angiogenic properties, bFGF is also implicated in the paracrine control of the development of the thecal vaculature in the preovulatory follicle (Gospodarowicz & Ferrara, 1989) (see also Chapter 7).

*Cytokines*

Immunoregulatory peptides produced by blood and immune cells (cytokines, or monokines/lymphokines for those factors produced by monocytes/lymphocytes) are modulators of the growth and differentiation of diverse non-immunological cell types (Green, 1989), including ovarian endocrine cells (Adashi, 1989). Several members of the interleukin, interferon and colony stimulating factor families of immunoregulatory peptides have been shown to influence granulosa cell growth and steroidogenesis *in vitro* (Fukuoka *et al.*, 1989; Kasson & Gorospe, 1989). Distinctions between 'cytokines' and 'growth factors' (i.e. peptidic regulatory factors produced by parenchymal cells) are becoming increasingly blurred as many growth factors (such as the TGFs and bFGFs) are now also recognized as cytokines (Harrison & Campbell, 1988).

*'Other factors'*

Other factors produced by ovarian cells which are likely to have local regulatory functions include plasminogen activators (Knecht, 1988) and inhibitors (Ny *et al.*, 1985), components of the renin−angiotensin system (Kim *et al.*, 1987; Do *et al.*, 1988; Pucell *et al.*, 1988), extracellular matrix (Amsterdam *et al.*, 1989), platelet-derived growth factor (Schomberg, 1988; Ross, 1989); MIF (Voutilainen & Miller, 1989), heparin-binding growth factors other than bFGF (Burgess & Maciag, 1989), and relaxin (Too *et al.*, 1984). Also implicated are various peptidic factors including GnRH-like peptide(s) (Jones, 1989; LaTouch *et al.*, 1989); substance P (Dees *et al.*, 1985); vasoactive intestinal peptide (Davoren & Hsueh, 1985; Trzeciak *et al.*, 1986; Ojeda *et al.*, 1989) oxytocin/arginine vasopressin (Verges *et al.*, 1986; Khan-Dawood & Dawood, 1989); POMC-derived peptides (Young *et al.*, 1989); and follistatin (Shimasaki *et al.*, 1989). Then there are diverse prostanoids, leukotrienes, catecholamines and nucleotides, all of which inevitably function in various ways in the follicular paracrine system.

## Summary

FSH plays a pivotal role as the primary (endocrine) stimulus of folliculogenesis via activation of specific FSH receptors on immature granulosa cells. The phenotypic expression of functional and morphological cellular changes in response to FSH is subject to a second (paracrine) level of control by steroidal and non-steroidal factors of thecal origin produced under endocrine control by LH. Interfollicular variations in the extent to which this paracrine system operates ultimately determine which follicle undegoes full preovulatory development and ovulates. FSH-induced (cAMP-mediated) granulosa cell development in this follicle entails increased responsiveness to FSH and LH and is associated with the increased expression of genes encoding proteins required for mature granulosa cell function such as LH receptors, steroidogenic enzymes (including aromatase), proteases and diverse regulatory peptides including IGFs and inhibin subunits. Steroids and growth factors produced by FSH-stimulated granulosa cells constitute a third (autocrine) level of control which culminates in terminal differentiation (luteinization) and the expression of LH-responsive endocrine function (progesterone, oestradiol and inhibin synthesis) by the corpus luteum.

# References

Adashi, E.Y. (1989) Cytokine-mediated regulation of ovarian function: encounters of a third kind. *Endocrinology*, **124**, 2043–5.

Adashi, E.Y. & Resnick, C.E. (1986) Antagonistic interactions of transforming growth factors in the regulation of granulosa cell differentiation. *Endocrinology*, **119**, 1879–81.

Adashi, E.Y., Resnick, C.E., D'Ercole, A.J., Svoboda, M.E. & Van Wyk, J.J. (1985) Insulin-like growth factors as intraovarian regulators of granulosa cell growth and function. *Endocr. Rev.*, **6**, 400–20.

Adashi, E.Y., Resnick, C.E., Hernandez, E.R., Svoboda, M.E. & Van Wyk, J.J. (1989) Potential relevance of insulin-like growth factor I to ovarian physiology: from basic science to clinical application *Semin. Reprod. Endocrinol.* **7**, 94–99.

Adashi, E.Y., Resnick, C.E., Svoboda, M.E. & Van Wyk, J.J. (1986) Follicle-stimulating hormone enhances Somatomedin C binding to cultured rat granulosa cells: evidence for cAMP dependence. *J. Biol. Chem.*, **261**, 3923–6.

Amsterdam, A.A., Koch, Y., Lieberman, M.E. & Lindner, H.R. (1975) Distribution of binding sites for human chorionic gonadotropin in the preovulatory follicle of the rat. *J. Biol. Chem.*, **67**, 894–900.

Amsterdam, A., Rotmensch, S., Furman, A., Venter, E.A. & Vlodavsky, I. (1989) Synergistic effect of human chorionic gonadotropin and extracellular matrix on *in vitro* differentiation of human granulosa cells: progesterone production and gap junction formation. *Endocrinology*, **124**, 1956–64.

Armstrong, D.T. & Dorrington, J.H. (1976). Androgens augment FSH-induced progesterone secretion by cultured rat granulosa cells. *Endocrinology*, **99**, 1411–14.

Armstrong, D.T. & Dorrington, J.H. (1979) Estrogen biosynthesis in the ovaries and testes. In Thomas, J.A. & Singhal, R.L. (eds) *Regulatory Mechanisms Affecting Gonadal Hormone Action*, Vol. 2, pp. 217–58. University Park Press, Baltimore.

Armstrong, D.T., & Papkoff, H. (1976) Stimulation of aromatization of exogenous and endogenous androgens in ovaries of hypophysectomized rats *in vivo* by follicle stimulating hormone. *Endocrinology*, **99**, 1144–51.

Armstrong, D.T., Siuda, A., Opavsky, M.A. & Chandrasekhara, Y. (1989) Bimodal effects of luteinizing hormone and role of androgens in modifying superovulatory responses of rats to infusion with purified follicle-stimulating hormone. *Biol. Reprod.*, **40**, 54–62.

Ascoli, M. & Segaloff, D.L. (1989) On the structure of the luteinizing hormone/chorionic gonadotropin receptor. *Endocr. Rev.*, **10**, 27–44.

Ax, R.L. & Ryan, K.J. (1979) FSH stimulation of $^3$H-glycosaminic incorporation into proteoglycans by porcine granulosa cells *in vitro*. *J. Clin. Endocrinol. Metab.*, **49**, 646.

Baird, D.T. (1977) Synthesis and secretion of steroid hormones by the ovary *in vivo*. In Zuckerman, S. & Weir, B.J. (eds) *The Ovary*, Vol. 3, 2nd edn., pp. 305–57. Academic Press, London.

Baird, A. & Hsueh, A.J.W. (1986) Fibroblast growth factor as an intraovarian hormone: differential regulation of steroidogenesis by an angiogenic factor. *Regul. Pept.*, **16**, 243–50.

Baird, D.T., Baker, T.G., McNatty, K.P. & Neal, P. (1975) Relationship between the secretion of the corpus luteum and the length of the follicular phase of the ovarian cycle. *J. Reprod. Fertil.*, **45**, 611–19.

Baird, D.T., Swanston, I.A. & McNeilly, A.S. (1981) Relationship between LH, FSH and prolactin concentration and the secretion of androgens and oestrogens by the preovulatory follicle in the ewe. *Biol. Reprod.*, **24**, 1013–25.

Barbieri, R.L., Makris, A., Randall, R.W., Daniels, G., Kistner, R.W. & Ryan, K.J. (1986) Insulin stimulates androgen accumulation in incubations of ovarian stroma obtained from women with hyperandrogenism. *J. Clin. Endocrinol. Metab.*, **62**, 904–10.

Barbieri, R.L., Makris, A. & Ryan, K.J. (1983) Insulin stimulates androgen accumulation in incubations of human ovarian stroma and theca. *Obstet. Gynecol.*, Suppl. **64**, 73–80S.

Beebe, S.J., Segaloff, D.L., Burks, D., Beasley-Leach, A., Limbird, L.L. & Corbin, J. (1989). Evidence that cyclic adenosine 3′,5′-monophosphate-dependent protein kinase activation causes pig ovarian granulosa cell differentiation, including increases in two type II subclasses of this kinase. *Biol. Reprod.*, **41**, 295−307.

Bendell, J.J. & Dorrington, J. (1988) Rat thecal/intersitial cells secrete a transforming growth factor-β-like factor that promotes growth and differentiation of rat granulosa cells. *Endocrinology*, **123**, 941−8.

Ben-Ze'ev, A. & Amsterdam, A. (1989) Regulation of heat shock protein synthesis by gonadotropins in cultured granulosa cells. *Endocrinology*, **124**, 2584−94.

Berridge, M.J. (1987a) Inositol triphosphate and diacylglycerol: two interacting second messengers. *Annu. Rev. Biochem.*, **56**, 159−93.

Berridge, M.J. (1987b) Inositol lipids and cell proliferation. *Biochim. Biophys. Acta*, **907**, 33−45.

Bicsak, T.A., Cajander, S.B., Vale, W. & Hsueh, A.J.W. (1988) Inhibin: studies of stored and secreted forms by biosynthetic labelling and immunodetection in cultured rat granulosa cells. *Endocrinology*, **122**, 741−8.

Bicsak, T.A. & Hsueh, A.J.W. (1988) Recent advances in inhibin research. In Stouffer, R.L. (ed.) *The Primate Ovary*, pp. 35−47. Plenum, London.

Birnbaumer, L. & Kirchik, H.J. (1983) Regulation of gonadotropic action: the molecular mechanisms of gonadotropin-induced activation of ovarian adenylyl cyclases. In Greenwald, G.S. & Terranova, P.F. (eds) *Factors Regulating Ovulation*, pp. 287−310. Raven Press, New York.

Bjersing, L. (1967) On the morphology and endocrine functions of granulosa cells in ovarian follicles and corpora lutea. Biochemical, histochemical, and ultrastructural studies on the porcine ovary with special reference to steroid hormone synthesis. *Acta Endocrinol. Copenh.*, Suppl. **125**.

Bomsel-Helmreich, O., Gougeon, A., Thebault, A., Salterelli, D., Milgrom, E., Frydman, R. & Papiernik, E. (1979) Healthy and atretic human follicles in the preovulatory phase: Differences in evolution of follicular morphology and steroid content of follicular fluid. *J. Clin. Endocrinol. Metab.*, **48**, 686−94.

Brailly, S., Gougeon, A., Milgrom, E., Bomsel-Helmreich, O. & Papiernik, E. (1981) Androgens and progestins in the human ovarian follicles: Differences in the evolution of preovulatory, healthy nonovulatory, and atretic follicles. *J. Clin. Endocrinol. Metab.*, **53**, 128−34.

Brown, J.B. (1978) Pituitary control of ovarian function − concepts derived from gonadotrophin therapy. *Aust. NZ. J. Obstet. Gynaecol.*, **18**, 47−54.

Burger, H.G. & Findlay, J.K. (1989) Potential relevance of inhibin to ovarian physiology. *Semin. Reprod. Endocrinol.* **7**, 69−78.

Burgess, W.H. & Maciag, T. (1989) The heparin-binding (fibroblast) growth factor family of proteins. *Annu. Rev. Biochem.*, **58**, 575−606.

Cara, J.F. & Rosenfield, R.L. (1988) Insulin-like growth factor I and insulin potentiate luteinizing hormone-induced androgen biosynthesis by rat ovarian theca-intersitial cells. *Endocrinology*, **123**, 733−9.

Channing, C.P. & Tsafriri, A. (1977) Mechanism of action of luteinizing hormone and follicle-stimulating hormone on the ovary *in vitro*. *Metabolism*, **26**, 413−68.

Daniel, S.A.J. & Armstrong, D.T. (1980) Enhancement of follicle-stimulating hormone induced aromatase activity by androgen in cultured rat granulosa cells. *Endocrinology*, **107**, 1027−33.

Daniel, S.A.J. & Armstrong, D.T. (1986) Androgens in the ovarian microenvironment. *Semin. Reprod. Endocrinol.*, **4**, 89−100.

Davis, J.S., Leigh, A.W. & Farese, R.V. (1984) Effects of luteinizing hormone on phosphoinosotide metabolism in rat granulosa cells. *J. Biol. Chem.*, **259**, 15028−34.

Davis, J.S., Tedesco, T.A., West, L.A., Maroulis, G.B. & Weakland, L.L. (1989) Effects of human chorionic gonadotropin, prostaglandin F-2-alpha and protein kinase C activators on the cyclic AMP and inositol phosphate 2nd messenger systems in cultured human granulosa-luteal cells. *Mol. Cell. Endocrinol.*, **65**, 187−94.

Davoren, J.B. & Hsueh, A.J.W. (1985) Vasoactive peptide: a novel stimulator of steroidogenesis by cultured rat granulosa cells. *Biol. Reprod.*, **33**, 37−52.

Dees, W.L., Kozlowski, G.P., Dey, R. & Ojeda, S.R. (1985) Evidence for the existence of substance P in the prepubertal rat ovary. II. Immunocytochemical localization. *Biol. Reprod.*, **33**, 471−6.

Dehennin, L., Blacker, C., Reifsteck, A. & Scholler, R. (1984) Estrogen 2-, 4-, 6- or 16-hydroxylation by human follicles shown by gas chromatography associated with stable isotope dilution. *J. Steroid Biochem.*, **20**, 465−71.

Dehennin, L., Jondet, L. & Scholler, R. (1987) Androgen and 19-nonsteroid profiles in human preovulatory follicles from stimulated cycles: an isotope dilution-mass spectrometric study. *J. Steroid Biochem.*, **26**, 399−405.

de Jong, F.H. (1988) Inhibin. *Physiol. Rev.*, **68**, 555−607.

Derynck, R. (1986) Transforming growth factor-α: structure and biological activities. *J. Cell. Biochem.*, **32**, 293−304.

Do, Y.S., Sherrod, A., Lobo, R., Paulson, R.J., Shinagawa, T., Chen, S., Kjos, S. & Hsueh W. (1988) Human ovarian theca cells are a source of renin. *Proc. Natl. Acad. Sci. USA*, **85**, 1957−61.

Dorrington, J., Chuma, A.V. & Bendell, J.J. (1988) Transforming growth factor β and follicle-stimulating hormone promote rat granulosa cell proliferation. *Endocrinology*, **123**, 353–9.

Dorrington, J.H., McKeracher, H.L., Chan, A.K. & Gore-Langton, R.E. (1983) Hormonal interactions in the control of granulosa cell differentiation. *J. Steroid Biochem.*, **19**, 17–32.

Ekstrom, R.C. & Hunzicker-Dunn, M. (1989) Homologous desensitization of ovarian luteinizing hormone/human chorionic gonadotropin-responsive adenylyl cyclase is dependent upon GTP. *Endocrinology*, **124**, 956–63.

Erickson, G.F. & Hsueh, A.J.W. (1978) Secretion of inhibin by rat granulosa cells *in vitro*. *Endocrinology*, **103**, 1960–3.

Erickson, G.F., Magoffin, D.A., Dyer, C.A. & Hofeditz, C. (1985) The ovarian androgen producing cells: a review of structure/function relationships. *Endocr. Rev.*, **6**, 371–99.

Esch, F.S., Shimasaki, S., Cooksey, K., Mercado, M., Mason, A.J., Ying, S.-Y., Ueno, N. & Ling, N. (1987) Complementary deoxyribonucleic acid (cDNA) cloning and DNA sequence analysis of rat ovarian inhibins. *Mol. Endocrinol.*, **1**, 388–96.

Eto, Y., Tsuji, Y., Takezawa, M., Takano, S., Yokogawa, Y. & Shibai, H. (1987) Purification and characterization of Erythroid Differentiation Factor (EDF) isolated from human leukemia cell line THP-1. *Biophys. Biochem. Res. Commun.*, **142**, 1095–103.

Falck, B. (1959) Site of production of oestrogen in rat ovary as studied in micro-transplants. *Acta Physiol. Scand.*, Suppl. 163, **47**, 1–101.

Feng, P., Catt, K. & Knecht, M. (1986) Transforming growth factor β regulates the inhibitory actions of epidermal growth factor during granulosa cell differentiation. *J. Biol. Chem.*, **261**, 14167–70.

Feng, P., Knecht, M. & Catt, K. (1987) Hormonal control of epidermal growth factor receptors by gonadotropins during granulosa cell differentiation. *Endocrinology*, **120**, 1121–6.

Filicori, M., Butler, J.P. & Crowley, W.F. (1984). Neuroendocrine regulation of the corpus luteum in the human. *J. Clin. Invest.*, **73**, 1638–47.

Forage, R.G., Ring, J.W., Brown, R.W., McInerey, B.V., Cobon, G.S., Gregson, R.P., Robertson, D.M. *et al.* (1986) Cloning and sequence analysis of cDNA species coding for the two subunits of inhibin from bovine follicular fluid. *Proc. Natl. Acad. Sci. USA*, **83**, 3091–5.

Fowler, R.E., Chan, S.T.H., Walters, D.E., Edwards, R.G. & Steptoe, P.C. (1977) Steroidogenesis in human follicles judged from assays of follicular fluid. *J. Endocrinol.*, **72**, 259–71.

Franchimont, P. (1986) Foreword. *Baillerés Clin. Endocrinol. Metab.*, **15**, ix–xiii.

Franchimont, P., Hazee-Hagelstein, M.T., Charlet-Renard, Ch. & Jasper, J.M. (1986) Effect of mouse epidermal growth factor on DNA and protein synthesis, progesterone and inhibin production by bovine granulosa cell cultures. *Acta Endocrinol. Copenh.*, **111**, 122–7.

Froesch, E.R., Schmid, Chr., Scwander, J. & Zapf, J. (1985) Actions of insulin-like growth factors. *Annu. Rev. Physiol.*, **47**, 443–67.

Fukuoka, M., Yasuda, K., Taii, S., Takakura, K. & Mori, T. (1989) Interleukin stimulates growth and inhibits progesterone secretion in cultures of porcine granulosa cells. *Endocrinology*, **124**, 884–90.

Funkenstein, B., Waterman, W.R. & Simpson, E.R. (1984) Induction of synthesis of cholesterol side-chain cleavage, cytochrome P450 and adrenodoxin by follicle-stimulating hormone, 8-bromo-cyclic AMP, and low-density lipoprotein in cultured bovine granulosa cells. *J. Biol. Chem.*, **259**, 8572–7.

Gaarenstroom, J.H. & de Jongh, S.E. (1946) A contribution to the knowledge of the influence of gonadotropic and sex hormones on the gonads of rats. In Houwink, R. & Ketelaar, J.A.A. (eds) *Monographs on the Progress of Research in Holland During the War*, Vol. 7, pp. 59–164. Elsevier, Amsterdam.

Gates, G.S., Bater, S., Seibel, M., Poretsky, L., Flier, J.S. & Moses, A.C. (1987) Characterization of insulin-like growth factor binding to human granulosa cells obtained during *in vitro* fertilization. *J. Receptor Res.*, **7**, 885–902.

Gill, G.N., Bertics, P.J. & Santon, J. (1987) Epidermal growth factor and its receptor. *Mol. Cell. Endocrinol.*, **51**, 169–86.

Gilman, A. (1987) G-proteins: transducers of receptor-generated signals. *Annu. Rev. Biochem.*, **56**, 615–49.

Glasier, A.F., Baird, D.T. & Hillier, S.G. (1989) FSH and the control of follicular development. *J. Steroid Biochem.*, **32** (1B), 167–170.

Goldenberg, R.L., Reiter, E.O. & Ross, G.T. (1973) Follicle response to exogenous gonadotropins: and estrogen-mediated phenomenon. *Fertil. Steril.*, **24**, 121–5.

Golos, T.G., Strauss, J.F. & Millier, W.L. (1987). Regulation of lipoprotein receptor and cytochrome P-450scc mRNA levels in human granulosa cells. *J. Steroid Biochem.*, **27**, 767–73.

Gonzalez-Manchon, C. & Vale, W. (1989) Activin-A, inhibin and transforming growth factor-β modulate growth of two gonadal cell lines. *Endocrinology*, **125**, 1666–72.

Gore-Langton, R.E. & Armstrong, D.T. (1988) Follicular steroidogenesis and its control. In Knobil, E. & Neill, J.D. (eds) *The Physiology of Reproduction*, Vol. 1, pp. 331–85. Raven Press, New York.

Gospodarowicz, D. & Balecki, H. (1979) Fibroblast and epidermal growth factors are mitogenic agents for cultured granulosa cells of rodent, porcine, and human origin. *Endocrinology*, **104**, 757–64.

Gospodarowicz, D. & Ferrara, N. (1989) Fibroblast growth factor and the control of pituitary and gonad development and function. *J. Steroid Biochem.*, **32**, 183–91.

Green, A.R. (1989) Peptide regulatory factors: multi-functional mediators of cellular growth and differentiation. *Lancet*, **i**, 705–7.

Gwynne, J.T. & Strauss, J.F. (1982) The role of lipoproteins in steroidogenesis and cholesterol metabolism in steroidogenic glands. *Endocr. Rev.*, **3**, 299–329.

Hammond, J.M., Baranao, J.L.S., Skaleris, D., Knight, A.B., Romanus, J.A. & Rechler, M.M. (1985) Production of insulin-like growth factors by ovarian granulosa cells. *Endocrinology*, **117**, 2553–5.

Hammond, J.M. & English, H.F. (1987) Regulation of deoxyribonucleic acid synthesis in cultured porcine granulosa cells by growth factors and hormones. *Endocrinology*, **120**, 1039–46.

Hammond, J.M., Hersey, R.M., Walega, M.A. & Weisz, J. (1986). Catecholestrogen production by porcine ovarian cells. *Endocrinology*, **118**, 2292–9.

Hammond, J.M., Hsu, C.-J., Mondschein, J.S. & Canning, S.H. (1988). Paracrine and autocrine functions of growth factors in the ovarian follicle. *J. Anim. Sci.*, **66**, 21–31.

Harlow, C.R., Hillier, S.G. & Hodges, J.K. (1986) Androgen modulation of follicle-stimulating hormone-induced granulosa cell steroidogenesis in the primate ovary. *Endocrinology*, **119**, 1403–5.

Harlow, C.R., Shaw, H.J., Hillier, S.G. & Hodges, J.K. (1988) Factors influencing FSH-induced steroidogenesis in marmoset granulosa cells: effects of androgens and stages of follicular development. *Endocrinology*, **122**, 2780–7.

Harrison, L.C. & Campbell, I.L. (1988) Cytokines: an expanding network of immuno-inflammatory hormones. *Mol. Endocrinol.*, **2**, 1151–6.

Hedin, L., McKnight, G.S., Lifka, J., Durica, J.M. & Richards, J.S. (1987) Tissue distribution and hormonal regulation of messenger ribonucleic acid for regulatory and catalytic subunits of adenosine 3′,5′-monophosphate-dependent protein kinases during ovarian follicular development in the rat. *Endocrinology*, **120**, 1928–35.

Henderson, K.M. & Franchimont, P. (1983) Inhibin production by bovine ovarian tissues *in vitro* and its regulation by androgens. *J. Reprod. Fertil.*, **67**, 291–8.

Hernandez, E.R., Resnick, C.E., Svoboda, M.E., Van Wyk, J.J., Payne, D.W. & Adashi, E.Y. (1988) Somatomedin-C/insulin-like growth factor I as an enhancer of androgen biosynthesis by cultured rat ovarian cells. *Endocrinology*, **122**, 1603–12.

Hickey, G.J., Chen, S., Besman, M.J., Shively, J.E., Hall, P.F., Gaddy-Kurten, D. & Richards, J.S. (1988) Hormonal regulation, tissue distribution, and content of aromatase cytochrome P450 messenger ribonucleic acid and enzyme in rat ovarian follicles and corpora lutea: relationship to estradiol biosynthesis. *Endocrinology*, **122**, 1426–36.

Hild-Petito, S., Stouffer, R.L. & Brenner, R.M. (1988)

Immunocytochemical localization of estradiol and progesterone receptors in the monkey ovary throughout the menstrual cycle. *Endocrinology*, **123**, 2896–905.

Hillier, S.G. (1981) Regulation of follicular oestrogen biosynthesis: a survey of current concepts. *J. Endocrinol.*, Suppl. **89**, 3–19P.

Hillier, S.G. (1985) Sex steroid metabolism and follicular development in the ovaries. *Oxf. Rev. Reprod. Biol.*, **7**, 168–222.

Hillier, S.G. & de Zwart, F.A. (1981) Evidence that induction/activation of granulosa cell aromatase activity by follicle-stimulating hormone is an androgen receptor-regulated process *in vitro*. *Endocrinology*, **109**, 1303–5.

Hillier, S.G., Harlow, C.R., Shaw, H.J., Wickings, E.J., Dixson, A.F. & Hodges, J.K. (1988) Cellular aspects of preovulatory folliculogenesis in primate ovaries. *Hum. Reprod.*, **3**, 507–11.

Hillier, S.G., Knazek, R.A. & Ross, G.T. (1977) Androgenic stimulation of progesterone production by granulosa cells from preantral ovarian follicles: further *in vitro* studies using replicate cell cultures. *Endocrinology*, **100**, 1539–49.

Hillier, S.G., Reichert, L.E.R. Jr. & van Hall, E.V. (1981) Control of preovulatory follicular estrogen biosynthesis in the human ovary. *J. Clin. Endocrinol. Metab.*, **52**, 847–56.

Hillier, S.G. & Ross, G.T. (1979) Effects of exogenous testosterone on ovarian weight, follicular morphology and intraovarian progesterone concentration in estrogen-primed, hypophysectomized immature female rats. *Biol. Reprod.*, **20**, 261–8.

Hillier, S.G., Saunders, P.T.K., White, R. & Parker, M.G. (1989) Oestrogen receptor mRNA and a related RNA transcript in mouse ovaries. *J. Mol. Endocrinol.*, **2**, 39–45.

Hillier, S.G., Trimbos-Kemper, T.C.M., Reichert, L.E. Jr. & van Hall, E.V. (1983) Gonadotropic control of human granulosa cell function: *in vitro* studies on aspirates of preovulatory follicles. In Greenwald, G.S. & Terranova, P.F. (eds) *Factors Regulating Ovulation*, pp. 49–54. Raven Press, New York.

Hillier, S.G., van den Boogaard, A.J.M., Reichert, L.E. Jr. & van Hall, E.V. (1980a) Intraovarian sex steroid hormone interactions and the control of follicular maturation: aromatization of androgens by human granulosa cells *in vitro*. *J. Clin. Endocrinol. Metab.*, **50**, 640–7.

Hillier, S.G., van Hall, E.V., van den Boogaard, A.J.M., de Zwart, F.A. & Keyzer, R. (1982) Activation and modulation of the granulosa cell aromatase system: experimental studies with rat and human ovaries. In Rolland, R., van Hall, E.V., Hillier, S.G., McNatty, K.P. & Schoemaker, J. (eds) *Follicular Maturation and Ovulation*, pp. 51–70. Amsterdam, Excerpta Medica.

Hillier, S.G. & Wickings, E.J. (1985). Cellular aspects

of corpus luteum function. In Jeffcoate, S.L. (ed.) *The Luteal Phase*, pp. 1−23. Wiley, London.

Hillier, S.G., Wickings, E.J., Saunders, P.T.K., Shimisaki, S., Reichert, L.E. Jr. & McNeilly, A.S. (1989) Hormonal control of inhibin production by primate granulosa cells. *J. Endocrinol.*, **123**, 65−73.

Hillier, S.G., Zeleznik, A.J., Knazek, R.A. & Ross, G.T. (1980b) Hormonal regulation of preovulatory follicle maturation in the rat. *J. Reprod. Fertil.*, **60**, 219−29.

Hillier, S.G., Zeleznik, A.J. & Ross, G.T. (1978) Independence of steroidogenic capacity and luteinizing hormone receptor induction in developing granulosa cells. *Endocrinology*, **102**, 937−46.

Hisaw, F.L. (1947) Development of the Graafian follicle and ovulation. *Physiol. Rev.*, **27**, 95−119.

Hofeditz, C., Magoffin, D.A. & Erickson, G.F. (1988) Evidence for protein kinase C regulation of ovarian theca−interstitial cell androgen biosynthesis. *Biol. Reprod.*, **39**, 873−81.

Hsueh, A.J.W. (1986) Paracrine mechanisms involved in granulosa cell differentiation. *Baillièrés Clin. Endocrinol. Metab.*, **15**, 117−34.

Hsueh, A.J.W., Adashi, E.Y., Jones, P.B.C. & Welsh, T.J. Jr. (1984) Hormonal regulation of the differentiation of cultured granulosa cells. *Endocr. Rev.*, **5**, 76−126.

Hsueh, A.J.W., Bicsak, T.A., Jia, X-C., Dahl, K.D., Fauser, B.C.J.M., Galway, A.B., Czekala, N., Pavlou, S.N., Papkoff, H., Keene, J. & Boime, I. (1989). Granulosa cells as hormone targets: the role of biologically active follicle-stimulating hormone in reproduction. *Recent Prog. Horm. Res.* **45**, 209−73.

Hsueh, A.J.W., Dahl, K.D., Vaughan, J., Tucker, E., Rivier, J., Bardin, C.W. & Vale, W. (1987) Heterodimers and homodimers of inhibin subunits have different paracrine action in the modulation of luteinizing hormone-stimulated androgen biosynthesis. *Proc. Natl. Acad. Sci. USA*, **84**, 5082−6.

Hudson, K.E. & Hillier, S.G. (1985) Catechol oestradiol control of FSH-stimulated granulosa cell steroidogenesis. *J. Endocrinol.*, **106**, R1−3.

Hutchison, L.A., Findlay, J.K., de Vos, F.L. & Robertson, D.M. (1987) Effects of bovine inhibin, transforming growth factor-β and bovine activin-A on granulosa cell differentiation. *Biochem. Biophys. Res. Commun.*, **146**, 1405−12.

Jia, X-C., Kalmijn, J. & Hsueh, A.J.W. (1986) Growth hormone enhances follicle-stimulating hormone-induced differentiation of cultured rat granulosa cells. *Endocrinology*, **118**, 1401−9.

Johnson, G.J. & Dhanasekaran, N. (1989) The G-protein family and their interaction with receptors. *Endocr. Rev.*, **10**, 317−31.

Jones, P.B.C. (1989) Potential relevance of gonadotropin-releasing hormone to ovarian physiology. *Semin. Reprod. Endocrinol.* **7**, 41−51.

Jones, P.B.C., Welsh, T.H. Jr. & Hsueh, A.J.W. (1982)

Regulation of ovarian progestin production by epidermal growth factor in cultured granulosa cells. *J. Biol. Chem.*, **257**, 11268−73.

Kasson, B.G., Conn, P.M. & Hsueh, A.J.W. (1985) Inhibition of granulosa cell differentiation by dioctanoylglycerol − a novel activator of protein kinase C. *Mol. Cell. Endocrinol.*, **42**, 29−37.

Kasson, B.G. & Gorospe, W.C. (1989) Effects of interleukins 1, 2 and 3 on follicle-stimulating hormone-induced differentiation of rat granulosa cells. *Mol. Cell. Endocrinol.*, **62**, 103−11.

Khan-Dawood, F.S. & Dawood, M.Y. (1989) Potential relevance of neurohypohysial hormones to ovarian physiology. *Semin. Reprod. Endocrinol.* **7**, 61−78.

Kim, I-C. & Schomberg, D.W. (1989) The production of transforming growth factor-β by rat granulosa cell cultures. *Endocrinology*, **124**, 1345−51.

Kim. S-J., Shinjo, M., Tada, M., Usuki, S., Fukamizu, A., Miyazaki, H. & Murakami, K. (1987) Ovarian renin gene expression is regulated by follicle-stimulating hormone. *Biochem. Biophys. Res. Commun.*, **146**, 989−95.

Knecht, M. (1988) Plasminogen activator is associated with the extracellular matrix of ovarian granulosa cells. *Mol. Cell. Endocrinol.*, **56**, 1−9.

Knecht, M. & Catt, K.J. (1983) Modulation of cAMP-mediated differentiation in ovarian granulosa cells by epidermal growth factor and platelet-derived growth factor. *J. Biol. Chem.*, **258**, 2789−94.

Knecht, M., Feng, P. & Catt, K.J. (1986) Transforming growth factor-beta regulates the expression of luteinizing hormone receptors in ovarian granulosa cells. *Biochem. Biophys. Res. Commun.*, **139**, 800−7.

Knecht, M., Feng, P. & Catt, K. (1987) Bifunctional role of transforming growth factor-β during granulosa cell development. *Endocrinology*, **120**, 1243−9.

Kudlow, J.E., Kobrin, M.S., Purchio, A.F., Twardzik, D.R., Hernandez, E.R., Asa, S.L. & Adashi, E.Y. (1987) Ovarian transforming growth factor-α gene expression: immunohistochemical localization to the theca-interstitial cells. *Endocrinology*, **121**, 1577−9.

Kudolo, G.B., Elder, M.G. & Myatt, L. (1984a) A novel oestrogen binding species in rat granulosa cells. *J. Endocrinol.*, **102**, 83−91.

Kudolo, G.B., Elder, M.G. & Myatt, L. (1984b) Further characterization of the second oestrogen-binding species of the rat granulosa cell. *J. Endocrinol.*, **102**, 93−102.

Kurten, R.C. & Richards, J.S. (1989) An adenosine 3′,5′-monophosphate-responsive deoxyribonucleic acid element confers forskolin sensitivity on gene expression by primary rat granulosa cells. *Endocrinology*, **125**, 1345−57.

LaTouche, J., Crumeyrolle-Arias, M., Jordan, D., Kopp, N., Augendre-Ferrante, B., Cedard, L. & Haour, F. (1989) GnRH receptors in human granulosa cells: anatomical localization and characterization by autoradiographic study. *Endocrinology*, **125**, 1739−41.

Leung, P.C.K. & Armstrong, D.T. (1980) Interactions of steroids and gonadotrophins in the control of steroidogenesis in the ovarian follicle. *Annu. Rev. Physiol.*, **42**, 71−82.

Leung, P.C.K. & Wang, J. (1989) The role of inositol lipid metabolism in the ovary. *Biol. Reprod.*, **40**, 703−8.

Ling, N., Ying, S.-Y., Ueno, N., Esch, F., Denoroy, L. & Guillemin, R. (1985) Isolation and partial characterization of a Mr 32 000 protein with inhibin activity from porcine follicular fluid. *Proc. Natl. Acad. Sci. USA*, **82**, 7217−21.

Ling, N., Ying, S.-Y., Ueno, N., Shimasaki, S., Esch, F., Hotta, M. & Guillemin, R. (1986) Pituitary FSH is released by a heterodimer of the β-subunits from the two forms of inhibin. *Nature*, **321**, 779−82.

Lischinsky, A., Khalil, M.W., Hobkirk, R. & Armstrong, D.T. (1983) Formation of androgen conjugates by porcine granulosa cells. *J. Steroid Biochem.*, **19**, 1435−40.

Louvet, J-P., Harman, S.M., Schreiber, J.R. & Ross, G.T. (1975) Evidence for a role of androgens in follicular maturation. *Endocrinology*, **97**, 366−72.

Lucky, A.W., Schreiber, J.R., Hillier, S.G., Schulman, J.D. & Ross, G.T. (1977) Progesterone production by cultured granulosa cells: stimulation by androgens. *Endocrinology*, **100**, 128−33.

McAllister, J.M., Kerin, J.F.P., Trant, J.M., Estabrook, R.W., Mason, J.I., Waterman, M.R. & Simpson, E.R. (1989) Regulation of cholesterol side-chain cleavage and 17α-hydroxylase/lyase activities in proliferating human theca interna cells in long term monolayer culture. *Endocrinology*, **125**, 1959−66.

McFarland, K.C., Sprengel, R., Phillips, H.S., Köhler, M., Rosemblit, N., Nikolocs, K., Segaloff, D.L. & Seeburg, P.H. (1989) Lutropin-choriogonadotropin receptor: an unusual member of the G-protein-coupled receptor family. *Science*, **245**, 494−9.

McNatty, K.P. (1981) Hormonal correlates of follicular development in the human ovary. *Aust. J. Biol. Sci.*, **34**, 249−68.

McNatty, K.P., Reinhold, V.N., DeGrazia, C., Osathanondh, R. & Ryan, K. (1979) Metabolism of androstenedione by human ovarian tissue *in vitro* with particular reference to reductase and aromatase activity. *Steroids*, **34**, 429−43.

Magoffin, D.A. (1989) Evidence that luteinizing hormone-stimulated differentiation of purified ovarian thecal-interstitial cells is mediated by both Type I and Type II adenosine 3′,5′-monophosphate-dependent protein kinases. *Endocrinology*, **125**, 1464−73.

Magoffin, D.A., Gancedo, B. & Erickson, G.F. (1989) Transforming growth factor-β promotes differentiation of ovarian thecal−interstitial cells but inhibits androgen production. *Endocrinology*, **125**, 1951−8.

Magoffin, D.A. Kurtz, K.M. & Erickson, G.F. (1990) Insulin-like growth factor-1 selectively stimulates cholesterol side-chain cleavage expression in ovarian theca-interstitial cells. *Mol. Endocrinol.* **4**, 489−96.

Marsh, J.M. (1976) The role of cyclic AMP in gonadal steroidogenesis. *Biol. Reprod.*, **14**, 30−53.

Mason, A.J., Hayflick, J.S., Ling, N., Esch, F., Ueno, N., Ying, S.-Y., Guillemin, R. *et al.* (1985) Complementary DNA sequences of ovarian follicular fluid inhibin show precursor structure and homology with transforming growth factor-β. *Nature*, **318**, 659−63.

Mason, A.J., Niall, H.D. & Seeburg, P.H. (1986) Structure of two human ovarian inhibins. *Biochem. Biophys. Res. Commun.*, **135**, 957−64.

Massagué, J. (1983) Epidermal growth factor-like transforming growth factor. II. Interaction with epidermal growth factor receptors in human placenta membranes and A431 cells. *J. Biol. Chem.*, **258**, 13614−20.

Massagué, J. (1987) The TGF-β family of growth and differentiation factors. *Cell*, **49**, 437−8.

Mayo, K.E., Cerelli, G.M., Spiess, J., Rivier, J., Rosenfeld, M.G., Evans, R.M. & Vale, W. (1986) Inhibin A-subunit cDNAs from porcine ovary and human placenta. *Proc. Natl. Acad. Sci. USA*, **83**, 5849−53.

Mendelson, C.R., Merrill, J.C., Steinkampf, M.P. & Simpson, E.R. (1988) Regulation of the synthesis of aromatase cytochrome P-450 in human adipose, stromal and ovarian granulosa cells. *Steroids*, **50**, 51−9.

Michell, R.H. (1989) Post-receptor signalling pathways. *Lancet*, **i**, 765−8.

Miller, W.L. (1988) Molecular biology of steroid hormone synthesis. *Endocr. Rev.*, **9**, 295−318.

Miyamoto, K., Hasegawa, Y., Fukuda, M., Nomura, M., Igarashi, M., Kangawa, K. & Matsuo, H. (1985) Isolation of porcine follicular fluid inhibin of 32K daltons. *Biochem. Biophy. Res. Commun.*, **129**, 396−403.

Mondschein, J.S., Canning, S.F., Miller, D.Q. & Hammond, J. (1989) Insulin-like growth factors (IGFs) as autocrine/paracrine regulators of granulosa cell differentiation and growth: studies with a neutralizing monoclonal antibody to IGF-1. *Biol. Reprod.*, **40**, 79−85.

Neufeld, G., Ferrara, N., Mitchell, R., Schweigerer, L. & Gospdarowicz, D. (1987) Granulosa cells produce basic fibroblast growth factor. *Endocrinology*, **121**, 597−603.

Nimrod, A. & Lindner, H.R. (1976) A synergistic effect of androgen on the stimulation of progesterone secretion by FSH in cultured rat granulosa cells. *Mol. Cell. Endocrinol.*, **5**, 315−20.

Nishizuka, Y. (1988) The molecular heterogeneity of protein kinase C and its implications for cellular regulation. *Nature*, **334**, 661−5.

Noland, T.A. & Domino, M.J. (1986) Characterization

and distribution of protein kinase C in ovarian tissue. *Biol. Reprod.*, **35**, 863–72.

Ny, T., Bjersing, L., Hsueh, A.J.W. & Loskutoff, D.J. (1985) Cultured granulosa cells produce two plasminogen activators and an antiactivator, each regulated differently by gonadotropins. *Endocrinology*, **116**, 1666–8.

O'Connell, M.L., Canipari, R. & Strickland, S. (1987) Hormonal regulation of tissue plasminogen activator secretion and mRNA levels in rat granulosa cells. *J. Biol. Chem.*, **262**, 2339–444.

Ohlsson, M., Hsueh, A.J.W. & Ny. T. (1988) Hormonal regulation of tissue type plasminogen activator messenger ribonucleic acid levels in rat granulosa cells: mechanisms of induction by follicle-stimulating hormone and gonadotropin hormone releasing hormone. *Mol. Endocrinol.*, **2**, 854–61.

Oliver, J.E., Aitman, T.J., Powell, J.F., Wilson, C.A. & Clayton, R.N. (1989) Insulin-like growth factor I gene expression in the rat ovary is confined to the granulosa cells of developing follicles. *Endocrinology*, **124**, 2671–9.

Opavsky, M.A. & Armstrong, D.T. (1989) Effects of luteinizing hormone on superovulatory and steroidogenic responses of rat ovaries to infusion with follicle-stimulating hormone. *Biol. Reprod.*, **40**, 12–25.

Poretsky, L, Grigorescu, F., Seibel, M., Moses, A.C. & Flier, J.S. (1985) Distribution and characterization of insulin and insulin-like growth factor receptors in normal human ovary. *J. Clin. Endocrinol. Metab.*, **61**, 728–34.

Pucell, A.G., Bumpus, F.M. & Husain, A. (1988) Regulation of angiotensin II receptors in cultured rat ovarian cells by follicle-stimulating hormone and angiotensin II. *J. Biol. Chem.*, **263**, 11954–61.

Ramasharma, K., Caberera, C.M. & Li, C.H. (1986) Identification of insulin-like growth factor II in human seminal and follicular fluids. *Biochem. Biophys. Res. Commun.* **140**, 536–42.

Ramasharma, K. & Li, C.H. (1987) Human pituitary and placental hormones control human insulin-like growth factors secretion in human granulosa cells. *Proc. Natl. Acad. Sci. USA*, **84**, 2643–7.

Readhead, R., Lobo, R.A. & Kletzky, O.A. (1983) The activity of 3β-hydroxysteroid dehydrogenase and $\Delta^{4-5}$ isomerase in human follicular tissue. *Am. J. Obstet. Gynecol.*, **145**, 491–5.

Rechler, M.M. & Nissley, S.P. (1985) The nature and regulation of the receptors for insulin-like growth factors. *Annu. Rev. Physiol.*, **47**, 425–42.

Richards, J.S. (1975) Estradiol receptor content in rat granulosa cells during follicular development: modification by estradiol and gonadotropins. *Endocrinology*, **97**, 1174–84.

Richards, J.S. (1980) Maturation of ovarian follicles: actions and interaction of pituitary and ovarian hormones on follicular differentiation. *Physiol. Rev.*, **60**, 51–89.

Richards, J.S., Jahnsen, T., Hedin, L., Lifka, J., Ratoosh, S.L., Durica, J.M. & Goldring, N.B. (1987) Ovarian follicular development: from physiology to molecular biology. *Recent Prog. Horm. Res.*, **43**, 231–70.

Rivier, J., Spiess, J., McClintock, R., Vaughan, J. & Vale, W. (1985) Purification and partial characterization of inhibin from porcine follicular fluid. *Biochem. Biophys. Res. Commun.*, **133**, 120–7.

Roberts, A.B., Flanders, K.C., Kondaiah, P., Thomson, N.L., Van Obberghen-Schilling, E., Wakefield, L., Rossi, P. *et al.* (1988) Transforming growth factor β: biochemistry and roles in embryogenesis, tissue repair and remodeling, and carcinogenesis. *Recent Prog. Horm. Res.*, **44**, 157–93.

Robertson, D.M., Foulds, L.M., Leversha, L., Morgan, F.J., Hearn, M.T.W., Burger, H.G., Wettenhall, R.E.H. & de Kretser, D.M. (1985) Isolation of inhibin from bovine follicular fluid. *Biochem. Biophys. Res. Commun.*, **126**, 220–6.

Roesler, W.J., Vandenbark, G.R. & Hanson, R.W. (1988) Cyclic AMP and the induction of eukaryotic gene transcription. *J. Biol. Chem.*, **263**, 9063–6.

Ross, G.T. and Schreiber, J.R. (1986). The ovary. In Yen, S.S.C. & Jaffe, R.B. (eds) *Reproductive Endocrinology*, 2nd edn., pp. 115–39. W.B. Saunders, London.

Ross, R. (1989) Platelet-derived growth factor. *Lancet*, **i**, 1179–82.

Ryan, K.J. (1979) Granulosa–thecal interaction in ovarian steroidogenesis. *J. Steroid Biochem.*, **11**, 799–800.

Saiduddin, S. & Zassenhaus, H.P. (1977) Estradiol-17β receptors in the immature rat ovary. *Steroids*, **29**, 197–213.

Sasano, H., Okamoto, M., Mason, J.I., Simpson, E.R., Mendelson, C.R., Sasano, N. & Silverberg, S.G. (1989) Immunolocalization of aromatase, 17α-hydroxylase and side-chain cleavage cytochromes P-450 in the human ovary. *J. Reprod. Fertil.*, **85**, 163–9.

Schomberg, D.W. (1988) Regulation of follicle development by gonadotropins and growth factors. In Stouffer, R.L. (ed.) *The Primate Ovary*, pp. 25–33. Plenum, London.

Schomberg, D.W., Stouffer, R.L. & Tyrey, L. (1976) Modulation of progestin secretion in ovarian cells by 17β-hydroxy-5α-androstan-3-one (dihydrotestosterone): a direct demonstration in monolayer culture. *Biochem. Biophys. Res. Commun.*, **68**, 77–85.

Schreiber, J.R. & Ross, G.T. (1976) Further characterization of a rat ovarian testosterone receptor with evidence for nuclear translocation. *Endocrinology*, **99**, 590–6.

Segaloff, D.L., Wang, H. & Richards, J.S. (1990) Hormone specific regulation of LH/CG receptor mRNA expression in rat ovarian follicles and corporalutea. *Proc. 72nd Annual Meeting of the Endocrine Society (abstr. 1064)*.

Shaw, H.J., Hillier, S.G., & Hodges, J.K. (1989) Developmental changes in luteinizing hormone/human chorionic gonadotropin steroidogenic responsiveness in marmoset granulosa cells: Effects of follicle-stimulating hormone and androgens. *Endocrinology*, **124**, 1669–77.

Shimasaki, S., Koga, M., Buscaglia, M.L., Simmons, D.M., Bicsak, T.A. & Ling, N. (1989) Follistatin gene expression in the ovary and extragonadal tissues. *Mol. Endocrinol.*, **3**, 651–9.

Shinohara, O., Knecht, M. & Catt, K.J. (1985) Inhibition of gonadotropin-induced granulosa cell differentiation by activation of protein kinase C. *Proc. Natl. Acad. Sci. USA*, **82**, 8518–22.

Short, R.V. (1962) Steroids in follicular fluid and the corpus luteum of the mare. A 'two-cell type' theory of ovarian steroid synthesis. *J. Endocrinol.*, **24**, 59–63.

Sibley, D.R., Benovic, J.L., Caron, M. & Lefkowitz, R.L. (1988) Phosphorylation of cell surface receptors: a mechanism for regulating signal transduction pathways. *Endocr. Rev.*, **9**, 38–56.

Skinner, M.K., Keski-Oja, J., Osteen, K.G. & Moses, H.L. (1987) Ovarian theca cells produce transforming growth factor-β which regulates granulosa cell growth. *Endocrinology*, **121**, 786–92.

Skinner, M.K., McKeracher, H.L. & Dorrington, J.H. (1985) Fibronectin as a marker of granulosa cell cytodifferentiation. *Endocrinology*, **117**, 886–92.

Slack, J.M.W. (1989) Peptide regulatory factors in embryonic development. *Lancet*, **i**, 1312–15.

Spicer, L.J., & Hammond, J.M. (1989) Catechol oestrogens inhibit proliferation and DNA synthesis of porcine granulosa cells *in vitro*: comparison with estradiol, 5α-dihydrotestosterone, gonadotropins and catecholamines. *Mol. Cell. Endocrinol.*, **64**, 119–26.

Sprengel, R., Braun, T., Nikolics, K., Segaloff, D.L. & Seeburg, P.H. (1990) The testicular receptor for follicle stimulating hormone: structure and functional expression of cloned cDNA. *Mol. Endocrinol.*, **4**, 525–30.

Steinkampf, M.P., Mendelson, C.R. & Simpson, E.R. (1987) Regulation by follicle-stimulating hormone of the synthesis of aromatase cytochrome P-450 in human granulosa cells. *Mol. Endocrinol.*, **1**, 465–71.

Steinkampf, M.P., Mendelson, C.R. & Simpson, E.R. (1988) Effects of epidermal growth factor and insulin-like growth factor I on the levels of mRNA encoding aromatase P-450 of human ovarian granulosa cells. *Mol. Cell. Endocrinol.*, **59**, 93–9.

Suikkari, A.M., Jalkanen, J., Koistinen, R., Bützow, R., Ritvos, O., Ranta, T. & Seppälä, M. (1989) Human granulosa cells synthesize low molecular weight insulin-like growth factor binding protein. *Endocrinology*, **124**, 1088–90.

Suzuki, T., Miyamoto, K., Hasegawa, Y., Abe, Y., Ui, M., Ibuki, Y. & Igarashi, M. (1987) Regulation of inhibin production by rat granulosa cells. *Mol. Cell.*

*Endocrinol.*, **54**, 185–95.

Tonetta, S.T. & DiZerega. G.S. (1989) Intragonadal regulation of follicular maturation. *Endocr. Rev.*, **10**, 205–29.

Too, C.K.L., Bryant-Greenwood, G. & Greenwood, F.C. (1984) Relaxin increases the release of plasminogen activator, collagenase, and proteoglycanase from rat granulosa cells *in vitro*. *Endocrinology*, **115**, 1043–50.

Trzeciak, W.H., Waterman, M.R. & Simpson, E.R. (1986) Synthesis of the cholesterol side-chain cleavage enzymes in cultured rat ovarian cells: induction by follicle-stimulating hormone and dibutyryl adenosine 3′,5′-monophosphate. *Endocrinology*, **119**, 323–30.

Trzeciak, W.H., Waterman, M.R., Simpson, E.R. & Ojeda, S.R. (1987) Vasoactive intestinal peptide regulates cholesterol side-chain cleavage cytochrome P-450 (P-450scc) gene expression in granulosa cells from immature ovaries. *Mol. Endocrinol.*, **1**, 500–4.

Tsang, B.K., Moon, Y.S., Simpson, C.W. & Armstrong, D.T. (1979) Androgen biosynthesis in human ovarian follicles: cellular source, gonadotropic control, and adenosine 3′,5′-monophosphate mediation. *J. Clin. Endocrinol. Metab.*, **48**, 153–8.

Tsonis, C.G., Hillier, S.G. & Baird, D.T. (1987) Production of inhibin bioactivity by human granulosa–lutein cells: stimulation by LH and testosterone *in vitro*. *J. Endocrinol.*, **112**, R11–14.

Tsonis, C.G. & Sharpe, R.M. (1986) Dual gonadal control of follicle-stimulating hormone. *Nature*, **321**, 724–5.

Turner, I.M., Saunders, P.T.K., Shimasaki, S. & Hillier, S.G. (1989) Regulation of inhibin subunit gene expression by FSH and estradiol in cultured rat granulosa cells. *Endocrinology*, **125**, 2790–2.

Ui, M., Shimonaka, M., Shimasaki, S. & Ling, N. (1989) An insulin-like growth factor binding protein in ovarian follicular fluid blocks follicle-stimulating hormone-stimulated steroid production by ovarian granulosa cells. *Endocrinology*, **125**, 912–16.

Vale, W., Rivier, C., Hsueh, A., Campen, C., Meunier, H., Bicsak, T., Vaughan, J. *et al.* (1988) Chemical and biological characterization of the inhibin family of protein hormones. *Recent Prog. Horm. Res.*, **44**, 1–30.

Vale, W., Rivier, J., Vaughan, J., McClintock, R., Corrigan, A., Woo, W., Karr, D. & Spiess, J. (1986) Purification and characterization of an FSH releasing protein from porcine ovarian follicular fluid. *Nature*, **321**, 776–9.

Van Noorden, S. & Polak, J.M. (1979) Hormones of the alimentary tract. In Barrington, E.J.W. (ed.) *Hormones and Evolution*, Vol. 2, pp. 791–828. Academic Press, London.

Veldhuis, J.D., Rodgers, R.J. & Fulanetto, R.W. (1986) Synergistic actions of estradiol and the insulin-like growth factor Somatomedin-C on swine ovarian (granulosa) cells. *Endocrinology*, **119**, 530–8.

Verges, B., Maurice, C., Cornet, D., Salat-Baroux, J. & Ardaillou, R. (1986) Arginine vasopressin in human follicular fluid. *J. Clin. Endocrinol. Metab.*, **63**, 928–30.

Voutilainen, R. & Miller, W.L. (1989) Potential relevance of Müllerian-inhibiting substance to ovarian physiology. *Semin. Reprod. Endocrinol.* **7**, 88–93.

Wang, C., Hsueh, A.J.W. & Erickson, G.F. (1981) LH stimulation of estrogen secretion by cultured rat granulosa cells. *Mol. Cell. Endocrinol.* **24**, 17–28.

Waterfield, M.D. (1989) Epidermal growth factor and related molecules. *Lancet* **1**, 1243–6.

Westergaard, L., Christensen, I.J. & McNatty, K.P. (1986) Steroid levels in ovarian follicular fluid related to follicle size and health status during the normal menstrual cycle in women. *Hum. Reprod.*, **1**, 227.

Wheeler, M.B. & Veldhuis, J. (1989) Facilitative actions of the protein kinase-C effector system on hormonally stimulated adenosine 3',5'-monophosphate production by swine luteal cells. *Endocrinology*, **125**, 2414–20.

Whitman, M. & Cantley, L. (1988) Phosphoinositide metabolism and the control of cell proliferation. *Biochim. Biophys. Acta.*, **948**, 327–44.

Wickings, E.J., Hillier, S.G. & Reichert, L.E. Jr. (1986) Gonadotrophic control of steroidogenesis in human granulosa–lutein cells. *J. Reprod. Fertil.*, **76**, 677–84.

Woodruff, T.K., D'Agostino, J.B., Schwartz, N.B. & Mayo, K.E. (1988) Dynamic changes in inhibin messenger RNAs in rat ovarian follicles during the reproductive cycle. *Science*, **239**, 1296–9.

Woodruff, T.K., Meunier, H., Jones, P.B., Hsueh, A.J.W. & Mayo, K.E. (1987) Rat inhibin: molecular cloning of α- and β-subunit complementary deoxyribonucleic acids and expression in the ovary. *Mol. Endocrinol.*, **1**, 561–9.

Wyne, K.L., Schreiber, J.R., Larsen, A.L. & Getz, G.S. (1989) Regulation of apolipoprotein E biosynthesis by cAMP and phorbol ester in rat ovarian granulosa cells. *J. Biol. Chem.*, **264**, 981.

Yanagashita, M., Hascall, V.C. & Rodbard, D. (1981) Biosynthesis of proteoglycans by rat granulosa cells cultured *in vitro*: modulation by gonadotropins, steroid hormones, prostaglandins and cyclic nucleotide. *Endocrinology*, **109**, 1641–9.

Yen, S.S.C. (1986). The human menstrual cycle. In Yen, S.S.C. & Jaffe R.B. (eds) *Reproductive Endocrinology*, 2nd edn., pp. 33–74. W.B. Saunders, New York.

Ying, S.-Y. (1988) Inhibins, activins, and follistatins: gonadal proteins modulating the secretion of follicle-stimulating hormone. *Endocr. Rev.*, **9**, 267–93.

Ying, S-Y., Becker, A., Ling, N., Ueno, N. & Guillemin, R. (1986) Inhibin and beta type transforming growth factor (TGFβ) have opposite modulating effects on the follicle stimulating hormone (FSH)-induced aromatase activity of cultured rat granulosa cells. *Biochem. Biophys. Res. Commun.*, **136**, 969–75.

Young, S.L., Nielsen, C.P., Lundblad, J.R., Roberts, J.L. & Melner, M.H. (1989) Gonadotropin regulation of the rat proopiomelanocortin promoter: characterization by transfection of primary ovarian granulosa cells. *Mol. Endocrinol.*, **3**, 15–21.

Yu, J., Shao, L., Lemas, V., Yu, A.L., Vaughan, J., Rivier, J. & Vale, W. (1987) Importance of FSH-releasing protein and inhibin in erythroid differentiation. *Nature*, **330**, 765–7.

Zeleznik, A.J. & Hillier, S.G. (1984) The role of gonadotropins in the selection of the preovulatory follicle. *Clin. Obstet. Gynecol.*, **27**, 927–40.

Zeleznik, A.J., Keyes, P.L., Menon, K.M.J., Midgley, A.R. Jr. & Reichert, L.E. Jr. (1977) Development-dependent responses of ovarian follicles to FSH and hCG. *Am. J. Physiol.*, **233**, E229–34.

Zeleznik, A.J., Schuler, H.M. & Reichert, L.E. Jr. (1981) Gonadotropin-binding sites in the rhesus monkey ovary: Role of the vasculature in the selective distribution of human chorionic gonadotropin to the preovulatory follicle. *Endocrinology*, **109**, 356–62.

Zhang, Z., Lee, V.W.K., Carson, R.S. & Burger, H.G. (1988) Selective control of rat granulosa cell inhibin production by FSH and LH *in vitro*. *Mol. Cell. Endocrinol.*, **56**, 35–40.

Zoller, L.C. & Weisz, J. (1978) Identification of cytochrome P-450, and its distribution in the membrana granulosa of the preovulatory follicle using quantitative cytochemistry. *Endocrinology*, **103**, 310–3.

# 4 Mammalian Oocyte Development

J.J. EPPIG

## Introduction

Ovarian follicles do not form in the absence of oocytes. Unlike the situation in males where testicular components including the seminiferous tubules with Sertoli cells develop in the absence of germ cells, there are no granulosa or theca cells in the absence of oocytes. The oocyte, therefore, is an essential participant in follicular development and, since the follicle is the source of factors essential for the full development and function of virtually all the components of the female reproductive system, there is little or no development or function of the female reproductive system in the absence of oocytes.

Oocytes originate outside the primitive gonad, probably in the hindgut region of the embryo and migrate as primordial germ cells to the genital ridge resulting in the formation of the primitive ovary (Hardisty, 1978). Once within the primitive ovary the primordial germ cells are called oogonia and they proliferate by mitotic division. Responding to an unknown signal, the oogonia enter meiosis, the process whereby the number of chromosomes is reduced from the diploid to the haploid number, and become secondary oocytes. Meiosis in oocytes is not a continuous process in the ovary, but rather is interspersed with stop and start signals (Fig. 4.1). The first stop signal in meiosis occurs at the diplotene stage of meiosis I. At this time the oocyte is situated in a primordial follicle consisting of a single layer of flattened pregranulosa cells surrounding the oocyte. The oocyte in a primordial follicle is 15–20 µm in diameter and can remain in this state for years, depending on the species, until it is recruited by unknown mechanisms into the pool of growing oocytes. As the oocytes near completion of growth, they become competent of resuming meiosis I, but do not do so at this time because the reinitiation of meiosis is held in abeyance by somatic components of the follicle. The preovulatory gonadotrophin surge induces the resumption of meiosis which proceeds to metaphase II where it is arrested for the last time. Upon completion of the first meiotic division, the oocyte becomes a secondary oocyte (ovum) or an egg*. Meiosis resumes in the egg upon penetration of the sperm. This chapter will concentrate on the mechanisms of oocyte development beginning with the growing oocyte. Although the emphasis will be on mammalian oocyte development in general, it is important to realize that relatively few mammalian species have actually been studied and that significant deviations in some aspects of oogenesis are possible.

## Co-ordination of oocyte and follicle development

### Co-ordination of oocyte growth with granulosa cell proliferation and antrum development

Oocyte growth and follicular development are generally initiated at about the same time, although atypical examples of oocyte growth without concomitant granulosa cell proliferation have been reported (Eppig, 1978). It is not known whether the oocyte is induced to enter the growth phase by signals from outside the oocyte or by an oocyte-autonomous programme. As the oocyte increases in size, the flattened granulosa cells become cuboidal and proliferate and enclose the growing oocyte within several layers of cells (Fig. 4.2). Oocyte growth and pre-antral follicular development are independent of gonadotrophin stimulation since they occur in hypophysectomized females and in females genetically deficient in circulating gonadotrophins (Fig. 4.3). Follicular antrum formation begins in many species as the oocyte nears completion

---

* When defined functionally as a gamete capable of being fertilized, a secondary oocyte is an egg, homologous to sperm. In the strictest sense, however, there are no known mammalian eggs since a secondary oocyte has not actually completed the second meiotic division at the time of penetration by a sperm. After penetration by a sperm, the secondary oocyte completes the second meiotic division and becomes a zygote. In this chapter secondary oocytes will be referred to as eggs.

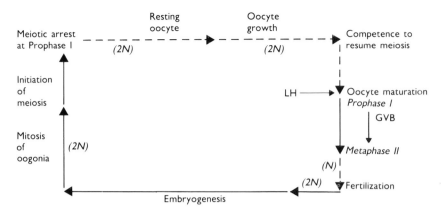

Fig. 4.1. 'Stop-and-go' pattern of meiosis during oocyte development. Meiosis is initiated after mitotic proliferation of oogonia in primitive ovary. Oocyte development with arrested meiosis is indicated by broken arrows. Meiosis is arrested in resting oocytes residing in primordial follicles, growing oocytes, and fully grown oocytes in non-atretic antral follicles. The preovulatory surge of LH triggers the resumption of meiosis which progresses from prophase I to metaphase II. Eggs (secondary oocytes) remain arrested in metaphase II until they are penetrated by a sperm; meiosis II is then completed with the production of the second polar body. N refers to the ploidy (2N=diploid, 1N=haploid).

of its growth phase. Two types of granulosa cells are distinguishable when the ovarian follicle has formed an antrum: cumulus cells that immediately enclose the oocyte, and mural cells which comprise the follicle wall centripetal to the basal lamina (Fig. 4.4). Before antrum formation, all of the somatic cells confined by the basal lamina, whether or not in contact with the oocyte, are simply called granulosa cells.

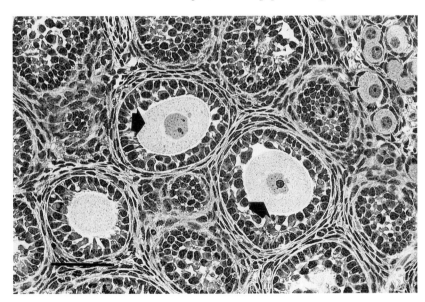

Fig. 4.2. Photomicrograph of primordial and preantral follicles in the ovary from an 8-day-old mouse. The primordial follicles (arrowheads) contain oocytes that have not entered growth phase while the preantral follicles (arrows) contain growing oocytes. Bar indicates 50 μm.

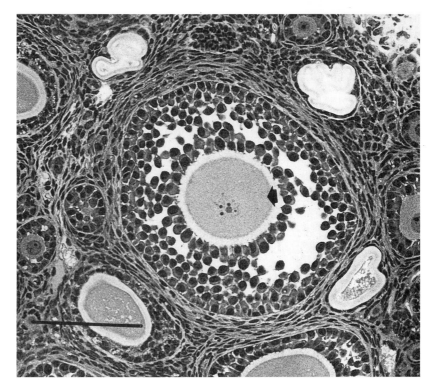

**Fig. 4.3.** Photomicrograph of a small antral follicle in the ovary of a mouse homozygous for the recessive gene hypogonadal which has undetectable levels of circulating gonadotrophins. Follicles do not develop beyond this stage. Note that the oocyte (arrow) is nearly fully grown despite gonadotrophin deficiency. Bar indicates 100 μm.

## Gap junctional communication and metabolic cooperativity

Gap junctions are membrane specializations that allow metabolic cooperativity between cells by permitting the transfer of low molecular weight metabolites from one cell to another. Homologous gap junctions couple cells of the same type while heterologous gap junctions couple cells of different types. Thus granulosa cells communicate with each other via homologous gap junctions (Albertini & Anderson, 1974) and granulosa cells communicate with the oocyte via heterologous gap junctions (Anderson & Albertini, 1976; Gilula *et al.*, 1978). Heterologous gap junctions mediate the transfer of low molecular weight signals by which one cell type regulates functions specific to the other (Lawrence *et al.*, 1978). Since gap junctions couple oocytes and their companion granulosa cells, and cumulus cells are coupled to mural granulosa cells, all the granulosa cells, cumulus and mural, and the oocyte constitute a functional syncytium mediated by gap junctions. The role of gap junctions in the regulation of oocyte development will be discussed below.

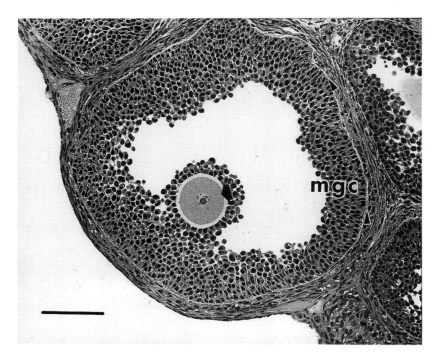

**Fig. 4.4.** Photomicrograph of a well developed antral follicle in a normal mouse. The granulosa cells that are tightly packed around the germinal vesicle-stage oocyte (arrow) are called cumulus cells while the granulosa cells that line the follicle wall are mural granulosa cells (mgc). The mural granulosa cells constitute a pseudostratified epithelium in contact with the basal lamina (arrowheads). Bar indicates 100 μm.

## Mucification of the cumulus oophorus

The cumulus oophorus undergoes a dramatic change while the oocyte is undergoing meiotic maturation. Before the preovulatory surge of gonadotrophins, the cumulus cells are tightly packed around the oocyte (Figs 4.4 and 4.5a). After the surge, the cumulus cells become dispersed in a mucus-like matrix (Fig. 4.5c) as a result of the synthesis and secretion of the non-sulphated glycosaminoglycan, hyaluronic acid. This process is often referred to as cumulus expansion or mucification and is completed by the time of ovulation. During cumulus expansion, the direct cytoplasmic communication between the cumulus cells and the maturing oocyte is disrupted. The purpose of cumulus expansion is not clearly understood, but it is possible that it facilitates the transfer of the egg into the oviduct and/or allows easier access of the sperm to the egg. The cumulus oophorus is dispersed by the sperm in the oviduct.

Cumulus expansion can also be stimulated in culture by follicle-stimulating hormone (FSH) after isolation of oocyte−cumulus cell complexes from the follicles (Figs 4.5 and 4.5d; Dekel & Kraicer, 1978; Eppig, 1979a,b; Hillensjo & Channing, 1980; Salustri & Siracusa, 1983;

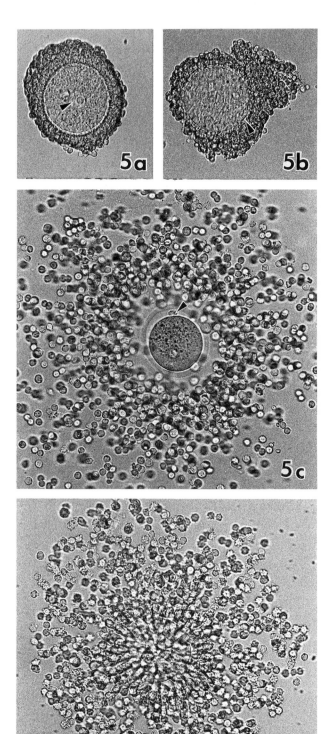

**Fig. 4.5.** Photomicrographs of oocytes and eggs isolated from mice. Bar indicates 50 μm. (a) A freshly isolated oocyte–cumulus cell complex. Note tightly packed cumulus cells and intact germinal vesicle (arrowhead). (b) An egg derived from an oocyte isolated at the germinal vesicle stage (as in (a)) and cultured in medium without gonadotrophins. The oocyte underwent germinal vesicle breakdown spontaneously, but the cumulus cells remain tightly packed around the oocyte. The arrowhead indicates the polar body. (c) An ovulated egg recovered from the oviduct. Note the dispersion of the cumulus cells which are embedded in a matrix of hyaluronic acid. The arrowhead indicates the polar body. (d) An egg derived from an oocyte isolated at the germinal vesicle stage (as in (a)) and cultured in medium containing FSH. The cumulus has dispersed similarly to that shown in the ovulated egg in (c).

Ball *et al.*, 1985). The action of FSH is probably mediated by cyclic adenosine monophosphate (cAMP) because membrane permeable analogues of cAMP induce cumulus expansion and FSH increases the cAMP levels in cumulus cells. Luteinizing hormone (LH) is generally less effective than FSH presumably because of fewer receptors for LH than FSH on the cumulus cells. LH, however, will stimulate cumulus expansion in intact follicles (Eppig, 1980). Thus cumulus expansion *in vivo* may be stimulated by LH via an indirect mechanism. Perhaps LH stimulates the elevation of cAMP in the mural granulosa cells, which have abundant LH receptors and the cAMP is passed to the cumulus cells through the gap junctions or LH could stimulate the production of some other substance by the mural granulosa cells that induces cumulus expansion. Alternatively, it is possible that LH promotes the loss of some factor(s) that prevents the cumulus cells from responding to FSH already present in the follicle. It is not clear why the cumulus oophorus does not respond to FSH present in the follicle before the LH surge. Perhaps FSH is not present in sufficient concentration in the follicle to induce cumulus expansion or there are factors that prevent the cumulus cells from responding to FSH.

Epidermal growth factor (EGF) also stimulates the expansion of isolated cumuli oophori (Downs, 1989). This response of the cumulus cells to EGF appears to be specific since the response to EGF was much greater than to any of the other growth factors tested. Actually, cumulus expansion in response to EGF was greater than that to FSH, although FSH stimulated the generation of much higher cAMP levels in cumulus cells than EGF did (Downs *et al.*, 1988). The physiological significance of these observations has yet to be resolved.

## Oocyte growth and the acquisition of competence to resume the first meiotic division

### Oocyte growth

During their growth phase, oocytes increase in size from *c.* 20 to *c.* 80 μm, or more, depending on the species. Oocyte growth is dependent upon gap junctional coupling to granulosa cells (Eppig, 1977, 1979a; Brower & Schultz, 1982); the rate of oocyte growth is directly related to the number of granulosa cells attached to the oocyte (Herlands & Schultz, 1984). The granulosa cells in effect increase the surface area of the oocyte and thereby decrease the surface to volume ratio of the oocyte. This increases the rate at which small molecules having nutritional or regulatory functions enter the oocyte. Moreover, the oocyte is apparently deficient in the transport systems required for the entry of some molecules. For example, although adenosine is readily taken up by granulosa cell-free oocytes, uridine is not (Heller & Schultz, 1980). Although oocytes establish gap junctional communication with other types of cells in culture, only granulosa cells will promote oocyte growth (Buccione *et al.*, 1987). Granulosa cells, moreover, affect both the pattern of protein synthesis and phosphorylation in growing oocytes (Colonna *et al.*, 1989). These changes do not occur when the oocytes are coupled to other cell types in culture. While it is not clear what specific aspects of oocyte development are related to the alterations in protein phosphorylation, it is clear that the granulosa cells have qualitative effects on growing oocytes and are not simply a conduit for nutritional molecules.

## Acquisition of competence to complete the first meiotic division

When fully grown oocytes are isolated from antral follicles and cultured, they spontaneously resume the first meiotic division (Fig. 4.5b; Pincus & Enzmann, 1935; Pincus & Saunders, 1939; Edwards, 1965). In contrast, growing oocytes isolated from preantral follicles do not resume meiosis. The first morphological indication that oocytes have resumed meiosis is the dissolution of the oocyte nucleus, or germinal vesicle. This process of dissolution is called germinal vesicle breakdown (GVB). Thus as the oocyte nears completion of its growth phase, it becomes competent to undergo GVB (Szybek 1972; Sorenson & Wassarman, 1976). The molecular basis for the acquisition of competence to undergo GVB is not known but maturation-related changes in protein phosphorylation in GVB-competent oocytes do not occur in incompetent oocytes (Bornslaeger *et al.*, 1988). It is not yet clear whether these specific changes in protein phosphorylation are causally related to GVB.

Both oocyte growth and acquisition of GVB-competence occur *in vitro* (Eppig, 1977). Oocyte–granulosa cell complexes from preantral follicles, wherein the oocyte is GVB-incompetent, can be cultured in the absence of gonadotrophins and most of the oocytes acquire GVB-competence as they near completion of growth. This result suggests that neither oocyte growth nor the acquisition of GVB-competence require gonadotrophic stimulation. In these experiments, however, the oocytes have completed about half of their growth phase *in vivo* and could have received sufficient exposure to gonadotrophin to promote the acquisition of GVB-competence before being placed in culture. Further evidence for oocyte growth and acquisition of GVB-competence being independent from gonadotrophic stimulation comes from studies using animals genetically deficient in circulating gonadotrophins. Mice homozygous for the mutation hypogonadal (*hpg/hpg*) do not have detectable levels of circulating gonadotrophins because of a defect in the production of gonadotrophin-releasing hormone (GnRH). The oocytes in these mutant mice, therefore, have not been exposed to detectable levels of gonadotrophins throughout postnatal life. Nevertheless, oocytes grow and *c.* 80% of them acquire competence to undergo GVB in the hypogonadal mice. Treatment of hypogonadal mice with gonadotrophin promotes the acquisition of competence to undergo GVB by virtually all of the oocytes (Schroeder & Eppig, 1989). Similar results have been reported using hypophysectomized immature rats. Hypophysectomy decreases the proportion of GVB-competent oocytes, but treatment with gonadotrophin or oestrogen normalizes this proportion (Bar-Ami *et al.*, 1983). These results indicate that while gonadotrophins are not essential for the acquisition of GVB-competence by oocytes, they have nevertheless a beneficial effect on this process. This effect is probably not exerted directly on the oocyte, since oocytes do not have gonadotrophin receptors, but is mediated by granulosa cells, possibly via an oestrogen-dependent process. Since oestrogen is thought to play an important role in granulosa cell development and function, and since normal development and function of granulosa cells is probably important for normal oocyte development, it is likely that oestrogen acts on oocyte development by promoting critical functions of granulosa cells (see Chapter 3).

Although oocyte growth depends upon gap junction-mediated coupling of the oocyte with its companion granulosa cells, and although oocytes normally acquire competence to undergo GVB as they near completion of their growth, acquisition of competence to undergo GVB is independent of oocyte growth. This was demonstrated by maintaining mid-growth phase oocytes denuded of granulosa cells on a monolayer of fibroblasts (Canipari *et al.*, 1984). The fibroblasts maintained oocyte viability but did not sustain oocyte growth. Nevertheless, these oocytes acquired competence to undergo GVB at the same time as age-matched oocytes *in vivo*. The developmental programme for the acquisition of GVB-competence, therefore, is sustained within the oocytes, is time-dependent, but independent of continued gap junctional associations with granulosa cells.

## Follicular components which participate in the maintenance of meiotic arrest

Oocytes that have acquired competence to undergo GVB are thought to be maintained in meiotic arrest by somatic cells within the follicle because the oocytes undergo spontaneous GVB when isolated from the follicle and cultured. Several different substances have been proposed to participate in the maintenance of meiotic arrest within the follicle. Since the oocyte-cumulus cell complex is bathed by follicular fluid, and because this fluid was reported to have the capacity to inhibit spontaneous maturation, substances present in follicular fluid have been subjected to extensive experimental scrutiny. There is evidence from work on oocyte maturation in amphibians that a decline in intracellular levels of cAMP, a molecule well studied in its role as a second-messenger for regulatory signals, is important in the initiation of GVB in these species. Subsequent studies on the potential role of cAMP in oocyte maturation in mammals also suggest that one way factors which maintain meiotic arrest could function is by maintaining elevated levels of cAMP in the oocyte.

## cAMP: evidence for participation in the maintenance of meiotic arrest and mechanism of action

Oocytes isolated from several mammalian species are reversibly prevented from undergoing spontaneous maturation by membrane permeable analogues of cAMP, such as dibutyrl cAMP, and by cAMP-phosphodiesterase inhibitors, such as 3-isobutyl-1-methyl xanthine (IBMX), that prevent hydrolysis of cAMP (Cho et al., 1974; Wassarman et al., 1976; Magnusson & Hillensjo, 1977; Dekel & Beers, 1978, 1980). Microinjection of oocytes with an inhibitor of the catalytic subunit of cAMP-dependent protein kinase A while the oocytes were incubated in dibutyryl cAMP or IBMX induces GVB, showing that these meiosis-arresting factors function via a typical cAMP-dependent protein phosphorylation mechanism (Fig. 4.6; Bornslaeger et al., 1986). Moreover, a decline in cAMP levels is associated with GVB in mouse and rat oocytes (Schultz et al., 1983; Racowsky, 1984). While these experiments and others indicate that cAMP within the oocyte participates in the maintenance of meiotic arrest in several mammalian species, it has been reported that sheep oocytes are refractory to cAMP-elevating agents (Crosby et al., 1985). Furthermore, a reduction in cAMP levels in sheep, hamster, and pig oocytes has not been detected (Moor & Heslop, 1981; Racowsky, 1985a,b; Hubbard, 1986). Thus caution should be used in assuming that the participation of a cAMP-dependent process in the maintenance of meiotic arrest is generally applicable to all mammalian species. Other intracellular systems may participate to varying extents depending on the species. One other pathway that warrants further investigation is the protein kinase C-dependent pathway since phorbol esters, activators of protein kinase C, suppress spontaneous GVB in some species (Urner & Schorderet-Slatkine, 1984; Bornslaeger et al., 1986).

Assuming that cAMP in the oocyte participates to some extent in the maintenance of meiotic arrest, it is important to determine how meiosis-arresting levels of cAMP are achieved within the oocyte. Some cAMP may be produced within the oocyte itself. This idea is supported by the cytochemical observation that adenylyl cyclase is in fact present in bovine oocytes (Kuyt et al., 1988) and that forskolin, an activator of the catalytic subunit of adenylyl cyclase, elevates cAMP levels and transiently maintains meiotic arrest in cumulus cell-free oocytes in vitro (Urner et al., 1983; Ekholm et al., 1984; Bornslaeger & Schultz, 1985a; Racowsky, 1985a,b). It is not clear, however, why cholera toxin, a

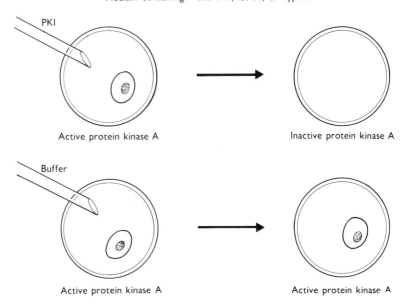

Medium containing:  dbcAMP, IBMX, or hypoxanthine

PKI

Active protein kinase A

Inactive protein kinase A

Buffer

Active protein kinase A

Active protein kinase A

**Fig. 4.6.** Diagram illustrating the relationship between maintenance of meiotic arrest, cAMP, hypoxanthine, and protein kinase A. Analogues of cAMP, such as dibutyryl cyclic (dbc)AMP, and cAMP-phosphodiesterase inhibitors, such as IBMX, maintain meiotic arrest unless microinjected with an inhibitor (PKI) of the catalytic subunit of cAMP-dependent protein kinase (protein kinase A). This shows that the action of dibutyryl cAMP and IBMX is mediated by protein kinase A. Similarly, microinjection of PKI into oocytes maintained in meiotic arrest by hypoxanthine, a purine found in preparations of pig and mouse follicular fluid, also induces germinal vesicle breakdown indicating that the action of hypoxanthine is mediated, at least in part, by protein kinase A and, therefore, by cAMP.

potent activator of adenylyl cyclase in many cell types, fails to affect cAMP levels or meiotic arrest in cumulus cell-free oocytes. Most likely there is an atypical regulatory subunit for oocyte adenylyl cyclase. This subunit is the site of action for cholera toxin via a ribosylation mechanism. It is also not clear why the action of forskolin on cumulus cell-free oocytes in culture is transient. This observation suggests that even if the oocyte is able to make some cAMP, it is not sufficient for maintaining meiotic arrest. It must be said, however, that the oocytes in these experiments are isolated from other ovarian factors that could augment the action of cAMP generated by oocyte adenylyl cyclase. One example of such a factor is the purine hypoxanthine, a naturally occurring phosphodiesterase inhibitor that has been found in preparations of ovarian follicular fluid. It is also important to ask how oocyte adenylyl cyclase could be stimulated *in vivo* since forskolin is not a normal component of ovarian follicles. Follicular purines may also participate in this aspect of maintaining meiosis-arresting levels of cAMP within the oocyte. The potential role of such purines will be discussed further in the next section.

Oocyte cAMP may also originate in mural and/or cumulus–granulosa cells and enter the oocyte via the heterologous gap junctions that couple cumulus cells with the oocyte. Small molecules with approximately the same molecular weight as cAMP, such as uridine and its phosphorylated derivatives, equilibrate freely between cumulus cell and oocyte compartments of the oocyte–cumulus cell complex, therefore there is no obvious physical reason why cAMP itself could not move between these compartments. Elevation of cAMP in cumulus cells results in elevation of cAMP in the oocyte under certain experimental conditions (Racowsky, 1984, 1985a,b; Bornslaeger & Schultz, 1985b) suggesting that the cAMP produced in the cumulus cells may have moved into the oocyte. This cAMP, however, did not equilibrate between the two cell types as do uridine and its derivatives. Moreover, the cAMP levels generated in the cumulus cells in these experiments far exceed those that occur in cumulus cells *in situ*. There is an alternative explanation for the observed increase in oocyte cAMP in these experiments. The cumulus cells may have been stimulated to produce some factor that promoted cAMP production within the oocyte. Such a factor may stimulate oocyte adenylyl cyclase or be a substrate for adenylyl cyclase, that is adenosine triphosphate (ATP). To recapitulate, while there is no obvious physical reason why cAMP could not move from cumulus cells to oocytes, and while there is some evidence that it does, such movement has not been unequivocally demonstrated.

## Purines: evidence for participation in the maintenance of meiotic arrest

Preparations of pig follicular fluid prevented the spontaneous maturation of oocytes isolated not only from pigs, but also from rats and mice (Tsafriri *et al.*, 1982; Downs & Eppig, 1984). It was proposed that the meiosis-arresting component of the pig follicular fluid was a low molecular weight peptide which was referred to as oocyte maturation inhibitor (OMI) (Tsafriri *et al.*, 1982). OMI, however, has not been purified to homogeneity. Moreover, it was found that the principal component of pig follicular fluid that maintained isolated mouse oocytes in meiotic arrest was not a peptide but rather the purine hypoxanthine (Downs *et al.*, 1985). Subsequently, hypoxanthine was also found in preparations of mouse follicular fluid as was another purine adenosine (Eppig *et al.*, 1985). These two purines act synergistically to maintain meiotic arrest in isolated mouse oocytes.

The concentrations of hypoxanthine detected in the preparations of pig and mouse follicular fluid were in the millimolar range; much higher than is normally measured in biological fluids. It is possible that these concentrations are actually higher than those in follicular fluid *in situ* and that conditions of isolation generated the higher concentrations measured. Nevertheless, hypoxia promotes the generation of hypoxanthine and the avascular structure of the follicle centripital to the basal lamina may foster hypoxia within the follicle and result in elevated hypoxanthine concentrations in follicular fluid.

Other evidence points to a role for purines in the maintenance of meiotic arrest *in vivo*; the evidence, however, points most convincingly in the direction of guanyl compounds. Injecting mice with inhibitors of inosine monophosphate (IMP) dehydrogenase (Fig. 4.7), which catalyses the conversion of IMP to guanosine monophosphate (GMP) via xanthyl monophosphate (XMP), induces maturation in almost all of the meiotically competent oocytes when injected 24 h after priming the animals with pregnant mares' serum gonadotrophin (Downs & Eppig, 1987). Interestingly, guanosine was the most active purine tested for maintaining meiotic arrest in mouse oocytes *in vitro* even though this purine was not found in mouse follicular fluid (Downs *et al.*, 1985; Eppig *et al.*, 1985). Inhibitors of IMP dehydrogenase also induced maturation in isolated cumulus cell-enclosed oocytes cultured in medium containing hypoxanthine suggesting that the presence of hypoxanthine in the medium promotes the production of the guanyl compounds that mediate the meiosis-arresting action of hypoxanthine (Downs *et al.*, 1986). It is not known whether hypoxanthine itself is metabolized to GMP via the hypoxanthine−guanosine phosphoribosyl transferase salvage pathway or whether hypoxanthine promotes GMP production via *de novo* purine synthesis (Fig. 4.7). Nevertheless, the observation that IMP dehydrogenase inhibitors induce maturation both *in vivo* and *in vitro* when meiotic arrest was maintained by hypoxanthine, suggests a common pathway for maintaining meiotic arrest under both conditions.

Hypoxanthine appears to act, at least in part, by maintaining a meiosis-arresting level of cAMP within the oocyte. This was concluded

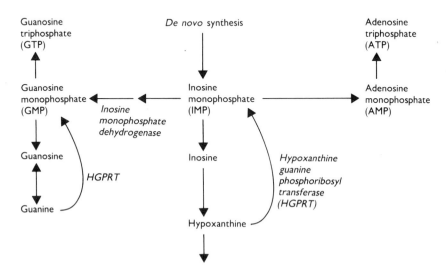

**Fig. 4.7.** Outline of the purine metabolic pathway.

because microinjection of an inhibitor of protein kinase A induced maturation of oocytes incubated in medium containing hypoxanthine (Fig. 4.6; Downs et al., 1989). This purine, like other xanthines, is an inhibitor of cAMP-phosphodiesterase (Downs et al., 1989). One way, therefore, that hypoxanthine could maintain meiosis-arresting levels of cAMP within oocytes is by preventing cAMP hydrolysis. It is also possible, however, that hypoxanthine affects cAMP levels by stimulating adenylyl cyclase activity via G proteins (regulatory proteins that bind GTP). As described above, hypoxanthine appears to act to some extent by promoting GMP production via IMP dehydrogenase activity. GMP could then be phosphorylated to GTP and subsequently bind to G proteins. Hypoxanthine or G proteins may also participate in the maintenance of meiotic arrest according to some other pathways.

As mentioned above, both hypoxanthine and adenosine are present in mouse follicular fluid and adenosine augments the meiosis-arresting action of hypoxanthine in vitro (Eppig et al., 1985). The effect of adenosine on oocyte maturation is very similar to that of forskolin; both transiently delay the time of GVB in both cumulus cell-enclosed and denuded oocytes (Urner et al., 1983; Ekholm et al., 1984; Bornslaeger et al., 1985a; Eppig et al., 1985; Salustri et al., 1988). The augmentation by adenosine of the meiosis-arresting action of hypoxanthine is stable, not transient (Eppig et al., 1985). Hypoxanthine and adenosine together raise the cAMP content of cumulus cell-enclosed oocytes higher than either of these purines alone (Downs et al., 1989). Although adenosine can be metabolized to ATP and, therefore, become a substrate for adenylyl cyclase, this metabolism is not necessarily the mechanism by which adenosine augments the meiosis-arresting action of hypoxanthine; poorly metabolized analogues of adenosine function the same as adenosine itself (Eppig et al., 1985). Similarly, these analogues of adenosine mimic the action of adenosine in potentiating the delay in the time of GVB in cumulus cell-denuded oocytes produced by forskolin (Salustri et al., 1988). Taken together these studies suggest that adenosine could function to maintain meiotic arrest physiologically in an environment containing hypoxanthine by stimulating adenylyl cyclase in oocytes via an adenosine receptor-mediated mechanism.

## Follicular regulation of gonadotrophin-induced oocyte maturation

Oocyte maturation in vivo is induced in ovarian follicles by the preovulatory surge of gonadotrophin. This induction is certainly indirect since oocytes do not have gonadotrophin receptors. An important question is whether oocyte maturation is stimulated by depriving the oocyte of meiosis-arresting factors or by a positive maturation-inducing signal produced by somatic cells in response to the preovulatory surge of gonadotrophin that overrides the blocking effect of meiosis-arresting substances, or both.

Depriving the oocyte of meiosis-arresting factors could occur in two ways which are not mutually exclusive. First, concentrations of the arresting factor in the follicle could be reduced by degradation, secretion, or both. The concentrations of cAMP, hypoxanthine, or adenosine do not decrease in the follicle as a result of gonadotrophic stimulation (Schultz et al., 1983; Eppig et al., 1985). Second, the pathway by which the factor is delivered to the oocyte could be dismantled or blocked. This pathway could be the gap junctions that couple granulosa cells, cumulus cells and the oocyte. There is no evidence for a significant decrease in gap junctional communication between the cumulus cells and the oocyte before the oocytes become committed to undergo GVB after gonadotrophic stimulation in vivo or in intact follicles in vitro (Moor et al., 1981; Eppig, 1982; Salustri & Siracusa, 1983; Eppig & Downs, 1988). There is, however, a decrease in the gap junctional area between cumulus cells and between mural granulosa cells induced by administration of gonadotrophins (Larsen et al., 1987). The junctions between cumulus cells appear to be lost more rapidly than those between mural granulosa cells. These observations led to the hypothesis that oocyte maturation could be induced by disrupting the passage of meiosis-arresting substances between the mural granulosa cells and the cumulus cells, thus depriving the oocyte−cumulus cell complex of these substances and inducing GVB. As described above, the meiosis-arresting substance most commonly thought to be transferred from the granulosa cells to the oocyte for maintaining meiotic arrest is cAMP. The concentration of cAMP in the intact oocyte−cumulus cell complex, however, does not decrease before the oocytes become committed to undergo GVB (Eppig & Downs, 1988). If disruption of communication between the granulosa cells and the oocyte−cumulus cell complex is the mechanism for depriving the oocyte of meiosis-arresting substances, the substance whose transfer is disrupted cannot be cAMP. This experiment, though, does not eliminate the possibility that the transfer of substances involved in cAMP generation within the oocyte−cumulus cell complex is reduced by loss of gap junctions or that the transfer of meiosis-arresting substances not related to cAMP is reduced.

Whether or not depriving the oocyte of maturation-arresting substances occurs as a result of the maturation-inducing surge of gonadotrophin, it is also possible that gonadotrophins stimulate the production of a positive maturation-inducing stimulus in mammals. Such a positive stimulus has been demonstrated in other species. Isolated cumulus cell-enclosed mouse oocytes maintained in meiotic arrest with hypoxanthine, analogues of cAMP, or synthetic phosphodiesterase inhibitors mature in response to FSH (Downs et al., 1988). FSH is, therefore, able to overcome the meiosis-arresting action of these substances. In these experiments, FSH was used to induce maturation in vitro because isolated cumuli oophori have few LH receptors. In conclusion, although cAMP is probably involved in the maintenance of meiotic arrest, and although a decrease in oocyte cAMP levels may be sufficient to induce oocyte maturation *in vitro* and may in fact occur in some species as a part of the maturation process *in vivo*, a decrease in oocyte cAMP may not actually be necessary because of the production of a maturation-inducing signal by granulosa cells in response to gonadotrophin. The nature of this signal is not known.

## Maturation promoting factor (MPF)

In the 1970s, it was shown that the positive signals from follicle cells that induced oocyte maturation in starfish and amphibians resulted in the generation of a GVB-inducing activity in the oocyte which, upon transfer to another oocyte, induced GVB in the recipient oocyte without prior stimulation by the signal originating in the follicle cells (Reynout & Smith, 1974; Kishimoto & Kanatani, 1976). This activity produced in the oocyte became known as 'maturation promoting factor', or MPF. MPF is present in mammalian oocytes and somatic cells as well as the oocytes from starfish and amphibians (Kishimoto *et al.*, 1982; Sorenson *et al.*, 1985). Since MPF appears to be ubiquitous in promoting the transition from G2 to metaphase of the cell cycle in both somatic and germ cells, it is now often referred to as 'M-phase promoting factor'.

MPF was demonstrated in mammalian oocytes by microinjecting cytoplasm from maturing mouse oocytes into amphibian or starfish oocytes and observing GVB in the recipient oocytes (Sorenson *et al.*, 1985; Hashimoto & Kishimoto, 1988). Cytoplasm from mouse oocytes arrested in the GV stage did not induce GVB in the recipient oocytes indicating that active MPF is not present in mouse oocytes that have not initiated the maturation process. Furthermore, fusion of maturing mouse oocytes with oocytes arrested in the GV stage with dibutyryl cAMP induced maturation in the arrested oocytes which indicates that a factor(s) in maturing oocytes can bypass the meiosis-arresting pathways sustained by dibutyryl cAMP (Clarke & Masui, 1985). Fusion of maturing mouse oocytes with small growing mouse oocytes induced maturation in these oocytes that had been incompetent of undergoing maturation before fusion (Balakier, 1978), suggesting that the inability of these oocytes to resume maturation may be due to a deficiency of MPF. Fusion of these small oocytes with GV-stage competent oocytes, however, prevented the initiation of maturation in these competent oocytes which should have readily undergone spontaneous maturation (Fulka, 1985), indicating that the small oocytes may contain a substance(s) that prevents the initiation of the processes that lead to activation of MPF, but once MPF is activated, as in maturing oocytes, the initiation-preventing substance has no action.

Inhibitors of protein synthesis, cycloheximide or puromycin, do not prevent GVB in mouse oocytes, but they do prevent the completion of maturation; the oocytes do not proceed past metaphase with bivalent chromosomes, and spindle formation does not occur (Wassarman et al., 1976; Hashimoto & Kishimoto, 1988). Therefore, de novo protein synthesis is not required for the initiation of maturation, GVB, and chromosome condensation in mouse oocytes. Since active MPF is produced in the presence of cycloheximide, it can be concluded that this initial production of the active MPF required for these processes does not require protein synthesis. MPF activity, however, declines in the continued presence of cycloheximide indicating that the maintenance of elevated levels of MPF activity requires protein synthesis. Production of active MPF is restored after removal of cycloheximide; spindle assembly and polar body production also occur upon restoration of protein synthesis (Hashimoto & Kishimoto, 1988). Thus the correlation of MPF activity with spindle assembly and polar body formation suggests a role for MPF in initiating these processes at metaphase I. MPF activity normally declines during anaphase I but increases again after polar body formation so that activity is high in metaphase II ova (Hashimoto & Kishimoto, 1988).

Changes in patterns of protein phosphorylation during oocyte maturation have suggested that the regulation of MPF activity could be the result of phosphorylation and that MPF itself has kinase activity that is essential for its functions. Blocking protein phosphorylation in mouse oocytes prevents GVB (Rime et al., 1989). To aid in assessing the properties and function of MPF, a cell-free system has been developed using extracts from frog eggs (Cyert & Kirschner, 1988; Lohka et al., 1988). Using the cell-free system, a pre-MPF has been identified that becomes activated independently of MPF itself. Pre-MPF is probably activated by phosphorylation which converts it to MPF. There also appears to be an inhibitor of the conversion of pre-MPF to MPF which itself is inactivated by a phosphatase (Cyert & Kirschner, 1988). The cell-free system for assaying MPF activity has facilitated the production of a highly purified preparation of MPF from frog oocytes. The active fraction contains two subunits with molecular masses of c. 45 and 32 kDa and has kinase activity that includes the 45 kDa subunit itself as a substrate (Lohka et al., 1988).

The product of the $cdc2^+$ gene identified in the fission yeast Schizosaccharomyces pombe regulates the initiation of mitosis. This protein is a kinase with a molecular weight estimated to be 34 kDa. Antibodies to S. pombe p34[cdc2] recognize the frog 32 kDa MPF subunit. This result indicates that the small subunit of frog MPF is the homologue of S. pombe p34[cdc2] (Gautier et al., 1988). Further support for this idea is provided by experiments showing that the 13 kDa product of the yeast suc1 gene, which binds to S. pombe p34[cdc2], binds to and inhibits frog MPF in cell-free extracts (Dunphy et al., 1988). These studies demonstrate that there are common components essential for entry into metaphase in both mitosis of somatic cells and meiosis of germ cells. It seems likely that there are other factors in common that regulate these processes. There is recent evidence that the protein encoded by the proto-oncogene c-*mos* is a cytostatic factor responsible for the maintenance of meiotic arrest in vertebrate eggs. The protein appears to maintain meiotic arrest by stabilizing MPF activity (Sagata *et al.*, 1989) and is apparently destroyed upon fertilization, allowing the eggs to enter anaphase (Watanabe *et al.*, 1989). Studies on the expression and function of c-*mos* in mouse oocytes are described below.

## Gene expression during oogenesis

RNA synthesis occurs during the growth of mouse oocytes, the only mammalian species in which gene expression during oogenesis has been studied in detail. Most of the RNA is stable so that the RNA accumulates during oocyte growth. These results have been reviewed in detail by Bachvarova (1985). The total RNA content of mouse oocytes decreases by *c.* 20% during oocyte maturation. Polyadenylated mRNA comprises *c.* 19% of the RNA content of fully grown immature oocytes and this is reduced to *c.* 10% in eggs suggesting an overall loss of polyadenylated mRNA of *c.* 9%. When the fate of a specific mRNA, that coding for actin, was assessed during oocyte maturation, it was found that the actin mRNA content does not decrease during oocyte maturation, but it is substantially deadenylated. This deadenylation coincides with a decrease in actin synthesis. Thus the decrease in actin synthesis appears to be the result of deadenylation of the actin mRNA rather than the degradation of this mRNA (Bachvarova *et al.*, 1985).

## Expression of genes encoding zona pellucida proteins

The zona pellucida is the acellular coat that encloses the oocyte and which, in the mouse, is composed of three sulphated glycoproteins synthesized by the oocyte: Zp1, Zp2 and Zp3 (Bleil & Wassarman, 1980; Shimizu *et al.*, 1983). The function of the zona pellucida is to provide sites for the binding sperm, promote the acrosome reaction and, after the penetration of a single sperm into the egg, prevent the penetration of additional sperm and thus prevent polyspermy. The oocyte begins to synthesize zona pellucida proteins shortly after it enters the growth phase and synthesis continues, albeit at reduced levels, in fully grown GV-stage oocytes (Fig. 4.8).

cDNA clones coding for Zp3 have been isolated and characterized and used as probes for assessing the developmental regulation of *Zp3* gene expression (Ringuette *et al.*, 1986; Philpott *et al.*, 1987). *Zp3* mRNA accounts for 0.1−0.2% of the total polyadenylated mRNA present

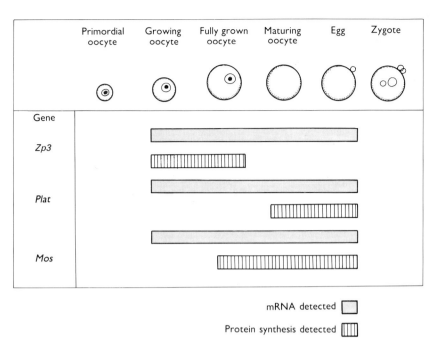

**Fig. 4.8.** Development-dependent expression of the *Zp3*, tPA (*Plat*) and c-*mos* (*Mos*) genes by mouse oocytes.

in growing oocytes. It is not found in primordial oocytes, but is detected shortly after the oocytes enter the growth phase. As the oocytes complete their growth and undergo maturation, there is a striking loss in the amount of *Zp3* mRNA (Fig. 4.8). This mRNA has not been detected in other tissues and, therefore, appears to be specific to the oocyte. Interestingly, the *Zp3* cDNA probe cross-hybridizes with DNA from several other species including human, indicating significant homology in this gene between species.

### Expression of the gene encoding tissue-type plasminogen activator (tPA) in mouse oocytes

tPA is a serine protease that is thought to be important in cell migration and tissue remodelling mechanisms, including ovulation (see Chapter 5). Surprisingly, tPA activity has been found in maturing oocytes (Huarte *et al.*, 1985). tPA-mediated zones of proteolysis were found to surround the maturing oocytes indicating that tPA is secreted by the oocyte, although its function is not known. In mouse oocytes, tPA activity is not detected in GV-stage oocytes, but is detected after 4 h in cultured mouse oocytes and activity increases rapidly to a peak after *c.* 10 h of culture. No activity was found in oocytes maintained in meiotic arrest with dibutyryl cAMP, indicating that oocyte maturation and not simply oocyte culture is required for the production of active tPA. In addition, no tPA activity was detected in fertilized eggs. The production of active tPA in oocytes is prevented by cycloheximide, an inhibitor of protein synthesis, but not by actinomycin D or α-amanitin, inhibitors of RNA synthesis, indicating that tPA mRNA is present in immature oocytes and that the initiation of oocyte maturation is required to promote translation of this mRNA. Northern blot analysis of RNA prepared from oocytes at various stages of development has shown that tPA mRNA is produced in a stable untranslated form in growing oocytes so that fully grown immature oocytes contain *c.* 10 000 copies of this mRNA (Huarte *et al.*, 1987). No tPA mRNA was detected in fertilized eggs (Fig. 4.8). The size of tPA mRNA increases during oocyte maturation, beginning before tPA activity is detected, and this increase in mRNA size is attributable to increased polyadenylation (Strickland *et al.*, 1988).

## Expression and function of the proto-oncogene c-*mos* in mouse oocytes

c-*mos* is the cellular homologue of v-*mos*, the transforming gene of Molony sarcoma virus. c-*mos* mRNA is found in increasing numbers in growing oocytes and appears stable in fully grown GV-stage oocyte but the number of transcripts decreases by *c.* 50% during oocyte maturation (Keshet *et al.*, 1988; Mutter *et al.*, 1988). Synthesis of p39$^{mos}$, the protein encoded by c-*mos*, occurs in fully grown GV-stage oocytes, maturing oocytes and metaphase II oocytes, but not in primordial or growing oocytes incompetent of undergoing oocyte maturation or in zygotes (Paules *et al.*, 1989) (Fig. 4.8). Microinjection of oligodeoxyribonucleotides (20-mer) antisense to c-*mos* transcripts into cumulus cell-enclosed GV-stage oocytes does not prevent GVB, but prevents polar body formation. Oocytes appeared to be arrested at or about metaphase I (Paules *et al.*, 1989). It therefore appears that p39$^{mos}$ functions during oocyte maturation and is apparently required for progress past metaphase I.

## Termination of gene expression during oogenesis

As illustrated in Fig. 4.8, transcripts of the genes coding for Zp3, tPA, and p39$^{mos}$ are detectable at the same stages of mouse oocyte development. Initiation of transcription of these genes apparently occurs at about the time the oocytes enter into the growth phase and some transcripts persist until fertilization. Initiation of synthesis of the proteins, however, appears differentially regulated. Zp3 synthesis occurs in growing oocytes while synthesis of tPA and p39$^{mos}$ apparently does not. p39$^{mos}$ is synthesized in GV-stage oocytes, but tPA is not. The molecular basis of the differential times of initiation of protein synthesis is not known but its resolution is critical for understanding mechanisms of oocyte development.

# Implications for reproductive medicine

This chapter began with the observation that the development and function of the female reproductive system is largely dependent upon the presence of oocytes because ovarian follicles do not form without an oocyte. This is in contrast to the situation in the testis where seminiferous tubules form in the absence of germ cells (Handel & Eppig, 1979). The impact of defective oocyte development on reproduction is not well evaluated. It is possible that some cases of unexplained reproductive failure in women result from defective oocyte development. It is well documented, however, that some birth defects such as Down's syndrome involve errors in meiotic chromosome segregation. Knowledge of the mechanisms that govern oocyte development could be put to medical use in the area of fertility control by either encouraging normal oocyte maturation to promote fecundity or by disruption of oocyte development for contraception. Contraception can also be achieved by exploiting a normal product of oocyte development, the zona pellucida; immunization against zona pellucida protein prevents conception (East et al., 1985).

The technology for oocyte development in vitro could have considerable impact on reproductive medicine. The area most likely to benefit from this technology is clinical in vitro fertilization (IVF). Current protocols for IVF involve drug and/or hormonal treatments to promote the maturation of as many oocytes as possible and retrieval of the ova just before ovulation. While evidence indicates that the chance of pregnancy increases with the number of embryos transferred, the drug and/or hormonal treatments are probably detrimental to the developmental capacity of the oocytes and to the development of the uterus (see Chapter 10). Cryopreservation of the embryos can allow the uterus to recover, but certainly does nothing to restore the developmental capacity of the embryos and can lead to ethical and legal problems regarding the fate of frozen embryos not transferred to mothers. Studies with several mammalian species have shown that oocytes undergoing maturation in vitro are competent of fertilization and development to live young (Van Blerkom & McGaughey, 1978; Shalgi et al., 1979; Schroeder & Eppig, 1984; Staigmiller & Moor, 1984; Goto et al., 1988; Sirard et al., 1988). Refinement and application of the technology for development of GV-stage oocytes in vitro could eliminate the need for hormone treatments. Oocytes isolated from mice at all stages of the oestrous cycle without hormone treatments have equivalent developmental capacity after maturation in vitro. Cryopreservation of eggs would eliminate the ethical problems associated with cryopreservation of embryos. Improvements in the protocols for oocyte development in vitro will depend upon a greater understanding of oocyte metabolism and the factors involved in the regulation of the various stages of oogenesis. Of particular importance is the understanding of oocyte—

granulosa cell interactions and the factors which regulate granulosa cell function (see Chapter 3), since the most important of these functions is the support of oocyte development.

## Acknowledgements

I thank Drs Roberto Buccione, Janan T. Eppig, Allen C. Schroeder, and Barbara C. Vanderhyden for their helpful suggestions in the preparation of this chapter. I also acknowledge the Public Health Service for their support of research in my laboratory through grants HD20575, HD21970, and HD23839 from the National Institutes of Health.

## References

Albertini, D.F. & Anderson, E. (1974) The appearance and structure of the intercellular connections during the ontogeny of the rabbit ovarian follicle with special reference to gap junctions. *J. Cell Biol.*, **63**, 234–50.

Anderson, E. & Albertini, D.F. (1976) Gap junctions between the oocyte and companion follicle cells in the mammalian ovary. *J. Cell Biol.*, **71**, 680–6.

Bachvarova, R. (1985a) Gene expression during oogenesis and oocyte development in mammals. In Browder, L.W. (ed.) *Developmental Biology — A Comprehensive Synthesis, Vol. 1 Oogenesis*, pp. 453–524. Plenum Press, New York.

Bachvarova, R., De Leon, V., Johnson, A., Kaplan, G. & Payton, B.V. (1985b) Changes in total RNA, polyadenylated RNA, and actin mRNA during meiotic maturation of mouse oocytes. *Dev. Biol.*, **108**, 325–31.

Balakier, H. (1978) Induction of maturation in small oocytes from sexually immature mice by fusion with meiotic or mitotic cells. *Exp. Cell Res.*, **112**, 137–41.

Ball, G.D., Wieben, E.D. & Byers, A.P. (1985) DNA, RNA, and protein synthesis by porcine oocyte–cumulus cell complexes during expansion. *Biol. Reprod.*, **33**, 739–44.

Bar-Ami, S., Nimrod, A., Brodie, A.M.H. & Tsafriri, A. (1983) Role of FSH and oestradiol-17β in the development of meiotic competence in rat oocytes. *J. Steroid Biochem.*, **19**, 965–71.

Bleil, J.D. & Wassarman, P.W. (1980) Synthesis of zona pellucida proteins by denuded and follicle-enclosed mouse oocytes during culture *in vitro*. *Proc. Natl. Acad. Sci. USA*, **77**, 1029–33.

Bornslaeger, E.A., Mattei, P.M. & Schultz, R.M. (1986) Involvement of cAMP-dependent protein kinase and protein phosphorylation in regulation of mouse oocyte maturation. *Dev. Biol.*, **114**, 453–62.

Bornslaeger, E.A., Mattei, P.M. & Schultz, R.M. (1988) Protein phosphorylation in meiotically competent and incompetent mouse oocytes. *Mol. Reprod. Dev.*, **1**, 19–25.

Bornslaeger, E.A., Poueymirou, W.T., Mattei, P. & Schultz, R.M. (1986) Effects of protein kinase C activators on germinal vesicle breakdown and polar body emission of mouse oocytes. *Exp. Cell Res.*, **165**, 507–17.

Bornslaeger, E.A. & Schultz, R.M. (1985a) Adenylate cyclase activity in zona-free mouse oocytes. *Exp. Cell Res.*, **156**, 277–81.

Bornslaeger, E.A. & Schultz, R.M. (1985b) Regulation of mouse oocyte maturation: effect of elevating cumulus cell cAMP levels. *Biol. Reprod.*, **33**, 698–704.

Brower, P.T. & Schultz, R.M. (1982) Intercellular communication between granulosa cells and mouse oocytes: existence and possible nutritional role during oocyte growth. *Dev. Biol.*, **90**, 144–53.

Buccione, R., Cecconi, S., Tatone, C., Mangia, F. & Colonna, R. (1987) Follicle cell regulation of mammalian oocyte growth. *J. Exp. Zool.*, **242**, 351–4.

Canipari, R., Palombi, F., Riminucci, M. & Mangia, F. (1984) Early programming of maturation competence in mouse oogenesis. *Dev. Biol.*, **102**, 519–24.

Cho, W.K., Stern, S. & Biggers, J.D. (1974) Inhibitory effect of dibutyryl cAMP on mouse oocyte maturation *in vitro*. *J. Exp. Zool.*, **187**, 383–6.

Clarke, H.J. & Masui, Y. (1985) Inhibition by dibutyryl cyclic AMP of the transition to metaphase of mouse oocyte nuclei and its reversal by cell fusion to metaphase oocytes. *Dev. Biol.*, **108**, 32–7.

Colonna, R., Cecconi, S., Tatone, C., Mangia, F. & Buccione, R. (1989) Somatic cell–oocyte interactions in mouse oogenesis: stage-specific regulation of mouse oocyte protein phosphorylation by granulosa cells. *Dev. Biol.*, **133**, 305–8.

Crosby, I.M., Moor, R.M., Heslop, J.P. & Osborn, J.C. (1985) cAMP in ovine oocytes: localization of synthesis and its action on protein synthesis, phosphorylation, and meiosis. *J. Exp. Zool.*, **234**, 307–18.

Cyert, M.S. & Kirschner, M.W. (1988) Regulation of MPF activity *in vitro*. *Cell*, **53**, 185–95.

Dekel, N. & Beers, W.H. (1978) Rat oocyte maturation *in vitro*: relief of cyclic AMP inhibition with gonadotropins. *Proc. Natl. Acad. Sci. USA*, **75**, 4369–73.

Dekel, N. & Beers, W.H. (1980) Development of the rat oocyte *in vitro*: inhibition and induction of maturation in the presence or absence of the cumulus oophorus. *Dev. Biol.*, **75**, 247–54.

Dekel, N. & Kraicer, P.F. (1978) Induction *in vitro* of mucification of rat cumulus oophorus by gonadotropins and adenosine 3′,5′-monophosphate. *Endocrinology*, **102**, 1797–802.

Downs, S.M. (1989) Specificity of epidermal growth factor action on maturation of the murine oocyte and cumulus oophorus *in vitro*. Biol. Reprod. **41**, 371–9.

Downs, S.M., Coleman, D.L. & Eppig, J.J. (1986) Maintenance of murine meiotic arrest: uptake and metabolism of hypoxanthine and adenosine by cumulus cell-enclosed and denuded oocytes. *Dev. Biol.*, **117**, 174–83.

Downs, S.M., Coleman, D.L., Ward-Bailey, P.F. & Eppig, J.J. (1985) Hypoxanthine is the principal inhibitor of murine oocyte maturation in a low molecular weight fraction of porcine follicular fluid. *Proc. Natl. Acad. Sci. USA*, **82**, 454–8.

Downs, S.M., Daniel, S.A.J., Bornslaeger, E.A., Hoppe, P.C. & Eppig, J.J. (1989) Maintenance of meiotic arrest in mouse oocytes by purines: modulation of cAMP levels and cAMP phosphodiesterase activity. *Gamete Res.* **23**, 323–34.

Downs, S.M., Daniel, S.A.J. & Eppig, J.J. (1988) Induction of maturation in cumulus cell-enclosed mouse oocytes by follicle-stimulating hormone and epidermal growth factor: evidence for a positive stimulus of somatic cell origin. *J. Exp. Zool.*, **245**, 86–96.

Downs, S.M. & Eppig, J.J. (1984) Cyclic adenosine monophosphate and ovarian follicular fluid act synergistically to inhibit mouse oocyte maturation. *Endocrinology*, **114**, 418–27.

Downs, S.M. & Eppig, J.J. (1987) Induction of mouse oocyte maturation *in vivo* by perturbants of purine metabolism. *Biol. Reprod.*, **36**, 431–7.

Dunphy, W.G., Brizuela, L., Beach D. & Newport J. (1988) The Xenopus *cdc2* protein is a component of MPF, a cytoplasmic regulator of mitosis. *Cell*, **54**, 423–31.

East, I.J., Gulyas, B.J. & Dean, J. (1985) Monoclonal antibodies to the murine zona pellucida protein with sperm receptor activity: effects on fertilization and early development. *Dev. Biol.*, **109**, 268–73.

Edwards, R.G. (1965) Maturation *in vitro* of mouse, sheep, cow, pig, rhesus monkey and human ovarian oocytes. *Nature*, **208**, 349–51.

Ekholm, C., Hillensjo, T., Magnusson, C. & Rosberg, S. (1984) Stimulation and inhibition of rat oocyte meiosis by forskolin. *Biol. Reprod.*, **30**, 537–43.

Eppig, J.J. (1977) Mouse oocyte development *in vitro* with various culture systems. *Dev. Biol.*, **60**, 371–88.

Eppig, J.J. (1978) Granulosa cell deficient follicles. Occurrence, structure, and relationship to ovarian teratocarcinogenesis in strain LT/Sv mice. *Differentiation*, **12**, 111–20.

Eppig, J.J. (1979a) A comparison between oocyte growth in coculture with granulosa cells and oocytes with granulosa cell–oocyte junctional contact maintained *in vitro*. *J. Exp. Zool.*, **209**, 345–53.

Eppig, J.J. (1979b) FSH stimulates hyaluronic acid synthesis by oocyte–cumulus cell complexes from mouse preovulatory follicles. *Nature*, **281**, 483–4.

Eppig, J.J. (1979c) Gonadotropin stimulation of the expansion of cumuli oophori isolated from mice: general conditions for expansion *in vitro*. *J. Exp. Zool.*, **208**, 345–53.

Eppig, J.J. (1980) Regulation of cumulus oophorus expansion by gonadotropins *in vivo* and *in vitro*. Biol. Reprod., **23**, 545–52.

Eppig, J.J. (1982) The relationship between cumulus cell–oocyte coupling, oocyte meiotic maturation, and cumulus expansion. *Dev. Biol.*, **89**, 268–72.

Eppig, J.J. & Downs, S.M. (1988) Gonadotropin-induced murine oocyte maturation *in vivo* is not associated with decreased cyclic adenosine monophosphate in the oocyte–cumulus cell complex. *Gamete Res.*, **20**, 125–31.

Eppig, J.J., Ward-Bailey, P.F. & Coleman, D.L. (1985) Hypoxanthine and adenosine in murine ovarian follicular fluid: concentrations and activity in maintaining oocyte meiotic arrest. *Biol. Reprod.*, **33**, 1041–9.

Fulka, J. (1985) Maturation-inhibiting activity of growing mouse oocytes. *Cell Diff.*, **17**, 45–8.

Gautier, J., Norbury, C., Lohka, M., Nurse, P. & Maller, J. (1988) Purified maturation-promoting factor contains the product of a Xenopus homolog of the fission yeast cell cycle control gene *cdc2+*. *Cell*, **54**, 433–9.

Gilula, N.B., Epstein, M.L. & Beers, W.H. (1978) Cell-to-cell communication and ovulation. A study of the cumulus–oocyte complex. *J. Cell Biol.*, **78**, 58–75.

Goto, K., Kajihara, Y., Kosaka, S., Koba, M., Nakanishi, Y. & Ogawa, K. (1988) Pregnancies after co-culture of cumulus cells with bovine embryos derived from in vitro fertilization of in vitro matured follicular oocytes. *J. Reprod. Fertil.*, **83**, 753–8.

Handel, M.A. & Eppig, J.J. (1979) Sertoli cell differentiation in the testis of mice genetically deficient in germ cells. *Biol. Reprod.*, **20**, 1031–8.

Hardisty, M.W. (1978) Primordial germ cells and the vertebrate germ line. In Jones, R.E. (ed.) *The Vertebrate Ovary — Comparative Biology and Evolution*, pp. 1–45. Plenum Press, New York.

Hashimoto, H. & Kishimoto, T. (1988) Regulation of meiotic metaphase by a cytoplasmic maturation-promoting factor during mouse oocyte maturation. *Dev. Biol.*, **126**, 242–52.

Heller, D.T. & Schultz, R.M. (1980) Ribonucleoside metabolism by mouse oocytes: metabolic cooperativity between fully grown oocytes and cumulus cells. *J. Exp. Zool.*, **214**, 355–64.

Herlands, R.L. & Schultz, R.M. (1984) Regulation of mouse oocyte growth: probable nutritional role for intercellular communication between follicle cells and oocytes in oocyte growth. *J. Exp. Zool.*, **229**, 317–25.

Hillensjo, T. & Channing, C.P. (1980) Gonadotropin stimulation of steroidogenesis and cellular dispersion in cultured porcine cumuli oophori. *Gamete Res.*, **3**, 223–40.

Huarte, J., Belin, D. & Vassalli, J.-D. (1985) Plasminogen activator in mouse and rat oocytes: induction during meiotic maturation. *Cell*, **43**, 551–8.

Huarte, J., Belin, D., Vassalli, A., Strickland, S. & Vassalli, J.-D. (1987) Meiotic maturation of mouse oocytes triggers the translation and polyadenylation of dormant tissue-type plasminogen activator mRNA. *Gene Dev.*, **1**, 1201–11.

Hubbard, C.J. (1986) Cyclic AMP changes in the component cells of Graafian follicles: possible influences on maturation in the follicle-enclosed oocytes of hamsters. *Dev. Biol.*, **118**, 343–51.

Keshet, E., Rosenberg, M.P., Mercer, J.A., Propst, F., Vande Woude, G.F., Jenkins, N.A. & Copeland, N.G. (1988) Developmental regulation of ovarian-specific *Mos* expression. *Oncogene*, **2**, 235–40.

Kishimoto, T. & Kanatani, H. (1976) Cytoplasmic factor responsible for germinal vesicle breakdown and meiotic maturation in starfish oocyte. *Nature*, **260**, 321–2.

Kishimoto, T., Kuriyama, R., Kondo, H. & Kanatani, H. (1982) Generality of the action of various maturation-promoting factors. *Exp. Cell Res.*, **137**, 121–6.

Kuyt, J.R.M., Kruip, T.A.M. & DeJong-Brink, M. (1988) Cytochemical localization of adenylate cyclase in bovine cumulus–oocyte complexes. *Exp. Cell Res.*, **174**, 139–45.

Larsen, W.J., Wert, S.E. & Brunner, G.D. (1987) Differential modulation of rat follicle gap junction populations at ovulation. *Dev. Biol.*, **112**, 61–71.

Lawrence, T.S., Beers, W.H. & Gilula, N.B. (1978) Transmission of hormonal stimulation by cell-to-cell communication. *Nature*, **272**, 501–6.

Lohka, M.J., Hayes, M.K. & Maller, J.L. (1988) Purification of maturation-promoting factor, an intracellular regulator of early mitotic events. *Proc. Natl. Acad. Sci. USA*, **85**, 3009–13.

Magnusson, C. & Hillensjo, T. (1977) Inhibition of maturation and metabolism of rat oocytes by cyclic AMP. *J. Exp. Zool.*, **201**, 138–47.

Moor, R.M. & Heslop, J.P. (1981) Cyclic AMP in mammalian follicle cells and oocytes during maturation. *J. Exp. Zool.*, **216**, 205–9.

Moor, R.M., Osborn, J.C., Cran, D.G. & Walters, D.E. (1981) Selective effect of gonadotrophins on cell coupling, nuclear maturation and protein synthesis in mammalian oocytes. *J. Embryol. Exp. Morphol.*, **61**, 347–65.

Mutter, G.L., Grills, G.S. & Wolgemuth, D.J. (1988) Evidence for the involvement of the proto-oncogene c-*mos* in mammalian meiotic maturation and possibly very early embryogenesis. *EMBO J.*, **7**, 683–9.

Paules, R.S., Buccione, R., Propst, F., Moschel, R.C., Vande Woude, G.F. & Eppig, J.J. (1989) Mouse *Mos* proto-oncogene is product is present and functions during oogenesis. *Proc. Natl. Acad. Sci. USA* **86**, 5395–9.

Philpott, C.C., Ringuette, M.J. & Dean, J. (1987) Oocyte-specific expression and developmental regulation of *ZP3*, and sperm receptor of the mouse zona pellucida. *Dev. Biol.*, **121**, 568–75.

Pincus, G. & Enzmann, E.V. (1935) The comparative behavior of mammalian eggs *in vivo* and *in vitro*. I. The activation of ovarian eggs. *J. Exp. Med.*, **62**, 655–75.

Pincus, G. & Saunders, B. (1939) The comparative behavior of mammalian eggs *in vivo* and *in vitro*. IV. The maturation of human ovarian ova. *Anat. Rec.*, **75**, 537–45.

Racowsky, C. (1984) Effect of forskolin on the spontaneous maturation and cyclic AMP content of rat oocyte–cumulus complex. *J. Reprod. Fertil.*, **72**, 107–16.

Racowsky, C. (1985a) Effect of forskolin on the spontaneous maturation and cyclic AMP content of hamster oocyte–cumulus complexes. *J. Exp. Zool.*, **234**, 87–96.

Racowsky, C. (1985b) Effect of forskolin on maintenance of meiotic arrest and stimulation of cumulus expansion, progesterone and cyclic AMP production by pig oocyte–cumulus complexes. *J. Reprod. Fertil.*, **74**, 9–21.

Reynhout, J.K. & Smith, L.D. (1974) Studies on the appearance and nature of a maturation-inducing factor in the cytoplasm of amphibian oocytes exposed to progesterone. *Dev. Biol.*, **38**, 394–400.

Rime, H., Neant, I., Guerrier, P. & Ozon, R. (1989) 6-Dimethylaminopurine (6-DMAP), a reversible inhibitor of the transition to metaphase during the first meiotic cell division of the mouse oocyte. *Dev. Biol.*, **133**, 169–79.

Ringuette, M.J., Sobieski, D.A., Chamow, S.M. & Dean, J. (1986) Oocyte-specific gene expression: molecular characterization of a cDNA coding for ZP-3, the sperm receptor of the mouse zona pellucida. *Proc. Natl. Acad. Sci. USA*, **83**, 4341–5.

Sagata, N., Watanabe, N., Vande Woude, G.F. & Ikawa, Y. (1989) The c-*mos* proto-oncogene product is a cytostatic factor responsible for meiotic arrest in vertebrate eggs. *Nature*, **342**, 512−8.

Salustri, A., Petrungaro, S., Conti, M. & Siracusa, G. (1988) Adenosine potentiates forskolin-induced delay of meiotic resumption by mouse denuded oocytes: evidence for an oocyte surface site of adenosine action. *Gamete Res.*, **21**, 157−68.

Salustri, A. & Siracusa, G. (1983) Metabolic coupling, cumulus expansion and meiotic resumption in mouse cumuli oophori cultured *in vitro* in the presence of FSH or dbcAMP or stimulated *in vivo* by hCG. *J. Reprod. Fert.*, **68**, 335−41.

Schroeder, A.C. & Eppig, J.J. (1984) The developmental capacity of mouse oocytes that matured spontaneously *in vitro* is normal. *Dev. Biol.*, **102**, 493−7.

Schroeder, A.C. & Eppig, J.J. (1989) Developmental capacity of mouse oocytes that undergo maturation *in vitro*: effect of the hormonal state of the oocyte donor. *Gamete Res.* **24**, 81−92.

Schultz, R.M., Montgomery, R. & Belanoff, J. (1983) Regulation of mouse oocyte maturation: implication of a decrease in oocyte cAMP and protein dephosphorylation in commitment to resume meiosis. *Dev. Biol.*, **97**, 264−73.

Shalgi, R., Dekel, N. & Kraicer, P.F. (1979) The effect of LH on the fertilizability and developmental capacity of rat oocytes matured *in vitro*. *J. Reprod. Fertil.*, **55**, 429−35.

Shimizu, S., Tsuji, M. & Dean, J. (1983) In vitro biosynthesis of three sulfated glycoproteins of murine zonae pellucidae by oocytes grown in follicle culture. *J. Biol. Chem.*, **258**, 5858−63.

Sirard, M.A., Parrish, J.J., Ware, C.B., Leibfried-Rutledge, M.L. & First, N.L. (1988) The culture of bovine oocytes to obtain developmentally competent embryos. *Biol. Reprod.*, **39**, 546−52.

Sorensen, R.A., Cyert, M.S. & Pedersen, R.A. (1985) Active maturation-promoting factor is present in mature mouse oocytes. *J. Cell Biol.*, **100**, 1637−40.

Sorensen, R.A. & Wassarman, P.M. (1976) Relationship between growth and meiotic maturation of the mouse oocyte. *Dev. Biol.*, **50**, 531−6.

Staigmiller, R.B. & Moor, R.M. (1984) Effect of follicle cells on the maturation and developmental competence of ovine oocytes matured outside the follicle. *Gamete Res.*, **9**, 221−9.

Strickland, S., Huarte, J., Belin, D., Vassalli, A., Rickles, R.J. & Vassalli, J.-D. (1988) Antisense RNA directed against the 3′noncoding region prevents dormant mRNA activation in mouse oocytes. *Science*, **241**, 680−4.

Szybek, K. (1972) In vitro maturation of oocytes from sexually immature mice. *J. Endocrinol.*, **54**, 527−8.

Tsafriri. A., Dekel, N. & Bar-Ami, S. (1982) The role of oocyte maturation inhibitor in follicular regulation of oocyte maturation. *J. Reprod. Fertil.*, **64**, 541−51.

Urner, F., Herrmann, W.L., Baulieu, E.E. & Schorderet-Slatkine, S. (1983) Inhibition of denuded mouse oocyte meiotic maturation by forskolin, an activator of adenylate cyclase. *Endocrinology*, **113**, 1170−2.

Urner, F. & Schorderet-Slatkine, S. (1984) Inhibition of denuded mouse oocyte meiotic maturation by tumor-promoting phorbol esters and its reversal by retinoids. *Exp. Cell Res.*, **154**, 600−5.

Van Blerkom, J. & McGaughey, R.W. (1978) Molecular differentiation of the rabbit ovum. II. During the preimplantation development of *in vivo* and *in vitro* matured oocytes. *Dev. Biol.*, **63**, 151−64.

Wassarman, P.M., Josefowicz, W.J. & Letourneau, G.E. (1976) Meiotic maturation of mouse oocytes *in vitro*: inhibition of maturation at specific stages of nuclear progression. *J. Cell Sci.*, **22**, 531−45.

Watanabe, N., Vande Woude, G.F., Ikawa, Y. & Sagata, N. (1989) Specific proteolysis of the *c-mos* proto-oncogene product by calpain on fertilization of *Xenopus* eggs. *Nature*, **342**, 505−11.

# 5 The Biochemistry of Ovulation

M. BRÄNNSTRÖM & P.O. JANSON

## Introduction

Ovulation is the central event in the ovarian cycle when the mature oocyte is discharged onto the surface of the ovary and passes into the oviduct where it may be fertilized. In developmental terms, it is the final step in the growth and differentiation of the preovulatory follicle and marks the onset of corpus luteum formation. In cyclic adult women, the ovulatory process is initiated by the spontaneous mid-cycle leuteinizing hormone (LH) surge. It can also be induced by giving exogenous human chorionic gonadotrophin (hCG; surrogate LH) after appropriate gonadotrophic priming of the preovulatory follicle(s).

The biochemistry of ovulation has most often been studied in rats or rabbits by observing the effects of treatment with agonists or antagonists of putative regulatory factors on follicular rupture *in vivo*. The results of such experiments have usually been difficult to interpret since they have not always distinguished between direct (intraovarian) or indirect (systemically-mediated) modes of action on the ovarian follicle. *In vitro* models based on the incubation of whole ovaries, isolated follicles or strips of follicular wall tissue provide less complex experimental systems to interpret but they cannot always distinguish between the physiological process of ovulation and rupture induced non-specifically by physical or biochemical artefacts created by the incubation conditions (cf. Neal & Baker, 1973; Baranzuk & Fainstat, 1976). A circulatory fluid supply to and from the follicle and an attendant positive capillary pressure appear to be necessary for ovulation to be induced and proceed normally *in vitro*. Systems for the long-term perfusion *in vitro* of isolated ovaries have therefore been developed to study ovulation in a number of species including man (Stähler *et al.*, 1974; Lambertsen *et al.*, 1976; Janson *et al.*, 1982; Koos *et al.*, 1984b; Brännström *et al.*, 1987a) (Fig. 5.1).

No *in vitro* model can fully mimic the conditions which prevail *in vivo* but use of ovarian perfusion systems has allowed direct experimental manipulation and visualization of the ovulatory process unconstrained by neural and systemic inputs (Plate 5.1). In this chapter we shall survey knowledge gained using the *in vitro* perfusion system and other experimental approaches to study the biochemistry of ovulation in laboratory animals and integrate that knowledge with the more limited information which is available concerning the biochemistry of follicular rupture in women.

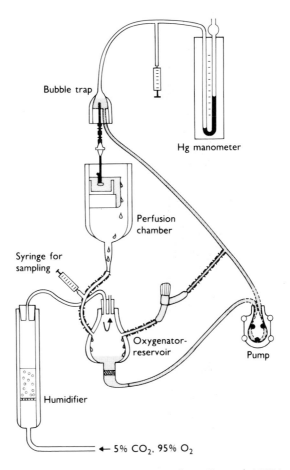

**Fig. 5.1.** The *in vitro* ovarian perfusion system (Brännström *et al.* 1987a).

## Preovulatory changes in follicular morphology and endocrine function

In addition to changes in the oocyte which allow it to become fertilizable by the time of follicular rupture (see Chapter 4), the gonadotrophin surge stimulates distinct structural and functional changes in the somatic cell layers of the follicular wall and the overlying ovarian surface. These changes facilitate the process of follicular rupture and transform the ovulatory follicle into a corpus luteum.

### Preovulatory follicular morphology

When the LH surge begins, the follicle(s) destined to ovulate is located in the ovarian cortex immediately beneath the tunica albuginea and surface epithelium. The follicle wall and overlying non-follicular tissues comprise several functionally and morphologically distinct cell layers and four discrete layers of collagen which, collectively, give the distended follicle its tensile strength (Fig. 5.2).

The changes in follicular and ovarian surface morphology which occur between the LH surge and follicular rupture have been most extensively studied in the rabbit (Bjersing & Cajander, 1974a–f) but are also well documented for small rodents (Parr, 1974; Reed *et al.*, 1979) and to a lesser extent for man (Okamura *et al.*, 1980). However, the architecture of the follicular wall appears to be similar in most mammalian species.

#### *Surface epithelium*

The ovarian surface is covered by a low cuboidal epithelium, which is

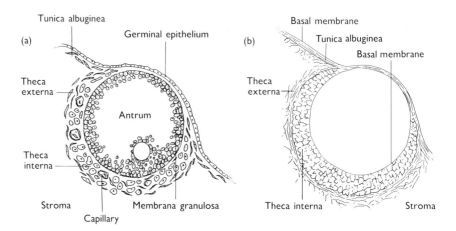

**Fig. 5.2.** Schematic structure of the ovary showing (a) the cellular composition of the follicle wall, and (b) its content of collagen fibres and layers. Reproduced with permission from Beers *et al.* (1975).

continuous with the peritoneal serosa. The surface epithelial cells have the usual content of cell organelles and also lysosome-like electron dense granules within the cytoplasm (Cajander & Bjersing, 1975; Rawson & Espey, 1977). These cells are attached to each other by so-called 'zona occludens' on their lateral surface (Espey, 1967a). On their apical surfaces there are large numbers of microvilli. After the preovulatory LH surge, epithelial cells situated on the apices of preovulatory follicles tend to flatten and lose their microvilli (Motta & van Blerkom, 1975). Sack-like blebs of various sizes develop on these apical cells prior to ovulation (Bjersing & Cajander, 1974b). At the same time there is a twofold increase in the density of electron-dense bodies within the cells which persists until rupture occurs (Rawson & Espey, 1977). The electron-dense bodies are probably lysosomes and it has been postulated that these cells produce proteolytic enzymes involved in the breakdown of the follicular wall (Cajander & Bjersing, 1975). Just before the wall ruptures, these surface epithelial cells appear to undergo degeneration or become detached from the underlying basal membrane (Bjersing & Cajander, 1974a).

## Tunica albuginea

The surface epithelium is separated from the tunica albuginea by a basal membrane rich in laminin and collagen Type IV which forms an open mesh-like structure. The tunica albuginea is composed of scattered fibroblasts and densely packed interstitial collagen fibres which are composed of collagen Types I and III (Palotie *et al.*, 1984). The metabolic activity of tunica cells has also been linked to follicular rupture since they contain multivesicular cytoplasmic structures which increase in concentration just before rupture occurs (Espey, 1971). During the ovulatory process, many of the fibroblasts in the apical portion of the tunica albuginea die and the collagen fibres in these regions fragment and become dissociated from each other (Bjersing & Cajander, 1974c).

## Theca externa

The outermost follicular compartment is the theca externa which is composed mainly of collagen fibres made up of collagen Types I and III. These fibres are spread throughout the ground substance and are less densely packed than in the tunica albuginea. The fibrous theca externa also contains four to seven layers of elongated fibroblasts and smooth muscle cells. The morphology of these cells is similar to that of fibroblasts but they have a greater density of surface microfilaments (Fumagalli *et al.*, 1971). The smooth muscle cells lie in close proximity to nerve terminals and it has been suggested that neurally mediated contractions of these cells may play a role in ovulation (Owman *et al.*, 1975). Ovulatory changes in the theca externa include disintegration of collagen fibres and elongation of fibroblasts and smooth muscle cells with no obvious necrosis (Bjersing & Cajander, 1974e). Multi-vesicular bodies accumulate within these fibroblasts, similar to the situation for fibroblasts in the tunica albuginea (Espey, 1971). The theca externa also contains a vascular network of arterioles and venules connected to a rich capillary plexus in the theca interna. Extravasation of blood cells in the theca externa occurs shortly before ovulation (Bjersing & Cajander, 1974e).

### Theca interna

The theca interna is one to three cell layers thick and highly vascularized by a dense capillary network. The theca interna cells are slightly elongated or polyhedral with oval nuclei. These cells are in close proximity to each other and embedded in a network of collagen fibres which is continuous with the fibrous part of the theca externa. After the preovulatory gonadotrophin surge, these cells increase in size and accumulate lipid droplets. The thecal vasculature also undergoes conspicuous ovulatory changes, including an increased fenestration of the endothelium leading to the formation of large intracellular and intercellular gaps (Bjersing & Cajander, 1974f). Dilatation of capillaries and venules also occurs (Kanzaki et al., 1982), constituting the morphological basis for the increased vascular permeability and oedematization which occurs shortly before ovulation (Bjersing & Cajander, 1974f; Okuda et al., 1980a; Tanaka et al., 1989) (see below). Extravasation of erythrocytes (Parr, 1974) and leukocytes (Bjersing & Cajander, 1974a) also occurs at this time, heralding the disruption of the perivascular basal membrane and breakdown of the 'blood−follicle' barrier.

### Membrana granulosa

Until shortly before follicular rupture, the highly vascularized theca interna is separated from the avascular membrana granulosa by a basal membrane, the lamina propria. The membrana granulosa is made up of a layer of about five to 10 layers of granulosa cells. Granulosa cells immediately adjacent to the basal membrane are columnar epithelioid in appearance while those which are centripetally located are more polyhedral in shape. These cells are connected to each other via gap junctions which allow the passage of nutritional and instructional substances between individual granulosa cells and between cumulus granulosa cells and the oocyte (see Chapter 4). After the LH surge, mitotic activity among these cells rapidly ceases and luteinization is initiated. The morphological signs of granulosa cell luteinization are accumulation of eosinophilic granules and lipid droplets, presence of mitochondria with tubular christae, and a large proportion of smooth endoplasmic reticulum consistent with the steriod synthesizing function of these cells. The number of granulosa cell gap junctions decrease after the LH surge and the cells become dissociated from each other due to intercellular accumulation of hyaluronic acid (Dekel & Kraicer, 1978). This is the biochemical basis of cumulus expansion in the oocyte–cumulus complex (see Chapter 4). Some granulosa cells bordering the follicular antrum become detached from the residual granulosa cell mass and 'free-float' in the follicular fluid (Parr, 1974). In the apical regions of the follicular wall, the granulosa cell layer becomes completely detached from the lamina basalis shortly before rupture. Elsewhere in the follicle, mural granulosa cells may penetrate the partially digested lamina propria, suggesting an outward migration of these cells as ovulation approaches.

### Preovulatory follicular endocrine function

Cellular mechanisms underlying the shift which occurs from oestrogen to predominantly progesterone secretion by the periovulatory follicle(s) are detailed elsewhere (see Chapters 2 and 3). Essential features of the c. 36-h interval between the onset of the LH surge and ovulation in women are activation of the granulosa potential for progesterone biosynthesis; suppression of theca cell androgen synthesis; and maintenance of granulosa cell aromatase activity. Thus in most mammalian species which have been examined, as ovulation approaches, the follicular fluid level and ovarian secretion rate of progesterone tend to rise whereas the production of aromatizable androgen, and hence oestrogen, declines. Implications which these changes may have for the mechanism of ovulation are considered later in this chapter.

## Mechanics and haemodynamics of follicular rupture

Active tissue-remodelling in the apical region of the follicle wall is of overriding importance to the ovulatory process. However, mechanical and hydrodynamic forces arising from within the follicle are also required to expel the cumulus–oocyte complex onto the surface of the ovary once the follicle has ruptured.

### Mechanics

Intrafollicular pressure recordings from ovulating rabbit follicles (Espey & Lipner, 1963; Rondell, 1964) have shown 'a slight fall in pressure as ovulation approaches, a sharp drop as fluid begins to leak from the follicle, then a transient rise in pressure and finally a stabilization at some low, positive value' (Rondell, 1970a). The slight preovulatory fall in pressure coincides with the small leak of follicular fluid observed several hours before the major rupture in perfused rat ovaries (Löfman *et al.*, 1989). The absence of any increase in pressure preceding rupture contradicts the 'endosmosis' theory which attempts to relate ovulation to changes in follicular pressure or volume and supports the 'enzyme' theory which proposes that enzymic or vascular processes result in deterioration and disruption of the follicle wall.

Rodbard (1968) analysed the mechanics of follicular rupture and constructed a mathematical model from which he concluded that because of possible changes in follicular volume and wall thickness, factors other than distensibility could be operative. However, Rondell (1970a) showed beyond doubt that the distensibilty of the follicle wall increases as ovulation approached. Similar findings were reported by Espey (1967b), working with strips of follicular wall from pig ovaries. Espey also showed that increased distensibility at the site of follicular rupture is caused by changes in collagen or the ground substances which binds collagen fibrils together. Similar increases in the distensibility of follicular strips can be induced by exposure *in vitro* to LH, cyclic adenosine monophosphate (cAMP), or progesterone (Rondell, 1970b).

## Haemodynamics

During preovulatory follicular growth the follicular microvasculature develops into a complex, multi-layered plexus or vascular wreath consisting of sinusoidal capillaries (Kanazaki, 1981; Kanazaki *et al.*, 1982). By the time of ovulation, this vascular system is sufficiently developed to sustain relatively high rates of blood flow to the rupturing follicle as compared with other parts of the ovary (Bruce & Moor, 1976; Zeleznik *et al.*, 1981; Janson, 1988; Murakami *et al.*, 1988). This is the morphological basis of the well-known ovarian hyperaemia which precedes ovulation (Zondek *et al.*, 1945; Ellis, 1961).

An increase in ovarian blood flow occurs due to arteriolar vasodilatation within minutes of LH administration to rats (Wurtman, 1964) and rabbits (Janson, 1975). hCG also causes dilatation and increased permeability of capillaries in the apex of the ovulating follicle, leading to the eventual breakdown of the 'blood−follicle' barrier (Lipner & Smith, 1971). Resin injection-corrosion casts made shortly before the expected time of follicular rupture have shown there to be capillary dilatation followed by leakage of resin into the interstitial space (Kanzaki *et al.*, 1982). Light and electron-microscopic studies on ovulating rabbit follicles have also shown an increase in the number of gaps and fenestrations in the capillary endothelium and in the number of pinocytotic vesicles present in the endothelial cells (Bjersing & Cajander, 1974a; Okuda *et al.*, 1980a). Carbon particles are able to pass through these endothelial gaps 10−12 h after administration of hCG (Okuda *et al.*, 1980b).

# Cellular basis of LH action

The action of LH on the preovulatory follicle is mediated by high-affinity binding of the hormone to specific receptors on the surface of thecal cells and mural granulosa cells (Amsterdam *et al.*, 1975). Expression of the granulosa cell LH receptor is a correlate of follicle-stimulating hormone (FSH)-induced cell differentiation in the preovulatory follicle whereas thecal cells express LH receptors throughout antral follicular development (see Chapter 3). At least three postreceptor signalling systems are implicated in the ovulation-inducing actions of LH and hCG: cAMP and cAMP-dependent protein kinase (protein kinase A), phosphoinositide (PI) metabolism and calcium-dependent protein kinase (protein kinase C) (Fig. 5.3), and metabolism of arachidonic acid (Fig. 5.4).

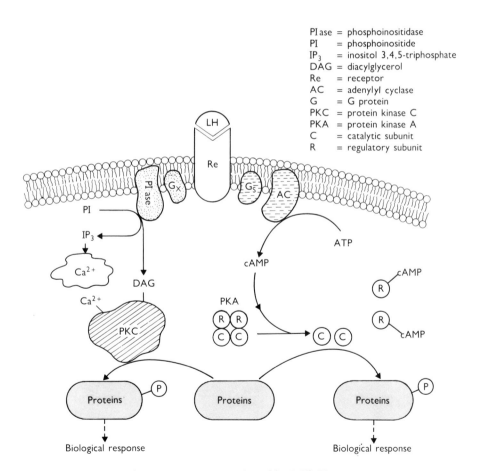

| | |
|---|---|
| PI ase | = phosphoinositidase |
| PI | = phosphoinositide |
| IP$_3$ | = inositol 3,4,5-triphosphate |
| DAG | = diacylglycerol |
| Re | = receptor |
| AC | = adenylyl cyclase |
| G | = G protein |
| PKC | = protein kinase C |
| PKA | = protein kinase A |
| C | = catalytic subunit |
| R | = regulatory subunit |

**Fig. 5.3.** Second-messenger systems activated by LH/hCG.

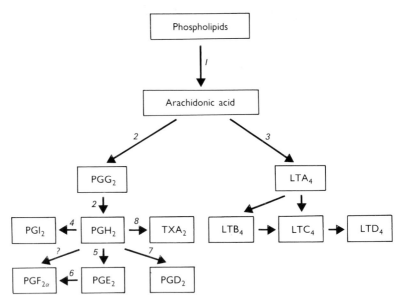

**Fig. 5.4.** Pathways of arachidonic acid metabolism. PG, prostaglandin; TX, thromboxane; LT, leukotriene. Enzymes: *1*, phospholipase; *2*, prostaglandin endoperoxide synthase (cyclooxygenase); *3*, lipoxygenase; *4*, prostacyclin synthase; *5*, 9-ketoisomerase; *6*, 9-ketoreductase; *7*, 11-ketoisomerase; *8*, thromboxane synthase.

### cAMP and protein kinase A

LH binding to its receptor activates the catalytic subunit of membrane associated adenylate cyclase to generate cAMP from ATP. The activation of adenylate cyclase is mediated by a stimulatory GTP-binding protein ($G_s$). cAMP binds to the regulatory subunits of cAMP-dependent protein kinase A, derepressing its catalytic subunits which phosphorylate and activate specific cytosolic and nuclear proteins involved in cellular function. Substrates of protein kinase A include a recently discovered cAMP response-element (CRE) binding-protein (Montminy & Bilezikjian, 1987) which mediates cAMP action at the level of gene expression.

There are at least two major types of ovarian protein kinase A: types I and II (Jahnsen *et al.*, 1985). These kinases are distinguished essentially by differences in their regulatory subunits (Robinson-Steiner & Corbin, 1983). The rat ovarian content of mRNA encoding the regulatory 'β'-subunit of Type II protein kinase A (RIIβ) is stimulated for up to 7 h after the administration of an ovulation-inducing dose of hCG, whereupon the level of mRNA subsides (Hedin *et al.*, 1987b). There is no corresponding change in the level of catalytic α-subunit mRNA (Hedin *et al.*, 1987b) so the increased preovulatory expression of RIIβ may regulate overall protein kinase A activity during this period. Other intracellular variables which would be expected to influence cellular responsiveness to LH via protein kinase A postreceptor signalling include the density of LH receptors on the cell surface, the type(s) and amount of GTP binding-protein(s) present, adenylyl cyclase levels, and the type(s) and amount of substrate available for phosphorylation by protein kinase A.

The ability of cAMP to stimulate ovulation has been demonstrated experimentally using isolated perfused rabbit (Holmes *et al.*, 1986) and rat ovaries (Brännström *et al.*, 1987b). Normal preovulatory increases in steroidogenesis and multiple ovulations were induced by addition to the perfusion medium of forskolin (non-hormonal activator of adenylyl cyclase) or dibutyryl cAMP (cell-membrane permeable analogue of cAMP) in the presence of a phosphodiesterase inhibitor. Inhibition of phosphodiesterase also enhanced the number of ovulations induced by a fixed dose of LH, highlighting the central role of cAMP in mediating LH-stimulated follicular rupture (Holmes *et al.*, 1986; Brännström *et al.*, 1989a).

### PI metabolism and protein kinase C

LH also activates the PI/protein kinase C system in granulosa cells (Davis *et al.*, 1984). LH stimulation probably results in a fast activation of protein kinase C since a rapid elevation of inositol 1,4,5-triphosphate ($IP_3$) levels (Davis *et al.*, 1986) and alteration in $Ca^{2+}$ flux (Veldhuis & Klase, 1982) have been demonstrated in LH-treated granulosa cells. However, to date, direct experimental evidence is still lacking that the PI/protein kinase C system is crucial to ovulation.

### Arachidonic acid metabolism

LH also stimulates release of arachidonic acid from phospholipids in follicular cell-surface membranes, presumably via activation of phospholipase C and/or $A_2$. Arachidonic acid is metabolized to prostaglandins, prostacyclins and thromboxanes via the cyclooxygenase pathway and to leukotrienes via the lipoxygenase pathway (Fig. 5.4). As discussed below, prostaglandin biochemistry is integral to the mechanism of follicular rupture. However, the exact functions of lipoxygenase products of arachidonic acid metabolism in the ovulatory process are less clear.

## Biochemical systems and follicular rupture

### Steroids

Steroid synthesis in preovulatory follicles is influenced dramatically by the ovulation-inducing LH surge. In particular, progesterone synthesis in luteinizing granulosa cells increases due to stimulation of the cholesterol side-chain cleavage system (P450scc), and androgen synthesis in the theca interna is suppressed due to inhibition of 17-hydroxylase/

C17,20-lyase (P450c17) (see Chapters 2 and 3). Although granulosa cell aromatase activity seems not to be suppressed by the LH surge, oestrogen synthesis declines due to the lack of available aromatase substrate. Thus, in the interval between onset of the LH surge and follicular rupture, progesterone levels in follicular fluid rise many-fold while androgen and oestradiol levels fall precipitately (Hillier, 1985).

Although it is well established that steroids serve paracrine regulatory functions in ovarian follicles (see Chapter 3), experimental evidence that they participate directly in the normal ovulatory process is controversial. However, a consensus is emerging from work with several animal species regarding the importance to ovulation of the preovulatory increase in follicular progesterone synthesis.

### Steroids and ovulation in rats

Early evidence for involvement of steroids in follicular rupture was based on the observation that administration of inhibitors of steroid synthesis also inhibited ovulation (Lipner & Greep, 1971; Lipner & Wendelken, 1971). However, the results of these experiments are difficult to interpret because the inhibitors which were used are now known to have non-specific effects on ovulation which cannot be reversed by steroid-replacement therapy (Bullock & Kappauf, 1973).

More recently, a specific local function for progesterone in ovulation in the rat has been established. hCG-induced ovulations in pregnant mare serum gonadotrophin (PMSG)-primed rats were inhibited by passive immunization against progesterone (Mori et al., 1977a) or by administering Epostane to specifically inhibit 3β-hydroxysteroid dehydrogenase (Snyder et al., 1984), the enzyme which converts pregnenolone to progesterone. In the in vitro perfused rat ovary model, another 'specific' 3β-hydroxysteroid dehydrogenase inhibitor (17α-(3'hydroxypropyl)-1,3,5,6,8(9)-oestropentaene-3,17β-diol) (Compound A) was shown to suppress progesterone levels in follicular fluid and markedly decrease the number of ovulations induced by LH (Brännström & Janson, 1989). The inhibition was reversed dosedependently by progesterone but not by testosterone. A progesterone receptor antagonist RU486 was also shown to partially block hCG-induced ovulation in vivo (Tsafriri et al., 1987).

Other experiments suggest that follicular androgen rather than progesterone is involved in ovulation in rats (Mori et al., 1977b; Peluso et al., 1980). A role for oestrogen appears to have been convincingly ruled out in vivo (Lipner & Wendelken, 1971) and in vitro (Koos et al., 1984a; Morioka et al., 1988a).

### Steroids and ovulation in rabbits

Studies with the in vitro perfused ovary system have revealed apparent differences between rats and rabbits concerning the role of steroids in follicular rupture. Inhibition of the cholesterol side-chain cleavage system by aminoglutethimide (Yoshimura *et al.*, 1986) and inhibition of 3β-hydroxysteroid dehydrogenase by cyanoketone (Yoshimura *et al.*, 1987a) or Compound A (Holmes *et al.*, 1985) did not inhibit ovulation in perfused rabbit ovaries. Rather, the proportion of isolated follicles which collapsed during incubation *in vitro* was increased by the presence of progesterone in the culture medium (Testart *et al.*, 1983). However, intrafollicular injections of progesterone antiserum blocked ovulation *in vivo* (Swanson & Lipner, 1977). Work with the *in vitro* perfused rabbit ovary appears to have ruled out an important direct role for oestrogen in the mechanism of follicular rupture (LeMaire *et al.*, 1982).

### Steroids and ovulation in sheep

Ovulation in the ewe was inhibited by administration of an inhibitor of progesterone synthesis (Murdoch *et al.*, 1986). There are few other data concerning direct steroid action and the ovulatory process in sheep.

### Steroids and ovulation in women

No firm data exist to demonstrate local steroid action in human ovulation. However, when pieces of follicular wall were incubated *in vitro*, presence of progesterone or androstenedione decreased the formation of collagen (Tjugum *et al.*, 1984). Were such effects to operate *in vivo* this could lead to an accelerated net loss of collagen fibres, thereby expediting follicular rupture. Preovulatory follicular fluid progesterone levels rise markedly following the LH surge or injection of hCG and it is possible that this preovulatory rise is essential to the ovulatory process. Administration of the antiprogesterone RU486 inhibited folliculogenesis and ovulation in women but it was not established if this effect was direct at the ovarian level or indirect mediated via decreased release of pituitary gonadotrophins (Luukainen *et al.*, 1988).

### Role of intrafollicular progesterone in ovulation

Several lines of evidence suggest that follicular progesterone affects the process of follicular rupture by influencing prostaglandin biochemistry (Espey, 1986). Follicular fluid prostaglandin levels begin to rise after the preovulatory increase in progesterone accumulation has begun, and inhibitors of progesterone synthesis (Lipner & Greep, 1971), or action (Swanson & Lipner, 1977; Tajima *et al.*, 1988) only inhibit ovulation if administered before the peak preovulatory prostaglandin level is attained (LeMaire *et al.*, 1975). In the rat ovary, maximal levels of prostaglandin endoperoxide (cyclooxygenase) synthase occur *c*. 7 h after an ovulation inducing dose of LH (Hedin *et al.*, 1987a). The implication that progesterone stimulates intraovarian prostaglandin formation is strengthened by recent evidence that treatment with progesterone increases uterine cyclooxygenase activity in sheep (Raw *et al.*, 1988). A positive association also exists between the levels of progesterone and prostaglandin $F_{2\alpha}$ found in human ovarian tissue (Vijayakumar & Walters, 1987). In the ovine ovary, progesterone may affect prostaglandin $E_2$-9-ketoreductase activity, the enzyme that converts prostaglandin $E_2$ to prostaglandin $F_{2\alpha}$ (Murdoch *et al.*, 1986). Locally produced steroids may also affect the production of prostaglandin $I_2$ (prostacyclin) by vascular tissue, thereby increasing ovarian blood flow (Roncaglioni *et al.*, 1979; Karpati *et al.*, 1980).

Not all experimental data support the idea that prostaglandin synthesis in the ovary is dependent on steroid synthesis. Inhibition of follicular steroidogenesis by treatment with aminoglutethimide *in vitro* (Bauminger *et al.*, 1975) or *in vivo* (Armstrong *et al.*, 1976) did not inhibit LH-induced increases in rat ovarian prostaglandin levels.

A direct action of progesterone on the synthesis of a proteolytic enzyme(s) involved in follicular rupture was suggested by the work of Rondell (1974) who showed that treatment with progesterone *in vitro* specifically increases the distensibility of porcine preovulatory follicular strips. More recently, steroids have been implicated in the regulation of plasminogen activator (PA) synthesis and the activation of collagenase, thereby facilitating breakdown of the follicle wall (Ohno & Mori, 1985). Oestradiol (Reich *et al.*, 1985b), progestins and androgens (Ny *et al.*, 1985) were shown to potentiate gonadotrophin-induced elevation of PA activity in rat preovulatory follicles and granulosa cells, respectively. Moreover, inhibition of progesterone synthesis in the ovine ovary resulted in suppression of the preovulatory rise in collagenolysis, possibly mediated by a decrease in PA activity (Murdoch *et al.*, 1986).

## Arachidonic acid metabolites

A number of biologically active eicosanoids have been detected in ovarian tissue which are likely to be involved in the mechanism of follicular rupture. These include the prostaglandins $E_2$, $F_{2\alpha}$ and $I_2$ and various leukotrienes (Fig. 5.4), all of which are implicated in the local mediation of LH/hCG action in the follicle wall.

### Prostaglandins

Follicular fluid levels of prostaglandins increase markedly in the preovulatory follicles of most mammalian species (Lipner, 1988). In the rat ovary, from the morning of pro-oestrus until just before ovulation, prostaglandin $E_2$ levels increase 30- to 70-fold and prostaglandin $F_{2\alpha}$ levels increase 6- to 20-fold (Bauminger & Lindner, 1975; LeMaire *et al.*, 1975). Increased plasma levels of prostaglandin $F_{2\alpha}$ have also been detected during the preovulatory period in rats (Iesaka *et al.*,1975). In *in vitro* perfused rat ovaries treated with LH or pharmacological stimulators of cAMP production, prostaglandin reaches a high level shortly before the expected time of ovulation (Brännström *et al.*, 1987b). In contrast to the situation in rats and sheep (Murdoch *et al.*, 1981), ovarian prostaglandin $F_{2\alpha}$ levels increase faster than do prostaglandin $E_2$ levels before ovulation in the rabbit (LeMaire *et al.*, 1973). The rise in follicular fluid prostaglandin levels is most pronounced in those follicles which are destined to ovulate (Yang *et al.*, 1974). Similar preovulatory changes in follicular fluid prostaglandin levels have been observed using *in vitro* perfused rabbit ovaries (Koos *et al.* 1983).

*Control of follicular prostaglandin synthesis*

The rate-limiting step in the conversion of arachidonic acid to prostaglandins and thromboxanes is catalysed by prostaglandin endoperoxide synthase, a haem-binding protein with both cyclooxygenase and peroxidase activities (Fig. 5.4). Immunohistochemical studies on rat ovaries have shown that prostaglandin endoperoxide synthase is induced by hCG (Hedin *et al.* 1987a; Huslig *et al.*, 1987). The enzyme appears to be localized to the granulosa cell surface membrane and is absent from thecal cells (Hedin *et al.*, 1987a). This is consistent with granulosa cells being primary intrafollicular cellular sites of prostaglandin synthesis (Clark *et al.*, 1978b; Triebwasser *et al.*, 1978).

LH-stimulated increases in follicular prostaglandin synthesis appear to be mediated both by cAMP/protein kinase A and PI/protein kinase C postreceptor signalling (Clark *et al.*, 1978a; Kawai & Clark, 1985). The role of cAMP in mediating prostaglandin synthesis has been confirmed in the *in vitro* perfused rat ovary system (Brännström *et al.*, 1978b; Brännström *et al.*, 1989b).

There is a 2−4 h lag between initiation of treatment with gonadotrophin and onset of elevated prostaglandin levels in the rat ovary (Bauminger & Lindner, 1975; Clark *et al.*, 1976). This reflects the need for *de novo* synthesis of proteins to sustain increased rates of prostaglandin synthesis in follicular cells (Clark *et al.*, 1976), including prostaglandin endoperoxide synthase (Hedin *et al.*, 1987a; Brännström *et al.*, 1989b).

*Evidence for involvement of prostaglandins in ovulation*

The first evidence that prostaglandins might play an obligatory role in the ovulatory process came from experiments in which the administration of aspirin or indomethacin, inhibitors of prostaglandin endoperoxide synthase, were shown to block ovulation in rats (Armstrong & Grinwich, 1972; Tsafriri *et al.*, 1973) and rabbits (Grinwich *et al.*, 1972).

These findings were subsequently extended to several other mammalian species, including primates (Armstrong, 1981). In women, the blockade of ovulation caused by indomethacin results in luteinized unruptured follicles (Killick & Elstein, 1987) (see Chapter 9).

Antiovulatory effects due to *in vivo* administration of indomethacin or other inhibitors of prostaglandin synthesis might be explained by drug action at hypothalamic and/or pituitary levels (Orczyk & Behrman, 1972), since prostaglandins are also involved in the mechanism of gonadotrophin releasing hormone (GnRH)-induced gonadotrophin release (Harms *et al.*, 1974). However, a direct ovarian action is suggested by the ability of these inhibitors to inhibit ovulation even when administered after the LH surge has begun but before the expected time of follicular rupture (Tsafriri *et al.*, 1973). Furthermore, experiments with *in vitro* perfused rabbit (Hamada *et al.*, 1977; Holmes *et al.*, 1983) and rat (Sogn *et al.*, 1987; Brännström *et al.*, 1987b) ovaries have demonstrated conclusively that indomethacin can block ovulation via direct action(s) on the ovary.

### Which prostaglandin causes ovulation?

There may be interspecies differences regarding the type of prostaglandin which is involved in ovulation. Rat granulosa cells synthesize and release prostaglandins $E_2$, $F_{2\alpha}$ (Clark *et al.*, 1981) and $I_2$ (Koos & Clark, 1982), but prostaglandin $E_2$ appears to be the major mediator of ovulation in this species (Tsafriri *et al.*, 1972, 1973; Sogn *et al.*, 1987). However, an action of prostaglandin $E_2$ via conversion to prostaglandin $F_{2\alpha}$ cannot be ruled out since ovarian tissue contains prostaglandin $E_2$-9-ketoreductase, the enzyme which converts prostaglandin $E_2$ to prostaglandin $F_{2\alpha}$ (Watson *et al.*, 1979) (see Fig. 5.4).

In rabbits, prostaglandin $F_{2\alpha}$ seems to be critical to ovulation. Concentrations of this prostaglandin in rabbit preovulatory follicular fluid increase more than 60-fold, whereas prostaglandin $E_2$ levels increase only 15-fold (LeMaire *et al.*, 1973). Moreover, treatment with prostaglandin $F_{2\alpha}$ induces ovulation in *in vitro* perfused rabbit ovaries (Holmes *et al.*, 1983) and is also effective in *in vivo* when given as a direct intrafollicular injection (Moon & Armstrong, 1974). In contrast, treatment with prostaglandin $E_2$ does not stimulate ovulation and even inhibits hCG- or LH-stimulated ovulation *in vitro* (Hamada *et al.*, 1977; Schmidt *et al.*, 1986a). Prostaglandin $F_{2\alpha}$ is also implicated as the ovulatory prostaglandin in sheep (Murdoch, 1985).

There is no direct evidence concerning the relative importance of prostaglandin $F_{2\alpha}$ and prostaglandin $E_2$ in human ovulation. Follicular fluid prostaglandin $F_{2\alpha}$ levels increase whereas prostaglandin $E_2$ levels decrease during the interval between onset of the LH surge and ovulation (Sechel *et al.*, 1984). In one study, prostaglandin $E_2$ was shown to decrease collagen synthesis in the apical area of incubated follicular wall tissue but the effect of prostaglandin $F_{2\alpha}$ was not examined (Dennefors *et al.*, 1982).

There could also be an active role for prostaglandin $I_2$ in ovulation since this substance is reported to induce ovulation directly in the isolated perfused rabbit ovary (Yoshimura *et al.*, 1988a). Production of prostaglandin $I_2$ by human granulosa cells can be stimulated by activation of protein kinase C *in vitro* (Ranta *et al.*, 1986).

### Mechanism of prostaglandin involvement in ovulation

Prostaglandins appear to exert multiple effects at various levels within the ovaries to influence the process of follicular rupture.

*Follicular blood flow.* Prostaglandins have profound effects on haemo-dynamics. Blood flow to the ovaries increases within minutes after gonadotrophin stimulation, probably because of arteriolar vasodilation (Janson, 1975). Ovarian prostaglandin levels do not begin to rise until $2-4$ h after LH stimulation. It is therefore unlikely that prostaglandins are responsible for the immediate increase in blood flow but they may be important for longer-term vasodilatation and increased vascular permeability. Prostaglandin $E_2$ is a potent stimulator of vasodilation (Kaley, *et al.*, 1972) and it also causes increased vascular permeability (Crunkhorn & Willis, 1975). Local production of prostaglandin $E_2$ appears to mediate the increase in vascular permeability caused by various inflammatory factors which might be involved in ovulation, including histamine and bradykinin (Johnson *et al.*, 1976). Prostaglandin $I_2$ is generally a much more effective vasodilator than prostaglandin $E_2$ (Moncada & Vane, 1979). In *in vitro* perfused rabbit ovaries, prosta-glandin $I_2$ has been shown to induce dilatation and increased perme-ability of blood vessels in the microvasculature of preovulatory follicles, suggesting a vasoactive function during ovulation (Yoshimura *et al.*, 1988a). Prostaglandin $F_{2\alpha}$ may also participate in follicular rupture via a vasoconstrictive action in the apical region of the follicle wall, thereby promoting tissue breakdown at the site of eventual follicular rupture and stigma formation (Murdoch, 1985).

The increased capillary permeability caused by prostaglandin $E_2$ and $I_2$ could be important in increasing the efflux of plasma proteins such as plasminogen and kininogens and the extravasation of blood cells which may participate in ovulation (reviewed by Espey, 1980). It would also allow hydrodynamic communication to begin between the fluid-filled antral cavity and the surrounding vasculature, thereby gen-erating the protracted driving force which leads to expulsion of the oocyte following follicular rupture.

*Chemotaxis.* Prostaglandins exert chemotactic effects on leukocytes (Kaley & Weiner, 1971) which may be of importance to the ovulatory process since leukocytes secrete proteases (Weissman *et al.*, 1973). There is a preovulatory rise in the ovarian content of neutrophilic leukocytes which can be suppressed by indomethacin (Abisogun *et al.*, 1988).

*Steroidogenesis.* Prostaglandins $E_2$ and $I_2$ can mimic the stimulatory effect of LH on steroid production by preovulatory follicles (Armstrong, 1981; Band *et al.*, 1986). The initial increase in steroid production induced by LH may be dependent on the small increase in prostaglandin production which precedes it (Mori *et al.*, 1980), although this is uncertain (Munalulu *et al.*, 1987). In the *in vitro* perfused rabbit ovary, prostaglandin $F_{2\alpha}$ can induce follicular rupture without causing a detectable increase in steroid production (Holmes *et al.*, 1983), indicating that prostaglandin-induced changes in steroid synthesis are not of major importance to ovulation.

*Plasminogen activator.* Prostaglandins of the E type can stimulate the production of PA in cultured granulosa cells (Strickland & Beers, 1976) and treatment with indomethacin *in vivo* or of follicles *in vitro* suppresses PA secretion by rat ovarian tissue (Canipari & Strickland, 1986; Liu & Cajander, 1988). Given the importance of proteolysis to the tissue-remodelling which precedes follicular rupture, increased PA activity in response to locally produced prostaglandin formation could be a significant factor in the overall mechanism of ovulation (see below).

*Collagenolysis.* Collagenase activity may also be regulated by prostaglandins (Reich *et al.*, 1985c). Prostaglandins do not appear to increase procollagenase synthesis; rather they enhance proteolytic conversion of the proenzyme to active collagenase, possibly by stimulating PA activity (Curry *et al.*, 1986) (see Fig. 5.5).

*Neuromusculature.* Adrenergic nerves and smooth muscle-like cells in the follicle wall may participate in the process of ovulation (Owman *et al.*, 1975) (see below). Prostaglandin $F_{2\alpha}$ has a direct stimulatory effect on ovarian contractility (Virutamasen *et al.*, 1972a) whereas prostaglandin $E_2$ seems to be inhibitory (Hamada *et al.*, 1977). Prostaglandin $F_{2\alpha}$ also potentiates the contractile response to electrical nerve stimulation (Hedqvist, 1977; Walles *et al.*, 1986), suggesting an influence on neurotransmitter release.

*Kallikreins.* Locally produced prostaglandins appear to regulate the activities of bradykinin-forming kallikrein enzymes, since treatment with indomethacin inhibits the rise in kinin generating capacity during preovulatory follicular development in the rat ovary (Espey *et al.*, 1985). However, prostaglandin synthesis does not seem to be required

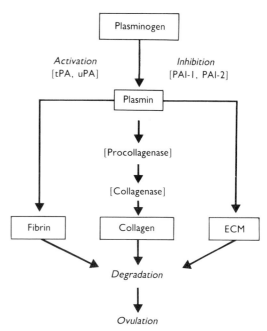

**Fig. 5.5.** The PA system and its proposed role in the disintegration of the follicle wall. The inactive proenzyme, plasminogen is produced in the liver and is present in follicular fluid at the same high concentrations as in plasma. The two PAs, urokinase (uPA) and tissue-type (tPA) are serine proteases produced by granulosa cells capable of cleaving plasminogen and converting it into plasmin which is an active trypsin-like enzyme with broad substrate specificity. Plasminogen activation probably reflects a balance between the actions of PAs and specific plasminogen activator inhibitors (PAI-1, PAI-2). Plasmin degrades fibrin and may be involved in collagenolysis (Types I, II and IV) by activating procollagenase. Plasmin also exerts a lytic effect on extracellular matrix (ECM) proteins such as laminin and fibronectin. Collectively, these proteolytic changes in the follicle wall are crucial to ovulation.

for exogenous bradykinin to exert its ovulation-inducing effect in the *in vitro* perfused rabbit ovary (Yoshimura *et al.*, 1988b).

### Leukotrienes

Products of the lipoxygenase pathway of arachidonic acid metabolism are also implicated in the ovulatory process. Lipoxygenase activity has been detected in the rat ovary (Reich *et al.*, 1985a) and human granulosa cells (Feldman *et al.*, 1986). The activity in rat preovulatory follicular extracts rose fivefold after hCG stimulation to induce ovulation (Reich *et al.*, 1985a). Furthermore, intrabursal injection of lipoxygenase inhibitors reduced the number of hCG-induced ovulations in PMSG-primed rats (Reich *et al.*, 1983). On the other hand, presence of lipoxygenase inhibitors increased the LH-induced ovulation rate in isolated perfused rabbit ovaries (Hellberg *et al.*, 1990).

Although the exact function of leukotrienes in ovulation is not clear, they are implicated in several ways. In rats, lipoxygenase inhibitors have been shown to inhibit hCG-induced collagenolysis (Reich *et al.*, 1985c) and suppress the preovulatory increase in ovarian content of neutrophil leukocytes (Abisogun *et al.*, 1988). Lipoxygenase products have been shown to affect non-ovarian tissues in various ways which would have implications for ovulation if they can be shown to operate in the ovary, including increased leukocytic chemotaxis (Ford-Hutchinson *et al.*, 1980), and increased vascular permeability and dilatation (Björk *et al.*, 1982; Ford-Hutchinson *et al.*, 1981), Leukotrienes C4 and D4 have been shown to stimulate synthesis of platelet-activating factor (PAF) in human endothelial cells (McIntyre *et al.*, 1986) and ovarian PAF activity is now strongly implicated in the process of follicular rupture.

## Platelet-activating factor

Ovulation has been likened to an inflammatory response (Espey, 1980) and factors which influence inflammation are thought to be involved in follicular rupture. PAF is a phospholipid released locally by a number of cell types during an inflammatory response. Recently, evidence was provided for the participation of PAF in ovulation (Abisogun *et al.*, 1989). In PMSG-primed rats, hCG-induced ovulation rate was dose-dependently decreased by intrabursal injection of a specific PAF antagonist. Moreover, the blockade of ovulation was reversed by concomitant administration of PAF. Ovarian PAF activity decreases during the process of follicular rupture, possibly due to local release of the factor. Changes in ovarian levels of PAF inhibitors have also been implicated in the local regulation of PAF activity (Espey *et al.*, 1989). Diverse cell types in the ovaries are likely sites of production and release of PAF, including fibroblasts (Michel *et al.*, 1988), endothelial cells (Henson, 1987) and mast cells (Mencia-Huerta *et al.*, 1983).

The precise role of PAF in ovulation is not clear. PAF activity may contribute to the preovulatory increase in vascular permeability (Humprey *et al.*, 1984; Rubin *et al.*, 1988), and it has also been associated with increased collagenolysis (Abisogun *et al.*, 1989). PAF may also stimulate prostaglandin production in the follicle wall, similar to its action on non-ovarian tissues (Weismann *et al.*, 1988). This is suggested by the evidence that blockade of hCG-induced ovulation in PMSG-primed rats due to treatment with indomethacin can be reversed by intrabursal injection of PAF (Abisogun *et al.*, 1989).

## Proteases

The structural and biochemical changes in the follicle wall which culminate in its rupture are largely the consequences of tissue remodelling brought about by the actions of hormonally regulated proteolytic enzymes such as PAs, collagenases and various kinins.

### *Plasminogen activators*

PAs are selective serine proteases which convert plasminogen, an inactive zymogen present in high concentrations in most extracellular fluids, including follicular fluid (Beers, 1975), into plasmin. Plasmin is a protease with broad substrate specificity and one of its main actions is to proteolytically activate collagenase by cleavage of extracellular procollagenase (Wooley, 1984) (Fig. 5.5).

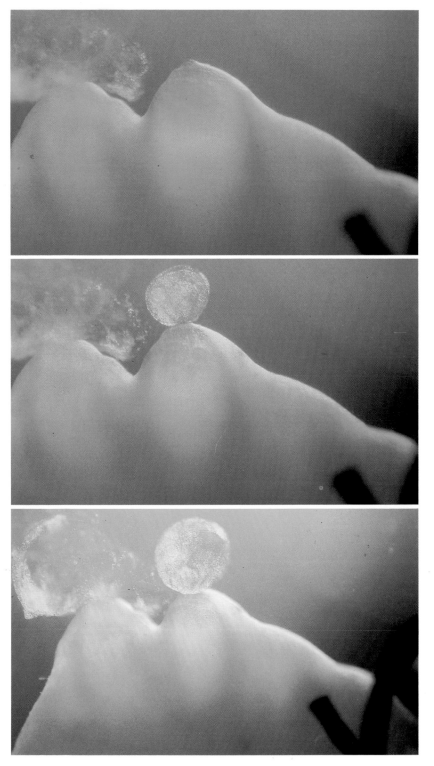

**Plate 5.1.** Ovulation in the *in vitro* perfused rabbit ovary. The time period covered in the figure is *c.* 3 min. From a cinematographic recording by Carl O. Löfman.

*Evidence for the involvement of PAs in ovulation*

The product of PA action, plasmin, decreases the tensile strength of the follicular wall (Beers, 1975). Various inhibitors of PA and plasmin activity and substances that inhibit the conversion of plasminogen to plasmin have been shown to inhibit ovulation *in vivo* (Akazawa *et al.*, 1982; Reich *et al.*, 1985b) and *in vitro* (Ichikawa *et al.*, 1983; Yoshimura *et al.*, 1987b; Morioka *et al.* 1988). Moreover, streptokinase, an exogenous PA, induces ovulation in the *in vitro* perfused rabbit ovary (Yoshimura *et al.*, 1987b) while intrabursal administration of antibodies to tissue PA suppresses ovulation rate in PMSG/hCG primed rats (Tsafriri *et al.* 1989).

In rat ovaries, a large (3−14-fold) preovulatory increase in PA activity occurs shortly before follicular rupture, after which the activity subsides (Espey *et al.*, 1985; Canipari & Strickland, 1985; Liu *et al.*, 1987a). This increase in PA activity has been localized to the apical region of preovulatory follicles where stigmata eventually develop (Akazawa *et al.*, 1983; Smokovits *et al.*, 1988).

*Hormonal control of PA activity*

Treatment with gonadotrophin *in vitro* stimulates PA activity in isolated follicles (Reich *et al.*, 1985b), granulosa cells (Beers *et al.*, 1975; Knecht, 1988), cumulus−oocyte complexes (Liu & Hsueh, 1987) and theca cells (Liu *et al.*, 1987a; Liu, 1988). FSH induces PA mRNA expression during granulosa cell differentiation and LH promotes PA activity in thecal and luteinized granulosa cells (O'Connell *et al.*, 1987; Ohlsson *et al.*, 1988). Other factors which enhance granulosa cell PA activity include GnRH (Hsueh *et al.*, 1988), relaxin (Too *et al.*, 1984), vasoactive intestinal peptide (Liu *et al.*, 1987b), prostaglandins $E_1$ and $E_2$ (Strickland & Beers, 1976), and epidermal growth factor (EGF) (LaPolt *et al.*, 1989). There is evidence that both the cAMP/protein kinase A (Beers *et al.*, 1975) and the PI/protein kinase C (Belin *et al.*, 1984) second-messenger systems are involved in induction of PA synthesis.

*Modulation of PA activity*

Stimulation of PA synthesis by gonadotrophins may be subject to modulation by locally produced steroids. Steroids by themselves do not induce granulosa cell PA production (Beers & Strickland, 1977) but oestradiol (Reich *et al.*, 1985b), androgens and progestins (Ny *et al.*, 1985) augment gonadotrophin-induced PA synthesis. Prostaglandins are also implicated as local modulators of PA production (Shimada *et al.*, 1983; Canipari & Strickland, 1986) although this seems to be equivocal (Reich *et al.*, 1985b; Espey *et al.*, 1985; Liu & Cajander, 1988).

Changes in PA inhibitor levels may also contribute to net PA activity during the preovulatory period (Liu, 1988). Specific PA inhibitors, PAI-1 and PAI-2, have been partially characterized and identified in several tissues including the ovary (Ny *et al.*, 1985). PA is also inhibited by general serine protease inhibitors such as $\alpha_2$-macroglobulin, $\alpha_1$-antitrypsin, antithrombin III, and $\alpha_2$-antiplasmin, although it seems unlikely that these substances play specific roles as inhibitors of PA activity in the follicle wall (Dano *et al.*, 1985).

### Which PA-type is involved in follicular rupture?

It is uncertain whether urokinase-type PA (uPA) or tissue-type PA (tPA) activity is involved in ovulation. tPA is strongly implicated because it is the main form of PA which accumulates in gonadotrophin-stimulated follicles (Reich *et al.*, 1986). Granulosa and theca/interstitial cells secrete maximal amounts of tPA but not uPA *in vitro* when harvested shortly before follicular rupture (Liu *et al.*, 1987a). Moreover, intrabursal injection of a specific tPA antibody has been shown to suppress ovulation in the rat (Tsafriri *et al.*, 1989). tPA is dependent on the presence of fibrin for its activity, therefore it might be involved in directional proteolysis (Dano *et al.*, 1988) during angiogenesis in the ruptured follicle when blood clots and fibrin are present.

uPA may also be important to ovulation because it is released in larger quantities than tPA by isolated preovulatory follicles (Canipari & Strickland, 1985). Moreover, treatment with indomethacin to block ovulation *in vivo* reduced subsequent follicular secretion *in vitro* of uPA, but not tPA (Canipari & Strickland, 1986).

### Collagenases

Collagenous layers provide the follicular wall with most of its tensile strength (Fig. 5.2) and the collagen fibres in these layers must be degraded by specific collagenase enzymes to permit rupture to occur. Extracellular collagen is initially acted upon by true collagenases: metalloproteinases which cleave native collagen at neutral pH (Gross & Lapière, 1962). The enzyme protein is secreted as a latent procollagenase, which can be activated through limited proteolysis by proteinases such as cathepsin B, kallikrein and plasmin (Eeckhout & Vaes, 1977). Collagenases cleave collagen at specific sites to yield polypeptide fragments which are susceptible to further degradation by several different proteinases (Wooley, 1984). Collagenase activity may be subject to negative regulation by several inhibitory factors including a serum $\alpha_2$-macroglobulin (Eisen *et al.*, 1971), a tissue inhibitor of metalloproteinase (TIMP: Cawston *et al.*, 1983) (see below) and a third inhibitor which has not yet been fully characterized (Woessner *et al.*, 1989).

*Evidence for activation of collagenase and collagenolysis in ovulation*

Dissociation and fragmentation of collagen and a threefold decrease in the density of collagen fibres occurs in the rabbit follicle wall near the time of ovulation (Espey, 1967). Similar preovulatory changes have also been observed in the tunica albuginea (Bjersing & Cajander, 1974e) and in the apical region of the follicle wall in mouse (Downs & Longo, 1983), hamster (Martin *et al.*, 1983) and rat (Tsujimoto *et al.*, 1982) ovaries. The amount of collagen in the rat preovulatory follicle also declines during the hours leading up to ovulation (Morales *et al.*, 1983; Reich *et al.*, 1985c).

A number of early studies failed to show a preovulatory increase in collagenase levels or enzyme activity (reviewed by Espey, 1974) and no conclusion could be drawn concerning the specific role of collagenases in ovulation. However, it is now known that ovulation in the *in vitro* perfused rat ovary is inhibited by the presence of a specific collagenase inhibitor, supporting the concept that collagenases have specific functions which contribute to the breakdown of the follicle wall before ovulation (Brännström *et al.*, 1988).

*Regulation of collagenase activity*

Tissue collagenolytic activity is influenced by a number of factors including changes in synthesis, activation and degradation of the enzyme as well as presence of collagenase inhibitors. Preovulatory increases in collagenase enzyme activity have been measured in ovarian and follicular extracts (Curry *et al.*, 1985; Reich *et al.*, 1985c) and the activity can be stimulated by treatment with hCG (Curry *et al.*, 1985; Palotie *et al.*, 1987). Gonadotrophic control of collagenase inhibition also occurs. Rat granulosa cells undertake LH-responsive production of the serine protease inhibitor TIMP *in vitro* (Slackman *et al.*, 1986), and ovarian TIMP activity increases (LeMaire *et al.*, 1987) at around the same time as collagenase levels do following stimulation *in vivo* with LH (Curry *et al.*, 1985). However, the LH-stimulated increase in TIMP appears to be less than the corresponding increase in collagenase synthesis, such that before ovulation a net increase occurs in the ovarian content of uninhibited collagenase enzyme.

Collagenolytic activity may also be regulated by prostaglandins (Dowsett *et al.*, 1976) and leukotrienes. Thus treatment *in vitro* with inhibitors of cyclooxygenase (Kawamura *et al.*, 1984, 1986) or lipoxygenase (Reich *et al.*, 1985c) suppress the preovulatory rise in ovarian collagenolytic activity as well as ovulation in rabbit and rat ovaries. The action of prostaglandin appears to be at the level of enzyme activation rather than synthesis of the procollagenase molecule (Curry *et al.*, 1986).

## Follicular localization of collagenases

The mechanism by which the digestion of collagen is localized to the apical portion of the follicle wall is not understood. Region-specific factors could: (1) increased production of procollagenase and/or PA; (2) raised levels of uPA receptors include; (3) reduced production of collagenase inhibitor(s). It is still uncertain if granulosa cells actually secrete procollagenase, although collagenolytic activity is present in rat (Too *et al.*, 1984) and human (Fukumoto *et al.*, 1981) granulosa cells as well as in human preovulatory follicular fluid (Puistola *et al.*, 1986). Other likely cellular sites of procollagenase formation in the ovaries are fibroblasts (Birkedahl-Hansen *et al.*, 1976a), germinal epithelial cells (Bjersing & Cajander, 1974a), capillary endothelial cells (Herron *et al.*, 1986), extravasated polymorphnuclear leukocytes (Kruze & Wojtecka, 1972), and macrophages (Birkedahl-Hansen *et al.*, 1976b).

## *Bradykinin*

Bradykinin and other kinins are small proteolytic peptides produced locally from circulating kininogens. Kinins are implicated in ovulation by the preovulatory rise in kallikreins (kinin-forming enzymes) which occurs in the rat ovary (Espey *et al.*, 1986; Smith & Perks, 1983a). A reciprocal decline in plasma kininogen levels occurs during the preovulatory period (McDonald & Perks, 1976; Smith & Perks, 1983b) and kinins have been detected in the follicular fluid of several species (Ramwell *et al.*, 1970). Moreover, experiments with *in vitro* perfused ovaries have shown that treatment with bradykinin induces ovulation in its own right (Yoshimura *et al.*, 1988b) and enhances the ovulatory response to LH (Brännström & Hellberg, 1989).

The mechanism through which bradykinin exerts its stimulatory effect on ovulation remains to be clarified. Bradykinin increases production of prostaglandins in ovarian (Yoshimura *et al.*, 1988b) and vascular tissues (Charo *et al.*, 1984) and this could be of importance in promoting preovulatory hyperaemia and vascular permeability in the ovaries. However, inhibition of prostaglandin synthesis by treatment with indomethacin does not block bradykinin-induced ovulation in the *in vitro* perfused rabbit ovary (Yoshimura *et al.*, 1988b).

Another possible mechanism of bradykinin action is to increase ovarian contractility at the time of follicular rupture. This is suggested by studies on the isolated rat ovary showing that exogenous bradykinin stimulates ovarian contractility and that sensitivity to bradykinin is highest during the period immediately before ovulation (Smith & Perks, 1984).

The preovulatory increase in ovarian kallikrein may also bring about increased tissue levels of PA, plasmin or collagenase, as well as inducing kinin production (Arrigoni-Martelli, 1977; Eeckhout & Vaes,

1977; Movat, 1979). Bradykinin has also been shown to stimulate histamine release by mast cells (Douglas, 1980), which could also have implications for follicular rupture, as discussed below.

## *Renin–angiotensin*

The ovaries also produce renin, a proteolytic enzyme which regulates local production of angiotensin II. This octapeptide, best known as a smooth muscle vasoconstrictor and stimulant of aldosterone production by the adrenals, is present in high concentrations in human follicular fluid (Culler *et al.*, 1986). Rat granulosa cells express receptors for angiotensin II (Hussain *et al.*, 1987) and there is evidence that the peptide negatively regulates progesterone synthesis in bovine luteal cells (Stirling *et al.*, 1990). However, the role (if any) of angiotensin in follicular rupture is uncertain.

## Histamine

Enzymic degradation of the follicular wall preceding ovulation is a form of controlled tissue damage. Histamine is released from tissues when they are injured causing capillary dilatation and increased blood flow, factors which are of great importance in the process of follicular rupture.

Histamine is stored in granules, mostly in tissue-bound mast cells and in circulating basophilic leukocytes and platelets. In the ovary, mast cells are present in the stroma around the blood vessels in the hilar region and are also present in the endothelial cells of small blood vessels (Jones *et al.*, 1980). Cyclic changes in ovarian histamine concentrations have been reported in women (Morikawa *et al.*, 1981), rabbits (Morikawa *et al.*, 1976), hamsters (Krishna & Terranova, 1985) and rats (Schmidt *et al.*, 1988b). In rat ovaries, there is a preovulatory decrease in histamine content (Szego & Gitin, 1964; Schmidt *et al.*, 1988b) which is associated with a corresponding reduction in the granulation of ovarian mast cells (Jones *et al.*, 1980). Additional evidence for the involvement of histamine in ovulation is that treatment with exogenous histamine induces ovulations in *in vitro* perfused rabbit (Kobayashi *et al.*, 1983) and rat (Schmidt *et al.*, 1986b) ovaries and is also effective *in vivo* (Batta, 1980). Moreover, LH-induced ovulation *in vitro* was partially suppressed by the presence of $H_1$ or $H_2$ receptor antagonists in the perfusion medium (Schmidt *et al.* 1988b).

Histamine could facilitate ovulation by causing a dilatation of precapillary arterioles and increasing the permeability of postcapillary venules, thereby facilitating the acute increase in ovarian blood flow which is initiated by the LH surge (Piacsek & Huth, 1971; Harvey & Owen, 1979).

# Neuromuscular mechanisms

Increased ovarian contractility has long been implicated in the process of follicular rupture and the extrusion of the oocyte (reviewed by Espey, 1978). Smooth muscle cells present in the theca externa and in the stroma surrounding ovarian follicles (Oswaldo-Decima, 1970; Okamura et al., 1972) and spontaneous ovarian contractions have been recorded in several species (Coutinho & Maia, 1972; Virutamasen et al., 1972b). Autonomic nerves form a network around individual ovarian follicles, localized to outer regions of the theca externa. The distance between nerve terminals and the smooth muscle cells is small enough to suggest that they are functionally linked (Owman et al., 1975). Studies with incubated follicular strips from bovine ovaries have shown that contraction of the follicle wall is mediated via $\alpha$-adrenergic receptors, and relaxation via $\beta$-adrenergic receptors (Walles et al., 1975). Intrabursal administration of $\alpha$-adrenergic agonists increases ovulation number in the rat ovary (Kannisto et al., 1985).

Prostaglandins also appear to influence ovarian contractility. Treatment in vitro with prostaglandin $F_{2\alpha}$ increases the spontaneous contractility of the rabbit ovary whereas prostaglandin $E_2$ is inhibitory (Virutamasen et al., 1972a). Other studies point to a role for serotonin in follicular rupture (Clausell & Soliman, 1977; Schmidt et al., 1988a) which may also entail an effect on ovarian contractility (Kannisto et al., 1987).

Evidence against a role of the ovarian neuromusculature in ovulation is that denervation of the ovary does not affect ovulation rate in the rat (Wylie et al., 1985). Moreover, inhibition of smooth muscle contractions by $Ca^{2+}$-deprivation (Kobayashi et al., 1984) or blockade of $Ca^{2+}$ channels (Kitai et al., 1985) does not affect hCG-induced ovulation number in the in vitro perfused rabbit ovary.

# Summary

Preovulatory follicular development culminates in rupture of the follicle wall and extrusion of the mature oocyte (Fig. 5.6). Ovulation is initiated by the mid-cycle LH surge and can be induced by the administration of exogenous hCG. The biochemical basis of ovulation induction by LH/hCG depends on the activation of diverse second-messenger systems in thecal and granulosa cells, leading to increases in proteolytic enzyme activities which reduce the tensile strength of the apical region of the follicle wall. Cellular events activated by LH/hCG include increased production of cAMP, steroids, prostaglandins, leukotrienes, PAF, kinins, PAs and collagenases. Locally produced prostaglandins appear to be primarily responsible for the increase in vascular permeability which sustains positive intrafollicular pressure during the period when follicular fluid begins to leak through the partially digested follicular wall. A

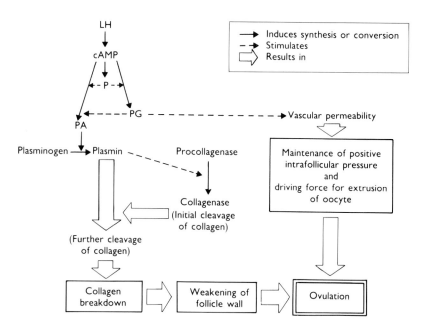

**Fig. 5.6.** Schematic outline of the ovulatory process.

gradual reduction in the tensile strength of the follicular wall eventually leads to its complete rupture; the flow of follicular fluid and vascular transudate then carries the cumulus-enclosed oocyte out of the follicle on to the surface of the ovary.

## Acknowledgements

This study was supported by grants from the Swedish Medical Research Council (projects 0027 and 4982).

## References

Abisogun, A.O., Braquet, P. & Tsafriri, A. (1989) The involvement of platelet activating factor in ovulation. *Science*, **243**, 381−3.

Abisogun, A.O., Daphna-Iken, D. & Tsafriri, A. (1988) Periovulatory changes in ovarian follicular neutrophils: modulation by eicosanoids. *Endocrinology*, Suppl. **122**, 291 (Abstr. 1083).

Akazawa, K., Matsuo, O., Kosugi, T., Mihara H. & Mori, N. (1982) The role of plasminogen activator in ovulation. *Acta Physiol. Pharmacol. Latinoam.* **33**, 105−10.

Akazawa, K., Mori, N., Kosugi, T., Matsuo, O. & Mihara, H. (1983) Localization of fibrinolytic activity in ovulation of the rat follicle as determined by the fibrin slide method. *Jpn. J. Physiol.*, **33**, 1011−18.

Armstrong, D.T. (1981) Prostaglandins and follicular functions. *J. Reprod. Fertil.*, **62**, 283−91.

Armstrong, D.T., Dorrington, J.H. & Robinson, J.

(1976) Effects of indomethacin and aminoglutethimide phosphate *in vivo* on luteinizing-hormone induced alterations of cyclic adenosine monophosphate, prostaglandin F and steroid levels in preovulatory rat ovaries. *Can. J. Biochem.*, **54**, 796−802.

Armstrong, D.T. & Grinwich, D.L. (1972) Blockade of spontaneous and LH-induced ovulation in rats by indomethacin, an inhibitor of prostaglandin biosynthesis. *Prostaglandins*, **1**, 21−8.

Amsterdam, A.A., Koch, Y., Lieberman, M.E. & Lindner, H.R. (1975). Distribution of binding sites for human chorionic gonadotropin in the preovulatory follicle of the rat. *J. Biol. Chem.* **67**, 894−900.

Arrigoni-Martelli, E. (1977) *Inflammation and Antiinflammatories*. Spectrum, New York.

Band, V., Kharbanda, S.M., Murugesan, K. & Farooq,

A. (1986) Prostacyclin and steroidogenesis in goat ovarian cell types *in vitro*. *Prostaglandins*, **31**, 509−25.

Baranczuk, R.J. & Fainstat, T. (1976) *In vitro* ovulation from adult hamster ovary. *Am. J. Obstet. Gynecol.*, **124**, 517−22.

Batta, S.K. (1980) Effect of histamine, phenycyclidine, phenoxybenzamine and gamma-aminobutyric acid on ovulation and quality of ova in rats. *Reproduction*, **4**, 99−107.

Bauminger, S., Lieberman, M.E. & Lindner, H.R. (1975) Steroid-independent effect of gonadotropins on prostaglandin synthesis in rat Graafian follicles *in vitro*. *Prostaglandins*, **9**, 753−64.

Bauminger, S. & Lindner, H.R. (1975) Periovulatory changes in ovarian prostaglandin formation and their hormonal control in the rat. *Prostaglandins*, **9**, 737−51.

Beers, W.H. (1975) Follicular plasminogen and plasminogen activator and the effect of plasmin on ovarian follicle wall. *Cell*, **6**, 379−86.

Beers W.H. & Strickland, S. (1977) Involvement of plasminogen activator in ovulation. In Spitman, C.W. & Wilks, J.W. (eds) *Novel Aspects of Reproductive Physiology*, pp. 13−36. Halstead Press, New York.

Beers, W.H., Strickland, S. & Reich, E. (1975) Ovarian plasminogen activator: relationship to ovulation and hormonal regulation. *Cell*, **6**, 387−94.

Belin, D., Godeau, F. & Vassalli, J.-D. (1984) Tumor promotor PMA stimulate the synthesis and secretion of mouse pro-urokinase in MSV transformed 3T3 cells: this is mediated by an increase in urokinase mRNA content. *EMBO J.*, **3**, 1901−6.

Birkedal-Hansen, H., Cobb, C.M., Taylor, R.E. & Fullmer, H.M. (1976a) Activation of fibroblasts procollagenase by mast cell proteases. *Biochem. Biophys. Acta*, **483**, 273−86.

Birkedal-Hansen, H., Cobb, C.M., Taylor R.E. & Fullmer, H.M. (1976b) Synthesis and release of procollagenase by cultured fibroblasts. *J. Biol. Chem.*, **251**, 3162−8.

Bjersing, L. & Cajander, S. (1974a) Ovulation and the mechanism of follicle rupture. I. Light microscopic changes in rabbit ovarian follicles prior to induced ovulation. *Cell. Tiss. Res.*, **149**, 287−300.

Bjersing, L. & Cajander, S. (1974b) Ovulation and the mechanism of follicle rupture. II. Scanning electron microscopy of rabbit germinal epithelium prior to induced ovulation. *Cell. Tiss. Res.*, **149**, 301−12.

Bjersing, L. & Cajander, S. (1974c) Ovulation and the mechanism of follicular rupture III. Transmission electron microscopy of rabbit germinal epithelium prior to induced ovulation. *Cell. Tiss. Res.*, **149**, 313−27.

Bjersing, L. & Cajander, S. (1974d) Ovulation and the mechanism of follicle rupture. IV. Ultrastructure of membrana granulosa of rabbit Graafian follicles prior to induced ovulation. *Cell. Tiss. Res.*, **153**, 1−14.

Bjersing, L. & Cajander, S. (1974e) Ovulation and the mechanism of follicle rupture. V. Ultrastructure of tunica albuginea and theca externa of rabbit Graafian follicles prior to induced ovulation. *Cell. Tiss. Res.*, **153**, 15−30.

Bjersing, L. & Cajander, S. (1974f) Ovulation and the mechanism of follicle rupture. VI. Ultrastructure of theca interna and the inner vascular network surrounding rabbit Graafian follicles prior to induced ovulation. *Cell. Tiss. Res.*, **153**, 31−44.

Björk, J., Hedqvist, P. & Arfors, K.-E. (1982) Increase in vascular permeability induced by leukotriene B4 and the role of polymorphnuclear leukocytes. *Inflammation*, **6**, 189−200.

Brännström, M., Boberg, B.M., Törnell, J., Janson, P.O. & Ahrén, K. (1989a) Effects of inhibitors of protein synthesis on the ovulatory process of the perfused rat ovary. *J. Reprod. Fertil.*, **85**, 451−9.

Brännström, M. & Hellberg, P. (1989) Bradykinin potentiates LH-induced follicular rupture in the *in vitro* perfused rat ovary. *Human Reprod.* **4**, 475−81.

Brännström, M. & Janson, P.O. (1989) Progesterone is a mediator in the ovulatory process of the *in vitro* perfused rat ovary. *Biol. Reprod.* **40**, 1170−8.

Brännström, M., Johansson, B.M., Sogn, J. & Janson, P.O. (1987a) Characterization of an *in vitro* perfused rat ovary model: ovulation rate, oocyte maturation, steroidogenesis and influence of PMSG priming. *Acta Physiol. Scand.*, **130**, 107−14.

Brännström, M., Koos, R.D., LeMaire, W.J. & Janson, P.O. (1987b) Cyclic adenosine 3′,5′-monophosphate-induced ovulation in the perfused rat ovary and its mediation by prostaglandins. *Biol. Reprod.*, **37**, 1047−53.

Brännström M., Larson, L., Basta, B. & Hedin, L. (1989b) Regulation of prostaglandin endoperoxide synthase by cyclic adenosine 3′,5′-monophosphate in the in vitro perfused rat ovary. *Biol. Reprod.* **41**, 513−21.

Brännström, M., Woessner, J.F., Koos, R.D., Sear, C.H.J. & LeMaire, W.J. (1988) Inhibitors of mammalian tissue collagenase and metalloproteinases suppress ovulation in the perfused rat ovary. *Endocrinology*, **122**, 1715-21.

Bruce, N.W. & Moor, R.M. (1976) Capillary blood flow to ovarian follicles, stroma and corpora lutea of anesthetized sheep. *J. Reprod. Fertil.*, **46**, 299−304.

Bullock, D.W. & Kappauf, B.H. (1973) Dissociation of gonadotropin-induced ovulation and steroidogenesis in immature rats. *Endocrinology*, **92**, 1625−8.

Cajander, S. & Bjersing, L. (1975) Fine structural demonstration of acid phosphatase in rabbit germinal epithelium prior to induced ovulation. *Cell. Tiss. Res.*, **164**, 279−89.

Canipari, R. & Strickland, S. (1985) Plasminogen activator in the rat ovary. Production and gonadotropin regulation of the enzyme in granulosa and thecal cells. *J. Biol. Chem.*, **260**, 5121−5.

Canipari, R. & Strickland, S. (1986) Studies on the hormonal regulation of plasminogen activator production in the rat ovary. *Endocrinology*, **118**, 1652−9.

Cawston, T.E., Murphy, G., Mercer, E., Galloway, W.A., Hazleman, B.L. & Reynolds, J.J. (1983) The interaction of purified rabbit bone collagenase with purified rabbit bone metalloproteinase inhibitor. *Biochem. J.*, **211**, 313−18.

Charo, I.F., Shak, S., Karasek, M.A., Davison, P.M. & Goldstein, I.M. (1984) Prostaglandin $I_2$ is not a major metabolite of arachidonic acid in cultured endothelial cells from human foreskin microvessels. *J. Clin. Invest.*, **74**, 914−19.

Clark, M.R., Hillensjö, T., Marsh, J.M. & LeMaire W.J. (1981) Hormonal regulation of prostaglandin synthesis in rat granulosa cells. In Mahesh & Muldoon (eds) *Functional Correlates of Hormone Receptors in Reproduction*, pp. 275−90. Elsevier North-Holland, Amsterdam.

Clark, M.R., Marsh, J.M. & LeMaire, W.J. (1976) The role of protein synthesis in the stimulation by LH of prostaglandin accumulation in rat preovulatory follicles *in vitro*. *Prostaglandins*, **12**, 209−16.

Clark, M.R., Marsh, J.M. & LeMaire, W.J. (1978a) Stimulation of prostaglandin accumulation in preovulatory rat follicles by adenosine 3',5'-monophosphate. *Endocrinology*, **102**, 39−44.

Clark, M.R., Marsh, J.M. & LeMaire, W.J. (1978b) Mechanism of luteinizing hormone regulation of prostaglandin synthesis in rat granulosa cells. *J. Biol. Chem.*, **253**, 7757−61.

Clausell, D.E. & Soliman, K.F.A. (1977) Ovarian serotonin content in relation to ovulation. *Experientia*, **34**, 410−11.

Coutinho, E.M. & Maia, H.S. (1972) Effects of gonadotrophins on motility of human ovary. *Nature*, **235**, 94−6.

Crunkhorn, P. & Willis, A.L. (1975) Actions and interactions of prostaglandins administered intradermally in rat and in man. *Br. J. Pharmacol.*, **36**, 216−17.

Culler, M.D., Tarlatzis, B.C., Lightman, A., Fernandez, L.A., DeCherney, A.H., Negro-Vilar, A. & Naftolin, F. (1986) Angiotensin II-like activity in human ovarian follicular fluid. *J. Clin. Endocrinol. Metab.*, **62**, 613−15.

Curry, T.E. Jr., Clark, M.R., Dean, D.D., Woessner, J.F. Jr. & LeMaire, W.J. (1986) The preovulatory increase in ovarian collagenase activity in the rat is independent of prostaglandin production. *Endocrinology*, **118**, 1823−8.

Curry, T.E. Jr., Dean, D.D., Woessner, J.F. Jr., & LeMaire, W.J. (1985) The extraction of a tissue collagenase associated with ovulation in the rat. *Biol. Reprod.*, **33**, 981−91.

Dano, K., Andreasen, P.A., Behrendt, N., Grondahl-Hansen, J., Kristensen, P. & Lund, L.R. (1988) Regulation of the urokinase pathway of plasmin-

ogen activation. In Parvinen, M., Huhtaniemi, I. & Pelliniemi, L.J. (eds) *Development and Function of the Reproductive Organs*, pp. 259−78. Raven Press, New York.

Dano, K., Andreasen, P.A., Grondahl-Hansen, J., Kristensen, P., Nielsen, L.S. & Skriver, L. (1985) A. Regulation of plasminogen activator synthesis. 1. Steroid hormones. *Adv. Cancer Res.*, **44**, 139−265.

Davis, J.S., Weakland, L.L., West, L.A. & Farese, R.V. (1986) Luteinizing hormone stimulates the formation of inositol trisphosphate and cyclic AMP in rat granulosa cells. Evidence for phospholipase C generated second messengers in the action of luteinizing hormone. *Biochem. J.*, **238**, 597−604.

Davis, J.S., West, L.A. & Farese, R.V. (1984) Effects of luteinizing hormone on phosphoinositide metabolism in rat granulosa cell. *J. Biol. Chem.*, **259**, 15028−34.

Dekel, N. & Kraicer, P.F. (1978) Induction *in vitro* of mucification of rat cumulus oophorus by gonadotrophins and adenosine 3',5'-monophosphate. *Endocrinology*, **102**, 1797−802.

Dennerfors, B., Tjugum, J., Norström, A., Janson, P.O., Nilsson, L., Hanberger, L. & Wilhelmsson, L. (1982) Collagen synthesis inhibition by prostaglandin $E_2$ within the human follicular wall − one possible mechanism underlying ovulation. *Prostaglandins*, **24**, 295−302.

Douglas, W.W. (1980) Polypeptides-angiotensin, plasma kinins and others. In Gilman, A.G., Goodman, L.S. & Gilman, A. (eds) *The Pharmacological Basis of Therapeutics*, pp. 659−63. MacMillan, New York.

Downs, S.M. & Longo, F.J. (1983) An ultrastructural study of preovulatory apical development in mouse ovarian follicles: effects of indomethacin. *Anat. Rec.*, **205**, 159−68.

Dowsett, M., Eastman, A.R., Easty, D.M., Easty, G.C., Powles, T.J. & Neville, A.M. (1976) Prostaglandin mediation of collagenase-induced bone resorption. *Nature*, **263**, 72−4.

Eeckhout, Y. & Vaes, G. (1977) Further studies on the activation of procollagenase, the latent precursor of bone collagenase. *Biochem. J.*, **166**, 21−31.

Eisen, A.Z., Bauer, E.A. & Jeffrey, J.J. (1971) Human skin collagenase. The role of serum alpha-globulins in the control of activity *in vivo* and *in vitro*. *Proc. Natl. Acad. Sci. USA*, **68**, 248−51.

Ellis, S. (1961) Bioassay of luteinizing hormone. *Endocrinology*, **68**, 334-40.

Espey, L.L (1967a) Ultrastructure of the apex of the rabbit Graafian follicle during the ovulatory process. *Endocrinology*, **81**, 267−76.

Espey, L.L. (1967b) Tenacity of porcine Graafian follicle as it approaches ovulation. *Am. J. Physiol.* **212**, 1397−401.

Espey, L.L. (1971) Decomposition of connective tissue in rabbit ovarian follicles by multivesicular structures of thecal fibroblasts. *Endocrinology*, **88**, 437−44.

Espey, L.L. (1974) Ovarian proteolytic enzymes and ovulation. *Biol. Reprod.*, **10**, 216–35.

Espey, L.L. (1978) Ovarian contractility and its relationship to ovulation: a review. *Biol. Reprod.*, **19**, 540–51.

Espey, L.L. (1980) Ovulation as an inflammatory reaction — a hypothesis. *Biol. Reprod.*, **22**, 73–106.

Espey, L.L. (1986) Simultaneous determination of ovarian prostaglandin $E_2$, prostaglandin $F_{2\alpha}$, 6-keto-prostaglandin $F_{1\alpha}$, β-estradiol and progesterone during ovulation in the PMSG/hCG primed immature rat. *Biol. Reprod.*, Suppl. **34**, Abstr. 125.

Espey, L.L. & Lipner, H. (1963) Measurements of intrafollicular pressures in the rabbit ovary. *Am. J. Physiol.*, **205**, 1067–72.

Espey, L.L., Miller, D.H. & Margolius, H.S. (1986) Ovarian increase in kinin-generating capacity in PMSG/hCG-primed immature rat. *Am. J. Physiol.*, **251**, 362–5.

Espey, L., Shimada, H., Okamura, H. & Mori, T. (1985) Effect of various agents on ovarian plasminogen activator activity during ovulation in pregnant mare's serum gonadotropin-primed immature rats. *Biol. Reprod.*, **32**, 1087–94.

Espey, L.L., Tanaka, N., Woodard, D.S., Harper, M.J.K. & Okamura, H. (1989) Decrease in ovarian platelet-activating factor during ovulation in the gonadotropin-primed immature rat. *Am. J. Physiol.* **257**, E1–7.

Feldman, E., Haberman, S., Abisogun, A.O., Reich, R., Levran, D., Masciach, S., Zuckerman, H. *et al.* (1986) Arachidonic acid metabolism in human granulosa cells: evidence for cyclooxygenase and lipoxygenase activity *in vitro*. *Hum. Reprod.*, **1**, 353–6.

Ford-Hutchinson, A.W., Bray, A.M. & Cunningham, F.M. (1981) Isomers of leukotriene B4 possess different biological activities. *Prostaglandins*, **21**, 143–52.

Ford-Hutchinson, A.W., Bray, M.A., Doig, M.V., Shipley, M.E. & Smith, M.J.H. (1980) Leukotriene B, a potent chemokinetic and aggregating substance released from polymorphnuclear leukocytes. *Nature*, **286**, 264–5.

Fukumoto, M., Yajima, Y., Okamura, H. & Midorikawa, O. (1981) Collagenolytic enzyme activity in human ovary: an ovulatory enzyme system. *Fertil. Steril.*, **36**, 746–50.

Fumagalli, Z., Motta, P. & Calvieri, S. (1971) The presence of smooth muscular cells in the ovary of several mammals as seen under the electron microscope. *Experientia*, **27**, 682–3.

Grinwich, D.L., Kennedy, T.G. & Armstrong, D.T. (1972) Dissociation of ovulatory and steroidogenic actions of luteinizing hormone in rabbits with indomethacin, an inhibitor of prostaglandin biosynthesis. *Prostaglandins*, **1**, 89–96.

Gross, J. & Lapière, C.M. (1962) Collagenolytic activity in amphibian tissues: A tissue culture assay.

*Proc. Natl. Acad. Sci. USA*, **48**, 1014–22.

Hamada, Y., Bronson, R.A., Wright, K.H. & Wallach, E.E. (1977) Ovulation in the perfused rabbit ovary: the influence of prostaglandins and prostaglandin inhibitors. *Biol. Reprod.*, **17**, 58–63.

Harms, P.G., Ojeda, S.R. & McCann, S.M. (1974) Prostaglandin-induced release of pituitary gonadotropins: central nervous system and pituitary sites of action. *Endocrinology*, **94**, 1459–64.

Harper, M.J.K. (1963) Ovulation in the rabbit: the time of follicular rupture and expulsion of the egg in relation to injection of luteinizing hormone. *J. Endocrinol.*, **26**, 307–16.

Harvey, C.A. & Owen, D.A.A. (1979) Effect of histamine on uterine vasculature in rats. *Eur. J. Pharmacol.*, **56**, 293–6.

Hedin, L., Gaddy-Kurten, D., Kurten, R., DeWitt, D.L., Smith, W.L. & Richards, J.S. (1987a) Prostaglandin endoperoxide synthase in rat ovarian follicles: content, cellular distribution, and evidence for hormonal induction preceding ovulation. *Endocrinology*, **121**, 722–31.

Hedin, L., McKnight, G.S., Lifka, J., Durica, J.M. & Richards, J.S. (1987b) Tissue distribution and hormonal regulation of messenger ribonucleic acid for regulatory and catalytic subunits of adenosine 3'5'-monophosphate-dependent protein kinases during ovarian follicular development and luteinization in the rat. *Endocrinology*, **120**, 1928–35.

Hedqvist, P. (1977) Basic mechanisms of prostaglandin action on autonomic neurotransmission. *Annu. Rev. Pharmacol. Toxicol.*, **1**, 259–79.

Hellberg, P., Holmes, P., Brännström, M., Janson, P.O. (1990) Inhibitors of lipoxygenase increase the ovulation rate in the in vitro perfused LH-stimulated rabbit ovary (in press).

Henson, P.M. (1987) Extracellular and intracellular activities of platelet activating factor. In Winslow, C.M. & Lee, M.L. (eds) *New Horizons in Platelet Activating Factor Research*, pp. 3–10. Wiley, New York,

Herron, G.S., Werb, Z., Dwyer, K. & Banda, M.J. (1986) Secretion of metalloproteinases by stimulated capillary endothelial cells. I. Production of procollagenase and prostromelysin exceeds expression of proteolytic activity. *J. Biol. Chem.*, **261**, 2810–13.

Hillier, S.G. (1985) Sex steroid metabolism and follicular development in the ovaries. *Oxf. Rev. Reprod. Biol.* **7**, 168–222.

Holmes, P.V., Hedin, L. & Janson, P.O. (1986) The role of cyclic adenosine 3',5'-monophosphate in the ovulatory process of the in vitro perfused rabbit ovary. *Endocrinology*, **118**, 2195–202.

Holmes, P.V., Janson, P.O., Sogn, J., Källfelt, B., LeMaire, W.J., Ahrén, K.B., Cajander, S. & Bjersing, L. (1983) Effects of prostaglandin-$F_{2\alpha}$ and indomethacin on ovulation and steroid production in the isolated perfused rabbit ovary. *Acta Endocrinol. Copenh.*, **104**, 233–9.

Homes, P.V., Sogn, J., Schillinger, E. & Janson, P.O.

(1985) Effects of high and low preovulatory concentrations of progesterone on ovulation from the isolated perfused rabbit ovary. *J. Reprod. Fertil.*, **75**, 393−9.

Hsueh, A.J.W., Liu, Y-X., Cajander, S., Peng, X-R., Dahl, K., Kristensen, P. & Ny, T. (1988) Gonadotropin-releasing hormone induces ovulation in hypophysectomized rats: studies on ovarian tissuetype plasminogen activator activity, messenger ribonucleic acid content, and cellular localization. *Endocrinology*, **122**, 1486−95.

Humphrey, D.M., McManus, L.M., Hanahan, D.J. & Pincard, R.N. (1984) Morphological basis of increased vascular permeability induced by acetyl glyceryl ether phosphorylcholine. *Lab. Invest.*, **50**, 16−25.

Huslig, R.L., Malik, A. & Clark, M.R. (1987) Human chorionic gonadotropin stimulation of immunoreactive prostaglandin synthase in the rat ovary. *Mol. Cell. Endocrinol.*, **50**, 237−46.

Hussain, A., Bumpus, F.M., De Silvia, P. & Speth, R.C. (1987) Localization of angiotensin II receptors in ovarian follicles and the identification of angiotensin II in rat ovaries. *Proc. Natl. Acad. Sci. USA*, **84**, 2489−93.

Ichikawa, S., Morioka, H., Ohta, M., Oda, K. & Murao, S. (1983) Effect of various proteinase inhibitors of ovulation of explanted hamster ovaries. *J. Reprod. Fertil.*, **68**, 407−12.

Iesaka, T., Sato, T. & Igarashi, M. (1975) Role of prostaglandin $F_{2\alpha}$ in ovulation. *Endocrinol. Jpn.*, **22**, 279−85.

Jahnsen, T., Lohmann, S.M., Walter, U., Hedin, L. & Richards, J.S. (1985) Purification and characterization of hormone-regulated isoforms of the regulatory subunit of type II cAMP-dependent protein kinase from rat ovaries. *J. Biol. Chem.*, **260**, 15980−7.

Janson, P.O. (1975) Effects of luteinizing hormone on blood flow in the follicullar rabbit ovary, as measured by radioactive microspheres. *Acta Endocrinol. Copenh.*, **79**, 122−33.

Janson, P.O (1988) Methodological and functional aspects of ovarian blood flow. In Ichinoe, K., Segal, S.J. & Mastrioanni, L. (eds) *Preservation of Tubo-Ovarian Function in Gynecologic Benign and Malignant Diseases*, pp. 163−76. Raven Press, New York.

Janson, P.O., LeMaire, W.J., Källfelt, B., Holmes, P.V., Cajander, S., Bjersing, L., Wiqvist, N. & Ahrén, K. (1982) The study of ovulation in the isolated perfused rabbit ovary. I. Methodology and pattern of steroidogenesis. *Biol. Reprod.*, **26**, 456−65.

Johnston, M.G., Hay, J.B. & Movat, H.Z. (1976) The modulation of enhanced vascular permeability by prostaglandins through alterations in blood flow (hyperemia). *Agents Actions*, **6**, 705−11.

Jones, R.E., Duvall, D. & Guiliette, L.J. Jr. (1980) Rat ovarian mast cells: distribution and cyclic changes. *Anat. Rec.*, **197**, 489−90.

Kaley, G., Messina, E.J., & Weiner, R. (1972) The role of prostaglandins in microcirculatory regulation and inflammation. In Ramwell, P.W. & Pharriss, B.B. (eds) *Prostaglandins in Cellular Biology*, pp. 309−27. Plenum Press, New York.

Kaley, G. & Weiner, R. (1971) Effect of prostaglandin $E_1$ on leukocyte migration. *Nature*, **234**, 114−15.

Kannisto, P., Owman, C., Schmidt, G. & Sjöberg, N.O. (1987) Characterization of presynaptic 5-HT receptors on adrenergic nerves supplying the bovine ovarian follicle. *Br. J. Pharmacol.*, **92**, 487−97.

Kannisto, P., Owman, C. & Walles, B. (1985) Involvement of local adrenergic receptors in the process of ovulation in gonadotrophin-primed immature rats. *J. Reprod. Fertil.*, **75**, 357−62.

Kanzaki, H. (1981) Scanning electron microscopic study of corrosion casts for rabbit ovarian follicle microvasculature during the ovulatory and luteinizing process. *Acta Obstet. Gynecol. Jpn.*, **33**, 1925−33.

Kanzaki, H., Okamura, H., Okuda Y., Takenaka, A., Morimoto, K. & Nishimura. T. (1982) Scanning electron microscopic study of rabbit ovarian follicle microvasculature using resin injection-corrosion casts. *J. Anat.*, **134**, 697−704.

Karpati, L., Chow, F.P.R., Woollard, M.L., Hutton, R.A. & Dandona, P. (1980) Prostacyclin-like activity in the female rat thoracic aorta and the inferior vena cava after ethinyloestradiol and norethisterone. *Clin. Sci.*, **59**, 369−72.

Kawai, Y. & Clark, M.R. (1985) Phorbol ester regulation of rat granulosa cell prostaglandin and progesterone accumulation. *Endocrinology*, **116**, 2320−6.

Kawamura, N., Himeno, N., Okamura, H. & Mori, T. (1984) Effect of indomethacin on collagenolytic enzyme activities in rabbit ovary. *Acta Obstet. Gynaec. Jpn.*, **36**, 2099−105.

Kawamura, N., Himeno, N., Okamura, H. & Mori, T. (1986) Effect of prostaglandin $F_{2\alpha}$ on ovulation and collagenolytic activities in the rabbit treated by indomethacin. *Acta Obstet. Gynaec. Jpn.*, **38**, 81−7.

Killick, S. & Elstein, M. (1987) Pharmacologic production of luteinized unruptured follicles by prostaglandin synthetase inhibitors. *Fertil. Steril*, **47**, 773−7.

Kitai, H., Santulli, R., Wright, K.H. & Wallach, E.E. (1985) Examination of the role of calcium in ovulation in the in vitro perfused rabbit ovary with use of ethyleneglycol-bis(*b*-aminoethyl ether)-n,n′-tetraacetic acid and verapamil. *Am. J. Obstet. Gynecol.*, 152, 705−8.

Knecht, M. (1988) Plasminogen activator is associated with the extracellular matrix of ovarian granulosa cells. *Mol. Cell. Endocrinol.*, **56**, 1−9

Kobayashi, Y., Kitai, H., Santulli, R., Wright, K.H. & Wallach, E.E. (1984) Influence of calcium and magnesium deprivation on ovulation and ovum maturation in the perfused rabbit ovary. *Biol.*

*Reprod.*, **31**, 287−95.

Kobayashi, Y., Wright, K.H., Santulli, R., Kitai, H. & Wallach, E.E. (1983) Effect of histamine and histamine blockers on the ovulatory process in the in vitro perfused rabbit ovary. *Biol. Reprod.*, **28**, 385−92.

Koos, R.D., & Clark, M.R. (1982) Production of 6-keto-prostaglandin $F_{1\alpha}$ by rat granulosa cells in vitro. *Endocrinology*, **111**, 1513−18.

Koos, R.D., Clark, M.R., Janson, P.O., Ahrén, K.E.B. & LeMaire, W.J. (1983) Prostaglandin levels in preovulatory follicles from rabbit ovaries perfused in vitro. *Prostaglandins*, **25**, 715−24.

Koos, R.D., Feiertag, M.A., Brodie, A.M.H. & LeMaire, W.J. (1984a) Inhibition of estrogen synthesis does not inhibit luteinizing hormone-induced ovulation. *Am. J. Obstet. Gynecol.*, **148**, 939−45.

Koos, R.D., Jaccarino, F.J., Magaril, R.A. & LeMaire, W.J. (1984b) Perfusion of the rat ovary *in vitro*: methodology, induction of ovulation, and pattern of steroidogenesis. *Biol. Reprod.*, **30**, 1135−41.

Krishna, A. & Terranova, P.F. (1985) Alterations in mast cell degranulation and ovarian histamine in the proestrous hamster. *Biol. Reprod.*, **32**, 1211−17.

Kruze, D. & Wojtecka, E. (1972) Activation of leucocyte collagenase proenzyme by rheumatoid synovial fluid. *Biochem. Biophys. Acta*, **285**, 436−66.

Lambertsen, C.J. Jr., Greenbaum, D.F., Wright, K.H. & Wallach, E.E. (1976) In vitro studies of ovulation in the perfused rabbit ovary. *Fertil. Steril*, **27**, 178−87.

LaPolt, P.S., Tsafriri, A., Bicsak, T.A., Ny, T. & Hsueh, A.J.W. (1989) Changes in tissue-type plasminogen activator levels during ovulation, oocyte maturation and early embryonic development. In Tsafriri, A. & Dekel, N. (eds) *Follicular Development and the Ovulatory Response*, pp. 159−68. Ares-Serono Symposia, Rome.

LeMaire, W.J., Curry, T.E. Jr., Morioka, N., Brännström, M., Clark, M.R., Woessner, J.F. & Koos, R.D. (1987) Regulation of ovulatory processes. In Stoufer, R.L. (ed.) *The Primate Ovary*, pp. 91−111. Plenum, New York.

LeMaire, W.J., Janson, P.O., Källfelt, B.J., Holmes, P.V., Cajander, S., Bjersing, L. & Ahrén K. (1982) The preovulatory decline in the follicular estradiol is not required for ovulation in rabbit. *Acta Endocrinol. Copenh.*, **101**, 452−7.

LeMaire, W.J., Leidner, R. & Marsh, J.M. (1975) Pre and post ovulatory changes in the concentration of prostaglandins in rat Graafian follicle. *Prostaglandins*, **9**, 221−9.

LeMaire, W.J., Yang, N.S.T., Behrman, H.H. & Marsh, J.M. (1973) Preovulatory changes in the concentration of prostaglandins in rabbit Graafian follicles. *Prostaglandins*, **3**, 367−76.

Lipner, H. (1988) Mechanism of mammalian ovulation. In Knobil, E. & Neill, J. (eds) *The Physiology of Reproduction*, pp. 447−88. Raven Press, New York.

Lipner, H. & Greep, R.O. (1971) Inhibition of steroidogenesis at various sites in the biosynthetic pathway in relation to induced ovulation. *Endocrinology*, **8**, 602−7.

Lipner, H. & Smith, M.S. (1971) A method for determining the distribution and source of protein in preovulatory rat ovaries. *J. Endocrinol.*, **50**, 1−14.

Lipner, H. & Wendelken, L. (1971) Inhibition of ovulation by inhibition of steroidogenesis in immature rats. *Proc. Soc. Exp. Biol. Med.*, **136**, 1141−5.

Liu, Y-X. (1988) Interaction and regulation of plasminogen activators and their inhibitor in rat follicles during periovulatory periods. *Sci. Sin. (B)*, **31**, 47−57.

Liu, Y-X. & Cajander, S. (1988) Indomethacin inhibits hCG and GnRH agonist-induced secretion of plasminogen activator by granulosa and theca interstitial cells of hypophysectomized rats. *Sci. Sin (B)*, **3**, 807−17.

Liu, Y-X., Cajander, S.B., Ny, T., Kristensen, P. & Hsueh, A.J.W. (1987a) Gonadotropin regulation of tissue-type and urokinase-type plasminogen activators in rat granulosa and theca−interstitial cells during the periovulatory period. *Mol. Cell. Endocrinol.*, **54**, 221−9.

Liu, Y-X., Kasson, B.G., Dahl, K.D., & Hsueh, A.J.W. (1987b) Vasoactive intestinal peptide stimulates plasminogen activator activity by cultured rat granulosa cells and cumulus−oocyte complexes. *Peptides*, **8**, 29−33.

Liu, Y-X. & Hsueh, A.J.W. (1987) Plasminogen activator activity in cumulus−oocyte complexes of gonadotropin-treated rats during the periovulatory period. *Biol. Reprod.*, **36**, 1055−62.

Löfman, C.O., Brännström, M., Holmes, P.V. & Janson, P.O. (1989) Ovulation in the isolated perfused rat ovary as documented by intravital microscopy. *Steroids*, **54**, 481−90.

Luukainen, T., Heikinheimo, O., Haukkamaa, M. & Lähtenmäki, P. (1988) Inhibition of folliculogenesis and ovulation by the antiprogesterone RU 486. *Fertil. Steril.*, **49**, 961−3.

McDonald, M. & Perks, A.M. (1976) Plasma bradykininogen and the reproductive cycles: studies during the oestrus cycle and pregnancy in the rat, and the human, menstrual cycle. *Can. J. Zool.*, **54**, 941−7.

McIntyre, T.M., Zimmerman, G.A. & Prescott, S.M. (1986) Leukotrienes C4 and D4 stimulate human endothelial cells to synthesize platelet-activating factor and bind neutrophils. *Proc. Natl. Acad. Sci. USA*, **83**, 2204−8.

Martin, G.G. & Miller-Walker, C. (1983) Vizualization of the three-dimensional distribution of collagen fibrils over preovulatory follicles in the hamster. *J. Exp. Zool.*, **225**, 311−19.

Mencia-Huerta, J.M., Lee, C.W., Lee, T.H., Razin, E., Corey, E.J., Lewis, R.A. & Austen, F. (1983) Platelet-activating factor (PAF-acether): Generation from mast cell subclass by an IgE-dependent mechanism. In Benveniste, J. & Arnoux, B. (eds) *Platelet-Activating Factor and Structurally Related Ether-Lipids*, pp. 101–88. Elsevier, Amsterdam.

Michel, L., Denizot, Y., Thomas, Y., Jean-Louis, F., Pitton, C., Benveniste, J. & Dbertret, L. (1988) Biosynthesis of PAF-acther factor by human skin fibroblasts *in vitro*. *J. Immunol.*, **141**, 948–53.

Moncada, S. & Vane, J.R. (1979) Arachidonic acid metabolites and the interactions between platelets and blood-vessel walls. *N. Engl. J. Med.*, **300**, 1142–7.

Montminy, M.R. & Bilezikjian, L.M. (1987) Binding of a nuclear protein to the cyclic-AMP response element of the somatostatin gene. *Nature*, **328**, 175–8.

Moon, Y.S. & Armstrong, D.T. (1974) Evidence for a role of prostaglandin $F_{2\alpha}$ in ovulation. *Fed. Proc.*, **33**, 281.

Morales, T.I., Woessner, J.F. Jr., Marsh, J.M. & LeMaire, W.J. (1983) Collagen, collagenase and collagenolytic activity in rat Graafian follicles during follicular growth and ovulation. *Biochim. Biophys. Acta*, **756**, 119–22.

Mori, T., Kohda, H., Kinoshita, Y., Ezaki, Y., Morimoto, N. & Nishimura, T. (1980) Inhibition by indomethacin of ovulation induced by human chorionic gonadotrophin in immature rats primed with pregnant mare serum gonadotropin. *J. Endocrinol.*, **84**, 333–41.

Mori, T., Suzuki, A., Nishimura, T. & Kambegawa, A. (1977a) Inhibition of ovulation in immature rats by antiprogesterone antiserum. *J. Endocrinol.*, **73**, 185–6.

Mori, T., Suzuki, A., Nishimura, T. & Kambegawa, A. (1977b) Evidence for androgen participation in induced ovulation in immature rats. *Endocrinology*, **101**, 623–6.

Morikawa, H., Okamura, H., Okazaki, T. & Nishimura, T. (1976) Changes in histamine in rabbit ovary during ovulation. *Acta Obstet. Gynecol. Jpn.*, **28**, 504–8.

Morikawa, H., Okamura, H., Takenaka, A., Morimoto, K. & Nishimura. T. (1981) Histamine concentration and its effect on ovarian contractility in humans. *Int. J. Fertil.*, **26**, 283–6.

Morioka, N., Brännström, M., Koos, R.D. & LeMaire, W.J. (1988a) Ovulation in the perfused ovary *in vitro*: further evidence that estrogen is not required. *Steroids*, **51**, 173–83.

Morioka, N., Zhu, C., Woessner, J.F. Jr. & LeMaire, W.J. (1988b) The effect of *trans*-4-(aminomethyl)-cyclohexanecarboxylic acid on ovulation in rat ovaries perfused *in vitro*. *Biol. Reprod.*, Suppl. 1, **38** (Abstr. 129).

Motta, P. & van Blerkom, J. (1975) A scanning electron microscopic study of the luteo-follicular complex. II. Events leading to ovulation. *Am. J. Anat.*, **143**, 241–64.

Movat, H. (1979) The kinin system and its relation to other systems. *Curr. Top. Pathol.*, **68**, 111–34.

Munalulu, B.M., Hillier, K. & Peddie, M.J. (1987) Effect of human chorionic gonadotrophin and indomethacin on ovulation, steroidogenesis and prostaglandin synthesis in preovulatory follicles of PMSG-primed immature rats. *J. Reprod. Fertil.*, **80**, 229–34.

Murakami, T., Ikebuchi, Y., Ohtsuka, A., Kikuta, A., Taguchi, T. & Ohtani, O. (1988) The blood vascular wreath of rat ovarian follicle, with special reference to its changes in ovulation and luteinization: a scanning electron microscopic study of corrosion casts. *Arch. Histol. Cytol.*, **4**, 299–311.

Murdoch, W.J. (1985) Follicular determinants of ovulation in the ewe. *Domest. Anim. Endocrinol.*, **2**, 105–21.

Murdoch, W.J., Dailey, R.A. & Inskeep, E.K. (1981) Preovulatory changes in prostaglandins $E_2$ and $F_{2\alpha}$ in ovine follicles. *J. Anim. Sci.*, **53**, 192–205.

Murdoch, W.J., Peterson, T.A., Van Kirk, E.A., Vincent, D.L. & Inskeep, E.K. (1986) Interactive roles of progesterone, prostaglandins and collagenase in the ovulatory mechanism of the ewe. *Biol. Reprod.*, **35**, 1187–94

Neal, P. & Baker, T.G. (1973) Response of mouse ovaries *in vivo* and in organ culture to pregnant mare's serum gonadotrophin and human chorionic gonadotrophin. I. Examination of critical time intervals. *J. Reprod. Fertil.*, **33**, 399–410.

Ny, T., Bjersing, L., Hsueh, A.J.W. & Loskutoff, D.J. (1985) Cultured granulosa cells produce two plasminogen activators and an antiactivator, each regulated differently by gonadotropins. *Endocrinology*, **116**, 1666–8.

O'Connell, M.L., Canipari, R. & Strickland, S. (1987) Hormonal regulation of tissue plasminogen activator secretion and mRNA levels in rat granulosa cells. *J. Biol. Chem.*, **262**, 2339–444.

Ohlsson, M., Hsueh, A.J.W. & Ny, T. (1988) Hormonal regulation of tissue type plasminogen activator messenger ribonucleic acid levels in rat granulosa cells: mechanisms of induction by follicle-stimulating hormone and gonadotrophin hormone releasing hormone. *Mol. Endocrinol.*, **2**, 854–61.

Ohno, Y. & Mori, T. (1985) Correlation between progesterone and plasminogen activator in rat ovaries during the ovulatory process. *Acta Obstet. Gynaec. Jpn.*, **37**, 247–56.

Okamura, H., Takenaka, A., Yajima, Y. & Nishimura, T. (1980) Ovulatory changes in the wall at the apex of the human Graafian follicle. *J. Reprod. Fertil.*, **58**, 153–5.

Okamura, H., Virutamasen, P., Wright, K.H. & Wallach E.E. (1972) Ovarian smooth muscle in the human being, rabbit and cat. *Am. J. Obstet. Gynec.*, **112**, 183–91.

Okuda, Y., Okamura, H., Kanzaki, H., Takenaka, A., Morimoto, K. & Nishimura, T. (1980a) An ultrastructural study of capillary permeability of rabbit follicles during ovulatory process. *Acta Obstet. Gynaecol. Jpn.*, **32**, 739−48.

Okuda, Y., Okamura, H., Kanzaki, H., Takenaka, A., Morimoto, K. & Nishimura, T. (1980b) An ultrastructural study of capillary permeability of rabbit ovarian follicles during ovulation using carbon tracer. *Acta Obstet. Gynaecol. Jpn.*, **7**, 859−67.

Orczyk, G.P. & Behrman, H.R. (1972) Ovulation blockade by aspirin or indomethacin − *in vivo* evidence for a role of prostaglandin in gonadotrophin secretion. *Prostaglandins*, **1**, 3−20.

Oswaldo-Decima, L. (1970) Smooth muscle in the ovary of the rat and monkey. *J. Ultrastruct. Mol. Struct. Res.*, **29**, 218−37.

Owman, C., Sjöberg, N.-O., Svensson, K.G. & Walles, B. (1975) Autonomic nerves mediating contractility in the human Graafian follicle. *J. Reprod. Fertil.*, **45**, 553−6.

Palotie, A., Peltonen, L., Foidart, J.M. & Rajaniemi, H. (1984) Immunohistochemical localization of basement membrane components and interstitial collagen types in preovulatory rat ovarian follicles. *Coll. Relat. Res.*, **4**, 279−87.

Palotie, A., Salo, T., Vihko, K.K., Peltonen, L. & Rajaniemi, H. (1987) Types I and IV collagenolytic and plasminogen activator activities in preovulatory ovarian follicles. *J. Cell. Biochem.*, **34**, 101−12.

Parr, E.L. (1974) Histological examination of the rat ovarian follicle wall prior to ovulation. *Biol. Reprod.*, **11**, 483−503.

Peluso, J.J., Stude, D. & Steger, R.W. (1980) Role of androgens in hCG-induced ovulation in PMSG-primed immature rats. *Acta Endocrinol. Copenh.*, **93**, 505−12.

Piacsek, B.E. & Huth, J.F. (1971) Changes in ovarian venous blood flow following cannulation: effects of luteinizing hormone (LH) and antihistamine. *Proc. Soc. Exp. Biol. Med.*, **138**, 1022−4.

Puistola, U., Salo, T., Martikainen, H. & Rönnberg, L. (1986) Type IV collagenolytic activity in human preovulatory follicular fluid. *Fertil. Steril.*, **45**, 578−580.

Ramwell, P.W., Shaw, J.E. & Jessup, S.J. (1970) Follicular fluid kinin and its action on Fallopian tubes. *Endocrinology*, **84**, 931−6.

Ranta, T., Huhtaniemi, I., Jalkanen, J., Koskimies, A., Laatikainen, T. & Ylikorkala, O. (1986) Activation of protein kinase-C stimulates human granulosa-luteal cell prostacyclin production. *J. Clin. Endocrinol. Metab.*, **63**, 513−15.

Raw, R.E., Curry, T.E. & Silvia, W.J. (1988) Effects of progesterone and estradiol on the concentration and activity of cyclooxygenase in the ovine uterus. *Biol. Reprod.*, Suppl. **38**, 104 (Abstr.).

Rawson, J.M.R. & Espey, L.L. (1977) Concentration of electron dense granules in the rabbit ovarian surface epithelium during ovulation. *Biol. Reprod.*, **17**, 561−6.

Reed, M., Burton, F.A. & Van Dienst, P.A. (1979) Ovulation in the guinea pig. I. The ruptured follicle. *J. Anat.*, **128**, 195−200.

Reich, R., Kohen, F., Naor, Z. & Tsafriri, A. (1983) Possible involvement of lipoxygenase products of arachidonic acid pathway in ovulation. *Prostaglandins*, **26**, 1011−20.

Reich, R., Kohen, F., Slager, R. & Tsafriri, A. (1985a) Ovarian lipoxygenase activity and its regulation by gonadotropin in the rat. *Prostaglandins*, **30**, 581−90.

Reich, R., Miskin, R. & Tsafriri, A. (1985b) Follicular plasminogen activator: involvement in ovulation. *Endocrinology*, **116**, 516−21.

Reich, R., Miskin, R. & Tsafriri, A. (1986) Intrafollicular distribution of plasminogen activators and their hormonal regulation *in vitro*. *Endocrinology*, **119**, 1588−93.

Reich, R., Tsafriri, A. & Mechanic, G.L. (1985c) The involvement of collagenolysis in ovulation in the rat. *Endocrinology*, **116**, 522−7.

Robinson-Steiner, A.M. & Corbin, J.D. (1983) Probable involvement of both intrachain cAMP binding sites in activation of protein kinase. *J. Biol. Chem.*, **258**, 1032−40.

Rodbard, D. (1968) Mechanics of ovulation. *J. Clin. Endocrinol. Metab.*, **28**, 849−61.

Roncaglioni, M.C., di Minno, G., Reyers, I., de Gaetano, G. & Donati, M.B. (1979) Increased prostacyclin-like activity in vascular tissues from rats on long-term treatment with an oestrogen−progestagen combination. *Thromb. Res.*, **14**, 793−7.

Rondell, P. (1964) Follicular pressure and distensibility. *Am. J. Physiol.*, **207**, 590−4.

Rondell, P. (1970a) Biophysical aspects of ovulation. *Biol. Reprod.*, **2**, 64−89.

Rondell, P. (1970b) Follicular processes in ovulation. *Fed. Proc.*, **29**, 1875−9.

Rondell, P. (1974) Role of steroid synthesis in the process of ovulation. *Biol. Reprod.*, **10**, 199−215.

Rubin, R.M., Samples, J.R. & Rosenbaum, J.T. (1988) Prostaglandin-independent inhibition of ocular vascular permeability by a platelet-activating factor antagonist. *Arch. Ophthalmol.*, **106**, 1116−20.

Schmidt, G., Holmes, P.V., Owman, C., Sjöberg, N.-O. & Walles, B. (1986a) The influence of prostaglandin E$_2$ and indomethacin on progesterone production and ovulation in the rabbit ovary perfused *in vitro*. *Biol. Reprod.*, **35**, 815−21.

Schmidt, G., Kannisto, P., Owman, C. & Sjöberg, N.-O. (1988a) Is serotonin involved in the ovulatory process of the rat ovary perfused *in vitro*? *Acta Physiol. Scand.*, **132**, 251−6.

Schmidt, G., Owman, C. & Sjöberg, N.-O. (1986b) Histamine induces ovulation in the isolated perfused rat ovary. *J. Reprod. Fertil.*, **78**, 159−66.

Schmidt, G., Owman, C. & Sjöberg, N.-O. (1988b) Cellular localization of ovarian histamine, its cyclic variations, and histaminergic effects on ovulation in rat ovary perfused *in vitro*. *J. Reprod. Fertil.*, **82**,

409−17.

Sechel, M.M., Swartz, S.L., Smith, D., Levesque, L. & Taymor, M.L. (1984) *In vivo* prostaglandin concentrations in human preovulatory follicles. *Fertil. Steril.*, **42**, 482−5.

Shimada, H., Okamura, H., Noda, Y., Suzuki, A., Tojo, S. & Takada. A. (1983) Plasminogen activator in rat ovary during the ovulatory process: independence of prostaglandin mediation. *J. Endocrinol.*, **97**, 201−5.

Slackman, R.L., LeMaire, W.J., Koos, R.D., Dean, D.D., Woessner, J.F. & Curry, T.E. (1986) Production of collagenase and a metalloprotease inhibitor by cultured rat ovarian tissues. *Endocrinology*, Suppl. **118**, 222 (Abstr.).

Smith, C. & Perks, A.M. (1983a) The kinin system and ovulation: changes in plasma kininogens, and in kinin-forming enzymes in the ovaries and blood of rats with 4-day estrous cycles. *Can. J. Physiol. Pharmacol.*, **61**, 736−42.

Smith, C. & Perks, A.M. (1983b) Changes in plasma kininogen levels in rats before ovulation, and after treatment with luteinizing hormone and oestradiol-17β. *Acta Endocrinol. Copenh.*, **104**, 123−8.

Smith, C. & Perks, A.M. (1984) The effects of bradykinin on the contractile activity of the isolated rat ovary. *Acta Endocrinol. Copenh.*, **106**, 387−92.

Smokovits, A., Kokolis, N. & Alexaki-Tzivanidu, E. (1988) The plasminogen activator activity is markedly increased mainly at the area of the rupture of the follicular wall at the time of ovulation. *Anim. Reprod. Sci.*, **16**, 285−94.

Snyder, B.W., Beecham, G.D. & Schane, H.P. (1984) Inhibition of ovulation in rats with epostane, an inhibitor of 3β-hydroxysteroid dehydrogenase (41865). *Proc. Soc. Exp. Biol. Med.*, **176**, 238−42.

Sogn, J.H., Curry, T.E. Jr, Brännström, M., LeMaire, W.J., Koos, R.D., Papkoff, H. & Janson, P.O. (1987) Inhibition of follicle-stimulating hormone-induced ovulation by indomethacin in the perfused rat ovary. *Biol. Reprod.*, **36**, 536−42.

Stähler, E., Spätling, L., Bethge, H.D., Daume, E. & Buchholz, R. (1974) Induction of ovulation in human ovaries perfused *in vitro*. *Arch. Gynaecol. Obstet.*, **217**, 1−15.

Stirling, D., Magness, R.R., Stone, R., Watreman, M.R. & Simpson, E.R. (1990) Angiotensin II inhibits luteinizing hormone-stimulated cholesterol side chain cleavage expression and stimulates basic fibroblast growth factor expression in bovine luteal cells in primary culture. *J. Biol. Chem.*, **265**, 5−8.

Strickland, S. & Beers, W.H. (1976) Studies on the role of plasminogen activator in ovulation. *In vitro* response of granulosa cells to gonadotropins, cyclic nucleotides, and prostaglandins. *J. Biol. Chem.*, **251**, 5694−702.

Swanson, R.J. & Lipner, H. (1977) Mechanism of ovulation: effect of intrafollicular progesterone

antiserum in rabbits. *Fed. Proc.*, **36**, 390 (Abstr.).

Szego, C.M. & Gitin, E.S. (1964) Ovarian histamine depletion during acute hyperaemic response to luteinizing hormone. *Nature*, **201**, 682−4.

Tajima, C., Kawano, T., Matsuura, K. & Okamura, H. (1988) Role of progesterone in the ovulatory process of PMSG−HCG treated immature female rats. *Proc. 8th Int. Congr. Endocrinol., Kyoto* (Abstr. 453).

Tanaka, N., Espey, L.L. & Okamura, H. (1989) Increase in ovarian blood volume during ovulation in the gonadotropin-primed immature rat. *Biol. Reprod.*, **40**, 762−8.

Testart, J., Thébault, A. & Lefévre, B. (1983) In-vitro ovulation of rabbit ovarian follicles isolated after the endogenous gonadotrophin surge. *J. Reprod. Fertil.*, **68**, 413−18.

Tjugum, J., Dennerfors, B. & Norström, A. (1984) Influence of progesterone, androstenedione and oestradiol-17b on the incorporation of [$^3$H]-proline in the human follicular wall. *Acta Endocrinol. Copenh.*, **105**, 552−7.

Too, C.K.L., Bryant-Greenwood, G. & Greenwood, F.C. (1984) Relaxin increases the release of plasminogen activator, collagenase, and proteoglycanase from rat granulosa cells *in vitro*. *Endocrinology*, **115**, 1043−50.

Triebwasser, W.F., Clark, M.R., LeMaire, W.J. & Marsh, J.M. (1978) Localization and in vitro synthesis of prostaglandins in components of rabbit preovulatory Graafian follicles. *Prostaglandins*, **16**, 621−32.

Tsafriri, A., Abisogun, A.O. & Reich, R. (1987) Steroids and follicular rupture at ovulation. *J. Steroid Biochem.*, **27**, 359−63.

Tsafriri, A., Bicsak, T.A., Cajander, S., Ny, T. & Hsueh, A.J.W. (1989) Suppression of ovulation rate by antibodies to tissue plasminogen activator and α2-antiplasmin. *Endocrinology*, **124**, 415−21.

Tsafriri, A., Koch, Y. & Lindner, H.R. (1973) Ovulation rate and serum LH levels in rats treated with indomethacin or prostaglandin E$_2$. *Prostaglandins*, **3**, 461−7.

Tsafriri, A., Lindner, H.R., Zor, U. & Lamprecht, S.A. (1972) In-vitro induction of meiotic division in follicle-enclosed rat oocytes by LH, cyclic AMP and prostaglandin E$_2$. *J. Reprod. Fertil.*, **31**, 39−50.

Tsuijimoto, D., Katayama, K., Tojo, S. & Mizoguti, H. (1982) Scanning electron microscopic studies on stigmas in rat ovaries. *Acta Obstet. Gynecol. Scand.*, **61**, 269−73.

Veldhuis, J.D. & Klase, P.A. (1982) Mechanisms by which calcium ions regulate the steroidogenic actions of luteinizing hormone in isolated ovarian cells *in vitro*. *Endocrinology*, **111**, 1−6.

Vijayakumar, R. & Walters, W.A.W (1987) Ovarian stromal and luteal tissue prostaglandins, 17β-estradiol, and progesterone in relation to the phases of the menstrual cycle in women. *Am. J. Obstet. Gynecol.*, **156**, 947−51.

Virutamasen, P., Wright, K.H. & Wallach, E.E. (1972a)

Effects of prostaglandins $E_2$ and $F_{2\alpha}$ on ovarian contractility in the rabbit. *Fertil. Steril.*, **23**, 675–82.

Virutamasen, P., Wright, K.H. & Wallach E.E. (1972b) Effects of catecholamines on ovarian contractility in the rabbit. *Obstet. Gynecol.*, **39**, 225–36.

Walles, B., Edvinsson, L., Falck, B., Owman, C.H., Sjöberg, N.-O. & Svensson, K.-G. (1975) Evidence for a neuromuscular mechanism involved in the contractility of the ovarian follicular wall: fluorescence and electron microscopy and effects of tyramine on follicle strips. *Biol. Reprod.*, **12**, 239–48.

Walles, B., Edvinsson, L., Owman, C., Sjöberg, N-O. & Svensson, K.-G. (1975) Mechanical response in the wall of ovarian follicles mediated by adrenergic receptors. *J. Pharmacol. Exp. Ther.*, **103**, 460–73.

Walles, B., Owman, C., Schmidt, G. & Sjöberg, N-O. (1986) Evidence for a role of prostaglandins in the adrenergic neuromuscular mechanism of the ovarian follicle wall. *Neuroendocrinology*, **43**, 18–23.

Watson, J., Shepherd, T.S. & Dodson, K.S. (1979) Prostaglandin E-2-9-ketoreductase in ovarian tissues, *J. Reprod. Fertil.*, **57**, 489–96.

Weisman, S.M., Freund, R.M., Felsen, D. & Vaughan, E.D. Jr. (1988). Differential effect of platelet-activating factor (PAF) receptor antagonists on peptide and PAF-stimulated prostaglandin release in unilateral ureteral obstruction. *Biochem. Pharmacol.*, **3**, 2927–32.

Weissmann, G., Zurier, R.B. & Hoffstein, S. (1973) Leukocytes as secretory organs of inflammation. *Agents Actions*, **3/5**, 370–9.

Woessner, J.F. Jr., Butler, T., LeMaire, W.J., Morioka, N., Mukaida, T. & Zhu, C. (1989) The role of collagenase in the perfused rat ovary. In Tsafriri, A. & Dekel, N. (ed.) *Follicular Development and the Ovulatory Response*, pp. 169–78. Ares-Serono Symposia, Rome.

Woolley, D.E. (1984). Mammalian collagenases. In Piez, K.A. & Reddi, A.H. (eds) *Extracellular Matrix Biochemistry*, pp. 119–57. Elsevier, New York.

Wurtman, R.J. (1964) An effect of luteinizing hormone on the fractional perfusion of the rat ovary. *Endo-crinology*, **75**, 927–33.

Wylie, S.N., Roche, P.J. & Gibson, W.R. (1985) Ovulation after sympathetic denervation of the rat ovary produced by freezing its nerve supply. *J. Reprod. Fertil.*, **75**, 369–73.

Yang, N.S.T., Marsh, J.M. & LeMaire, W.J. (1974) Post ovulatory changes in the concentration of prostaglandins in rabbit Graafian follicles. *Prostaglandins*, **6**, 37–44.

Yoshimura, Y., Dharmarajan, A.M., Gips, S., Adachi, T., Hosoi, Y., Atlas, S.J. & Wallach, E.E. (1988a) Effects of prostacyclin on ovulation and microvasculature of the *in-vitro* perfused rabbit ovary. *Am. J. Obstet. Gynecol.*, **159**, 977–82.

Yoshimura, Y., Espey, L., Hosoi, Y., Adachi, T., Atlas, S.J., Ghodgaonkar, R.B., Dubin, N.H. & Wallach, E.E. (1988b) Effects of bradykinin on ovulation and prostaglandin production by the perfused rabbit ovary. *Endocrinology*, **122**, 2540–6.

Yoshimura, Y., Hosoi, Y., Atlas, S.J., Bongiovanni, A.M., Santulli, R. & Wallach, E.E. (1986) The effect of ovarian steroidogenesis on ovulation and fertilizability in the *in vitro* perfused rabbit ovary. *Biol. Reprod.*, **35**, 943–82.

Yoshimura, Y., Hosoi, Y., Bongiovanni, A.M., Santulli, R., Atlas, S.J. & Wallach, E.E. (1987a) Are ovarian steroids required for ovum maturation and fertilization? Effects of cyanoketone on the *in vitro* perfused rabbit ovary. *Endocrinology*, **120**, 2555–61.

Yoshimura, Y., Santulli, R., Atlas, S.J., Fujii, S. & Wallach, E.E. (1987b) The effects of proteolytic enzymes on *in vitro* ovulation in the rabbit. *Am. J. Obstet. Gynecol*, **157**, 468–75.

Zeleznik, A.J., Schuler, H.M. & Reichert, L.E. Jr. (1981) Gonadotropin-binding sites in the rhesus monkey ovary: role of the vasculature in the selective distribution of human chorionic gonadotropin to the preovulatory follicle. *Endocrinology*, **109**, 356–62.

Zondek, K.B., Sulman, F. & Black, R. (1945) The hyperemia effect of gonadotropins on the ovary. *J. Am. Med. Assoc.*, **128**, 939–44.

# 6 Control of Luteal Endocrine Function

A.J. ZELEZNIK

## Introduction

The luteal phase of the menstrual cycle commences in response to the mid-cycle gonadotrophin surge with the rupture of the Graafian follicle and the transformation of the follicular granulosa cells into luteal cells, a process called luteinization. Once formed, the corpus luteum has a finite lifespan of 14−16 days during which its major secretory products progesterone and oestradiol are required for the preparation of a secretory endometrium in anticipation of the implantation of the blastocyst and the maintenance of the endometrium until the placenta assumes this responsibility. In non-fertile menstrual cycles, steroid secretion continues during the functional lifespan of the corpus luteum following which the tissue ceases to synthesize steroids and luteal cells undergo death and removal from the ovary. If pregnancy occurs, the functional lifespan of the corpus luteum is prolonged by the trophoblastic hormone, chorionic gonadotrophin (CG). Thus, the corpus luteum provides an example of a tissue that undergoes synchronous development (luteinization), followed by co-ordinated control of cellular function (steroid biosynthesis and release) and synchronous cell death (luteolysis).

The goal of this chapter is to present current views regarding regulation *in vivo* of the corpus luteum of the primate menstrual cycle with particular emphasis on the control of the synthesis of steroid hormones, the control of the lifespan of the corpus luteum and the control of luteal cell death. This chapter primarily emphasizes recent data obtained from human and subhuman primates; references to other species are made where relevant primate data are not available.

Comprehensive reviews are available on comparative aspects of luteal function (Auletta & Flint, 1988; Keyes & Wiltbank, 1988; Niswender & Nett, 1988).

## The corpus luteum as an endocrine gland

### Structural characteristics

Luteinization of the Graafian follicle in response to the mid-cycle gonadotrophin surge is characterized by major structural reorganizations at the cellular level. The most obvious change is granulosa cell hypertrophy. Associated with this hypertrophy are marked changes in the presence of intracellular organelles, including an increase in smooth endoplasmic reticulum and an increase in the number of mitochondria with tubular cristae. By the fifth day following ovulation, cellular reorganization is complete and granulosa–lutein cells assume the full morphological characteristics of steroid-secretory endocrine cells. During this period there is extensive proliferation of capillaries into the luteinizing granulosa cell layer as the corpus luteum acquires its blood supply.

Commencing during the mid-luteal phase, c. Day 7–8, luteal cells begin to shrink due to the loss of cytoplasmic volume and this shrinkage continues for the remainder of the luteal phase. By Day 9–10, luteal cell nuclei exhibit chromatin condensation which is followed by nuclear pyknosis (Corner, 1956; Adams & Hertig, 1969). Interestingly, while luteal cells show degenerative changes during the late luteal phase, fibroblasts within the central core of the corpus luteum proliferate. This morphogenetic pattern indicates that the cellular death associated with luteal regression is not due to hypoxia or other manifestations of reduced nutrient delivery since this would be likely to affect all cells uniformly.

### Functional characteristics

The classical description of the corpus luteum as an endocrine gland is based upon the ability of this structure to produce the female sex steroid hormones progesterone and oestradiol-17$\beta$. Peripheral plasma progesterone concentrations during the luteal phase of the menstrual cycle are commonly measured to indicate the functional status of the corpus luteum.

The production of progesterone and oestradiol by luteal cells is regulated by separate steroidogenic pathways (Fig. 6.1; see also Chapter 2). Luteal cells are able to synthesize progesterone directly from cholesterol. However, although luteal cells have the ability to manufacture cholesterol *de novo* from acetate, the corpus luteum relies extensively on low-density lipoprotein (LDL)-associated cholesterol for use as precursor to synthesize progesterone *in vivo*. The dependence of normal

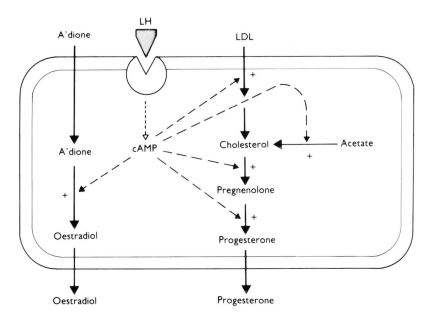

**Fig. 6.1.** Control by LH of luteal steroid synthesis. LH acts through its receptor on granulosa—lutein cells to stimulate cyclic adenosine monophosphate (cAMP)-dependent steps in steroidogenesis: LDL uptake; LDL-cholesterol ester hydrolysis; cholesterol synthesis from acetate; cholesterol metabolism to progesterone; and aromatization of androstenedione (A′dione). Production of oestradiol is limited by the availability of aromatizable $C_{19}$ androgen (testosterone and androstenedione) which is not produced by granulosa—lutein cells. Substrate for aromatization must therefore be provided by theca—lutein cells in an extension of the 'two-cell, two gonadotrophin' model of follicular oestradiol biosynthesis. Reproduced with permission from Hillier (1990).

luteal steroid secretion on LDL-associated cholesterol was highlighted by the finding of abnormally low plasma progesterone levels during pregnancy in a woman with hypobetalipoproteinaemia, a metabolic disorder characterized by low plasma concentrations of LDL (Parker *et al.*, 1986) (see Chapter 9).

Synthesis of oestradiol only proceeds if an appropriate $C_{19}$ steroid (androstenedione or testosterone) is available as aromatase substrate. Because granulosa—lutein cells do not express 17-hydroxylase/C-17,20-lyase (P450c17) (see Chapter 2), they cannot metabolize $C_{21}$ steroids to aromatizable androgens and therefore depend upon other cell types for the provision of substrate for aromatization. In the maturing follicle, thecal cells provide $C_{19}$ androgens for aromatization by granulosa cells (Hillier, 1990). Luteinized thecal (theca—lutein) cells presumably fulfil a similar function for granulosa—lutein cells in the corpus luteum.

Clinical studies and experimental work using non-human primates indicate that as well as steroid hormones, the corpus luteum synthesizes and releases a variety of protein hormones including relaxin (Weiss *et al.*, 1976), oxytocin (Khan-Dawood *et al.*, 1989), and inhibin (Bassett *et al.*, 1990). Inhibin in particular has received a great deal of attention because of its possible role in controlling secretion of follicle-stimulating hormone (FSH) by the pituitary gland (Steinberger & Ward, 1988) (see Chapter 1).

Because inhibin was isolated and purified from follicular fluid, and because bioassayable plasma inhibin levels were shown to parallel oestradiol during the follicular phase of the menstrual cycle, it was initially believed that the developing follicle was a major source of secreted inhibin (McLachlan et al., 1987). More recent studies using both bioassay and radioimmunoassay indicate that inhibin is present in blood during the luteal phase of the menstrual cycle at concentrations which markedly exceed those seen during the follicular phase. Moreover, various lines of evidence indicate that the primary source of circulating inhibin during the luteal phase of the menstrual cycle is the corpus luteum. Northern blot analysis has shown that the human corpus luteum expresses both inhibin $\alpha$- and $\beta_A$-subunit mRNAs (Davis et al., 1987), and in-situ hybridization studies on macaque ovaries have localized the $\alpha$- and $\beta_A$-subunit mRNAs (but not $\beta_B$ mRNA) to luteal cells present during the early and mid-luteal phases of the menstrual cycle (Schwall et al., 1990). In vivo studies have shown that removal of the corpus luteum during early, mid- and late luteal phases of the menstrual cycle results in a rapid and sustained fall in the plasma concentration of inhibin (Bassett et al., 1990). The secretion of inhibin during the luteal phase appears to be under gonadotrophic control because the administration of gonadotrophin-releasing hormone (GnRH) antagonists to block pituitary gonadotrophin secretion during the luteal phase results in a fall in inhibin concentrations (Fraser et al., 1989). To date, physiological functions of inhibin during the luteal phase have not been elucidated. It is possible that inhibin and related proteins are involved in the control of pituitary gonadotrophin secretion and/or serve local regulatory functions within the ovary itself.

## Preovulatory determinants of luteal function

The interval between the formation of the corpus luteum following ovulation and its demise at the conclusion of non-fertile menstrual cycles is c. 14–16 days. This period is usually referred to as the functional lifespan of the corpus luteum. When one considers that the corpus luteum is derived from the remnants of the ovulated Graafian follicle, the true lifespan of the cells which comprise the corpus luteum is actually the time it takes for a primordial follicle to develop to the preovulatory stage. In human beings, this period has been estimated to be as long as 150 days (Gougeon, 1982). During this interval, granulosa cells in the primordial follicle replicate, and as the follicle grows these cells undergo differentiation in anticipation of their function as luteal cells after ovulation. As discussed in Chapter 3, the primary hormone involved in the differentiation of granulosa cells is FSH. In response to stimulation by FSH during the follicular phase of the menstrual cycle, granulosa cells gain the capacity to produce both oestrogen and progesterone through the acquisition of steroidogenic enzymes and cell-surface receptors for luteinizing hormone (LH). In essence, the potential for these cells to undertake luteal-type differentiated function is acquired during the final stages of preovulatory follicular growth. Upon follicular rupture, granulosa−lutein cells are thereby immediately able to commence production of progesterone.

The importance of FSH to luteal cell function by way of its effect on granulosa cell development in the preovulatory follicle is evident from *in vivo* studies on primates in which the normal pattern of FSH secretion is disturbed during the follicular phase of the menstrual cycle by treatment with oestrogen or porcine follicular fluid, a source of inhibin and folliculostatin. Such studies have convincingly shown that reducing FSH concentrations during the follicular phase of the menstrual cycle leads to abnormal luteal phases characterized by inadequate progesterone production (Stouffer & Hodgen, 1980; Dierschke *et al.*, 1985). These findings have led clinical investigators to propose that the pathophysiology of inadequate luteal phases in humans may be secondary to inadequate stimulation of follicles by FSH during the follicular phase of the cycle (DiZerega & Hodgen, 1981). Indeed, one treatment for inadequate luteal phase is administration of clomiphine citrate during the follicular phase of the cycle, the theory being that elevated FSH concentrations due to the antioestrogenic effects of clomiphene on the hypothalamo−pituitary axis during the follicular phase may improve the quality of the granulosa cells prior to ovulation, leading subsequently to improved luteal cell function following ovulation and luteinization (see Chapter 9). Although it has been shown that treatment with clomiphene during the follicular phase is able to increase serum progesterone concentrations during the subsequent luteal phase and correct out-of-phase endometrial biopsies, it has recently been suggested that the increased serum progesterone concentrations seen during these luteal phases may be related more to the presence of two or more corpora lutea rather than improved quality of a single corpus luteum (Guzik & Zeleznik, 1990).

## Postovulatory determinants of luteal function

Daily serum progesterone concentrations during the luteal phase of a typical 28-day menstrual cycle are illustrated in Fig. 6.2. Based upon this pattern, the luteal phase can be separated into three periods. For the first 7−8 days after the mid-cycle LH peak (early luteal phase), serum progesterone concentrations rise progressively; between Days 9 and 12 (mid-luteal phase), serum progesterone values are maximal; and from Days 12 to 16 (late luteal phase), progesterone levels fall progressively and menstruation ensues.

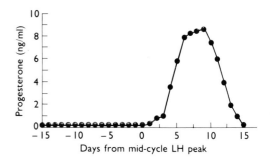

**Fig. 6.2.** Plasma concentrations of progesterone during the luteal phase of the non-fertile menstrual cycle in rhesus monkeys.

The fundamental question regarding control of luteal function is whether the temporal pattern of progesterone secretion during the luteal phase is primarily due to inherent changes in luteal cell function accompanying cellular ageing or to alterations in trophic stimulation of the corpus luteum. This question has been addressed using *in vitro* and *in vivo* experimental approaches. The benefit of *in vitro* analysis is that it permits luteal function to be assessed under defined experimental conditions independent of changing patterns of gonadotrophin secretion, luteal perfusion, or availability of precursor cholesterol substrate such as occur *in vivo*. It allows absolute steroidogenic capacity to be defined in relation to luteal development and permits comparisons to be made of the relative effects of various trophic factors on steroid synthesis. *In vivo* studies do not allow such stringent experimental control but they do permit analysis to be made of luteal function under physiological conditions. Recent results obtained using both approaches have provided novel information regarding both the control of luteal steroid secretion as well as the maintenance of the lifespan of the corpus luteum by gonadotrophic hormones.

### *In vitro* studies

The *in vitro* approach has revealed that the major, if not sole, luteotrophin that regulates luteal cell steroidogenesis is LH. Measurements of adenylyl cyclase activity in luteal cell membranes and intact luteal cells have failed to demonstrate significant stimulation of enzyme activity or progesterone synthesis by FSH (Eyster & Stouffer, 1985; Fisch *et al.*, 1989). In contrast, LH and human chorionic gonadotrophin (hCG) are both effective in stimulating adenylyl cyclase activity in luteal cell membranes as well as stimulating progesterone secretion by intact luteal cells in tissue culture (Eyster & Stouffer, 1985; Fisch *et al.*, 1989). The observation that LH is the major pituitary gonadotrophin which regulates luteal cell steroidogenesis greatly simplifies the examination of whether the gland's transient functional lifespan during the non-fertile menstrual cycle is caused by changes in gonadotrophin secretion or by changes in luteal cell responsiveness to gonadotrophic stimulation.

Possible determinants of luteal cell responsiveness to LH throughout the luteal phase are the density and affinity of LH receptors and the level of LH-sensitive adenylyl cyclase in luteal cell membranes. In rhesus monkey corpora lutea, the concentration of unoccupied LH receptors on luteal cell membranes increases by c. 30% between the early and mid-luteal phases, declining thereafter by 75% at the time of menstruation. Although the decline in serum progesterone concentrations during the late luteal phase is accompanied by a decrease in LH receptors, a direct cause−effect relationship between LH receptor levels and luteolysis has not been adduced because in some animals the reduction in serum progesterone concentration precedes the reduction in luteal LH receptor level (Cameron & Stouffer, 1982b).

By obtaining corpora lutea at defined stages of the menstrual cycle, it has been possible to examine basal and gonadotrophin-responsive luteal cell steroidogenesis in relation to luteal development. Surprisingly, the capacity of isolated luteal cells to produce progesterone in vitro does not correlate well with the pattern of plasma progesterone concentrations seen in vivo. Cellular capacities for basal synthesis of progesterone and oestradiol are maximal for corpora lutea obtained during the early luteal phase, with values declining thereafter in proportion to luteal age (Fisch et al., 1989). As basal steroidogenic capacity declines, cellular responsiveness to hCG increases such that the response (fold-increase over basal) elicited by treatment with a fixed concentration of hCG becomes greatest during the mid−late luteal phase. However, despite their increased sensitivity to hCG, the absolute amount of progesterone secreted by hCG-treated luteal cells obtained during the mid−late luteal phase is minimal compared with the amount of steroid produced basally by cells obtained during the early luteal phase. These findings indicate that as determined under well-defined conditions in vitro, the absolute steroidogenic capacity of luteal cells peaks shortly after ovulation and, like an uncharged battery, declines thereafter with a finite half-life. However, the fact that circulating serum progesterone concentrations do not correlate with the steroidogenic capacity of isolated luteal cells in vitro indicates that additional factors must influence steroid secretion by the corpus luteum in vivo.

A likely explanation for divergent patterns of progesterone secretion by the corpus luteum in vivo and luteal cells in vitro is that during the early luteal phase, the corpus luteum has yet to become fully vascularized. Delivery of blood-borne LDL-cholesterol to steroidogenic luteal cells is therefore restricted, serving to rate-limit progesterone synthesis in vivo. Supporting this explanation are the findings that addition of LDL-cholesterol to cultures of human luteal cells significantly increases hCG-stimulated progesterone production by these cells in vitro (Carr et al., 1982) (see Fig. 9.6). Factors influencing vascularization of the corpus luteum are discussed in detail in a later section of this chapter.

### *In vivo* studies

Although *in vitro* studies have provided important information regarding the hormonal control of steroidogenesis as well as the responsiveness of luteal cells as a function of age of the corpus luteum, major questions remain unanswered regarding control of luteal function *in vivo*. Notably, is luteal function at any stage of the luteal phase independent of gonadotrophic support, and does a change in the pattern of LH secretion cause onset of luteal regression if pregnancy does not occur?

### *Role of LH*

The notion that the corpus luteum might function independently of gonadotrophic support arose from studies in which hypophysectomized women were treated with gonadotrophins to stimulate follicular growth and ovulation was induced with hCG (Gemzell, 1965). These studies demonstrated that a single injection of an ovulatory dose of hCG was sufficient to maintain the secretory activity of the corpus luteum for its normal lifespan of 14–16 days. However, Vande Wiele *et al.* (1969) showed that when ovulation was induced by injecting LH instead of hCG, the corpus luteum regressed within 4–5 days unless additional LH was administered. The greater efficacy of hCG in maintaining the lifespan of the corpus luteum in hypophysectomized women appears to be due to its significantly longer half-life in plasma as compared with LH (Rizkallah *et al.*, 1969).

Recent studies in macaque monkeys have resurrected the hypothesis that the primate corpus luteum functions independently of gonadotrophic support. In these experiments, administration of a GnRH antagonist to suppress spontaneous gonadotrophin secretion during the luteal phase of the cycle did not result in premature luteal regression, despite the fact that plasma immunoactive LH levels became undetectable (Borghi *et al.*, 1983).

The responsiveness of the corpus luteum to gonadotrophin can be examined systematically using an experimental model in which macaque monkeys are rendered anovulatory by placement of radiofrequency lesions in the medial basal hypothalamus (MBH). This interrupts spontaneous secretion of GnRH, and hence LH (Wildt *et al.*, 1981). In such animals, pituitary gonadotrophin secretion and menstrual cycles can be restored by infusing synthetic GnRH intravenously in a pusatile fashion and the pattern of gonadotrophin secretion can be varied by altering the pattern of GnRH infusion. Figure 6.3 illustrates the pattern of serum progesterone concentrations in MBH-lesioned rhesus monkeys whose menstrual cycles were restored by the pulsatile infusion of synthetic GnRH at a frequency of one pulse per hour. The luteal-phase pattern of serum progesterone levels and the lifespan of the corpus

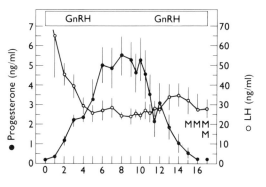

**Fig. 6.3.** Plasma concentrations of progesterone and LH in rhesus monkeys with lesions of the MBH that abolish the secretion of endogenous GnRH. Menstrual cycles were restored by intravenous pulsatile infusion of synthetic GnRH at a fixed frequency of one pulse an hour. Progesterone concentrations and luteal-phase length are indistinguishable from those of normal, spontaneous luteal phases.

luteum in these animals are indistinguishable from those of spontaneously cyclic animals.

Using this experimental system, the dependence of luteal progesterone production on pituitary secretion of LH was tested directly by terminating the infusion of GnRH and thereby interrupting secretion of LH at defined stages of the luteal phase (Hutchison & Zeleznik, 1984). Figure 6.4 illustrates the consequences of terminating the GnRH infusion during the early (a), and (b) mid-luteal phases of the menstrual cycle. In each case there was a prompt and sustained fall in serum concentrations of LH and progesterone when the GnRH infusion was stopped, and menstruation ensued shortly thereafter. These observations directly dispel the notion that existence of the corpus luteum is independent of pituitary gonadotrophic support. Others have shown in spontaneously

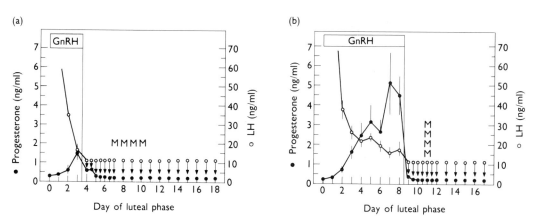

**Fig. 6.4.** Effects of terminating the infusion of GnRH in MBH-lesioned rhesus monkeys during early and mid-luteal phases of the menstrual cycle. In (a) plasma concentrations of LH and progesterone are shown before and after terminating the infusion of GnRH on Day 3 of the luteal phase; (b) shows the effects of terminating the infusion of GnRH on Day 9 of the luteal phase. In each case, plasma LH and progesterone concentrations fall rapidly when the infusion of GnRH is stopped; premature menstruation is observed in all animals. Reproduced from Hutchison and Zeleznik (1984).

cyclic women and macaques that the administration of potent GnRH antagonists during the early or late luteal phases of the menstrual cycle results in a prompt and sustained fall in serum progesterone concentration followed by premature menstruation (Fraser *et al.*, 1985; Mais *et al.*, 1986). This is further evidence that secretion of progesterone by the corpus luteum depends absolutely upon LH throughout the entire luteal phase of the primate menstrual cycle.

The demonstration that progesterone levels fall if infusion of GnRH is stopped during the early luteal phase is not consistent with *in vitro* data obtained using luteal cells isolated from human corpora lutea (Fisch *et al.*, 1989). Luteal cells from corpora lutea removed during the early luteal phase undertake high rates of basal progesterone secretion which are relatively refractory to the addition of hCG to the culture medium. This finding suggests that steroidogenic cells in the newly formed corpus luteum are already stimulated maximally by the preceding LH surge and/or that the function of the early luteal-phase corpus luteum is expressed independently of the prevailing degree of stimulation by LH. If this property of luteal cells were also manifest *in vivo* withdrawal of luteal support by LH during the early luteal phase of the cycle would not be expected to cause luteal progesterone secretion to cease. The reason for this discrepancy between *in vivo* and *in vitro* findings remains to be determined.

### Role of the pattern of LH secretion

One of the major unanswered questions regarding the function of the corpus luteum is whether changes in LH secretion cause the onset of luteal regression in non-fertile menstrual cycles. It is well known that the pattern of LH secretion varies throughout the luteal phase, such that during the early luteal phase episodes of LH secretion occur at a frequency of approximately one pulse per hour while during the mid−late luteal phase the pulse-frequency of LH secretion slows to one pulse per 4−8 h (Ellinwood *et al.*, 1984; Filicori *et al.*, 1984). In view of the aforementioned absolute dependence of luteal function on LH, it has been suggested that the decline in LH pulse-frequency could cause onset of luteal regression by reducing the trophic drive to the corpus luteum. This hypothesis has been tested directly using MBH-lesioned, GnRH-replaced rhesus monkeys. Because secretion of LH in this model is controlled by the administration of exogenous GnRH, the frequency of pulsatile LH release can be regulated directly by adjusting the frequency at which exogenous GnRH is given (Hutchison *et al.*, 1986). Results in Fig. 6.5 show that when an LH pulse-frequency of once per 8 h (i.e. that which usually occurs in spontaneously cyclic animals during the period of luteal regression) is provided during the early luteal phase, luteal function is not adversely affected. In fact, serum progesterone concentration increases progressively towards the mid-

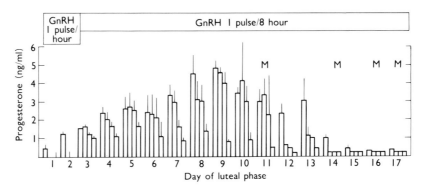

**Fig. 6.5.** Plasma progesterone concentrations in rhesus monkeys following a reduction in GnRH pulse-frequency from one pulse an hour to one every 8 h on Day 3 of the luteal phase. The GnRH pulse-frequency was reduced, and blood drawn 30, 60, 120 and 240 min after the a.m. pulse of GnRH; progesterone concentrations at each of these time-points are illustrated by individuals bars on each day. The letter M indicates the first day of menstrual bleeding in each of the animals. Reproduced from Hutchison and Zeleznik (1986).

luteal phase in the presence of a slow pulse frequency, which is exactly what occurs during the early–mid-luteal phase in spontaneous cycles or 'normal' cycles induced by giving GnRH at a frequency of one pulse per hour. The fact that luteal regression occurs at a normal time regardless of whether the pulse-frequency is fixed at once per hour or once per 8 h argues strongly that changes in the pattern of LH secretion do not cause luteal regression.

Interestingly, when the rate of GnRH-infusion is reduced further to a frequency of one pulse per 24 h, a premature drop in serum progesterone concentration and early menstruation does occur in MBH-lesioned animals (Hutchison *et al.*, 1986). However, an LH pulse-frequency as low as once every 24 h would not usually occur during spontaneous menstrual cycles and is therefore unlikely to account for spontaneous luteal regression. However, in MBH-lesioned monkeys receiving such low rates of pulsatile GnRH-infusion, the pattern of serum progesterone levels resembles that in women with so-called 'short luteal phases' (Jones *et al.*, 1974), suggesting that abnormal patterns of LH secretion might be a cause of this clinical disorder (see Chapter 9).

### Steroidal control of luteal function

Studies in both monkeys and women have demonstrated that administration of exogenous oestrogen during the luteal phase of the menstrual cycle causes premature regression of the corpus luteum (Gore *et al.*, 1973; Karsch *et al.*, 1973). These *in vivo* findings have been extended by *in vitro* observations that addition of oestradiol at high concentrations to cultures of rhesus monkey luteal cells results in suppression of progesterone secretion (Stouffer *et al.*, 1977b).

That endogenous oestrogen is a physiological luteolysin is an attractive hypothesis in view of the temporal relationship which exists in non-fertile menstrual cycles between onset of luteal demise and rising concentrations of oestrogen in luteal tissue and peripheral blood (Butler *et al.*, 1975). However, the mechanism by which oestrogen causes luteal regression is uncertain. Early studies concluded that oestrogen acts directly on the corpus luteum, since radioimmunoassay did not reveal any change in LH concentration during treatment with oestrogen (Karsch & Sutton, 1976; Schoonmaker *et al.*, 1981). However, more recent studies in which LH was measured by bioassay have indicated that plasma LH concentrations are suppressed during oestrogen-induced luteolysis (Schoonmaker *et al.*, 1982).

MBH-lesioned monkeys given pulsatile GnRH-infusion to induce ovulatory menstrual cycles have been used to determine whether oestrogen exerts its luteolytic effect indirectly via the hypothalamo−pituitary axis or directly at the level of the ovary (Hutchison *et al.*, 1987). Because input to the pituitary is provided by exogenous GnRH in this model, potential effects of oestrogen on hypothalamic GnRH secretion are ruled out. Results shown in Fig. 6.6 demonstrate that the administration of a luteolytic dose of exogenous oestradiol does not cause premature luteal regression in rhesus monkeys receiving pulsatile administration of exogenous GnRH to maintain secretion of endogenous gonadotrophin. These findings demonstrate that the luteolytic actions of oestradiol in spontaneously cyclic animals are due to inhibition of pituitary gonadotrophin secretion and not to a direct action on the ovary. This conclusion is consistent with the failure to observe oestrogen receptors in the primate corpus luteum by immunocytochemistry (Hild-Petito *et al.*, 1988).

The question as to whether the luteal secretion of oestrogen is still ultimately responsible for luteal regression remains unanswered. However, studies in both monkeys and baboons have shown that administration of oestrogen antagonists during the luteal phase of the cycle does not prolong the lifespan of the corpus luteum, suggesting that the luteolytic actions of oestrogen in primates may be pharmacological rather than physiological (Albrecht *et al.*, 1981; Westfahl & Resko, 1982). Interestingly, although immunocytochemical studies have failed to demonstrate the presence of oestrogen receptors in primate luteal cells, these cells have been shown to contain nuclear receptors for progesterone (Hild-Petito *et al.*, 1988). In view of the high levels of progesterone present within the corpus luteum, it will be interesting to see if the luteal progesterone receptor exhibits an affinity for progesterone similar to that of the 'classic' (i.e. endometrial) progesterone receptor. To-date, a specific progesterone-regulated luteal cell function has not been identified.

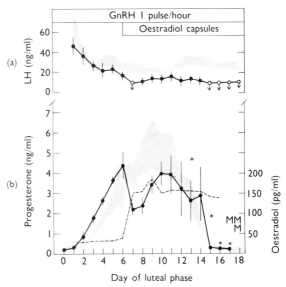

**Fig. 6.6.** Effects of exogenous oestradiol on plasma levels of (a) LH and (b) progesterone levels during luteal phase of the menstrual cycle induced by pulsatile infusion of GnRH in MBH-lesioned rhesus monkeys. Shaded areas denote mean (±SE) plasma hormone concentrations in control (non-oestrogen-treated) animals; solid lines indicate plasma hormone concentrations in animals which received oestradiol-filled Silastic implants placed subcutaneously on the days shown at the top of the figure. The interrupted line in (b) denotes mean plasma oestradiol concentrations before and after insertion of the oestradiol implants. Reproduced from Hutchison *et al.* (1986).

### Prolactin

Prolactin is a major luteotrophin in rats and mice (Hilliard, 1973). Whether this hormone plays a similar role in primates is less clear. Perhaps the most compelling evidence against this are the observations of Vande Wiele *et al.* (1969) that 'normal' luteal phases occur in gonadotrophin-treated, hypophysectomized women in the absence of exogenous prolactin. Similarly, del Pozo *et al.* (1975) have demonstrated that bromocriptine suppression of prolactin secretion does not affect normal luteal function. Although prolactin may not be an essential luteotrophin in primates, high prolactin concentrations may sustain the corpus luteum beyond its typical lifespan of 14–16 days. Richardson *et al.* (1985) noted that in some MBH-lesioned rhesus monkeys, serum prolactin concentrations were elevated to 100–800 ng/ml whereas in other animals they were normal (5–30 ng/ml). In animals with overt hyperprolactinaemia, serum progesterone concentrations during the early and mid-luteal phases were similar to those in animals with normal prolactin levels. However, unlike euprolactinaemic animals, progesterone concentrations in hyperprolactinaemic animals did not fall to undetectable concentrations at the expected time of luteolysis but remained elevated (at *c.* 1 ng progesterone/ml) for at least a week longer. Treatment with bromocriptine resulted in a rapid fall in both prolactin and progesterone concentrations and normal ovulatory menstrual cycles ensued. These findings point to a vestigial effect of prolactin on the primate corpus luteum and could be of relevance to the aetiology of hyperprolactinaemia-associated amenorrhoea (see Chapter 8).

## Luteal haemodynamics

The preovulatory follicle receives its entire blood supply by capillaries that perfuse the theca cell layer. Because granulosa cells are not in direct contact with follicular capillaries, their metabolism must be served solely by diffusion of nutrients across the follicular basement membrane. In addition to the restricted access of granulosa cells to capillary blood, the permeability properties of the follicular capillaries and basement membrane are such that a 'blood–follicle' barrier is created that excludes large protein molecules, such as LDL (Shalgi *et al.*, 1973). Secretion of progesterone by the corpus luteum *in vivo* is dependent on the supply of LDL-associated cholesterol as a steroidogenic substrate (Carr *et al.*, 1982). Accordingly, adequate vascularization of the corpus luteum is essential for the production of progesterone. The incisive experiments of Gospodarowicz and Thakral (1978) demonstrated that the newly ovulated follicle produces angiogenic factors that direct capillary proliferation into the luteinizing tissue. Although the specific angiogenic factor or factors produced by the luteinizing granulosa cells have not been identified with certainty, the recent findings that bovine luteal cells contain mRNA for basic fibroblast growth factor (bFGF) and that LH stimulates bFGF mRNA levels in luteal cells *in vitro* may help provide an explanation for the neovascularization of the newly formed corpus luteum (Stirling *et al.*, 1990) (see also Chapter 7).

In addition to the importance of neovascularization in the development of the corpus luteum and the provision of precursor cholesterol for steroidogenesis, the maintenance of blood flow to the corpus luteum throughout the luteal phase is essential for normal luteal function. Indeed, on a tissue-weight basis, blood flow to the corpus luteum is among the greatest of any tissue in the body (Abdul-Karim & Bruce, 1973). The possibility that changes in luteal blood flow during the luteal phase may directly influence the function and regression of the corpus luteum has received much attention (Niswender *et al.*, 1976). However, this hypothesis is confounded by two problems. First, the issue of cause vs. effect: does the corpus luteum regress because of a reduction in blood flow or is the reduction in blood flow secondary to luteal regression? Second, there is marked interspecies variation in the mechanisms which are seemingly responsible for luteal regression. In sheep, it is well documented that luteal regression is due to the luteolytic effects of prostaglandin $F_{2\alpha}$ produced by the uterus, and that administration of this prostaglandin results in a reduction in ovarian blood flow (Ellinwood *et al.*, 1978). However, in rabbits, experimental withdrawal of oestrogenic stimulation results in premature luteal regression and a fall in progesterone secretion with no concomitant fall in blood flow to the corpus luteum (Wiltbank *et al.*, 1989). Moreover, it has recently been shown that rabbit corpora lutea of pseudopregnancy lack vascular smooth muscle, rendering it doubtful if blood flow within the lupine corpus luteum could be influenced directly by factors which induce vasoconstriction or vasodilation (Wiltbank *et al.*, 1990). In primates, the role of blood flow in the regulation of the corpus luteum is even less clear. It is certain that the luteolytic signal does not originate in the uterus of these species (Neill *et al.*, 1969), but changes in luteal blood flow due to locally produced vasoactive substances, including prostaglandins, have yet to be ruled out.

## Rescue of the corpus luteum by CG

The corpus luteum of a non-fertile menstrual cycle has a finite lifespan of 14–16 days. However, its secretory activity is prolonged in the event of pregnancy due to the secretion of hCG by trophoblastic cells of the placenta. hCG and LH are structurally similar glycoprotein hormones which apparently interact with the same cell-surface receptor on primate luteal cells to stimulate adenylyl cyclase (Cameron & Stouffer, 1982a; Eyster & Stouffer, 1985). It is therefore assumed that the fundamental mechanism responsible for the rescue of the corpus luteum involves prolonged gonadotrophic stimulation of luteal cells by hCG. The recent cloning of the LH/hCG receptor should permit a definitive answer to the question of whether there is a single receptor that binds both LH and hCG (McFarland *et al.*, 1989).

The puzzling question regarding the role of gonadotrophins and rescue of the corpus luteum is why the gland regresses in the presence of LH whereas hCG, a similar glycoprotein hormone, is stimulatory. Regression of the corpus luteum in the non-fertile menstrual cycle may be a consequence of stimulation by LH at reduced intensity during the late luteal phase. However, a reduction in LH pulse-frequency, the most obvious alteration in gonadotrophin secretion at this time, has been ruled out as the sole cause of luteal regression, as discussed earlier (see Fig. 6.5).

The most notable difference between LH and hCG is the greater degree of glycosylation of the hCG molecule. Its extensive glycosylation explains why hCG has a much longer half-life in plasma than LH (Rizkallah *et al.*, 1969). In addition, data obtained with sheep corpora lutea indicate that the rate of internalization of receptor-bound hCG is nearly 50 times slower than the internalization of receptor-bound LH (Niswender *et al.*, 1985). These two differences between hCG and LH favour prolonged and more intense cellular stimulation by hCG. Thus, hCG may rescue the corpus luteum by providing an unrelenting stimulus to luteal cells during the mid–late luteal phase, as opposed to the periods of episodic stimulation given by LH (Monfort *et al.*, 1989). This possibility is supported by the observation that administration of large amounts of LH to women during the late luteal phase of the menstrual cycle is able to prolong the functional lifespan of the human corpus luteum (Hanson *et al.*, 1971). However, it should be recalled that maintenance of a rapid (once an hour) LH pulse-frequency throughout the entire luteal phase is not sufficient to prolong the lifespan of the monkey corpus luteum (Fig. 6.3). Therefore, the increasing dependence of the corpus luteum on gonadotrophic support when it begins to undergo functional regression during the mid−late luteal phase of the cycle is most likely due to changes which are occurring at the luteal cell level (see Chapter 7).

Stouffer *et al.* (1977a) have demonstrated that rhesus monkey luteal cells isolated during the late luteal phase show reduced responsiveness to hCG *in vitro*, as compared with cells isolated at earlier stages of luteal development. There is also evidence for a development-dependent change in the responsiveness of the primate corpus luteum to hCG *in vivo*. Ottobre & Stouffer (1984) gave rhesus monkeys 10 days of treatment with hCG, starting treatment at different times in the luteal phase. They noted that when the treatment with hCG was initiated 5 days after the mid-cycle LH surge, progesterone secretion increased throughout the entire 10 days of therapy with hCG. However, when the same hCG treatment-regimen was started 8 days after the mid-cycle gonadotropin surge, the increase in progesterone secretion was transient in that serum progesterone concentrations only rose over the first 2−3 days of treatment with hCG treatment and declined thereafter, despite continued administration of hCG. These observations indicate that there is a point in time during the lifespan of the corpus luteum beyond which hCG cannot induce a sustained increase in luteal steroidogenesis. Whether changing luteal-cell responsiveness to gonadotrophin is an intrinsic feature of luteal ageing or whether it is caused by direct actions of locally produced factors (e.g. prostaglandins) remain to be determined.

There is a paucity of basic information regarding roles of gonadotrophins in controlling luteal cell function. Virtually all of our knowledge is confined to the acute regulatory action of LH on progesterone synthesis. Are gonadotrophins simply responsible for the acute mobilization of cholesterol and its metabolism to progesterone in terminally differentiated luteal cells, or are they also responsible for longer-term maintenance of differentiated cell function via the regulation of steady-state levels of steroidogenic enzymes and the mRNAs which encode them (see Chapter 2)? Answers to these fundamental questions are essential to fully understand LH action and discover how hCG prolongs the lifespan of this ephemeral steroid-secretory gland.

## Cyclic luteal regression: a model of programmed cell death?

In non-fertile menstrual cycles, the corpus luteum produces progesterone for a period of 14−16 days. One of the most interesting questions in ovarian physiology is the mechanism responsible for the synchronous loss of cellular function and subsequent cell death that occurs during luteolysis. While it is certain that LH is absolutely required for the moment-to-moment control of progesterone secretion by the corpus luteum, the extent to which LH is involved in the maintenance of the viability of luteal cells is poorly understood. Use of progesterone secretion as an index of luteal cell viability indicates that LH is involved acutely in the maintenance of the lifespan of luteal cells since withdrawal of LH support results in rapid cessation of luteal progesterone secretion and onset of premature menses (Fig. 6.4). However, as shown in Fig. 6.7, the regulatory action of LH on luteal progesterone secretion can be dissociated from its influence on luteal cell lifespan. In these studies using MBH-lesioned rhesus monkeys, pulsatile infusion of exogenous GnRH to induce a normal menstrual cycle was interrupted for 3 days during the early, mid- or late luteal phases of the cycle, and

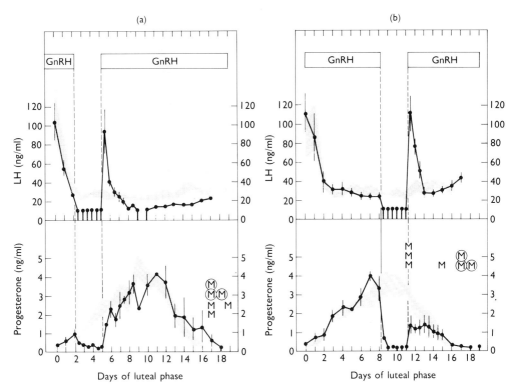

**Fig. 6.7.** Effect of transient withdrawal of pituitary gonadotrophin secretion on luteal function in rhesus monkeys. In (a) responses are shown by animals in which infusion of GnRH was terminated on Day 3 of the luteal phase and restored on Day 6. In (b) responses are shown by animals in which infusion of GnRH was terminated on day 8 of the luteal phase and restored on Day 11. The upper portion of each graph shows plasma LH concentrations; the bottom portion, plasma progesterone concentrations. Shaded areas denote control values (±SE). Solid lines represent hormone values in the animals in which infusion of GnRH infusion was stopped and then restarted 3 days later. The letter M signifies the first day of menstrual bleeding in the experimental animals, the encircled M shows the first day of menstrual bleeding in the control animals. Reproduced from Hutchison and Zeleznik (1985).

progesterone concentrations were measured as an index of luteal cell function (Hutchison & Zeleznik, 1985). As expected, withdrawal of GnRH led to a fall in plasma LH concentrations followed by a cessation of progesterone production by the corpus luteum, again demonstrating that the acute control of progesterone secretion by the corpus luteum is absolutely dependent on LH (see earlier). However, when LH secretion was restored by resuming GnRH-infusion, secretion of progesterone by the corpus luteum was reinitiated. Moreover, the overall length of the luteal phase was unaffected by the 3-day period of withdrawn gonadotrophic support. As seen in Fig. 6.7a, stopping the GnRH-infusion on Day 3 of the luteal phase and reinitiating it on day 5 was followed by a period of resumed progesterone secretion which effectively completed the tissue's full lifespan of 14−16 days. Similarly, as shown in Fig. 6.7b, terminating the GnRH-infusion on Day 9 of the luteal phase resulted in a rapid fall in serum progesterone concentrations and premature onset of menses on day 10. Restarting the GnRH-infusion on Day 12 resulted in a period of resumed progesterone secretion of sufficient duration to complete the length of a normal luteal phase. These data demonstrate that withdrawal of gonadotrophic support for 3 days does not result in an irreversible loss in the steroidogenic potential of the corpus luteum. Most remarkably, nor does it alter the timing of the onset of functional luteal regression. Thus although LH is clearly involved in the moment-to-moment regulation of luteal progesterone secretion, the gonadotrophin does not appear to tightly regulate the rate at which the mainspring of the 'luteal clock' unwinds. This raises the intriguing possibility that regulation by LH of the biosynthetic pathways responsible for steroidogenesis is somehow superimposed upon another more fundamental regulatory mechanism which governs cell viability.

An early theory to explain the invariance of luteal-phase length was that, in the absence of hCG production by the conceptus, the corpus luteum has an inherently programmed lifespan of 14−16 days. Although this theory has received little attention in recent years, current studies in other organ systems have described a specific pattern of programmed cell death, called apoptosis, that is associated with cell death occurring in differentiated tissues (Kerr *et al.*, 1972). This type of cell death is characterized by a specific pattern of morphological change. First, cells dying by apoptosis manifest an initial reduction in cytoplasmic volume. A loss of cell volume is opposite to the situation which would hold if cell death were caused by nutrient deficiency or hypoxia, because in these cases, cell volume would increase due to the impaired ability of $Na^+/K^+$ ATPase to maintain intracellular ion concentrations. The second characteristic of apoptotic cell death is condensation of nuclear chromatin followed by nuclear pyknosis. Thereafter, macrophages invade the tissue and phagocytose the dying cells, giving rise to cellular fragments composed of organelles termed apoptotic bodies.

This type of cell death was initially proposed as providing a mechanism by which tissue mass is maintained, that is to counterbalance cells added by mitosis. Subsequent studies show that this pattern of cell death occurs during embryogenesis as well as after withdrawal of hormonal support from hormone-dependent tissues in the endocrine system.

Corner (1956), in his description of the histological changes that occur in the human corpus luteum throughout the luteal phase, described morphological changes in luteal cells that are remarkably similar to those that occur during apoptosis. On c. Day 9 of the luteal phase, luteal cells begin to shrink and the cytoplasm begins to vacuolate. By Day 11 of the luteal phase, cell shrinkage is very pronounced and nuclear chromatin condensation and nuclear pyknosis becomes evident. By Day 13, the presence of a new type of cell was evident that was termed a 'mulberry' cell. The cytological description of the mulberry cell is remarkably similar to that of the apoptotic body that is a hallmark of cells undergoing cell death by apoptosis.

The process of luteal regression most likely begins 5–6 days before onset of menses when serum progesterone concentrations begin to decline from their mid-luteal phase peak (i.e. when functional luteolysis begins). This decline in serum progesterone concentration is associated with a reduction in luteal weight and appears to correlate temporally with shrinkage of luteal cells. Moreover, the ability of the corpus luteum to be rescued by CG appears to be temporally associated with the initial reduction in luteal cell volume. Thus, as described earlier, Ottobre and Stouffer (1984) noted that hCG was only effective in causing a sustained increase in progesterone production when it was administered prior to Day 8 of the luteal phase; delaying the treatment with hCG beyond that time resulted in only a transient increase in luteal progesterone production. If cell shrinkage is an early event in the process of luteal cell death, it would appear that once this process is initiated, there is an irreversible commitment to luteolysis that cannot be overcome by CG.

Studies on the mechanism of cell death by apoptosis have indicated that an early event in this process is the degradation of genomic DNA by a $Ca^{2+}/Mg^{2+}$-dependent endonuclease that cleaves DNA at internucleosomal sites. This endonuclease appears to be induced upon terminal cell differentiation and has been associated with the cell-death that occurs during glucocorticoid-induced lymphocytolysis and castration induced involution of the prostate (Wyllie, 1980; Kyprianou & Isaacs, 1988). Recent studies in rats have shown that this endonuclease is induced upon terminal differentiation of granulosa cells (Zeleznik et al., 1989). As shown in Fig. 6.8, nuclei obtained from undifferentiated granulosa cells in preantral ovarian follicles do not possess $Ca^{2+}/Mg^{2+}$-dependent endonuclease activity. However, nuclei from granulosa cells obtained from differentiated granulosa cells in preovulatory follicles exhibit marked DNA-degradation in the presence of $Ca^{2+}$ and $Mg^{2+}$

**Fig. 6.8.** Endogenous endonuclease activity in nuclear preparations from rat granulosa and luteal cells. In (a) results shown were obtained from undifferentiated granulosa cells [i.e. from preantral–early antral follicles in the ovaries of diethylstilboestrol (DES)-treated rats]; (b) shows results obtained from functionally differentiated granulosa cells [i.e. from preovulatory follicles in the ovaries of rats treated with DES and pregnant mare's serum gonadotrophin (PMSG)]; (c) shows results for luteal cells (i.e. from follicles and corpora lutea obtained after treatment with DES and PMSG, followed by hCG to induce luteinization). For each group of animals, solid bars represent nuclease activity at $t_0$ in the presence of 1 mM $Ca^{2+}$; stippled bars show activity measured under the same conditions at $t=10$ min. The cross-hatched bars represent nuclease activity at $t_0$ in the presence of 1 mM $Ca^{2+}$ and 5 mM $Mg^{2+}$; open bars show activity measured under the same conditions at $t=10$ min. Reproduced from Zeleznik *et al.* (1989)

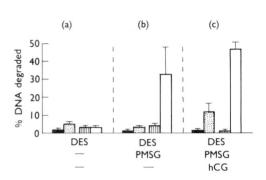

and this endonuclease activity is retained after ovulation and luteinization has been stimulated by hCG. Figure 6.9 shows that the degraded DNA migrates on agarose gels as discrete fragments of multiples of c. 180 nucleotide base pairs, typical of DNA cleaved intranucleosomally.

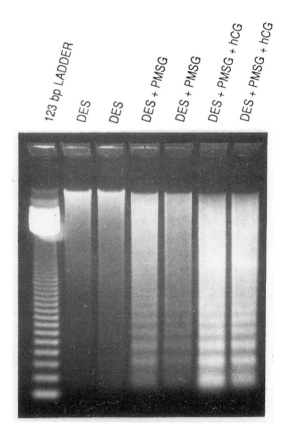

**Fig. 6.9.** Electrophoretic profile of low molecular weight DNA after assay for $Ca^{2+}/Mg^{2+}$-sensitive endonuclease activity. Letters at the top of the photograph identify the hormone treatments given *in vivo* (see legend to Fig. 6.8). A 123 base-pair nucleosomal ladder is shown in the left-hand lane. Reproduced from Zeleznik *et al.* (1989).

Although it has yet to be shown that this endonuclease contributes to luteolysis *in vivo*, the similarities between luteal regression and apoptosis suggest analogies between luteal cell death and cell death in other tissues. As an example, it has been shown recently that glucocorticoid-induced lymphocytolysis can be blocked by the removal of calcium from the incubation medium, by buffering intracellular calcium concentrations or by inhibiting calmodulin action (McConkey *et al.*, 1989), suggesting that an acute increase in intracellular free calcium concentration may serve to activate the $Ca^{2+}/Mg^{2+}$-dependent endonuclease and initiate degradation of DNA and cell death. Berman *et al.* in Chapter 7 discuss other important aspects of the role of calcium-mobilization in structural luteolysis.

The mid-luteal phase corpus luteum occupies *c.* 50% of the total ovarian volume. If mechanisms were not available to remove luteal tissue from the ovary after non-fertile cycles, by the menopause (after nearly 500 ovulations) the size of the ovaries would be immense. Teleologically, there must be a mechanism by which non-functional luteal cells are removed from the ovary. The attractiveness of the model of apoptosis is that it provides such a mechanism.

# References

Abdul-Karim, R.W. & Bruce, N. (1973) Blood flow to the ovary and corpus luteum at different stages of gestation in the rabbit. *Fertil. Steril.*, **24**, 44−7.

Albrechet, E.D., Haskins, A.L., Hodgen, G.D. & Pepe, G.C. (1981) Luteal function on baboons with administration of the anti-estrogen ethamoxytiphetol (MER-25) throughout the luteal phase of the menstrual cycle. *Biol. Reprod.*, **25**, 451−7.

Auletta, F.J. & Flint, A.P.F. (1988) Mechanisms controlling corpus luteum function in sheep, cows, non-human primates and women especially in relation to the time of luteolysis. *Endocr. Rev.*, **9**, 88−105.

Bassett, S.G., Winters, S.J., Keeping, H.J. & Zeleznik, A.J. (1990) Serum immunoreactive inhibin levels before and after lutectomy in the cynomolgus monkey. *J. Clin. Endocrinol. Metab.* (in press).

Borghi, M.R., Nievisky, R., Balcemeda, J.P., Coy, D.H., Schally, A.V. & Asch, R.H. (1983) Administration of luteinizing hormone − releasing hormone antagonist delays ovulation without affecting luteal function in rhesus monkeys. *Fertil. Steril.*, **40**, 678.

Butler, W.R., Hotchkiss, J. & Knobil, E. (1975) Functional luteolysis in the rhesus monkey: ovarian estrogen and progesterone during the luteal phase of the menstrual cycle. *Endocrinology*, **96**, 1509−12.

Cameron, J.L. & Stouffer, R.L. (1982a) Gonadotropin receptors of the primate corpus luteum. I. Characterization of $^{125}$-I labeled hLH and hCG binding to luteal membranes from the rhesus monkey. *Endocrinology*, **110**, 2059−67.

Cameron, J.L. & Stouffer, R.L. (1982b) Gonadotropin receptors of the primate corpus luteum. II. Changes in available luteinizing hormone and chorionic gonadotropin binding sites in macaque luteal membranes during the non-fertile menstrual cycle. *Endocrinology*, **110**, 2068−73.

Carr, B.R., MacDonald, P.C. & Simpson, E.R. (1982) The role of lipoproteins in the regulation of progesterone secretion by the corpus luteum. *Fertil. Steril.*, **38**, 303−11.

Corner, G.W. Jr. (1956) The histological dating of the human corpus luteum of menstruation. *Am. J. Anat.*, **98**, 37−65.

Davis, S.R., Krozowski, Z., McLachlan, R.I. & Burger, H.G. (1987) Inhibin gene expression in the human corpus luteum. *J. Endocrinol.*, **115**, R21−3.

del Pozo, E., Goldstein, M., Friesewn, H., Brun del Re, H. & Eppenberger, U. (1975) Lack of action of prolactin suppression in the regulation of the human menstrual cycle. *Am. J. Obstet. Gynecol.*, **123**, 719−23.

Dierschke, D.J., Hutz, R.J. & Wolf, R.C. (1985) Induced follicular atresia in rhesus monkeys: strength−duration relationship of the estrogen stimulus. *Endocrinology*, **117**, 1397−403.

DiZerega, G.S. & Hodgen, G.D. (1981) Luteal phase dysfunction: a sequel to abberent folliculogenesis. *Fertil. Steril.*, **35**, 489−99.

Ellinwood, W.E., Nett, T.M. & Niswender, G.D. (1978)

Ovarian vasculature: structure and function. In Jones, R.E. (ed.) *The Vertebrate Ovary*, pp. 583–614. Plenum Press, New York.

Ellinwood, W.E., Norman, R.L. & Spies, H.G. (1984) Changing frequency of pulsatile luteinizing hormone and progesterone secretion during the luteal phase of the menstrual cycle of rhesus monkeys. *Biol. Reprod.*, **31**, 714–22.

Eyster, K.M. & Stouffer, R.L. (1985) Adenylate cyclase in the corpus luteum of the rhesus monkey. II. Sensitivity to nucleotides, gonadotropins, catecholamines and non-hormonal activators. *Endocrinology*, **116**, 1552–8.

Filicori, M., Butler, J.P., Crowley, W.F. Jr. (1984) Neuroendocrine regulation of the corpus luteum in the human: evidence for pulsatile progesterone secretion. *J. Clin. Invest.*, **73**, 1638–47.

Fisch, B., Margara, R.A., Winston, R.M.L. & Hillier, S.G. (1989) Cellular basis of luteal steroidogenesis in the human ovary. *J. Endocrinol.*, **122**, 303–11.

Fraser, H.M., Baird D.T., McRae, G.T., Nestor, T.J. & Vickery, B.H. (1985) Suppression of luteal progesterone secretion in the stump tailed macaque by an antagonist of luteinizing hormone-releasing hormone. *J. Endocrinol.*, **104**, R1–4.

Fraser, H.M., Robertson, D.M. & de Kretser, D.M. (1989) Immunoreactive inhibin concentrations in serum throughout the menstrual cycle of the macaque: Suppression of inhibin during the luteal phase after treatment with an LHRH antagonist. *J. Endocrinol.*, **121**, R9–12.

Gemzell, C. (1965) Induction of ovulation with human gonadotropins. *Recent Prog. Horm. Res.*, **21**, 79–96.

Gore, B.Z., Caldwell, B.V. & Speroff, L. (1973) Estrogen-induced human luteolysis. *J. Clin. Endocrinol. Metab.*, **36**, 613–17.

Gospodarowicz, D. & Thakral, K.K. (1978) Production of a corpus luteum angiogenic factor responsible for proliferation of capillaries and neovascularization of the corpus luteum. *Proc. Natl. Acad. Sci. USA*, **75**, 847–51.

Gougeon, A. (1982) Rate of follicular growth in the human ovary. In Rolland, R. *Follicular Maturation and Ovulation*, pp. 155–63. Excerpta Medica, Amsterdam.

Guzik, D.S. & Zeleznik, A.J. (1990) Efficacy of clomiphene citrate in the treatment of luteal phase deficiency: quantity vs quality of preovulatory follicles. *Fertil. Steril.* (in press).

Hanson, F.W., Powell, J.E. & Stevens, V.C. (1971) Effects of hCG and human pituitary LH on steroid secretion and functional lifespan of the human corpus luteum. *J. Clin. Endocrinol. Metab.*, **32**, 211.

Hild-Petito, S., Stouffer, R.L. & Brenner, R.M. (1988) Immunocytochemical localization of estradiol and progesterone receptors in the monkey ovary throughout the menstrual cycle. *Endocrinology*, **123**, 2896.

Hilliard, J. (1973) Corpus luteum function in guinea pigs, mice and rabbits. *Biol. Reprod.*, **8**, 203–21.

Hillier, S.G. (1990) Ovarian steroid hormones. In Philipp, E. & Setchell, M.E. (eds) *Scientific Foundations of Obstetrics and Gynaecology*, 4th edn. Heinemann, London (in press).

Hutchison, J.S., Kubik, C.J., Nelson, P.B. & Zeleznik, A.J. (1987) Estrogen induces premature luteal regression in rhesus monkeys during spontaneous menstrual cycles but not in cycles driven by exogenous gonadotropin-releasing hormone. *Endocrinology*, **121**, 466–74.

Hutchison, J.S., Nelson, P.B. & Zeleznik, A.J. (1986) Effects of different gonadotropin pulse frequencies on corpus luteum function during the menstrual cycle of rhesus monkeys. *Endocrinology*, **119**, 1964–71.

Hutchison, J.S. & Zeleznik, A.J. (1984) The rhesus monkey corpus luteum is dependent on pituitary gonadotropin secretion throughout the luteal phase of the menstrual cycle. *Endocrinology*, **115**, 1780–6.

Hutchison, J.S. & Zeleznik, A.J. (1985) The corpus luteum of the primate menstrual cycle is capable of recovering from a transient withdrawal of pituitary gonadotropin support. *Endocrinology*, **117**, 1043–9.

Jones, G.S., Askel, S. & Wentz, C.A. (1974) Serum progesterone values in luteal phase defects: effects of chorionic gonadotropin. *Obstet. Gynecol.*, **44**, 26.

Kahn-Dawood, F.S., Goldsmith, L.T., Weiss, D. & Dawood, M.Y. (1989) Human corpus luteum secretion of relaxin, oxytocin and progesterone. *J. Clin. Endocrinol. Metab.*, **68**, 627–31.

Karsch, F.J., Krey, L.C., Weich, R.F., Dierschke, D.J. & Knobil, E. (1973) Functional luteolysis in the rhesus monkey: role of estrogen. *Endocrinology*, **92**, 1148–52.

Karsch, F.J. & Sutton, G.P. (1976) An intra-ovarian site for the luteolytic action of estrogen in the rhesus monkey. *Endocrinology*, **98**, 553–61.

Kerr, J.F.R., Wyllie, A.H. & Currie, A.R. (1972) Apoptosis: a basic biological phenomenon with wide-ranging implications in tissue kinetics. *Br. J. Cancer*, **26**, 239–57.

Keyes, P.L. & Wiltbank, M.C. (1988) Endocrine regulation of the corpus luteum. *Annu. Rev. Physiol.*, **50**, 465–82.

Kyprianou, N. & Isaacs, J.T. (1988) Activation of programmed cell death in the ventral rat prostate after castration. *Endocrinology*, **122**, 552–62.

McConkey, D.J., Nicotera, P., Hartzell, P., Bellomo, G., Wyllie, A.H. & Orresius, S. (1989) Glucocorticoids activate a suicide process in thymocytes through an elevation in cytosolic $Ca^{2+}$ concentrations. *Arch. Biochem. Biophys.*, **269**, 365–70.

McFarland, K.C., Sprengell, R., Phillips, H.S. *et al.* (1989) Lutropin–choriogonadotropin receptor: an unusual member of the G protein-coupled receptor family. *Science*, **245**, 494–9.

McLachlan, R.I., Robertson, D.M., Healy, D.L., Burger, H.G. & De Kretser, D.M. (1987) Circulating immunoreactive inhibin during the normal human menstrual cycle. *J. Clin. Endocrinol. Metab.*, **65**, 954−61.

Mais, V., Kazer, R.R., Cetel, N.S., Rivier, J., Vale, W. & Yen, S.S.C. (1986) The dependency of folliculogenesis and corpus luteum function on pulsatile gonadotropin secretion in cycling women using a gonadotropin releasing antagonist as a probe. *J. Clin. Endocrinol. Metab.*, **62**, 1250−5.

Monfort, S.L., Hess, D.L., Hendrickx, A.G. & Lasley, B.L. (1989) Absence of regular pulsatile gonadotropin secretion during implantation in the rhesus macaque. *Endocrinology*, **125**, 1766−73.

Neill, J.D., Johansson, E.D.B. & Knobil, E. (1969) Failure of hysterectomy to influence the normal pattern of cyclic progesterone secretion in the rhesus monkey. *Endocrinology*, **84**, 464−71.

Niswender, G.D. & Nett, T.M. (1988) The corpus luteum and its control. In Knobil, E. & Neill, J.D. (eds) *The Physiology of Reproduction*, pp. 489−525. Raven Press, New York.

Niswender, G.D., Reimers, T.J., Diekmasn, M.A. & Nett, T.M. (1976) Blood flow: a mediator of ovarian function. *Biol. Reprod.*, **14**, 64−81.

Niswender, G.D., Schwall, R.H., Fitz, T.A., Faren, C.E. & Sawyer, H.R. (1985) Regulation of luteal function in domestic ruminants: new concepts. *Recent Prog. Horm. Res.*, **41**, 101−51.

Ottobre, J.S. & Stouffer, R.L. (1984) Persistent versus transient stimulation of the macaque corpus luteum during prolonged exposure to hCG; a function of the age of the menstrual cycle. *Endocrinology*, **114**, 2175−82.

Parker, C.R., Illingworth, D.R., Bissonnette, J. & Carr, B.R. (1986) Endocrine changes during pregnancy in a patient with homozygous familial hypobetalipoproteinemia. *N. Engl. J. Med.*, **314**, 2557.

Richardson, D.W., Goldsmith, L.T., Pohl, C.R., Schallenberger, E. & Knobil, E. (1985) The role of prolactin in the regulation of the primate corpus luteum. *J. Clin. Endocrinol. Metab.*, **60**, 501−6.

Rizkallah, T., Gurpide, E. & Vande Wiele, R.L. (1969) Metabolism of hCG in man. *J. Clin. Endocrinol. Metab.*, **29**, 92−7.

Schoonmaker, J.N., Bergman, K.S., Steiner, R.A. & Karsch, F.J. (1982) Estradiol-induced luteal regression in the rhesus monkey: evidence for an extra-ovarian site of action. *Endocrinology*, **110**, 1708−15.

Schoonmaker, J.N., Victery, W. & Karsch, F.J. (1981) A receptive period for estradiol-induced luteolysis in the rhesus monkey. *Endocrinology*, **108**, 1874−7.

Schwall, R.S., Mason, A, J., Wilcox, J.N., Bassett, S.G. & Zeleznik, A.J. (1990) Localization of inhibin/activin subunit mRNA's within the primate ovary. *Mol. Endocrinol.*, **4**, 75−9.

Shalgi, R., Kraicer, P., Rimon, A., Pinto, M., & Soferman, N. (1973) Proteins of human follicular fluid: the blood−follicle barrier. *Fertil. Steril.*, **24**, 429−34.

Steinberger, A. & Ward, D.N. (1988) Inhibin. In Knobil, E. & Neill, J.D. (eds) *The Physiology of Reproduction*, pp. 567−83. Raven Press, New York.

Stirling, D., Magness, R.R., Stone, R., Waterman, M.R. & Simpson, E.R. (1990) Angiotensin II inhibits luteinizing hormone-stimulated cholesterol side chain cleavage expression and stimulates basic fibroblast growth factor expression in bovine luteal cells in primary culture. *J. Biol. Chem.*, **265**, 5−8.

Stouffer, R.L. & Hodgen, G.D. (1980) Induction of luteal phase defects in rhesus monkeys by follicular fluid administration at the onset of the menstrual cycle. *J. Clin. Endocrinol. Metab.*, **51**, 669−71.

Stouffer, R.L, Nixon, W.E., Gulyas, B.J. & Hodgen, G.D. (1977a) Gonadotropin-sensitive progesterone production by rhesus monkey luteal cells *in vitro*: a function of age of the corpus luteum during the menstrual cycle. *Endocrinology*, **100**, 506−12.

Stouffer, R.L., Nixon, W.E. & Hodgen, G.D. (1977b) Estrogen inhibition of basal and gonadotropin stimulated progesterone production by rhesus monkey luteal cells *in vitro*. *Endocrinology*, **101**, 1157.

Vande Wiele, R.L., Bogumil, J., Dyrenfurth, I., *et al.* (1969) Mechanisms regulating the menstrual cycle in women. *Recent Prog. Horm. Res.*, **26**, 63−92.

Weiss, G., O'Byrne, E.M. & Steinetz, B.G. (1976) Relaxin: a product of the human corpus luteum of pregnancy. *Science*, **194**, 948−9.

Westfahl, P.K. & Resko, J.A. (1982) The effects of clomiphene on luteal function in the nonpregnant cynomolgus macaque. *Biol. Reprod.*, **29**, 963−9.

Wildt, L., Hausler, A., Marshall, G., Hotchkiss, J.S., Plant, T.M., Belchetz, P.E. & Knobil, E. (1981) Frequency and amplitude of gonadotropin-releasing hormone stimulation and gonadotropin secretion in the rhesus monkey. *Endocrinology*, **109**, 367−85.

Wiltbank, M.C., Gallagher, K.P., Christensen, A.K., Brabec, R.K. & Keyes, P.L. (1990) Physiological and immunocytochemical evidence for a new concept of blood flow regulation in the corpus luteum. *Biol. Reprod.*, **42**, 139−51.

Wiltbank, M.C., Gallagher, K.P., Dysko, R.C. & Keyes, P.L. (1989) Regulation of blood flow to the rabbit corpus luteum: effects of estradiol and chorionic gonadotropin. *Endocrinology*, **124**, 605−11.

Wyllie, A.H. (1980) Glucocorticoid-induced thymocyte apaotosis is associated with endogenous endonuclease activation. *Nature*, **284**, 555−6.

Zeleznik, A.J., Ihrig, L.L. & Bassett, S.G. (1989) Developmental expression of $Ca^{++}/Mg^{++}$ sensitive endonuclease activity in rat granulosa and luteal cells. *Endocrinology*, **125**, 2218−20.

# 7 Cell-to-Cell Interactions in Luteinization and Luteolysis

H.R. BEHRMAN, R.F. ATEN & J.R. PEPPERELL

## Introduction

The corpus luteum is composed of more than steroidogenic parenchymal cells, and cell-to-cell interactions involving endothelial cells, blood cells and cells of the immune system must also contribute fundamentally to the cyclic formation, function and regression of this endocrine gland.

The aim of this chapter is to highlight the roles played by non-parenchymal cell types in luteal formation and regression. We survey the histogenetic composition of the corpus luteum and identify diverse angiogenic factors, growth factors and cytokines which are likely to mediate cell-to-cell interaction in the corpus luteum. We consider the evidence that purines (adenosine), prostaglandins and reactive oxygen species are vital components of the luteal paracrine system. Finally, we integrate this knowledge into a provisional framework which helps explain the cellular basis of luteolysis in primate and non-primate ovaries.

# Cellular composition of the corpus luteum

Several cell types make up the corpus luteum of bovine, ovine and porcine species (Lemon & Loir, 1977; Lemon & Mauleon, 1982; Rodgers *et al.*, 1983; Farin *et al.*, 1989). More than half are steroidogenic parenchymal cells; the remainder are fibroblasts and capillary endothelial cells (Rodgers *et al.*, 1984; Farin *et al.*, 1986, 1989), and cells associated with the immune response (Table 7.1).

## Endocrine cells

The human corpus luteum contains two main steroidogenic cell types: granulosa–lutein and theca–lutein cells, denoting their origins as follicular granulosa and thecal cells, respectively. The corpus luteum in domestic animal species contains at least two morphologically distinct steroidogenic cell types: 'small' and 'large'. Early studies suggested that small luteal cells originate from thecal cells whereas large luteal cells differentiate from granulosa cells (O'Shea *et al.*, 1979). More recent studies suggest that fibroblasts may differentiate into small luteal cells which become transformed into large cells in response to stimulation by leuteinizing hormone (LH) (Alila & Hannsel, 1984; Schwall *et al.*, 1986; Farin *et al.*, 1989).

General properties of bovine, ovine and porcine small and large luteal cells are listed in Table 7.1. Small luteal cells are stellate in shape with diameters ranging from 12 to 22 μm; they contain abundant smooth endoplasmic reticulum, mitochondria, and lipid droplets (O'Shea *et al.*, 1979; Fitz *et al.*, 1982; Rodgers *et al.*, 1984). Large luteal cells are polyhedral with diameters ranging from 25 to 35 μm and have numerous mitochondria, lipid droplets, and membrane-bound granules (McClellan *et al.*, 1975; O'Shea *et al.*, 1979). Both cell types contain adenylyl cyclase systems coupled to steroid synthesis, but only small cells are responsive to LH (Fitz *et al.*, 1982; Hoyer & Niswender, 1985; Harrison *et al.*, 1987). However, LH-non-responsive large luteal cells have receptors for prostaglandins ($F_{2\alpha}$ and $E_2$) and oestrogen (Fitz *et al.*, 1982; Alilia *et al.*, 1988; Davis *et al.*, 1988).

**Table 7.1.** General characteristics of steroidogenic cells in the corpora lutea of ruminant animal species

|  | Small | Large |
|---|---|---|
| Origin | Theca | Granulosa |
| Diameter (μm) | 12–18 | 25–35 |
| Basal steroidogenic capacity | Low | High |
| Responsiveness to LH | High | Low |
| Responsiveness to prostaglandin $F_{2\alpha}$ | Low | High |

Relative proportions of small and large luteal cells in ruminant corpora lutea vary with endocrine status, possibly reflecting a continuum in cell development and differentiation. During the oestrous cycle, small luteal cells appear to increase in number, but not size, whereas large cells increase in size, but not number (O'Shea et al., 1979; Rodgers et al., 1984; Farin et al., 1986, 1989). LH may stimulate the transformation of small luteal cells into large luteal cells (Farin et al., 1988, 1989). When LH/hCG (human chorionic gonadotrophin) was administered during the follicular phase of the bovine oestrous cycle, small luteal cells diminished in number whereas the number of large luteal cells increased; neither cell type changed in size. Administration of a luteolytic agent also affected luteal cell populations. Following administration of prostaglandin $F_{2\alpha}$, small luteal cells diminished in number but not size, and large cells were reduced in size, but not number (Braden et al., 1988).

Endothelial cells, but not fibroblasts, also diminish in number following administration of prostaglandin. During pregnancy, both small and large luteal cells increase in size and small cells lose their responsiveness to LH (Harrison et al., 1987; Farin et al., 1989). In the ferret, pregnancy increases the size, but not the number of all luteal cells and no discrete cell populations (i.e. small vs. large) are observed (Joseph & Mead, 1988). In other species, such as the rat, pregnancy increases the size, but not the number, of both small and large luteal cells (Meyer & Bruce, 1979).

## Non-endocrine cells

Cells involved in immuno-inflammatory responses are also present in the corpus luteum, for example endothelial cells, macrophages, neutrophils, fibroblasts and thymocytes (Bulmer, 1964; Adams & Hertig, 1969; Gillim, 1969; Meyer & Bruce, 1980; Kirsch et al., 1981; Azmi & O'Shea, 1984; Bagavandoss, 1988). As discussed later, growth factors and cytokines produced by these cells are increasingly implicated in the control of luteinization and luteolysis.

### Endothelial cells

The classic function of the endothelium is to serve as a lining of the vascular lumen which separates the blood from muscular and fibrous tissues in blood vessel walls. Nowadays, the endothelial cell is seen not so much as a barrier but as an interactive organ with functions which impinge upon circulating blood and immune cells as well as the surrounding parenchyma. Endothelial cells serve as the sources and sites of action of multiple humoral agents, and as such are integral components of the luteal paracrine system (DiCorletto & Fox, 1989).

## Vascular homeostasis

A major function of the endothelial cell is maintenance of normal vascular homeostasis, achieved partly through production of prostanoids. Prostacyclin (prostaglandin $I_2$) is an antithrombolytic agent which is also a potent vasodilator and inhibitor of platelet aggregation (Pace-Asciak & Gryglewski, 1983). Endothelial cells secrete prostacyclin in response to stimulation by various agents, including histamine, thrombin, bradykinin and adenosine triphosphate (ATP) (Weksler et al., 1978; Hong, 1980; Pearson et al., 1983; McIntyre et al., 1985). Histamine and thrombin also cause endothelial cells to contract which could increase vascular permeability (Rotrosen & Gallin, 1986), thereby allowing humoral agents direct access to the basement membrane and adjacent parenchyma.

Vascular homeostasis is also regulated by atrial naturetic peptide (ANP). High-affinity receptors for ANP are found in membrane preparations of luteal tissue obtained during various stages of the oestrous cycle and pregnancy (Vollmar et al., 1988). In addition, guanylyl cyclase activity is stimulated when ANP is added to particulate luteal fractions, a finding consistent with the presence of ANP receptors. ANP is also found in acidic extracts of the corpus luteum (Vollmar et al., 1988). However, a specific function for ANP in the corpus luteum, such as modulation of production or release of progesterone remains to be demonstrated.

## Endothelial–immune cell interaction

Endothelial cells interact with and influence functions of immune cells which, in turn, influence endothelial cell function. Cultured endothelial cells secrete cytokines which modulate immune cell function. Such factors include colony-stimulating factor (CSF) (Quesenberry et al., 1980; Gerson et al., 1985), interleukin-1 (IL-1) (Miossec et al., 1986), interferon (IFN) (Einhorn et al., 1985) and chemoattractants for neutrophils and monocytes (Mercandetti et al., 1984; Berliner et al., 1986). Some of these factors are also secreted by lymphocytes and hence are 'lymphokines'. IFN-γ, produced by activated T-lymphocytes, stimulates the expression of class II major histocompatability complex (MHC) in endothelial cells which, in turn, stimulates the proliferation of T-cells (Pober, 1989). IL-1 is produced by macrophages and causes endothelial cells to become adhesive for neutrophils (Bevilaqua et al., 1985; Cavender et al., 1986). Tumor necrosis factor (TNF), produced by macrophages, also induces neutrophil adhesion to endothelial cells (Pohlman et al., 1986) and stimulates secretion of IL-1 by endothelial cells (Nawroth et al., 1986). Thus, IFN-γ, IL-1 and TNF are functionally interrelated, sharing actions which in some circumstances are synergistic (Pober, 1989).

Locally synthesized prostacyclin and platelet-activating factor (PAF) seem to mediate inflammatory responses shown by endothelial cells (Moncada *et al.*, 1976; Camussi *et al.*, 1983). Prostanoids, leukotrienes and membrane-derived phospholipids such as phosphatidic acid may also regulate endothelial antigenicity and adherence of leukocytes. For example, cyclooxygenase-derived products downregulate endothelial class II MHC antigen, and lipoxygenase-derived products influence adherence of leukocytes to endothelium (Leszczynski & Hayry, 1989).

Endothelial cells produce a factor similar to platelet-derived growth factor (PDGF) (DiCorletto, 1984). This factor, termed PDGFc, is secreted by cultured endothelial cells and binds to PDGF receptors on fibroblasts and smooth muscle cells (DiCorletto & Bowen-Pope, 1983). PDGFc production is modulated by a number of factors which include IL-1, TNF, thrombin and activators of protein kinase C. PDGFc is chemotactic for monocytes (Deuel *et al.*, 1982). It also seems likely that PDGFc modulates the function of neighbouring parenchymal cells although no direct evidence is available to indicate that it affects luteal function.

## Angiogenesis and luteal endocrine function

### Angiogenesis

After follicular rupture, newly formed blood vessels invade the granulosa cell layer and move towards the centre of ruptured follicles. Eventually, a dense network of highly permeable capillaries is established, bringing each luteal cell in close proximity to the vascular system (Moriss & Sass, 1966). The development of the luteal vasculature continues until the mid-luteal phase which is when maximal rates of luteal progesterone secretion are also attained. The importance of the luteal vasculature in supplying steroidogenic luteal cells with amounts of precursor cholesterol adequate to sustain luteal progesterone secretion is discussed further in Chapters 6 and 9.

Cellular mechanisms of angiogenesis are incompletely understood. New vessels originate as shoots or sprouts from small capillaries rather than from larger blood vessels. Initially, the basement membrane of the endothelium is broken down and endothelial cells migrate as a cord towards the angiogenic stimulus. The endothelial cord then begins to develop a lumen by either cell curvature or vacuole formation. Mitosis then begins, also regulated by angiogenic factors, and growth occurs just behind the tip of the advancing vessel. Individual shoots anastamose to form the new blood vessel which is initially highly permeable. Formation of the vessel is completed by the laying down of a basement membrane and migration of pericytes along the length of the vessel (Schor & Schor, 1983; Folkman, 1985).

## Angiogenic factors

Angiogenic factors characteristically have chemotactic and/or mitogenic properties (Folkman & Klagsbrun, 1987a,b; D'Amore & Braunhut, 1989). They can be classified into two groups on the basis of their molecular size: low molecular weight (often non-peptidic) factors and higher molecular weight polypeptide growth factors.

### Low molecular weight angiogenic factors

Some low molecular weight factors stimulate angiogenesis by promoting mitosis. Such factors include: pyrimidine nucleosides; histamine; selenium compounds; polyamines (spermine, spermidine and putrescine); and adipocyte-derived angiogenic factor. Other low molecular weight factors stimulate angiogenesis through modification of the basement membrane or by stimulating the mobilization of endothelial cells. Factors in this category include: adenosine diphosphate (ADP); heparin; copper and ceruloplasmin; prostaglandins of the E series; lactic acid; hyaluronic acid; and proteolytic fragments of fibronectin/heparin.

### Angiogenic peptide growth factors

Polypeptide growth factors with angiogenic properties can be classified according to their ability to bind heparin.

#### Heparin-binding growth factors

The heparin-binding family of growth factors is ubiquitous. It includes basic and acidic forms of fibroblastic growth factor (bFGF and aFGF), endothelial cell growth factor (ECGF), and tumour angiogenic factor. All are structurally related proteins which regulate cell growth (Findlay, 1986).

bFGF has been isolated from pituitary and brain (Bohlen *et al.*, 1984; Gospodarowicz *et al.*, 1984), placenta (Gospodarowicz *et al.*, 1985b), kidney (Baird *et al.*, 1985) and the corpus luteum (Gospodarowicz *et al.*, 1985a); aFGF has been isolated predominantly from neural tissue (D'Amore & Braunhut, 1989). Both forms of FGF are angiogenic (Davidson *et al.*, 1985; Shing *et al.*, 1985; Lobb *et al.*, 1985), and both stimulate endothelial cell mitosis and migration *in vitro* (Azizkhan *et al.*, 1983; Maciag *et al.*, 1984; Montesano *et al.*, 1986). The FGFs which have been isolated from the ovary and other tissues share a common molecular structure (Baird *et al.*, 1986; Folkman & Klagsbrun, 1987a). Considerable sequence homology exists between aFGF and bFGF (Esch *et al.*, 1985; Gimenez-Gallego *et al.*, 1985) which may explain their overlapping biological activities. Also included in the family of heparin-binding factors is ECGF, which is an aFGF precursor (Jaye *et al.*, 1986).

The amino acid sequence of FGF does not contain the 'signal' sequence which usually characterizes a secretory protein (Abraham *et al.*, 1986; Jaye *et al.*, 1986). Thus bFGF may not be actively secreted but released in times of vascular crisis or during angiogenesis when ischaemic conditions promote cell damage. FGFs are present in the basement membrane and may be deposited in association with heparin-like glycosaminoglycans (GAGs) to form a constitutive part of the extracellular matrix (Baird & Ling, 1987). One mechanism by which FGF activity is released from the basement membrane may involve heparinase-like enzymes secreted by proximal parenchymal cells (Baird & Ling, 1987).

Endothelial cell numbers increase during luteal development in the oestrous cycle (sheep) and gestation (rat) (Farin *et al.*, 1986; Meyer & Bruce, 1979). bFGF produced by luteal endothelial cells may therefore effect positive autocrine control over the development of the luteal endothelium.

Ovarian cell types other than endothelial cells are also affected by bFGF (Schreiber *et al.*, 1985; Olwin & Hauschuka, 1986). This growth factor stimulates mitotic activity in bovine granulosa cells (Gospodarowicz *et al.*, 1985a) and also influences progesterone production by luteal cells (Tapanainen *et al.*, 1987). bFGF also stabilizes the phenotypic expression of cultured cells and delays their senescence *in vitro* (Baird *et al.*, 1986). This property of bFGF might affect the functional lifespan of the corpus luteum.

*Non-heparin-binding growth factors*

Non-heparin-binding growth factors which participate in angiogenesis include angiogenin; epidermal growth factor (EGF); transforming growth factors (TGFs); insulin and insulin-like growth factors (IGFs); cytokines, including TNF; PDGF; thrombin; and lipoproteins. These are structurally unrelated factors which appear to influence angiogenesis by mechanisms different from that of FGF.

Angiogenin has considerable sequence homology with ribonucleases and also has intrinsic ribonuclease activity (Shapiro *et al.*, 1986). This factor is secreted and is a potent angiogenic agent *in vivo* (Fett *et al.*, 1985). However, no stimulation of endothelial cell proliferation by angiogenin was seen *in vitro* (Folkman & Klagsbrun, 1987a). It is not yet known if the ribonuclease activity of angiogenin constitutes the basis for its angiogenic action.

EGF and TGFα share considerable sequence homology and both stimulate endothelial cell proliferation (Schreiber *et al.*, 1986). EGF is also a granulosa cell mitogen. The human corpus luteum contains receptors for EGF (Ayyagari *et al.*, 1987) and TGFα binds to the EGF receptor (Schreiber *et al.*, 1986). Either factor could thereby contribute to the local control of luteal neovascularization.

The newly formed corpus luteum is an intrinsic source of at least three other potential angiogenic factors due to the presence of the blood clot which forms after ovulation. Platelets and thrombin are both involved in the clotting process. Thrombin seems to have angiogenic properties while platelets are a source of TGFβ and various other angiogenic growth factors. Thrombin selectively binds to endothelial cells (Awbrey *et al.*, 1979) but there is conflicting evidence as to whether it is actually mitogenic (D'Amore & Braunhut, 1989). TGFβ stimulates angiogenesis *in vivo* (Folkman & Klagsburn, 1987b), and TGFβ released by platelets promotes wound healing by inducing blood vessel ingrowth (Sporn *et al.*, 1986). However, TGFβ inhibits mitogenesis and migration of cultured endothelial cells *in vitro* (Baird & Durkin, 1986; Heimark *et al.*, 1986). The reason for this apparent paradox is uncertain but could be due to the culture conditions used. When endothelial cells are cultured in a three-dimensional gel matrix they form tube-like structures which become more complex in the presence of TGFβ, and cell proliferation is not inhibited (Madri *et al.*, 1988). Thus extracellular matrix is likely to exert a major influence on the expression of endothelial phenotype and mitotic activity in response to angiogenic factors (Ignotz & Massague, 1986; Muller *et al.*, 1987).

In addition to TGFβ, a number of unidentified factors which stimulate endothelial mitosis have been isolated from platelets. These factors include a low molecular weight factor which apparently supports the angiogenic activity of FGF (Clemmons *et al.*, 1983), and at least two high molecular weight factors which may be conjugated forms of FGF (D'Amore & Braunhut, 1989). Recently, a unique endothelial cell PDGF was also identified (Ishikawa *et al.*, 1989).

## Growth factors and luteal endocrine function

Various locally or trophoblastically derived growth factors appear to be involved in the control of luteal endocrine function. The actions which these factors have on luteal function fall into three major areas: promotion of granulosa cell luteinization or enhancement of luteal cell function; inhibition of luteinization or suppression of luteal cell function; and maintenance of the corpus luteum of pregnancy.

### Promoters of luteinization and luteal cell function

Insulin-like growth factor-I (IGF-I) promotes luteinization and stimulates the production of progesterone and oxytocin by cultured bovine granulosa cells (Schams, 1989). Whether IGF-I has direct effects on luteal cells is less certain. McArdle and Holtorf (1989) reported that treatment with IGF-I and insulin, but not IGF-II, stimulated oxytocin and progesterone release by bovine luteal cells in serum-free culture. Prostaglandin dose-dependently reduced the stimulatory effect of IGF-I on the release of oxytocin but not progesterone. However, Schams *et al.* (1988) failed to observe stimulatory effects of IGF-I, EGF or FGF on secretion of either oxytocin or progesterone by dispersed bovine luteal cells.

TGFβ is implicated in the follicular paracrine system as a modulator of granulosa cell growth and steroid synthesis (see Chapter 3). However, it has yet to be established if this factor plays a local regulatory role in the control of luteal cell function. Proteins related structurally to TGFβ such as inhibin and activin are also produced by the corpus luteum, but again their intraluteal regulatory functions, if any, are still uncertain.

PDGF from human platelets was initially reported to promote granulosa cell luteinization *in vitro* (Mondschein & Schomberg, 1981) but this effect may have been due to the presence of contaminating TGFβ (Schomberg, 1988). A role of the PDGF molecule *per se* in the control of luteal function therefore remains to be established.

## Inhibitors of luteinization and luteal cell function

The human corpus luteum produces EGF (Khan-Dawood, 1987) which is implicated as a negative regulator of granulosa cell luteinization, serving to inhibit LH-stimulated progesterone production (Fukuoka *et al.*, 1988). In bovine granulosa cell cultures, EGF stimulates cell growth, inhibits production of inhibin and progesterone, and increases secretion of oxytocin. These effects are likely to be receptor-mediated since EGF binding-sites are present on bovine granulosa and luteal cells (Schams, 1989). EGF also inhibits follicle-stimulating hormone (FSH)-induced differentiation of cultured rat granulosa cells, including progesterone synthesis and development of LH receptors (Jones *et al.*, 1982; Adashi & Resnick, 1986; Dodson & Schomberg, 1987). In human granulosa-lutein cell cultures, EGF stimulates cell growth and enhances basal production of progesterone (Tapanainen *et al.*, 1987).

EGF appears to inhibit transformation of granulosa cells into luteal cells by stimulating mitosis. Porcine granulosa cells synthesize DNA and proliferate in serum-free media supplemented with EGF (May *et al.*, 1988). In these cells, IGF-I enhances EGF-stimulated DNA synthesis and replication whereas TGFβ enhances EGF-stimulated DNA synthesis but inhibits cell proliferation. Although EGF inhibits granulosa cell luteinization, there is no direct evidence to suggest that it affects the function of luteal cells *per se*.

Although the foregoing *in vitro* results suggest that EGF prevents luteinization, infusion of EGF into ewes during the follicular phase of the oestrous cycle did not diminish the rise in plasma progesterone level due to follicular luteinization. However, it did block the prooestrus rise in plasma oestradiol level as well as the ovulatory LH surge. Infusion of EGF during the luteal phase had no effect on plasma progesterone (Shaw *et al.*, 1985).

Arginine vasopressin (AVP) and oxytocin are present in luteal extracts (Titzel *et al.*, 1988) and have the potential to inhibit luteal cell function. In porcine luteal cell cultures, these peptides suppress basal and LH-stimulated production of progesterone without affecting production of oestradiol. The potency of AVP in this regard is *c.* 10 000-fold that of oxytocin. Specific AVP/oxytocin receptor antagonists block the antigonadotrophic effects of both peptides.

The cytokine IL-1 appears to inhibit granulosa cell luteinization. Basal and LH-stimulated progesterone production by porcine and rat luteinizing granulosa cells are both inhibited by this factor (Fukuoka *et al.*, 1988; Gottschall *et al.*, 1988). Morphological luteinization is also inhibited by IL-1 (Fukuoka *et al.*, 1989). Large amounts of IL-1-like activity have been found in human ovarian follicular fluid (Khan *et al.*, 1988). The activity could be neutralized by specific IL-1 antibodies but its physiochemical characteristics differed from macrophage-derived IL-1. Production of IL-1 by macrophages increases during treatment with progesterone or oestradiol *in vitro* (Cannon & Dinarello, 1985). Furthermore, plasma levels of IL-1 activity are higher in women during the luteal phase than during the follicular phase of the menstrual cycle, pointing to a luteal source of this peptide (Cannon & Dinarello, 1985).

TNFα is another luteal growth factor/cytokine with the potential to suppress granulosa cell luteinization. Both newly formed and regressing corpora lutea from rabbit ovaries secrete TNFα when treated with lipopolysaccharide *in vitro* (Bagavandoss *et al.*, 1988). Furthermore, regressing corpora lutea produce significantly more macrophage-derived TNFα than do functional corpora lutea. In rat granulosa cell cultures, TNFα inhibits FSH-induced aromatase activity (Emoto & Baird, 1988). However, low doses of TNFα stimulate progesterone synthesis in intact preovulatory follicles without affecting oestradiol production (Roby & Terranova, 1988).

## Pregnancy-related luteotrophins

The essential role of trophoblastic chorionic gonadotrophin (CG) in rescuing luteal function during early pregnancy in primates is well established (see Chapter 6). However, domestic animals such as sheep, cows and pigs do not produce a recognizable CG, indicating that other factors contribute to the maintenance of luteal function during pregnancy in these species.

Embryo-derived platelet-activating factor (PAF) may contribute to the maintenance of pregnancy by stimulating platelet-derived factors which maintain or promote luteal function. It has been suggested that serotonin and PDGF, released due to stimulation by embryo-derived PAF, promote progesterone synthesis in the bovine corpus luteum (Hansel *et al.*, 1989).

A trophoblast-derived *c.* 18 kDA acidic protein known as oTP-1 (Godkin *et al.*, 1982) or trophoblastin (Martal *et al.*, 1979) has anti-luteolytic actions in sheep (Bazer *et al.*, 1989). oTP-1 inhibits uterine production of luteolytic amounts of prostaglandin $F_{2\alpha}$ in response to stimulation by oestradiol and oxytocin. Bovine conceptuses secrete bovine TP-1 (bTP-1) which also exerts an antiluteolytic action via the uterus by modulating oxytocin-stimulated secretion of prostaglandin $F_{2\alpha}$ (Thatcher *et al.*, 1989).

Infusion of IFN-$\alpha$ into cows delays luteolysis (Plante *et al.*, 1988). Although not identical in structure to IFN-$\alpha$, oTP-1 and bTP-1 appear to be members of the same family of proteins. The amino acid sequences of IFN-$\alpha$ and bTP-1 are not identical and, unlike IFN-$\alpha$, bTP-1 is not glycosylated (Thatcher *et al.*, 1989). However, the amino acid and cDNA nucleotide sequences of IFN-$\alpha$ and oTP-1 share considerable homology and their molecular weights are also similar (17−18 kDa) (Stewart *et al.*, 1989). Furthermore, IFN-$\alpha$ and oTP-1 also compete with each other for the same binding sites on sheep endometrial membranes.

Other as yet unidentified factors may also participate in luteal rescue. Bovine allantoic fluid contains a 68 kDa glycoprotein which stimulates progesterone production by the bovine corpus luteum (Hickey *et al.*, 1989). Bovine fetal cotyledon granules contain material which inhibits binding of hCG to rat testis membranes and stimulates pro-duction of progesterone by bovine luteal cells (Izhar & Shemesh, 1989). Rabbit placenta contains a luteotrophic factor with an apparent mol-ecular weight of 6−8 kDa that stimulates progesterone production by rabbit granulosa−lutein cells (Gadsby, 1989).

Thus multiple growth factors and cytokines are involved in the luteinization process. Stimulators of luteinization include IGF-1 and insulin, and possibly TGFβ and related proteins. Inhibitors of luteiniz-ation include members of the EGF/TGFα family of proteins, AVP, oxytocin, IL-1, and TNFα. Various regulatory substances (other than CG in primates) may participate in rescuing the corpus luteum of pregnancy. In this regard, potential luteotrophins include PAF and members of the interferon family of proteins.

Non-peptidic factors, such as adenine purines, prostaglandins and reactive oxygen species are also likely to play important local roles in the control of luteinization and luteolysis, as discussed in the remaining sections of this chapter.

# Purines and luteal cell function

Adenine purines are molecules which serve fundamental regulatory and signal-transducing functions in many animal tissues. Here, we examine evidence implicating adenosine in the local control of endocrine and non-endocrine cell functions in the corpus luteum (Behrman et al., 1986). Pathways of purine metabolism and possible roles of purines in the control of oocyte maturation have been dealt with in Chapter 4.

Adenosine has been found in the low micromolar concentration range in follicular fluid (Behrman et al., 1988). Its levels in luteal tissue have not been determined. The origin of adenosine within tissues is uncertain but few tissues other than the liver are capable of producing purines in amounts adequate to meet cellular demands. Xanthine and hypoxanthine produced by the liver are taken up by red blood cells where they are metabolized and transported to peripheral tissues, primarily as ATP (Lajtha & Vane, 1958; Henderson & LePlage, 1959; Majer et al., 1967). In peripheral tissues, ATP is released from erythrocytes mainly as hypoxanthine. The erythrocyte is probably a target for specific products of endothelial and ovarian cells which stimulate the release of adenine purines.

Purines may influence endothelial and parenchymal luteal cell function directly, or be accumulated and released later to serve regulatory or nutritive functions. Upon their release from red blood cells, purines interact initially with endothelial cells. Purines can be stored within endothelial and other non-parenchymal cells as adenine nucleotides. Such cells can thereby act as reservoirs for the release of adenosine as well as serving to capture and reuse purines released by parenchymal cells. Purines released from red blood cells may also have direct access to luteal cells via endothelial clefts, possibly regulated by local agents such as prostaglandins (Behrman et al., 1978).

Ischaemia and hypoxia, factors in luteal regression (see below), are universal promoters of adenosine release (Murray et al., 1970; Fox & Kelly, 1978; Baer & Drummond, 1979; Arch & Newsholme, 1980; Burnstock & Brown, 1981). Neural stimulation causes adenosine release from nerve-endings as well as from innervated tissues (Haulica et al., 1973; Baer & Drummond, 1979; Arch & Newsholme, 1980; Fredholm & Hedquist, 1980; Burnstock & Brown, 1981; Spielman & Thompson, 1982; Monaco et al., 1984; Rommerts et al., 1984). Catecholamines play a role in the release of adenosine in innervated tissues such as the heart (Arch & Newsholme, 1980; Wangler et al., 1984) and probably the ovaries (Bahr & Ben Jonathan, 1981; Jordan, 1981; Kawakami et al., 1981).

Cellular release of adenine increases as ATP levels decline, for example due to decreased oxidative phosphorylation during hypoxia, increased energy demand, production of cyclic adenosine monophosphate (cAMP) or direct release of adenosine (Murray et al., 1970; Fox

& Kelly, 1978; Baer & Drummond, 1979; Arch & Newsholme, 1980; Burnstock & Brown, 1981; Spielman & Thompson, 1982). Tissues such as the corpus luteum (Cross *et al.*, 1987) which contain low levels of creatine phosphate show the most pronounced decreases in ATP levels because creatine phosphate serves to stabilize cellular levels of ATP. Soodak *et al.* (1988a) found that LH produces a prompt and marked depletion of ATP in the rat corpus luteum. A similar response was seen in regressing luteal tissue. Thus, with each pulse of LH, a burst of adenosine release is likely to occur which could influence both endocrine and non-endocrine cell function in the corpus luteum.

*In vitro*, adenosine promotes a marked increase in LH-responsive production of cAMP and progesterone by rat luteal cells (Hall *et al.*, 1981). Adenosine also prevents the inhibition by prostaglandin $F_{2\alpha}$ of LH-stimulated cAMP accumulation (Behrman *et al.*, 1982). Both rat and human luteal cells respond to adenosine in a similar manner (Polan *et al.*, 1983). These responses to adenosine are rapid in onset and are elicited with similar potencies and kinetics by ATP, ADP, and AMP, probably reflecting extracellular conversion of these substances into adenosine. Inosine, hypoxanithine and adenine are also agonists of LH action, but with lower potencies than adenosine (Behrman *et al.*, 1983; Brennan *et al.*, 1983).

## Mechanisms of adenosine action

Mechanisms by which adenosine influences cell function are poorly understood and several processes seem likely to be involved. One is a form of metabolic coupling by which adenosine acts to elevate levels of ATP (Arch & Newsholme, 1980). This appears to be a major mechanism of action of adenosine in the luteal cell. A second mechanism of adenosine action is via cell-membrane associated receptors coupled to adenylyl cyclase, resulting in either inhibition (via $A_1$ or $R_i$ receptors) or activation (via $A_2$ or $R_a$ receptors) of enzyme activity (Daly, 1982). Both granulosa and luteal cells appear to express stimulatory receptors for adenosine (Billig & Rosberg, 1988). Another adenosine binding-site (P site) has been proposed which is an intracellular inhibitory site intimately linked to the catalytic subunit of adenylyl cyclase (Londos *et al.*, 1978). In addition, there may be other receptors associated with the ion channels that interact with ATP and adenosine (Brown & Burnstock, 1981).

The major site of adenosine action in luteal cells is intramitochondrial (Soodak & Behrman, 1988), linked to increased formation of ATP (Hall *et al.*, 1981; Behrman *et al.*, 1983; Brennan *et al.*, 1983). However, elevated levels of ATP *per se*, do not seem to mediate adenosine action because adenosine and ATP do not cause comparable increases in cAMP production by isolated luteal cell membranes. Augmentation by adenosine of cAMP production by luteal cells seems to be selective for stimulation by LH since the purine effects only modest amplification of responses to isoproterenol, cholera toxin or forskolin (Soodak *et al.*, 1988b).

Adenosine may exert a protective effect against the release of reactive oxygen species by neutrophils (Nathan, 1989). These highly reactive products cause cell injury and are implicated in the cellular mechanism of luteolysis (see later). Release of adenosine within the follicle and corpus luteum, possibly in response to gonadotrophic stimulation, may therefore constitute a defence against cell damage, thereby promoting luteal function.

## Adenosine and cell-to-cell interaction in the corpus luteum

Based on the foregoing considerations, a hypothetical role is proposed for adenosine in co-ordinating interactions between endocrine and non-endocrine cells in the corpus luteum (Fig. 7.1). Adenosine produced *de novo* by the liver, is transported to the ovaries in red blood cells. Endothelial cells may respond to adenosine via receptor-mediated processes and can also serve as a conduit for the transport of adenosine into luteal cells. In luteal cells, a major effect of adenosine is to elevate ATP levels and amplify adenylyl cyclase-mediated postreceptor responses to LH. cAMP released by LH-stimulated luteal cells is degraded enzymically to extracellular adenosine. LH thereby promotes increased formation of adenosine which can act as a paracrine/autocrine regulator of luteal steroid synthesis, influence endothelial cell function, and prevent the activation of resident neutrophils. Through these actions, adenosine may enhance luteal function and prevent luteolysis.

## Reactive oxygen species and luteal cell function

Ischaemia sets in motion chemotaxis, adherence, extravasation and activation of macrophages and neutrophils, leading to the production

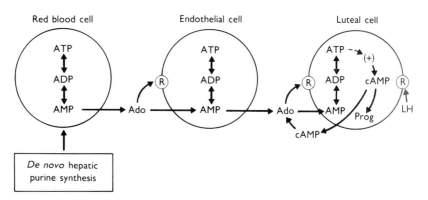

**Fig. 7.1.** Roles of adenosine in mediating interactions between red blood cells, endothelial cells and parenchymal luteal cells.

of reactive oxygen species which cause cell damage. In the ovaries, tissue infiltration by leukocytes, macrophages and thymocytes is a hallmark of luteal regression (Bulmer, 1964; Adams & Hertig, 1969; Gillim et al., 1969; Kirsch et al., 1981). Phagocytosis with production of TNF (Bagavandoss et al., 1988) also occurs during luteal regression. Thus reactive oxygen species produced by luteal non-endocrine cells are inextricably linked to the process of luteolysis.

Luteal endocrine cells, with their prolific mitochondrial and microsomal metabolism steroid precursors, are also likely sites of free-oxygen radical production. This would seem to be particularly likely during intense gonadotrophic stimulation when radical-mediated oxidation of cholesterol and other intermediates occurs during the synthesis of progesterone.

## Reactive oxygen species and cellular damage

The exact nature of the reactive oxygen species which cause cell damage in biological systems is uncertain, but superoxide ($O_2^{\pm}$), hydroxyl radical (OH$^{\cdot}$) and $H_2O_2$ are clearly implicated (Chance et al., 1979; Elstner et al., 1980; Fridovich, 1988; Halliwell, 1988; Imlay & Linn, 1988). The hydroxyl radical is extremely reactive and cell injury produced by this species is believed to occur at, or very near, the origin of production in a site-specific manner (Fridovich, 1986). Both $O_2^{\pm}$ (which can also produce damage directly) and $H_2O_2$, derived from $O_2^{\pm}$, participate in the production of the extremely toxic hydroxyl radical. The hydroxyl radical is therefore thought to mediate many of the destructive reactions of $O_2^{\pm}$ and $H_2O_2$.

## Production of reactive oxygen species by luteal non-parenchymal cells

### Neutrophils and macrophages

Other sources of reactive oxygen species that may adversely influence ovarian cells are neutrophils and macrophages, cellular elements of the non-specific immune response. Phagocytic leukocytes have a remarkable plasma membrane NADPH oxidase which upon activation produces a burst-release of reactive oxygen species of sufficient magnitude to cause cell injury (Gabig et al., 1978; Forman et al., 1980; Baboir et al., 1988).

Processes which regulate chemotaxis, adherence, and extravasation of phagocytic leukocytes in tissues, and which activate the respiratory burst-release of oxygen radicals are only just beginning to be understood. Ischaemia is well known to initiate infiltration of neutrophils (Simpson et al., 1988). Superoxide, produced in response to ischaemia, induces chemotaxis of neutrophils (Ward et al., 1988) by several mechanisms including production of leukotriene B4. Many cytokines are chemotactic and formyl-methionyl-leucyl-phenylanine (FMLP) is a well known chemotactic peptide. Neutrophil chemotactic factor (NCF), which also stimulates extravasation (Strieter *et al.*, 1989), may be similar to neutrophil-activating protein (NAP-1), which has both chemotactic and activating effects on neutrophils (Larsen *et al.*, 1989). Endothelial cells produce NCF in response to stimulation by TNF and IL-1 which are both produced by activated macrophages (Streiter *et al.*, 1989).

Injured endothelial cells become targets for attack by macrophages, presumably due to increased expression of cell-surface antigens. Macrophages, in turn, produce TNF and IL-1 which induce neutrophil adhesion and expression of antigen on the neutrophil surface. Adherence of activated neutrophils appears to be necessary for their production of reactive oxygen species. Neutrophils also became adherent to endothelial cells which are exposed to reactive oxygen species. Complement components, expression of receptors for gamma globulin (Fc), as well as adhesion-promoting receptors all seem to be involved in the adhesion process (Simpson *et al.*, 1988).

Activators of protein kinase C produce a respiratory burst-release of reactive oxygen species from phagocytic cells (Johnston *et al.*, 1978; Kano *et al.*, 1987; Christansen *et al.*, 1988). The principal macrophage activator is thought to be IFN-$\gamma$, a product of T-lymphocytes (Nathan *et al.*, 1983). Interestingly, TGF$\beta$, a product of parenchymal ovarian cells, deactivates macrophages (Tsunawaki *et al.*, 1988), hinting at a possible mechanism for terminating the production of reactive oxygen species and thereby limiting damage in such cells.

Cytokines (TNF and IL-1) produced by activated macrophages stimulate neutrophils and monocytes to generate oxygen radicals (Ward *et al.*, 1988). Oxygen radicals, in turn, stimulate TNF production by macrophages which initiates a positive feedback loop for continued production of reactive oxygen species (Clark *et al.*, 1988). However TNF only stimulates peroxide release from neutrophils if they are adherent. Colony-stimulating factors (CSF), produced by endothelial cells, fibroblasts, thymocytes, and macrophages, bind to specific receptors on neutrophils and also stimulate a respiratory burst if the neutrophils are adherent (Nathan, 1989). Physiological levels of adenosine suppress CSF-induced respiratory burst-release of reactive oxygen species by neutrophils (Nathan, 1989). This is interesting in view of the apparent positive regulatory actions of adenosine on luteal cell function discussed earlier. The chemotactic peptide FMLP also stimulates production of free oxygen radicals by neutrophils (Nathan, 1989). PAF produced by injured endothelial cells also promotes adherence and activates neutrophils (Jacob & Vercellotti, 1988).

In addition to oxygen radicals, activated neutrophils release elastase and collagenase (Jacob & Vercellotti, 1988). These degradative enzymes are normally inhibited by $\alpha_2$-macroglobulin and $\alpha_1$-antiproteinase, but reactive oxygen species prevent such inhibition. Consequently, extra-cellular matrix is degraded and endothelial cells become dislodged from the vascular lining. A similar sequence of events may occur during the degeneration of parenchymal luteal tissue in the ovaries.

### Endothelial cells

Endothelial cells produce reactive oxygen species and are phagocytic (Ryan, 1988; Gorog et al., 1988; Zweier et al., 1988). Release of reactive oxygen species by endothelial cells occurs in response to anoxia followed by reoxygenation (Zweier et al., 1988), stimulation of phagocytosis (Gorog et al., 1988), stimulation by cytokines (IL-1 and IFN-γ), or activation of protein kinase C (Matsubara & Ziff, 1986a,b). Injury due to ischaemia and reperfusion occurs in many tissues, apparently due to the release of reactive oxygen species by endothelial cells, as well as to invasion and activation of phagocytic cells of the immune system (Halliwell, 1987).

## Production of reactive oxygen species by luteal endocrine cells

LH-stimulable peroxidase (Agrawal & Laloraya, 1977) and superoxide dismutase (Laloraya et al., 1988) activities are present in the ovaries. LH induces increases in superoxide dismutase activity which correspond with its ability to increase superoxide levels in luteal tissue (Laloraya et al., 1988). Such effects of LH would be expected to lead to increased production of peroxide within the corpus luteum. Significantly, plasma membranes from regressing rat corpora lutea produce superoxide (Sawada & Carlson, 1989) and show an increase in lipid peroxidation (Sawada & Carlson, 1985) in vitro. The presence of enzymes which detoxify superoxide and peroxide, and the fact that LH increases the activity of these enzymes suggests that these reactive products are readily produced by luteal tissue in vivo.

## Actions of hydrogen peroxide in luteal cells

A direct luteolytic action of peroxide has been demonstrated in isolated rat luteal cells (Behrman & Preston, 1989a,b). A striking feature of this action of peroxide is the sensitivity and rapidity of its effect. Peroxide dose-dependently depletes cellular levels of ATP, blocks the ability of LH to stimulate cAMP accumulation, and inhibits LH-dependent pro-gesterone synthesis (Fig. 7.2). Peroxide-induced depletion of ATP in luteal cells appears to be due to DNA damage by a process similar, if not identical, to that seen in other tissues where tissue damage by free radical formation is known to occur (Schraufstatter et al., 1986). The induction of ATP-depletion by peroxide occurs independently of its inhibitory effect on cAMP accumulation and progesterone synthesis in

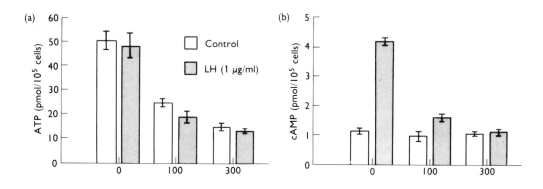

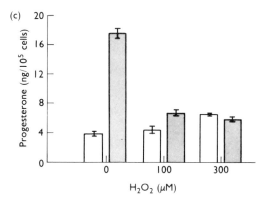

**Fig. 7.2.** Luteolytic actions of peroxide on rat luteal cells: dose-responsive suppression by $H_2O_2$ of cellular levels of (a) ATP, (b) cAMP and (c) progesterone in control and LH-stimulated rat luteal cells. Values are mean $\pm$ SE. The cells were preincubated with $H_2O_2$ for 60 min, followed by a 10-min incubation with catalase before incubation for a further 60 min with or without LH (1 µg/ml). Reproduced with permission from Behrman and Preston (1989b).

response to LH (Behrman & Preston, 1989a). Interestingly, the mechanism by which peroxide blocks the action of LH appears to be similar to that of prostaglandin $F_{2\alpha}$ (Thomas *et al.*, 1978), in that binding of LH to its receptor and adenylyl cyclase activity are unaffected. Peroxide does not, however, increase production of prostaglandin $F_{2\alpha}$ by luteal cells. Such antigonadotrophic actions of peroxide uniquely suit it as a cellular mediator of luteolysis.

## Antioxidant vitamins and luteal cell function

Follicles and corpora lutea have long been known to contain high levels of the antioxidant vitamin ascorbic acid (Hoch-Ligeti & Bourne, 1948; Deane, 1952). An early bioassay for LH was based on the ability of this gonadotrophin to deplete ovarian levels of ascorbic acid (Parlow, 1972). In the rat corpus luteum, depletion of ascorbic acid by LH is inversely related to activation of peroxidase and superoxide dismutase, and production of superoxide (Agrawal & Laloraya, 1977; Laloraya *et al.*, 1988). An LH-stimulated increase in production of free oxygen radicals (see above) could therefore constitute the biochemical basis of LH-induced ascorbic acid depletion.

Intraluteal levels of ascorbic acid (Hoch-Ligeti & Bourne, 1948) and ATP (Soodak *et al.*, 1988) fall during luteal regression; reactive oxygen species deplete cellular levels of both ascorbic acid and ATP; and plasma membranes from regressing corpora lutea produce superoxide *in vitro* (Sawada & Carlson, 1989). These findings strongly imply a role for free oxygen radicals in luteolysis. Paradoxically, the fact that LH can stimulate luteal depletion of ascorbic acid suggests that the gonadotrophin may itself have the potential to act as a luteolysin (see below).

### Reactive oxygen radicals, cytokines and luteolysis

Interactions between luteal endocrine and non-endocrine cells likely to involve locally produced reactive oxygen species and cytokines are summarized in Fig. 7.3. Oxygen radicals are generated by endothelial cells, phagocytic leukocytes, and by luteal cells. In endothelial cells,

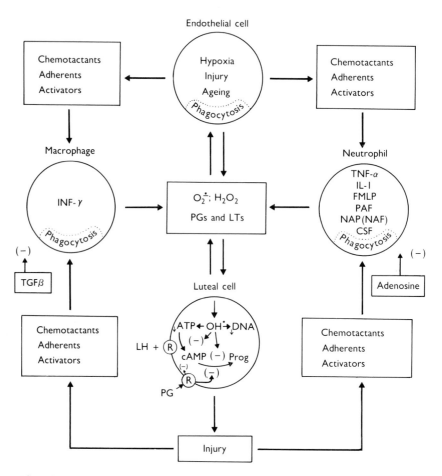

**Fig. 7.3.** Oxygen radicals, cytokines and luteolysis: postulated interactions between immune cells, endothelial cells and parenchymal luteal cells.

injury caused by hypoxia or oxygen radicals produced by luteal cells, results in the generation of chemotactic factors and presentation of adherence molecules on the cell surface and extracellular matrix. As a consequence, macrophages and neutrophils adhere, become activated and generate reactive oxygen species. Phagocytosis may be induced in endothelial cells, also generating reactive oxygen species. Cytokines are intimately involved in this sequence of events. Macrophages activated by IFN-γ release IL-1 and TNF which, in turn, activate neutrophils. Chemotaxis, adherence and activation of neutrophils are also stimulated by numerous other factors produced by macrophages, endothelial cells and probably also luteal cells. Interestingly, adenosine and TGFβ inhibit neutrophil and macrophage activation, pointing to an intraluteal mechanism for restricting the production of reactive oxygen species. Injury of luteal cells by oxygen radicals has been shown to be mediated by the hydroxyl radical, but the superoxide radical is also implicated. Oxygen radicals inhibit luteal cell responsiveness to LH by blocking the activation of adenylyl cyclase and inhibiting cAMP-dependent progesterone synthesis. Cellular depletion of ATP and damage to DNA also occur. Luteal cell injury may, in turn, lead to further production of the chemotactic and adherent factors that activate phagocytosis and cause generation of reactive oxygen species.

# Luteolysis

We have seen that the steroid-secretory function of the corpus luteum is completely dependent on LH/hCG but that spontaneous regression of the gland in non-fertile menstrual cycles cannot be explained simply by inadequate luteal stimulation by LH (Chapter 6). It therefore follows that luteolysis is likely to be a function of altered luteal cell responsiveness to LH.

## Luteolysis in non-primates

In domestic animal species such as sheep, pigs and cows, spontaneous luteolysis appears to be induced by prostaglandin $F_{2\alpha}$ released by the oestrogen-primed, non-gravid uterus in response to stimulation by luteal oxytocin (for reviews see Thatcher *et al.*, 1986 and Auletta & Flint, 1988). Luteolysis in these species is therefore initiated by an endocrine signal (oxytocin) emanating from within the corpus luteum itself (Fig. 7.4).

### Prostaglandin $F_{2\alpha}$ as an antigonadotrophic agent

The discovery of prostaglandin $F_{2\alpha}$ and the finding that this eicosanoid causes luteolysis in the laboratory rat (Pharriss & Wyngarden, 1969) marked the beginning of an era in the study of luteolysis. Prostaglandin

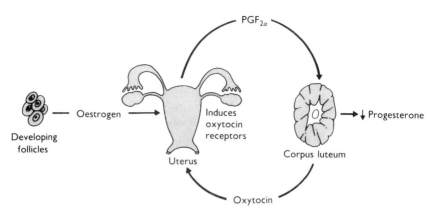

**Fig. 7.4.** The utero−ovarian interaction which regulates onset of functional luteolysis in non-primate animal species.

$F_{2\alpha}$ has since been shown to cause luteal regression in various non-primates and is generally regarded as the major physiological uterine luteolysin in domestic animal species (Thatcher *et al.*, 1986).

Prostaglandin $F_{2\alpha}$ acts directly as a luteolysin via a receptor-mediated mechanism in luteal cells (Behrman *et al.*, 1971, 1978; Wright *et al.*, 1980; Pang & Behrman, 1981), effectively blocking the luteotrophic action of LH (Behrman *et al.*, 1974; Lahav *et al.*, 1976; Thomas *et al.*, 1978; Behrman, 1979).

One way in which prostaglandin $F_{2\alpha}$ blocks the action of LH on the rat corpus luteum is to induce a loss of LH receptors (Behrman *et al.*, 1978). Since luteal progesterone secretion falls hours before LH receptor content does (Grinwich *et al.*, 1976), loss of LH receptors is probably a consequence rather than the cause of prostaglandin-induced luteolysis. However, the attendant loss of LH receptors probably ensures that the process of luteal regression, once initiated, is irreversible.

Another way in which prostaglandin $F_{2\alpha}$ blocks the luteotrophic action of LH is to inhibit gonadotrophin delivery to luteal cells, an effect that is rapid and seen only *in vivo* (Behrman & Hichens, 1976; Behrman *et al.*, 1978). Treatment *in vivo* with prostaglandin $F_{2\alpha}$ also inhibits uptake of prolactin by rat luteal tissue (Behrman *et al.*, 1978). The time-courses of inhibition of luteal gonadotrophin uptake and progesterone secretion by prostaglandin $F_{2\alpha}$ are similar (Behrman & Hichens, 1976). The prostaglandin does not interfere with uptake of LH by isolated luteal cells (Thomas *et al.*, 1978; Dorflinger *et al.*, 1984) or luteal plasma membranes (Behrman *et al.*, 1978; Thomas *et al.*, 1978; Dorflinger *et al.*, 1983). Since the prostaglandin does not acutely affect luteal blood flow (Behrman *et al.*, 1971; Pang & Behrman, 1981) its inhibitory effect on LH uptake may be due to impaired capillary transfer, possibly due to closure of endothelial clefts in the luteal vasculature (see above).

The third mechanism by which prostaglandin $F_{2\alpha}$ abrogates the action of LH is interference with postreceptor signalling. Physiological concentrations of prostaglandin $F_{2\alpha}$ acutely inhibit cAMP production and steroid synthesis in LH-stimulated luteal cells without stimulating degradation of cAMP (Lahav et al., 1976; Thomas et al., 1978; Dorflinger et al., 1983). The inhåbitory action of prostaglandin on cAMP production appears to depend on cellular integrity since no inhibition occurs from LH-sensitive adenylyl cyclase activity in isolated luteal membranes (Thomas et al., 1978).

The luteolytic action of prostaglandin $F_{2\alpha}$ is associated with acute changes in the microaggregation of LH receptors on the luteal cell plasma membrane. Lateral movements of LH receptors and changes in their distribution over the cell surface appear to be important for the expression of luteal cell responsiveness to LH. Upon association with LH, LH receptors rapidly gather into small aggregates which become larger as binding of LH and production of progesterone increase (Luborsky et al., 1984a,b). Acute exposure of rat luteal cells to prostaglandin $F_{2\alpha}$ reduces membrane fluidity, prevents receptor aggregation and interferes with the activation of adenylyl cyclase (Luborsky et al., 1984b). Reductions in membrane fluidity occur during luteal regression and can be induced in response to treatment with prostaglandin $F_{2\alpha}$, as confirmed by fluorescent-probe analysis (Carlson et al., 1981). The decrease in luteal cell membrane fluidity is associated with an increase in phospholipase $A_2$ activity (Riley et al., 1989).

The foregoing considerations indicate that prostaglandin $F_{2\alpha}$ blocks LH action by an indirect mechanism that is rapid in onset and requires an intact cell. An intracellular mediator of prostaglandin $F_{2\alpha}$ action is therefore likely to be involved, serving somehow to block activation of adenylyl cyclase by the occupied LH receptor.

### Intracellular mediation of prostaglandin $F_{2\alpha}$ action

There is increasing evidence that actions of prostaglandin $F_{2\alpha}$ on luteal cells involve postreceptor signalling mediated by products of inositol lipid metabolism in the plasma membrane. The importance of this intracellular signal transmission system in the context of cell-to-cell interaction in the ovarian follicle has already been discussed (see Chapter 3).

Early evidence suggested that calcium derived from intracellular sources might mediate the action of prostaglandin $F_{2\alpha}$ (Dorflinger et al., 1983; Gore and Behrman, 1984). An acute rise in intracellular calcium levels occurs in bovine and rat luteal cells treated with the prostaglandin (Davis et al., 1987; Pepperell et al., 1989). However, the antigonadotrophic action of prostaglandin $F_{2\alpha}$ in rat luteal tissue still occurs when the intracellular increase in $Ca^{2+}$ is completely blocked, suggesting that $Ca^{2+}$ per se is not a critical mediator.

Recent studies indicate that products of phosphatidylinositol (PI) turnover, such as inositol-1,4,5 triphosphate (IP$_3$) may serve a role in mediating the hormone-induced release of sequestered calcium from microsomes of liver cells (Burgess *et al.*, 1984). Prostaglandin F$_{2\alpha}$ stimulates phosphoinositide (PI) turnover and increased formation of IP$_3$ in rat luteal cells, presumably due to activation of phospholipase C (Raymond *et al.*, 1983; Leung *et al.*, 1986). Treatment of bovine luteal cells with prostaglandin F$_{2\alpha}$ stimulates release of IP$_3$ within 10 seconds, and this response is followed by a sustained increase in intracellular calcium levels which lasts for several minutes (Davis *et al.*, 1987, 1988).

Activation of phospholipase C to stimulate inositol lipid metabolism and increased PI turnover also gives rise to increased production of diacylglycerol, leading to activation of calcium-dependent protein kinase (protein kinase C) (Takai *et al.*, 1979). Protein kinase C is present in the ovaries (Davis & Clark, 1983) and its activation in swine granulosa cells causes antigonadotrophic effects (Veldhuis & Demers, 1986). In rat luteal cells treatment with phorbol esters which mimic the stimulatory action of diacylglycerol on protein kinase C (Van Duuren & Sivak, 1968) elicits antigonadotrophic effects similar to those of prostaglandin F$_{2\alpha}$ (Sender Baum & Rosberg 1987; Sender Baum, 1989). However, there is still uncertainty as to whether all the antigonadotrophic actions of prostaglandin F$_{2\alpha}$ are mediated by postreceptor signalling via the diacylglycerol/protein kinase C pathway (Musicki *et al.*, 1990) (Fig. 7.5).

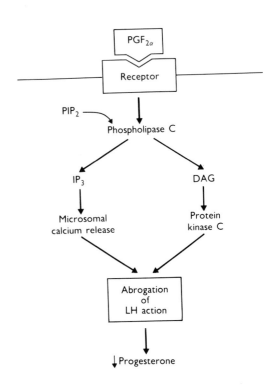

**Fig. 7.5.** Likely mediators of prostaglandin F$_{2\alpha}$ action in luteal cells: *PIP$_2$*, phosphatidyl 4,5-biphosphate; *IP$_3$*, inositol 1,4,5,-triphosphate; *DAG*, diacylglycerol.

## Luteolysis in primates

In women and non-human primates, ovarian cyclicity is not disrupted by hysterectomy, ruling out the uterus as a site of production of luteolytic prostaglandin. However, the primate corpus luteum is known to produce oestradiol (see Chapter 6) and there is evidence that oxytocin and prostaglandin $F_{2\alpha}$ (other components of the luteolytic utero–ovarian feedback loop active in non-primates) might also be produced and act locally in the primate corpus luteum.

The primate ovary contains oxytocin (Schaeffer *et al.*, 1984), and oxytocin has been reported to be luteolytic in these species (Auletta *et al.*, 1984). However, an endocrine role for luteal oxytocin in causing luteolysis in primates is not apparent since presence or absence of the uterus does not influence luteal-phase duration (Neill *et al.*, 1969). This does not, however, preclude the possibility of an intraovarian action of oxytocin which might result in the local release of a luteolytic agent(s) such as prostaglandin (Tan *et al.*, 1982).

The human corpus luteum contains prostaglandin $F_{2\alpha}$ (Challis *et al.*, 1976) and prostaglandin $F_{2\alpha}$ receptors (Powell *et al.*, 1974). Moreover, inhibitory effects of prostaglandin $F_{2\alpha}$ on hCG-stimulated progesterone production have been observed *in vitro* using minced luteal tissue (Dennefors *et al.*, 1982) and dispersed luteal cells (Khan-Dawood *et al.*, 1989) from mid-luteal phase human corpora lutea. However, little or no luteolytic action of prostaglandin has been observed *in vivo*. Even direct intraluteal administration of prostaglandin $F_{2\alpha}$ produces only a transient suppression of progesterone secretion in women (Korda *et al.*, 1975). In monkeys, a luteolytic effect of prostaglandin $F_{2\alpha}$ is seen following its injection into the ovarian artery (Auletta *et al.*, 1973), and treatment with indomethacin to inhibit prostaglandin biosynthesis extends the luteal phase (Aulete *et al.*, 1973). However, treatment of women with inhibitors of prostaglandin biosynthesis has little effect on the duration of the luteal phase (Gibson & Auletta, 1986).

Zeleznik in Chapter 6 has discussed evidence which apparently rules out luteal oestrogen as an important luteolysin in women. It nevertheless remains possible that locally produced oestrogen could somehow influence the release and/or modulate the action of intra-ovarian oxytocin; or perhaps induce the synthesis and/or release of other potentially luteolytic substances, such as reactive oxygen species.

## Initiation of structural luteolysis

Reduced vascularization of the corpus luteum with an attendant loss of endothelial cells occurs in the mid–late luteal phase of non-fertile cycles. Endothelial cells are deleted from the corpus luteum at this time by apoptosis (see Chapter 6). This mechanism of cell death leads to tissue-invasion by macrophages and phagocytosis, processes associated with neutrophil activation and free-oxygen radical formation (see above). Activated neutrophils can disrupt endothelial cell monolayers *in vitro* by proteolysis involving the action of elastase (Weiss & Regiani, 1984; Smedley, 1986). Thus, proteolytic degradation of the basement membrane by activated neutrophils appears to initiate endothelial cell loss and hence structural regression of the corpus luteum (Johnson & Varani, 1981; Weiss & Regiani, 1984).

## Cellular depletion of ATP: the fundamental event leading to structural luteolysis?

Whichever endocrine or paracrine signal(s) initiates functional luteolysis (i.e. cessation of progesterone synthesis), changes in intracellular levels of ATP and calcium seem to be instrumental in bringing about structural luteolysis (i.e. luteal cell death). ATP is critical for the optimal functioning of all cells because most, if not all, of their vital metabolic reactions are driven by this essential substrate. Under conditions which deplete cellular ATP levels (e.g. hypoxia) a cascade of reactions occurs leading to production of reactive oxygen species and elevation of intracellular calcium levels. The source of this calcium includes release from microsomes and mitochondria, as well as influx from the extracellular fluid. The increase in intracellular calcium level activates phospholipases $A_1$, $A_2$ and C, further elevating calcium and ultimately causing cell death (Hochachka, 1986). This sequence of events is illustrated schematically in Fig. 7.6. Note that increased intracellular calcium levels would also be expected to initiate DNA-degradation and apoptosis through the activation of $Ca^{2+}/Mg^{2+}$-dependent endonuclease, as discussed by Zeleznik in Chapter 6.

As mentioned earlier, there is evidence that luteal ATP levels are particularly susceptible to marked fluctuations due to the low creatine phosphate content of this tissue. After onset of spontaneous luteal regression in rats, luteal ATP levels are significantly reduced coincident with a rise in the serum level of LH (Soodak & Behrman, 1988b). Luteal ATP depletion also occurs within 5 min of injecting rats with exogenous LH. This effect becomes maximal within 30 min and is sustained for up to 24 h. The fall in ATP is not directly linked to initiation of functional luteolysis since no depletion occurs within 2 h of administering prostaglandin $F_{2\alpha}$ or within 24 h of hypophysectomy (Soodak et al., 1988b). Treatment *in vitro* with peroxide (but not LH or prostaglandin $F_{2\alpha}$) also depletes isolated luteal cells of ATP (Behrman & Preston, 1989a).

These experimental observations indicate that levels of ATP in mid- and late luteal stage rat corpora lutea are acutely susceptible to negative regulation by LH. The peripheral serum LH level becomes elevated once functional luteolysis is initiated due to withdrawal of negative

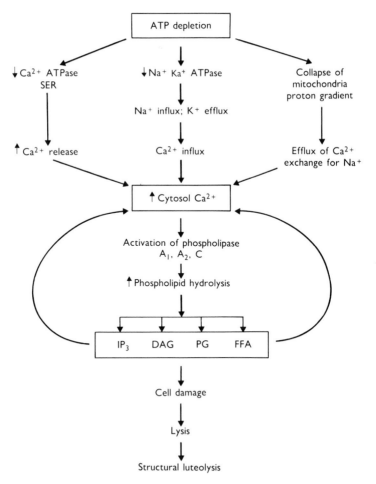

**Fig. 7.6.** Metabolic consequences of luteal cell ATP-depletion. $Ca^{2+}$ *ATPase* high-affinity calcium pump; *SER* smooth endoplasmic reticulum; $IP_3$, inositol 1,4,5-triphosphate; *DAG*, diacylglycerol; *PG*, prostaglandin; *FFA*, free fatty acid.

feedback control by progesterone. Increased stimulation by LH depletes luteal cells of ATP and renders them incapable of maintaining low levels of calcium. Once subcritical calcium levels are reached (see above), luteal cell death and structural luteolysis ensue. This situation would be expected to prevail until the serum LH level subsides, LH receptors are depleted, or luteal-cell responsiveness to LH is totally abated. It must be emphasized that to-date evidence for LH-induced depletion of luteal ATP levels has come exclusively from experimental work on rats. To our knowledge, such an effect of LH has yet to be sought in any other species.

## An overview

Our current overall concept of cell-to-cell interactions which underlie functional and structural luteolysis in mammalian ovaries is illustrated schematically in Fig. 7.7. Functional luteolysis in non-primates is initiated by prostaglandin $F_{2\alpha}$, resulting in a cascade of biochemical changes among which the most physiologically relevant is inhibition of progesterone synthesis. This action of the prostaglandin entails its binding to specific receptors on steroidogenic luteal cells and is mediated, at least in part, by intracellular signalling via formation of diacylglycerol and activation of protein kinase C. Other paracrine factors and post-receptor signalling systems are also likely to be involved. The factor(s) responsible for initiating luteolysis in primates is unknown. However, in primates as in non-primates, increased production of reactive oxygen species is likely to be crucial. The decrease in progesterone secretion associated with functional luteolysis results in loss of feedback-inhibition of pituitary gonadotrophin secretion, leading to increased blood levels of LH. Functional luteolysis also causes changes in endothelial cells which lead to increased phagocytic infiltration and activation. Reactive oxygen species are generated by activated macrophages, neutrophils and endothelial cells as well as by luteal cells responding to stimulation by LH. Locally produced oxygen radicals act directly to abolish luteal progesterone synthesis and luteal responsiveness to LH. Oxygen radicals

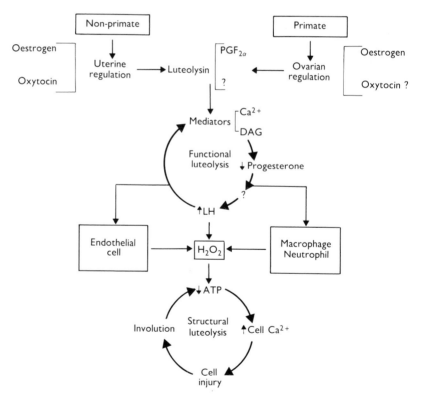

**Fig. 7.7.** Cellular bases of functional and structural luteolysis. A provisional framework accommodating interactions believed to occur between luteolysins, endothelial cells, immune cells and reactive oxygen species.

also deplete luteal cells of ATP, thereby triggering structural luteolysis and ultimately involution of the corpus luteum.

## Acknowledgements

This work was supported by NIH-HD-10718. The authors express their appreciation to Ms Cindy Davis for preparation of the manuscript, to Tradescript for editorial assistance, and to Mrs Nancy Chapman for artwork.

# References

Abraham, J.A., Mergia, A., Whang, J.L., Tumulo, A., Friedman, J., Hjerrild, K.A., Gospodarowicz, D. & Fiddes, J.C. (1986) Nucleotide sequence of a bovine clone encoding the angiogenic protein, basic fibroblast growth factor. *Science*, **233**, 545−8.

Adams, E.C. & Hertig, A.T. (1969) Studies on the human corpus luteum. I. Observations on the ultrastructure of development and regression of the luteal cells during the menstrual cycle. *J. Cell. Biol.*, **41**, 696−715.

Adashi, E.Y. & Resnick, C.E. (1986) Antagonistic interactions of growth factors in the regulation of granulosa cell differentiation. *Endocrinology*, **119**, 1879−81.

Agrawal, P. & Laloraya, M. (1977) Induction of peroxidase in corpora lutea of rat ovary by lutropin. *Biochem. J.*, **166**, 1040−5.

Alila, H.W. & Hansel, W. (1984) Origin of different cell types in the bovine corpus luteum as characterized by specific monoclonal antibodies. *Biol. Reprod.*, **31**, 1015−25.

Alila, H.W., Dowd, J.P., Corradino, R.A., Harris, W.V. & Hansel, W. (1988) Control of progesterone production in small and large bovine luteal cells separated by flow cytometry. *J. Reprod. Fertil.*, **82**, 645−55.

Arch, J.R.S. & Newsholme, E.A. (1980) The control of the metabolism and the hormonal role of adenosine. In Campbell, P.N. & Dickens, S. (eds) *Essays in Biochemistry*, pp. 82−123. Academic Press, New York.

Auletta, F.J. & Flint, A.P.F. (1988) Mechanisms controlling corpus luteum function in sheep, cows, nonhuman primates and women especially in relation to the time of luteolysis. *Endocr. Rev.*, **9**, 88−105.

Auletta, F.J., Paradis, D.K., Wesley, M. & Duby, R.T. (1984) Oxytocin is luteolytic in the rhesus monkey (*Macaca mulatta*). *J. Reprod. Fertil.*, **72**, 401−6.

Auletta, F.J., Speroff, L. & Caldwell, B.V. (1973) Prostaglandin F$_{2\alpha}$ induced steroidogenesis and luteolysis in the primate corpus luteum. *J. Clin. Endocrinol. Metab.*, **36**, 405−7.

Awbrey, B.J., Hoak, J.C. & Owen, W.G. (1979) Binding of human thrombin to cultured endothelial cells. *J. Biol. Chem.*, **254**, 4092−5.

Ayyagari, R.R. & Khan-Dawood, F.S. (1987) Human corpus luteum: presence of epidermal growth receptors and binding characteristics. *Am. J. Obstet. Gynecol.*, **156**, 942−6.

Azizkhan, J., Sullivan, R., Azizkhan, R., Zetter, B.R. & Klagsbrun, M. (1983) Stimulation of increased capillary endothelial cell motility by chondro-sarcoma cell-derived factors. *Cancer Res.*, **43**, 3281−6.

Azmi, T.I. & O'Shea, J.D. (1984) Mechanism of deletion of endothelial cells during regression of the corpus luteum. *Lab. Invest.*, **51**, 206−17.

Baboir, B.M., Curnutte, J.T. & Okamura, N. (1988) The respiratory burst oxidase of the human neutrophil. In Halliwell, B. (ed.) *Oxygen Radicals and Tissue Injury*, pp. 43−8. FASEB, Bethesda.

Baer, H.P. & Drummond, G.I. (1979) *Physiological and Regulatory Functions of Adenosine and Adenine Nucleotides*. Raven Press, New York.

Baird, A., Bohlen, P., Esch, F. & Gospodarowicz, D. (1985) Characterization and biological properties of fibroblast growth factor isolated from bovine kidney; homology with corpus luteum-derived fibroblast growth factor. *Regul. Pept.*, **12**, 201−13.

Baird, A. & Durkin, T. (1986) Inhibition of endothelial cell proliferation by type beta-transforming growth factor: interactions with acidic and basic fibroblast growth factors. *Biochem. Biophys. Res. Commun.*, **138**, 476−82.

Baird, A., Esch, F., Mormede, P., Ueno, N., Ling, N., Bohlen, P., Ying, S.-Y., Wehrenberg, W.B. & Guillemin, R. (1986) Molecular characterization of fibroblast growth factor: Distribution and biological activities in various tissues. *Rec. Prog. Horm. Res.*, **42**, 143−203.

Baird, A. & Ling, N. (1987) Fibroblast growth factors are present in the extracellular matrix produced by endothelial cells *in vitro*: Implications for a role of heparinase-like enzymes in the neovascular response. *Biochem. Biophys. Res. Comm.*, **142**, 428−35.

Bagavandoss, P., Kunkel, S.L., Wiggins, R.C. & Keyes, P.L. (1988) Tumor necrosis factor-α (TNF-α). Production and localization of macrophages and T lymphocytes in the rabbit corpus luteum. *Endocrinology*, **122**, 1185–7.

Bahr, J.M. & Ben-Jonathan, N. (1981) Preovulatory depletion of ovarian catecholamines in the rat. *Endocrinology*, **108**, 1815–20.

Bazer, F.W., Vallet, J.L., Harney, J.P., Gross, T.S. & Thatcher, E.W. (1989) Comparative aspects of maternal recognition of pregnancy between sheep and pigs. *J. Reprod. Fertil.*, Suppl. **37**, 85–9.

Behrman, H.R. (1979) Prostaglandins in hypothalamo-pituitary and ovarian function. *Annu. Rev. Physiol.*, **41**, 685–700.

Behrman, H.R., Aten, R.F., Luborsky, J.L., Polan, M.L., Miller, J.G.O. & Soodak, L.K. (1986) Purines, prostaglandins and peptides: Nature and mechanisms of local assist and assassin agents in the ovary. *J. Anim. Sci.*, **62** (Suppl. 2), 14–24.

Behrman, H.R., Grinwich, D.L., Hichens, M. & Macdonald, G.J. (1978) Effect of hypophysectomy, prolactin and PGF2α on LH and prolactin binding *in vivo* and *in vitro* in the corpus luteum. *Endocrinology*, **103**, 349–447.

Behrman, H.R., Hall, A.K., Preston, S.L. & Gore, S.D. (1982) Antagonistic interactions of adenosine and PGF2α modulate acute responses of luteal cells to LH. *Endocrinology*, **110**, 38–46.

Behrman, H.R. & Hichens, M. (1976) Rapid block of gonadotrophin uptake by corpora lutea *in vivo* induced by PGF2α. *Prostaglandins*, **12**, 83–95.

Behrman, H.R., Macdonald, G.J. & Greep, R.O. (1971) Regulation of ovarian cholesterol esters: evidence for the enzymatic sites of prostaglandin-induced loss of corpus luteum function. *Lipids*, **6**, 791–6.

Behrman, H.R., Ng, T.S. & Orzcyk, G.P. (1974) Interactions between prostaglandins and gonadotropins on corpus luteum function. In Moudgal, N.R. (ed.) *Gonadotropins and Gonadal Function*, pp. 332–44. Academic Press, New York.

Behrman, H.R., Ohkawa, R., Preston, S.L. & Macdonald, G.J. (1983) Transport and selective utilization of adenosine as a prosubstrate for LH-sensitive adenylate cyclase in the luteal cell. *Endocrinology*, **113**, 1132–40.

Behrman, H.R. & Preston, S.L. (1989a) Luteolytic actions of peroxide in rat ovarian cells. *Endocrinology*, **124**, 2895–900.

Behrman, H.R. & Preston, S.L. (1989b) Peroxide inhibits progesterone production in response to LH, forskolin and cyclic AMP in rat luteal cells. *Biol. Reprod.*, Suppl. **40**, 100 (abstr.).

Behrman, H.R., Preston, S.L., Pellicer, A. & Parmer, T.G. (1988) Oocyte maturation is regulated by modulation of the action of FSH in cumulus cells. In Haseltine, F.P. & First, N.L. (eds) *Meiotic Inhibition: Molecular Control of Meiosis*, pp. 115–35. Alan R. Liss, New York.

Berliner, J.A., Territo, M., Almada, L., Carter, A., Shafonsky, E. & Fogelman, A.M. (1986) Monocyte chemotactic factor produced by large vessel endothelial cells *in vitro*. *Arteriosclerosis*, **6**, 254.

Bevilaqua, M.P., Pober, J.S., Wheeler, M.A., Mendrick, D., Cotran, R.S. & Gilbrone, M.A. (1985) Interleukin-1 acts on cultured human vascular endothelial cells to increase the adhesion of polymorphonuclear leukocytes, monocytes and related leukocyte cell lines. *J. Clin. Invest.*, **76**, 2003–11.

Billig, H. & Rosberg, S. (1988) Evidence for A2 adenosine receptor-mediated effects on adenylate cyclase activity in rat ovarian membranes. *Mol. Cell. Endocrinol.*, **56**, 205–10.

Bohlen, P., Baird, A., Esch, F., Ling, N. & Gospodarowicz, D. (1984) Partial molecular characterization of pituitary fibroblast growth factor. *Proc. Natl. Acad. Sci. USA*, **81**, 5364–8.

Braden, T.D., Gamboni, F. & Niswender, G.D. (1988) Effects of prostaglandin F-2α-induced luteolysis on the populations of cells in the ovine corpus luteum. *Biol. Reprod.*, **39**, 245–53.

Brennan, T., Ohkawa, R., Gore, S.D. & Behrman, H.R. (1983) Adenine-derived purines increase ATP levels in the luteal cell: evidence that cell levels of ATP may limit the stimulation of cyclic AMP accumulation by LH. *Endocrinology*, **112**, 499–508.

Brown, C.M. & Burnstock, G. (1981) Evidence in support of the P1/P2 purinoceptor hypothesis in the guinea-pig taenia coli. *Br. J. Pharmacol.*, **73**, 617–24.

Bulmer, D. (1964) The histochemistry of ovarian macrophages in the rat. *J. Anat.*, **98**, 313–19.

Burgess, G.M., Godfrey, P.P., Mckinney, J.S., Berridge, M.J., Irvine, R.F. & Putney, J.W. (1984) The second messenger linking receptor activation to internal calcium release in liver. *Nature*, **309**, 63–6.

Burnstock, G. & Brown, C.M. (1981) Purinergic receptors. In Burnstock, G. (ed.) *Receptors and Recognition*, Series B, Vol. 12, p. 1. Chapman & Hall, New York.

Camussi, G., Aglietta, M., Malavasi, F., Tetta, C., Piacibello, W., Sanavio, F. & Bussolino, F. (1983) The release of platelet-activating factor from human endothelial cells in culture. *J. Immunol.*, **131**, 2397–403.

Cannon, J.G. & Dinarello, C.A. (1985) Increased plasma interleukin-1 activity in women after ovulation. *Science*, **227**, 1247–9.

Carlson, J.C., Buhr, M.M., Gruber, M.Y. & Thompson, J.E. (1981) Compositional and physical properties of microsomal membrane lipids from regressing rat corpora lutea. *Endocrinology*, **108**, 2124–8.

Cavender, D.E., Haskard, D.O., Joseph, B. & Ziff, M. (1986) Interleukin-1 increases the binding of human B and T lymphocytes to endothelial cell monolayers. *J. Immunol.*, **136**, 203–7.

Challis, J.R.G., Calder, A.A., Dilley, S., *et al.* (1976) Production of prostaglandins E and F by corpora lutea, corpora albicantes and stroma of the human ovary. *J. Endocrinol.*, **68**, 401–8.

Chance, B., Sies, H. & Boveris, A. (1979) Hydroperoxide metabolism in mammalian organs. *Physiol. Rev.*, **59**, 527−605.

Christiansen, N., Larsen, C. & Esmann, V. (1988) A study on the role of protein kinase C and intracellular calcium in the activation of superoxide generation. *Biochim. Biophys. Acta*, **971**, 317−24.

Clark, I.A., Thumwood, C.M., Chaudri, G., Cowden, W.B. & Hunt, N.H. (1988) Tumor necrosis factor and reactive oxygen species: implications for free-radical induced tissue injury. In Halliwell, B. (ed.) *Oxygen Radicals and Tissue Injury*, pp. 122−9. FASEB, Bethesda.

Clemmons, D.R., Isley, W.C. & Brown, M.T. (1983) Dialyzable factor in human serum of platelet origin stimulates endothelial cell replication and growth. *Proc. Natl. Acad. Sci. USA*, **80**, 1641−5.

Cross, J.C., Soodak, L.K. & Behrman, H.R. (1987) Absence of phosphocreatine in rat luteal cells. *Am. J. Physiol.*, **253**, E391−4.

Daly, J.W. (1982) Adenosine receptors: targets for future drugs. *J. Med. Chem.*, **25**, 197−207.

D'Amore, P.A & Braunhut, S.J. (1989) Stimulatory and inhibitory factors in vascular growth control. In Ryan, U.S. (ed.) *Endothelial Cells*, Vol. II., pp. 13−36. CRC Press: Florida.

Davidson, J., Klagsbrun, M., Hill, K., Buckley, A., Sullivan, R., Brewer, P. & Woodward, S.C. (1985) Accelerated wound repair, cell proliferation and collagen accumulation are produced by a cartilage-derived growth factor. *J. Cell Biol.*, **100**, 1219−27.

Davis, J.S., Alila, H.W., West, L.A., Corradino, R.A. & Hansel, W. (1988) Acute effects of prostaglandin F-2α on inositol phospholipid hydrolysis in the large and small cells of the bovine corpus luteum. *Mol. Cell. Endocrinol.*, **58**, 43−50.

Davis, J.S. & Clark, M.R. (1983) Activation of protein kinase in the bovine corpus luteum by phospholipid and $Ca^{2+}$. *Biochem. J.*, **214**, 569−74.

Davis, J.S., Weakland, L.L., Weiland, D.A., Farese, R.V. & West, L.A. (1987) Prostaglandin $F_{2\alpha}$ stimulates phosphatidyl 4,5-biphosphate hydrolysis and mobilizes intracellular $Ca^{2+}$ in bovine luteal cells. *Proc. Natl. Acad. Sci. USA*, **84**, 3728−32.

Deane, H. (1952) Histochemical observations on the ovary and oviduct of the albino rat during the estrous cycle. *Am. J. Anat.*, **291**, 363−93.

Dennefors, B., Sjören, A. & Hamberger, L. (1982) Progesterone and 3′,5′-monophosphate formation by isolated human corpora lutea of different ages. Influence of human chorionic gonadotropin and prostaglandins. *J. Clin. Endocrinol. Metab.*, **55**, 102.

Deuel, T., Senior, R.M., Huang, J.S. & Griffin, G.L. (1982) Chemotaxis of mononucleocytes and neutrophils to platelet derived growth factor. *J. Clin. Invest.*, **69**, 1046−9.

DiCorletto, P.E. (1984) Cultured endothelial cells produce multiple growth factors for connective tissue cells. *Exp. Cell Res.*, **153**, 167−72.

DiCorletto, P.E. & Bowen-Pope, D.F. (1983) Cultured endothelial cells produce a platelet-derived growth factor-like protein. *Proc. Natl. Acad. Sci. USA*, **80**, 1919−23.

DiCorletto, P.E. & Fox, P.L. (1989) Growth factor production by endothelial cells. In Ryan, U.S. (ed.) *Endothelial Cells*, Vol. II, pp. 51−61. CRC Press Inc: Florida.

Dodson, W.C. & Schomberg, D.W. (1987) The effect of transforming growth factor-beta on follicle-stimulating hormone-induced differentiation of cultured rat granulosa cells. *Endocrinology*, **120**, 512−16.

Dorflinger, L.J., Albert, P.J., Williams, A.T. & Behrman, H.R. (1984) Calcium is an inhibitor of LH-sensitive adenylate cyclase in the luteal cell. *Endocrinology*, **114**, 1208−15.

Dorflinger, L.J., Luborsky, J.L., Gore, S.D. & Behrman, H.R. (1983) Inhibitory characteristics of PGF2α in the rat luteal cell. *Mol. Cell Endocrinol.*, **33**, 225−41.

Einhorn, S., Eldor, A., Vlodavsky, I., Fuks, Z. & Panet, A. (1985) Production and characterization of interferon from endothelial cells. *J. Cell. Physiol.*, **122**, 200−4.

Elstner, E., Osswald, W. & Konze, J. (1980) Reactive oxygen species: electron donor-hydrogen peroxide complex instead of free radical OH radicals? *FEBS Lett.*, **121**, 219−21.

Emoto, N. & Baird, A. (1988) The effect of tumor necrosis factor/cachectin on follicle-stimulating hormone-induced aromatase activity in cultured rat granulosa cells. *Biochem. Biophys. Res. Commun.*, **153**, 792−8.

Esch, F., Ueno, N., Baird, A., Hill, F., Denoroy, L., Ling, N., Gospodarowicz, D. & Guillemin, R. (1985) Primary structure of bovine brain acidic FGF. *Biochem. Biophys. Res. Commun.*, **133**, 554−62.

Farin, C.E., Moeller, C.L., Mayan, H., Gamboni, F., Sawyer, H.R. & Niswender, G.D. (1988) Effect of LH and hCG on cell populations in the ovine corpus luteum. *Biol. Reprod.*, **38**, 413−21.

Farin, C.E., Moeller, C.L., Sawyer, H.R., Gamboni, F. & Niswender, G.D. (1986) Morphometric analysis of cell types in the ovine corpus luteum throughout the estrous cycle. *Biol. Reprod.*, **35**, 1299−308.

Farin, C.E., Sawyer, H.R. & Niswender, G.D. (1989) Analysis of cell types in the corpus luteum of the sheep. *J. Reprod. Fertil.*, Suppl. **37**, 181−7.

Fett, J.W., Strydom, D.J., Lobb, R.F., Alderman, E.M., Bethune, J.L., Riordan, J.F. & Vallee, B.L. (1985) Isolation and characterization of angiogenin, an angiogenic protein from human carcinoma cells. *Biochemistry*, **24**, 5480−5.

Findlay, J.K. (1986) Angiogenesis in reproductive tissues. *J. Endocrinol.*, **111**, 357−66.

Fitz, T.A., Mayan, M.H., Sawyer, H.R. & Niswender, G.D. (1982) Characterization of two steroidogenic cell types in the ovine corpus luteum. *Biol. Reprod.*, **27**, 703−11.

Folkman, J. (1985) Tumor angiogenesis. *Adv. Cancer Res.*, **43**, 175−203.

Folkman, J. & Klagsbrun, M. (1987a) A family of angiogenic factors. *Nature*, **329**, 671−2.

Folkman, J. & Klagsbrun, M. (1987b) Angiogenic factors. *Science*, **235**, 442−7.

Forman, H.J., Nelson, J. & Fisher, A.B. (1980) Rat alveolar macrophages require NADPH for superoxide production in the respiratory burst. *J. Biol. Chem.*, **255**, 9879−83.

Fox, I.H. & Kelly, W.N. (1978) The role of adenosine and 2′-deoxyadenosine in mammalian cells. *Annu. Rev. Biochem.*, **47**, 655−86.

Fredholm, B.B. & Hedqvist, P. (1980) Modulation of neurotransmission by purine nucleotides and nucleosides. *Biochem. Pharmacol.*, **29**, 1635−43.

Fridovich, I. (1986) Biological effects of the superoxide radical. *Arch. Biochem. Biophys.*, **247**, 1−11.

Fridovich, I. (1988) The biology of oxygen radicals: General concepts. In Halliwell B. (ed.) *Oxygen Radicals and Tissue Injury*, pp. 1−8, FASEB, Bethesda.

Fukuoka, M., Mori, T., Tali, S. & Yasuda, K. (1988) Interleukin-1 inhibits luteinization of porcine granulosa cells in culture. *Endocrinology*, **122**, 367−9.

Fukuoka, M., Yasuda, K., Taii, S., Takakura, K. & Mori, T. (1989) Interleukin-1 stimulates growth and inhibits progesterone secretion in the cultures of porcine granulosa cells. *Endocrinology*, **124**, 884−90.

Gabig, T.G., Kipnes, R.S. & Baboir, B.M. (1978) Solubilization of the $O^{2-}$-forming activity responsible for the respiratory burst in human neutrophils. *J. Biol. Chem.*, **253**, 6663−5.

Gadsby, J.E. (1989) Control of corpus luteum function in the pregnant rabbit. *J. Reprod. Fertil.*, Suppl. **37**, 45−54.

Gerson, S.L., Friedman, H.M. & Cinnes, D.B. (1985) Viral infection of vascular endothelial cells alters production of colony stimulating activity. *J. Clin. Invest.*, **76**, 1382−90.

Gibson, M. & Auletta, F.J. (1986) Effect of prostaglandin synthesis inhibition on human corpus luteum function. *Prostaglandins*, **31**, 1023−8.

Gillim, S., Christensen, K. & McLennan, C. (1969) Fine structure of the human menstrual corpus luteum at its stage of maximum secretory activity. *Am. J. Anat.*, **126**, 409−28.

Gimenez-Gallego, G., Rodkey, J., Bennet, C., Rios-Candelora, M., DiSalvo, J. & Thomas, K. (1985) Brain derived acidic fibroblast growth factor: complete amino acid sequence and homologies. *Science*, **230**, 1385−8.

Godkin, J.D., Bazer, F.W., Moffatt, J., Sessions, F. & Robberts, R.M. (1982) Purification and properties of a major low molecular weight protein released by the trophoblast of sheep at Day 13−21. *J. Reprod. Fertil.*, **65**, 141−50.

Gore, S.D. & Behrman, H.R. (1984) Alteration of transmembrane sodium and potassium gradients inhibits the action of LH in the luteal cell. *Endocrinology*, **114**, 2020−31.

Gorog, P., Pearson, J. & Kakkar, V. (1988) Generation of reactive oxygen metabolites by phagocytosing endothelial cells. *Artherosclerosis*, **72**, 19−27.

Gospodarowicz, D., Cheng, J., Lui, G-M., Baird, A. & Bohlen, P. (1984) Isolation by heparin-sepharose affinity chromatography of brain fibroblast growth factor: identity with pituitary fibroblast growth factor. *Proc. Natl. Acad. Sci. USA*, **81**, 6963−7.

Gospodarowicz, D., Cheng, J., Lui, G-M., Baird, A., Esch, F. & Bohlen, P. (1985a) Corpus luteum angiogenic factor is related to fibroblast growth factor. *Endocrinology*, **117**, 2283−91.

Gospodarowicz, D., Cheng, J., Lui, G-M., Fuji, D.K., Baird, A. & Bohlen, P. (1985b) Fibroblast growth factor in the human placenta. *Biochem. Biophys. Res. Commun.*, **128**, 5545−62.

Gottschall, P.I., Katsuura, G., Dahl, R.R., Hoffman, S.T. & Arimura, A. (1988) Discordance in the effects of interleukin-1 on rat granulosa cell differentiation induced by follicle-stimulating hormone or activators of adenylate cyclase. *Biol. Reprod.*, **39**, 1074−85.

Grinwich, D.L., Hichens, M. & Behrman, H.R. (1976) Control of the LH receptor by prolactin and $PGF_{2\alpha}$ in rat corpora lutea. *Biol. Reprod.*, **14**, 212−18.

Hall, A.K., Preston, S.L. & Behrman, H.R. (1981) Purine amplification of luteinizing hormone actions in ovarian luteal cells. *J. Biol. Chem.*, **256**, 10390−8.

Halliwell, B. (1987) Oxidants and human disease: some new concepts. *FASEB J.*, 1358−64.

Halliwell, B. (1988) *Oxygen Radicals and Tissue Injury*. FASEB, Bethesda.

Hansel, W., Stock, A. & Battista, P.J. (1989) Low molecular weight lipid soluble luteotrophic factors(s) produced by conceptuses in cows. *J. Reprod. Fertil.*, Suppl. **37**, 11−17.

Harrison, L.M., Kenny, N. & Niswender, G.D. (1987) Progesterone production, LH receptors, and oxytocin secretion by ovine luteal cell types on Day 25 of pregnancy. *J. Reprod. Fertil.*, **79**, 539−48.

Haulica, I., Ababei, L., Branisteanu, D. & Topoliceanu, F. (1973) Preliminary data on the possible hypnogenic role of adenosine. *J. Neurochem.*, **21**, 1019−20.

Heimark, R.L., Twardzik, D.R. & Schwartz, S.M. (1986) Inhibition of endothelial regeneration by type-beta transforming growth factor from platelets. *Science*, **233**, 1078−80.

Henderson, J.F. & LePage, G.A. (1959) Transport of adenine-8$^{14}$C among mouse tissues by red blood cells. *J. Biol. Chem.*, **234**, 3219−23.

Hickey, G.J., Walton, J.S. & Hansel, W. (1989) Identification of a luteotrophic protein in bovine allantoic fluid. *J. Reprod. Fertil.*, Suppl. **37**, 29−35.

Hochachka, P.W. (1986) Defence strategies against hypoxia and hypothermia. *Science*, **231**, 234−41.

Hoch-Ligeti, C. & Bourne, G. (1948) Changes in the

concentration and histological distribution of the ascorbic acid in ovaries, adrenals and livers of rats during oestrous cycles. *Br. J. Pathol.*, **29**, 400–7.

Hong, S.L. (1980) Effect of bradykinin and thrombin on prostacyclin synthesis in endothelial cells from calf and pig aorta and human umbilical cord vein. *Thromb. Res.*, **18**, 787–95.

Hoyer, P.B. & Niswender, G.D. (1985) The regulation of steroidogenesis is different in the two types of ovine luteal cells. *J. Physiol. Pharmacol.*, **63**, 240–8.

Ignotz, R.A. & Massague, J. (1986) Transforming growth factor-beta stimulates the formation of fibronectin and collagen and their incorporation into the extracellular matrix. *J. Biol. Chem.*, **261**, 4337–45.

Imlay, J. & Linn, S. (1988) DNA damage and oxygen radical toxicity. *Science*, **240**, 1302–9.

Ishikawa, F., Miyazono, K., Hellman, U., Drexler, H., Wernstedt, C., Hagiwara, K., Usuki, K. *et al.* (1989) Identification of angiogenic activity and the cloning and expression of platelet-derived endothelial cell growth factor. *Nature*, **338**, 557–62.

Izhar, M. & Shemesh, M. (1989) Partial purification of a luteotrophic substance from bovine fetal cotyledon granules. *J. Reprod. Fertil.*, Suppl. **37**, 37–44.

Jacob, H.S. & Vercelotti, G.M. (1988) Granulocyte-mediated endothelial injury: oxidant damage amplified by lactoferrin and platelet activating factor. In Halliwell, B. (ed.) *Oxygen Radicals and Tissue Injury*, pp. 57–61. FASEB, Bethesda.

Jaye, M., Howk, R., Burgess, W., Ricca, G.A., Chin, I-M., Ravera, M.W., O'Brien, S.J. *et al.* (1986) Human endothelial cell growth factor: cloning, nucleotide sequence and chromosome localization. *Science*, **233**, 541–5.

Johnson, K.J. & Varani, J. (1981) Substrate hydrolysis by immune complex-activated neutrophils: effect of physical presentation of complexes and protease inhibitors. *J. Immunol.*, **127**, 1875–9.

Johnston, R., Godzik, C. & Cohn, Z. (1978) Increased superoxide anion production by immunologically activated and chemically elicited macrophages. *J. Exp. Med.*, **148**, 115–27.

Jones, P.B.C., Welsh, T.H. Jr. & Hsueh, A.J.W. (1982) Regulation of ovarian progestin production by epidermal growth factor in cultured rat granulosa cells. *J. Biol. Chem.*, **257**, 11268–73.

Jordan, A.W. (1981) Changes in ovarian β-adrenergic receptors during the estrous cycle of the rat. *Biol. Reprod.*, **24**, 245–8.

Joseph, M.M. & Mead, R.A. (1988) Size-distribution of ferret luteal cells during pregnancy. *Biol. Reprod.*, **39**, 1159–69.

Kano, S., Iizuka, T., Ishimura, Y., Fujiki, H. & Sugimura, T. (1987) Stimulation of superoxide anion formation by the non-TPA type tumor promoters palytoxin and thapsigargin in porcine and human neutrophils. *Biochem. Biophys. Res. Commun.*, **143**, 672–7.

Kawakami, M., Kubo, K., Uemura, T., Nagase, M. & Hayashi, R. (1981) Involvement of ovarian innervation in steroid secretion. *Endocrinology*, **109**, 136–45.

Khan, S.A., Schmidt, K., Hallin, P., Di Pauli, R., DeGeyter, Ch. & Nieschlag, E. (1988) Human testis cytosol and ovarian follicular fluid contain high amounts of interleukin-1-like factor(s). *Mol. Cell. Endocrinol.*, **58**, 221–30.

Khan-Dawood, F.S. (1987) Human corpus luteum: immunocytochemical localization of epidermal growth factor. *Fertil. Steril.*, **47**, 916–19.

Khan-Dawood, F.S., Huang, J-C. & Dawood, M.Y. (1989) Effect of human chorionic gonadotropin and prostaglandin $F_{2\alpha}$ on progesterone production by human luteal cells. *J. Steroid Biochem.*, **33**, 941–7.

Kirsch, T., Friedman, A., Vogel, R. & Flickinger, G. (1981) Macrophages in corpora lutea of mice: characterization and effects on steroid secretion. *Biol. Reprod.*, **25**, 629–38.

Korda, A.R., Shutt, D.A., Smith, I.D., Shearman, R.P. & Lyneham, R.C. (1975) Assessment of possible luteolytic effect of intraovarian injection of prostaglandin $F_{2\alpha}$ in the human. *Prostaglandins*, **9**, 443–9.

Lahav, M., Freud, A. & Lindner, H.R. (1976) Abrogation by prostaglandin $F_{2\alpha}$ of LH-stimulated cyclic AMP accumulation in isolated rat corpora lutea of pregnancy. *Biochem. Biophys. Res. Commun.*, **68**, 1294–300.

Lajtha, L.G. & Vane, J.R. (1958) Dependence of bone marrow cells on the liver for purine supply. *Nature*, **182**, 191–2.

Laloraya, M., Kumar, G.P. & Laloraya, M. (1988) Changes in the levels of superoxide anion radical and superoxide dismutase during the estrous cycle of *Rattus norvegicus* and induction of superoxide dismutase in rat ovary by lutropin. *Biochem. Biophys. Res. Commun.*, **157**, 146–53.

Larsen, C., Anderson, A., Appella, E., Oppenheim, J. & Matsushima, K. (1989) The neutrophil-activating protein (NAP-1) is also chemotactic for T lymphocytes. *Science*, **243**, 1464–6.

Lemon, M. & Loir, M. (1977) Steroid release *in vitro* by two luteal cell types in the corpus luteum of the pregnant sow. *J. Endocrinol.*, **72**, 351–9.

Lemon, M. & Mauleon, P. (1982) Interaction between two luteal cells types from the corpus luteum of the sow in progesterone synthesis *in vitro*. *J. Reprod. Fertil.*, **64**, 315–23.

Leszczynski, D. & Hayry, D. (1989) Eicosanoids are regulatory molecules in γ-interferon-induced endothelial antigenicity and adherence for leucocytes. *FEBS Lett.*, **242**, 383–6.

Leung, P.C.K., Minegishi, T., Ma, F., Zhou, F. & Ho-Yeun, B. (1986) Induction of polyphosphoinositide breakdown in rat corpus luteum by prostaglandin $F_{2\alpha}$. *Endocrinology*, **119**, 12–18.

Lobb, R.R., Alderman, E.M. & Fett, J.W. (1985) Induction of angiogenesis by bovine brain-derived class I heparin binding growth factor. *Biochemistry*, **24**, 4969–73.

Londos, C., Cooper, D.M.F., Schlegel, W. & Rodbell, M. (1978) Adenosine analogs inhibit adipocyte adenylate cyclase by a GTP-dependent process: basis for actions of adenosine and methylxanthines on cyclic AMP production and lipolysis. *Proc. Natl. Acad. Sci. USA*, **75**, 5362–6.

Luborsky, J.L., Dorflinger, L.J., Wright, K. & Behrman, H.R. (1984a) Prostaglandin $F_{2\alpha}$ inhibits luteinizing hormone (LH)-induced increase in LH receptor binding to isolated rat luteal cells. *Endocrinology*, **115**, 2210–16.

Luborsky, J.L., Slater, W.T. & Behrman, H.R. (1984b) Luteinizing hormone (LH) receptor aggregation: Modification of ferritin-LH binding and aggregation by prostaglandin $F_{2\alpha}$ and ferritin-LH. *Endocrinology*, **115**, 2217–26.

McArdle, C.A. & Holtorf, A-P. (1989) Oxytocin and progesterone release from bovine corpus luteal cells in culture: effects of insulin like growth factor I, insulin, and prostaglandins. *Endocrinology*, **124**, 1278–86.

McClellan, M.C., Diekman, M.A., Abel, J.H., Jr. & Niswender, G.D. (1975) Luteinizing hormone, progesterone and the morphological development of normal and superovulated corpora lutea in sheep. *Cell Tiss. Res.*, **164**, 291–307.

McIntyre, T.M., Zimmerman, G.A., Satoh, K. & Prescott, S.M. (1985) Cultured endothelial cells synthesize both platelet-activating factor and prostacyclin in response to histamine, bradykinin and adenosine. *J. Clin. Invest.*, **76**, 271–80.

Maciag, T., Mehlmen, T., Friesel, R. & Schreiber, A.B. (1984) Heparin binds endothelial growth factor, the principal mitogen in the bovine brain. *Science*, **225**, 932–5.

Madri, J.A., Pratt, B.M. & Tucker, A.M. (1988) Phenotypic modulation of endothelial cells by transforming growth factor-beta depends upon the composition and organization of the extracellular matrix. *J. Cell. Biol.*, **106**, 1375–84.

Majer, J., Hershko, A., Zeitlin-Beck, R., Shoshani, T. & Razin, A. (1967) Turnover of purine nucleotides in rabbit erythrocytes I. Studies *in vivo*. *Biochem. Biophys. Acta*, **149**, 50–8.

Martal, J., Lacroix, M.C., Loudes, C., Saunier, M. & Witenberger-Torres, S. (1979) Trophoblastin, an antiluteolytic protein present in early pregnancy in sheep. *J. Reprod. Fertil.*, **56**, 63–7.

Matsubara, T. & Ziff, M. (1986a) Superoxide anion release by human endothelial cells: synergism between a phorbol ester and a calcium ionophore. *J. Cell. Physiol.*, **127**, 207–10.

Matsubaru, T. & Ziff, M. (1986b) Increased superoxide anion release from human endothelial cells in response to cytokines. *J. Immunol.*, **137**, 3295–8.

May, J.V., Frost, J.P. & Schomberg, D.W. (1988) Differential effects of epidermal growth factor, somatomedin-C/insulin-like growth factor I, and transforming growth factor-β on porcine granulosa cell deoxyribonucleic acid synthesis and cell proliferation. *Endocrinology*, **123**, 168–79.

Mercandetti, A.J., Lane, T.A. & Colmerauer, M.E.M. (1984) Cultured human endothelial cells elaborate neutrophil chemoattractants. *J. Lab. Clin. Med.*, **104**, 370–80.

Meyer, G.T. & Bruce, N.W. (1979) The cellular pattern of corpus luteal growth during pregnancy in the rat. *Anat. Rec.*, **193**, 823–30.

Miossec, P., Cavender, D. & Ziff, M. (1986) Production of interleukin-1 by human endothelial cells. *J. Immunol.*, **136**, 2486–91.

Monaco, L., Toscano, M.V. & Conti, M. (1984) Purine modulation of the hormonal response of the rat Sertoli cell in culture. *Endocrinology*, **15**, 1616–24.

Moncada, S., Gryglewski, R., Bunting, S. & Vane, J.R. (1976) An enzyme isolated from arteries transforms prostaglandin endoperoxides to an unstable substance that inhibits platelet aggregation. *Nature*, **263**, 663–5.

Mondschein, J.S. & Schomberg, D.W. (1981) Platelet-derived growth factor enhances granulosa cell luteinizing hormone receptor induction by follicle stimulation hormone and serum. *Endocrinology*, **109**, 325–7.

Montessano, R., Vassalli, J-D., Baird, A., Guillemin, R. & Orci, L. (1986) Basic fibroblast factor induced angiogenesis *in vitro*. *Proc. Natl. Acad. Sci. USA*, **83**, 7297–301.

Morris, B. & Sass, M.B. (1966) The formation of lymph in the ovary. *Proc. R. Soc. Lond. (Biol.)*, **164**, 577–91.

Muller, G., Behrens, J., Nussbaumer, U., Bohlen, P. & Birchmeier, W. (1987) Inhibitory action of transforming growth factor-β on endothelial cells. *Proc. Natl. Acad. Sci. USA*, **84**, 5600–4.

Murray, A.W., Elliott, D.C. & Atkinson, M.R. (1970) Nucleotide biosynthesis from preformed purines in mammalian cells: regulatory mechanisms and biological significance. *Prog. Nucleic Acid Res. Mol. Biol.*, **10**, 87–119.

Musicki, B., Aten, R.F. & Behrman, H.R. (1990) The antigonadotropic actions of prostaglandin $F_{2\alpha}$ and phorbol ester are mediated by separate processes in rat luteal cells. *Endocrinology*, **126**, 1388–95.

Nathan, C. (1989) Respiratory burst in adherent human neutrophils: triggering by colony-stimulating factors CSF-GM and CSF-G. *Blood*, **73**, 301–6.

Nathan, C.F., Murray, H.W., Wiebe, M.E. & Rubin, B.Y. (1983) Identification of interferon-γ as the lymphokine that activates human macrophage oxidative metabolism and antimicrobial activity. *J. Exp. Med.*, **158**, 670–89.

Nawroth, P.O., Bank, I., Handley, D., Cassimeris, J., Chess, L. & Stern, D. (1986) Tumor necrosis factor/cachectin interacts with endothelial cell receptors to induce release of interleukin-1. *J. Exp. Med.*, **163**, 1363–75.

Neill, J.D., Johansson, E.D. & Knobil, E. (1969) Failure of hysterectomy to influence the normal pattern of cyclic progesterone secretion in the Rhesus monkey. *Endocrinology*, **84**, 464–7.

Olwin, B.B. & Hauschka, S.D. (1986) Identification of the fibroblast growth factor-receptor of Swiss 3T3 cells and mouse skeletal muscle myoblasts. *Biochemistry*, **25**, 3487–92.

O'Shea, J.D., Cran, D.G. & Hay, M.F. (1979) The small luteal cell of the sheep. *J. Anat.*, **128**, 239–51.

Pace-Asciak, C. & Gryglewski, R. (1983) The prostacyclins. In Pace-Asciak, C. & Granstrom, E. (eds) *Prostaglandins and Related Substances*, Vol. 5, pp. 95–126. Elsevier, Amsterdam.

Pang, C.Y. & Behrman, H.R. (1981) Acute effects of prostaglandin $F_{2\alpha}$ on ovarian and luteal blood flow, luteal gonadotropin uptake *in vivo* and gonadotropin binding *in vitro*. *Endocrinology*, **108**, 2239–44.

Parlow, A. (1972) Influence of differences in the persistence of luteinizing hormones in blood on their potency in the ovarian ascorbic acid depletion bioassay. *Endocrinology*, **91**, 1109–12.

Pearson, J.D., Slakey, L.L. & Gordon, J.L. (1983) Stimulation of prostaglandin production through purinoreceptors on cultured porcine endothelial cells. *Biochem. J.*, **214**, 273–6.

Pepperell, J., Preston, S.L. & Behrman, H.R. (1989) The antigonadotropic action of prostaglandin $F_{2\alpha}$ is not mediated by elevated cytosolic calcium levels in rat luteal cells. *Endocrinology*, **125**, 144–51.

Pharriss, B.B. & Wyngarden, L.J. (1969) The effect of prostaglandin $F_{2\alpha}$ on the progestagen content of ovaries from pseudopregnant rats. *Proc. Soc. Exp. Biol. Med.*, **130**, 92–4.

Plante, C., Hansen, P.J. & Thatcher, W.W. (1988) Prolongation of luteal lifespan in cows by intrauterine infusion of recombinant bovine alpha-interferon. *Endocrinology*, **122**, 2342–4.

Pober, J.S. (1989) Lymphokine modulation of endothelial cell morphology and surface antigens. In Ryan U.S. (ed.) *Endothelial Cells*, Vol. II, pp. 259–70. CRC Press, Florida.

Pohlman, T.H., Stanness, K.A., Beatley, P.G., Ochs, H.D. & Harlan, J.M. (1986) An endothelial cell surface factor(s) induced *in vitro* by lipopolysaccharide, interleukin-1 and tumor necrosis factor-$\alpha$ increases neutrophil adherence by a CDw18-dependent mechanism. *J. Immunol.*, **136**, 4547–53.

Polan, M.L., DeCherney, A.H., Haseltine, F.P., Mezer, H. & Behrman, H.R. (1983) Adenosine amplifies FSH action in granulosa cells and LH action in luteal cells of the rat and the human. *J. Clin. Endocrinol. Metab.*, **56**, 288–94.

Powell, W.S., Hammerstrom, S., Samuelsson, B. & Sjoberg, B. (1974) Prostaglandin $F_{2\alpha}$ receptor in human corpora lutea. *Lancet*, **i**, 1120.

Quesenberry, P.J. & Gibvrone, M.A., Jr. (1980) Vascular endothelium as a regulator of granulopoiesis: production of colony-stimulating activity by cultured endothelial cells. *Blood*, **56**, 1060–7.

Raymond, V., Leung, P.C.K. & Labrie, F. (1983) Stimulation by prostaglandin $F_{2\alpha}$ of phosphatidic acid-phosphatidyl inositol turnover in rat luteal cells. *Biochem. Biophys. Res. Commun.*, **116**, 39–46.

Riley, J.C.M., Cziraki, S.E. & Carlson, J.C. (1989) The effects of prolactin and prostaglandin $F_{2\alpha}$ on plasma membrane changes during luteolysis in the rat. *Endocrinology*, **124**, 1564–70.

Roby, K.S., Terranova, P.F. (1988) Tumor necrosis factor alpha alters follicular steroidogenesis *in vitro*. *Endocrinology*, **123**, 2952–4.

Rodgers, R.J., O'Shea, J.D. & Bruce, N.W. (1984) Morphometric analysis of the cellular composition to the ovine corpus luteum. *J. Anat.*, **138**, 757–69.

Rodgers, R.J., O'Shea, J.D. & Findlay, J.K. (1983) Progesterone production *in vitro* by small and large ovine luteal cells. *J. Reprod. Fertil.*, **69**, 113–24.

Rodgers, R.J., O'Shea, J.D., Findlay, J.K., Flint, A.P.F. & Sheldrick, E.L. (1983) Large luteal cells the source of oxytocin in the sheep. *Endocrinology*, **113**, 2302–4.

Rommerts, F.F., Molenaar, R., Hoogerbrugge, J.W. & van der Molen H.J. (1984) Development of adenosine responsiveness after isolation of Leydig cells. *Biol. Reprod.*, **30**, 842–7.

Rotrosen, D. & Gallin, J.I. (1986) Histamine type 1 receptor occupancy increases endothelial cytosolic calcium, reduces F-actin and promotes albumin diffusion across cultured endothelial monolayers. *J. Cell Biol.*, **103**, 2379–87.

Ryan, U.S. (1988) *Endothelial Cells*, Vol. II. CRC Press, Miami.

Sawada, M. & Carlson, J.C. (1985) Association of lipid peroxidation during luteal regression in the rat and natural aging in the Rotifer. *Exp. Gerontol.*, **20**, 179.

Sawada, M. & Carlson, J.C. (1989) Superoxide radical production in plasma membrane samples from regressing corpora lutea. *Can. J. Physiol. Pharmacol.* **67**, 465–71.

Schaeffer, J.M., Liu, J. & Hseuh, A.J.W. (1984) Presence of oxytocin and arginine-vasopressin in human ovary, oviduct and follicular fluid. *J. Clin. Endocrinol. Metab.*, **59**, 970–3.

Schams, D. (1989) Ovarian peptides in the cow and sheep. *J. Reprod. Fertil.*, Suppl. **37**, 225–31.

Schams, D., Koll, R. & Li, C.H. (1988) Insulin-like growth factor-1 stimulates oxytocin and progesterone production by bovine granulosa cells in culture. *J. Endocrinol.*, **116**, 97–100.

Schomberg, D.W. (1988) Regulation of follicle development by gonadotropins and growth factors. In Stouffer, R.L. (ed.) *The Primate Ovary*, pp. 25–33. Raven Press, New York.

Schor, A. & Schor, S.L. (1983) Tumor angiogensis. *J.*

*Pathol.*, **141**, 385–413.

Schraufstatter, I., Hyslop, P., Hinshaw, D., Spraag, R., Sklar, L. & Cochrane, C. (1986) Hydrogen peroxide-induced injury of cells and its prevention by inhibitors of poly (ADP-ribose) polmerase. *Proc. Natl. Acad. Sci. USA*, **83**, 4908–12.

Schreiber, A.B., Kenny, J., Kowalski, W.J., Friesel, R., Mehlman, T. & Maciag, T. (1985) Interaction of endothelial cell growth factor with heparin: characterization by receptor and antibody recognition. *Proc. Natl. Acad. Sci. USA*, **82**, 6138–42.

Schreiber, A.B., Winkler, M.E. & Derynk, R. (1986) Transforming growth factor alpha: a more potent angiogenic mediator than epidermal growth factor. *Science*, **232**, 1250–3.

Schwall, R.H., Sawyer, H.R. & Niswender, G.D. (1986) Differential regulation by LH and prostaglandins of steroidogenesis in small and large luteal cells of the ewe. *J. Reprod. Fertil.*, **76**, 821–9.

Sender Baum, M. (1989) Prostaglandin $F_{2\alpha}$ administered *in vivo* induces $Ca^{2+}$-dependent protein phosphorylation in rat luteal tissue. *Endocrinology*, **124**, 555–7.

Sender Baum, M. & Rosberg, S. (1987) A phorbol ester, phorbol 12-myristate 13-acetate, and a calcium inophore, A23187, can mimic the luteolytic effect of prostaglandin $F_{2\alpha}$ in isolated luteal cells. *Endocrinology*, **120**, 1019–26.

Shapiro, R., Riodan, J.F. & Vallee, B.L. (1986) Characteristic ribonucleolytic activity of human angiogenin. *Biochemistry*, **25**, 3527–32.

Shaw, G., Jorgensen, G.I., Tweedale, R., Tennison, M. & Waters, M.J. (1985) Effect of epidermal growth factor on reproductive function of ewes. *J. Endocrinol.*, **107**, 429–36.

Shing, Y., Folkman, J., Haudenschild, C., Lund, D., Crum, R. & Klagsburn, M. (1985) Angiogenesis is stimulated by a tumor-derived endothelial cell factor. *J. Cell Biochem.*, **29**, 275–87.

Simpson, P.J., Fantone, J.C. & Lucchesi, B.R. (1987) Myocardial ischemia and reperfusion injury: oxygen radicals and the role of the neutrophil. In Halliwell, B. (ed.) *Oxygen Radicals and Tissue Injury*, pp. 63–77. FASEB, Bethesda.

Smedly, L.A., Tonnensen, M.G., Sandhaus, R.A., Haslett, C., Guthri, L.A., Johnston, R.B., Henson, P.M. & Worthen, G.S. (1986) Neutrophil-mediated injury to endothelial cells. Enhancement by endotoxin and essential role of neutrophil elastase. *J. Clin. Invest.*, **77**, 1233–43.

Soodak, L.K. & Behrman, H.R. (1988) Mitochondria mediate amplification of LH action by adenosine in luteal cells. *Endocrinology*, **122**, 1308–13.

Soodak, L.K., MacDonald, G. & Behrman, H.R. (1988a) Luteolysis is linked to LH-induced depletion of ATP *in vivo*. *Endocrinology*, **122**, 187–93.

Soodak, L.K., Musicki, B. & Behrman, H.R. (1988b) Selective amplification of luteinizing hormone by adenosine in rat luteal cells. *Endocrinology*, **122**,

847–54.

Spielman, W.S. & Thompson, C.I. (1982) A proposed role for adenosine in the regulation of renal hemodynamics and renin release. *Am. J. Physiol.*, **242**, F423–35.

Sporn, M.B., Roberts, A.B., Wakefield, I.M. & Assoian, R.K. (1986) Transforming growth factor-β: biological function and chemical structure. *Science*, **233**, 532–4.

Stewart, H.J., Flint, A.P.F., Lamming, G.E., McCann, S.H.E. & Parkinson, T.J. (1989) Antiluteolytic effects of blastocyst-secreted interferon investigated *in vitro* and *in vivo* in the sheep. *J. Reprod. Fertil.*, Suppl. **37**, 127–38.

Strieter, R., Kinkel, S., Showell, H., Remick, D., Phan, S., Ward, P. & Marks, R. (1989) Endothelial cell gene expression of a neutrophil chemotactic factor by TNF-α, LPS, and IL-IB. *Science*, **243**, 1467–9.

Takai, Y., Kishimoto, A., Kikkawa, U., Mori, T. & Nishizuka, Y. (1979) Unsaturated diacylglycerol as a possible messenger for the activation of calcium-activated, phospholipid-dependent protein kinase system. *Biochem. Biophys. Res. Commun.*, **91**, 1218–24.

Tan, G.J.S., Tweedale, R. & Biggs, J.S.G. (1982) Oxytocin may play a role in the control of the human corpus luteum. *J. Endocrinol.*, **95**, 65–70.

Tapanainen, J., Leinonen, P.J., Tapanainen, P., Yamamoto, M. & Jaffe, R.B. (1987) Regulation of human granulosa-luteal cell progesterone production and proliferation by gonadotrophins and growth factors. *Fertil. Steril.*, **48**, 576–80.

Thatcher, W.W., Bazer, F.W., Sharp, D.C. & Roberts, R.M. (1986) Interrelationships between uterus and conceptus to maintain corpus luteum function in early pregnancy: Sheep, cattle, pigs and horses. *J. Anim. Sci.*, **62**, (Suppl. 2), 25–46.

Thatcher, W.W., Hansen, P.J., Gross, T.S., Helmer, S.D., Plante, C. & Bazer, F.W. (1989) Antiluteolytic effects of bovine trophoblast protein-1. *J. Reprod. Fert.*, Suppl. **37**, 91–9.

Thomas, J.P., Dorflinger, L.J. & Behrman, H.R. (1978) Mechanism of the rapid antigonadotropic action of prostaglandins in cultured luteal cells. *Proc. Natl. Acad. Sci. USA*, **75**, 1344–48.

Titzel, L., Probst, I., Jarry, H. & Wuttke, W. (1988) Inhibitory effect of oxytocin and vasopressin on steroid release by cultured porcine luteal cells. *Endocrinology*, **122**, 1780–5.

Tsunawaki, S., Sporn, M., Ding, A. & Nathan, C. (1988) Deactivation of macrophages by transforming growth factor-β. *Nature*, **334**, 260–2.

Van Duuren, B.L. & Sivak, A. (1968) Tumor-promoting agents from croton tiglium L and their mode of action. *Cancer Res.*, **28**, 2349–56.

Veldhuis, J.D. & Demers, L.M. (1986) An inhibitory role for the protein kinase C Pathway in ovarian steroidogenesis. *Biochem. J.*, **239**, 505–11.

Vollmar, A.M., Mytzka, C., Arendt, R.M. & Schulz, R.

(1988) Atrial natriuretic peptide in bovine corpus luteum. *Endocrinology*, **123**, 762–7.

Wangler, R.D., DeWitt, D.F. & Sparks, H.V. (1984) Effect of β-adrenergic blockade on nucleoside release from the hypoperfused isolated heart. *Am. J. Physiol.*, **247**, H330–6.

Ward, P.A., Johnson, K.J., Warren, J.S. & Kunkel, R.G. (1988) Immune complexes, oxygen radicals and lung injury. In Halliwell, B. (ed.) *Oxygen Radicals and Tissue Injury*, pp. 107–14. FASEB, Bethesda.

Weis, S.J. & Regiani, S. (1984) Neutrophils degrade subendothelial matrices in the presence of alpha-1-proteinase inhibitor. Cooperative use of lysomal proteinases and oxygen metabolites. *J. Clin. Invest.*, 1297–303.

Weksler, B.B., Ley, C.W. & Jaffe, E.A. (1978) Stimulation of endothelial prostacyclin production by thrombin, trypsin and the ionophore A23187. *J. Clin. Invest.*, **62**, 923–30.

Wright, K., Pang, C.Y. & Behrman, H.R. (1980) Luteal membrane binding of prostaglandin$_{2\alpha}$ and sensitivity of corpora lutea to prostaglandin$_{2\alpha}$-induced luteolysis in pseudopregnant rats. *Endocrinology*, **106**, 1333–7.

Zweier, J., Kuppusamy, P. & Lutty, G. (1988) Measurement of endothelial cell free-radical generation: Evidence for a central mechanism of free radical injury in postischemic tissues. *Proc. Natl. Acad. Sci. USA*, **85**, 4046–50.

# 8 Diagnosis and Treatment of Anovulation

S. FRANKS

## Introduction

It is perhaps not surprising that anovulation is a common clinical problem given the complexity of the interacting processes that control normal ovulation. Anovulation is the principle cause of infertility in about one-third of couples presenting with this symptom and is one of the major causes of menstrual dysfunction (Hull, 1981; Franks *et al.*, 1985a). Recent advances in the understanding of the physiology of ovarian function have had important implications in understanding the basis of ovulatory disorders and in allowing the development of more successful methods of treatment. Such developments in diagnosis and treatment have been enhanced by the use of high resolution ultrasound imaging of the ovaries and uterus.

## Causes and presentation

The causes of anovulation may be divided broadly into those associated with primary ovarian failure and those due to deficiency or disorded hypothalamic regulation of gonadotrophins (Table 8.1). In women presenting with secondary amenorrhoea the latter group is very much the larger. It may be further subdivided into specific disorders of the hypothalamus or pituitary (such as a prolactin secreting pituitary tumour) or those which occur as a function of an underlying disorder such as anorexia nervosa. One very important cause of anovulation

**Table 8.1.** Causes of anovulation

*Primary ovarian failure*
Genetic (e.g. Turner)
Autoimmune
Others (e.g. cytotoxic chemotherapy)

*Secondary ovarian dysfunction*
1 Disorders of gonadotrophin regulation
  (a) Specific
     Hyperprolactinaemia
     Kallmann's
  (b) Functional
     Weight loss
     Exercise
     Idiopathic
2 Gonadotrophin deficiency
  Pituitary tumour
3 Disorder of gonadotrophin action
  Polycystic ovary syndrome

which does not fit comfortably into any of these categories is polycystic ovary syndrome (PCOS). In this case there may be a problem with gonadotrophin action at the ovarian level, as will be discussed in detail below.

Anovulation may present either as amenorrhoea, irregular menses or oligomenorrhoea, that is an intermenstrual interval of greater than 6 weeks.

In women with primary amenorrhoea there is a somewhat higher proportion of subjects who fail to ovulate as a result of primary ovarian dysfunction of which the most important cause is gonadal dysgenesis. In general, however, the spectrum of causes of anovulation is similar to that in women presenting with secondary amenorrhoea; thus the investigation and management follows the same principles as outlined below.

Tables 8.2 and 8.3 list the causes of anovulation in consecutive patients presenting to a single gynaecological endocrine clinic at the Samaritan Hospital for Women (St. Mary's Hospital group) with either secondary amenorrhoea or oligomenorrhoea (Adams *et al.*, 1986; Franks, 1987). The most common cause of secondary amenorrhoea in this series was a weight-loss-related disorder of gonadotrophin secretion. This was closely followed by PCOS, which as can be seen in Table 8.3 was by far the most common cause of anovulatory menses. Of the other important causes of secondary amenorrhoea, hyperprolactinaemia and primary ovarian failure accounted for 11% each and an unexplained disorder of gonadotrophin regulation was found in 9%. Note that despite a reported association of thyroid disorders with anovulation (Burrow, 1978) none of the subjects in this series had thyroid disease as a suspected cause of anovulation. Although women with thyroid

**Table 8.2.** Diagnosis in 100 consecutive patients with secondary amenorrhoea attending gynaecological clinic at the Samaritan Hospital for Women (St. Mary's Hospital group)

| Diagnosis | No. of patients |
|---|---|
| Amenorrhoea related to weight loss | 35 |
| Polycystic ovary syndrome | 32 |
| Hyperprolactinaemia | 11 |
| Primary ovarian failure | 11 |
| Hypogonadotrophic hypogonadism (not weight related) | 9 |
| Aschermann's syndrome | 2 |

**Table 8.3.** Diagnosis and classification of 75 women with anovulation and oligomenorrhoea

| Diagnosis | No. | (%) |
|---|---|---|
| Women with oligomenorrhoea ($n=75$) | | |
|   Hyperprolactinaemia | 1 | (1) |
|   Obese (no polycystic ovaries) | 3 | (4) |
|   Perimenopausal | 2 | (3) |
|   Recovered weight loss | 1 | (1) |
|   Unknown | 3 | (4) |
|   Polycystic ovaries | 65 | (87) |

disorders are thought to be vulnerable to menstrual disturbances (and both hyper- and hypothyroidism have been suggested as possible mechanisms for anovulation in thyroid tissue — Burrow 1978) the author is not aware of any systematic studies which have been performed to determine the prevalence of menstrual disorders in women presenting with thyroid disease.

## Mechanisms underlying ovulatory disorders

### Primary ovarian failure

This represents a spectrum of ovarian pathology associated with elevated serum concentrations of follicle-stimulating hormone (FSH) which signify a primary problem in folliculogenesis. Such patients present with amenorrhoea (or occasionally oligomenorrhoea) and may have symptoms of oestrogen deficiency such as hot flushes or vaginal dryness. The ovarian appearance on ultrasound or on biopsy is variable, ranging from no (or very few) primordial follicles to multiple antral follicles (Jones & De Moraes-Ruehsen, 1969; Van Campenhout et al., 1972; Board et al., 1979; O'Herlihy et al., 1980; Menon et al., 1984). This has lead to the use of the terms 'premature menopause' for the former, and 'resistant ovary syndrome' for the latter (Jones & De Moraes-Ruehsen, 1969; Board *et al.*, 1979; Menon *et al.*, 1984). In fact there is probably a continuum between these extremes and the descriptions are not very useful either prognostically or as an insight into the underlying pathophysiology (Menon *et al.*, 1984).

Specific causes of primary ovarian failure include chromosomal abnormalities — classically ovarian dysgenesis due to an XO genotype — external radiation (or cytotoxic chemotherapy) and autoimmune disorders of the ovary (Menon *et al.*, 1984; Hague *et al.*, 1987). In a recent study *c.* 50% of subjects with primary ovarian failure were found to have evidence of autoimmune endocrinopathy (Hague *et al.*, 1987) (principally with thyroid autoantibodies) and although much fewer had specific evidence of ovarian autoantibodies this is more likely to reflect the limitation of currently available techniques for their identification rather than the absence of such antibodies. It has been proposed that the resistant ovary is due to specific antibodies to gonadotrophin receptors but as yet the evidence for this is limited.

## Disorders of gonadotrophin regulation

### Specific disorders

#### Hyperprolactinaemia

This is the most common of the specific disorders of pituitary function in patients presenting with amenorrhoea (Franks *et al.*, 1975; Glass *et al.*, 1975; Pepperall, 1981; Franks & Jacobs, 1983). Many of these subjects have radiological evidence of a pituitary tumour but the prevalence of prolactinomas varies from 30 to 90% in different series depending partly on the sophistication of imaging techniques used for diagnosis of pituitary abnormalities (Lancet editorial, 1980; Burrow *et al.*, 1981; Jung *et al.*, 1982; von Werder *et al.*, 1985; Franks & Jacobs, 1983). The typical presentation is with oestrogen-deficient amenorrhoea with or without galactorrhoea (Jacobs, 1976; Hague *et al.*, 1987). The prevalence of galactorrhoea varies in different series from 30 to 90% (Franks & Jacobs, 1983) but the important clinical point is that whereas most patients with amenorrhoea and galactorrhoea are likely to have hyperprolactinaemia, the absence of galactorrhoea does not exclude the diagnosis; hence the importance of direct measurements of prolactin as indicated below.

There has always been some controversy regarding the mechanism of anovulation in women with hyperprolactinaemic amenorrhoea (Franks & Jacobs, 1983; Jacobs *et al.*, 1976; Thorner & Besser, 1977; Van Look *et al.*, 1977). *In vitro* studies in which it was demonstrated that addition of high concentrations of prolactin to human luteal cells inhibited progesterone synthesis (McNatty *et al.*, 1977) have been interpreted as evidence for a direct deleterious effect of hyperprolactin-aemia on the ovary (Thorner & Besser, 1977). However, the normal levels of gonadotrophins and the normal gonadotrophin response to gonadotrophin releasing-hormone (GnRH) in the face of low oestrogen concentrations strongly suggested a hypothalamic disorder of gonado-trophin secretion (Jacobs et al., 1976; Faglia et al., 1977). Bohnet and Schneider (1976) were the first to demonstrate abnormal pulsatile patterns of gonadotrophin secretion in hyperprolactinaemic amenor-rhoea. These results were confirmed by other authors (Leyendecker et al., 1980a; Moult et al., 1981), and in recent studies further evidence for a hypothalamic disorder has been provided by the demonstration that administration of pulsatile GnRH results in induction of ovulation (and indeed pregnancy) in the face of persistent hyperprolactinaemia (Leyendecker et al., 1980a; Bergh et al., 1984; Polson et al., 1986) (Fig. 8.1).

It is still not clear how excessive prolactin secretion affects hypo-thalamic release of GnRH. The mechanism is mediated by endogenous opiates (Quigley et al., 1980; Lamberts et al., 1981; Grossmann et al., 1982; Franks & Jacobs, 1983) but this gives little insight into how the abnormality is triggered. Data from animal models suggest that there is a secondary increase in dopamine turnover in the hypothalamus (Fuxe et al., 1981) which then inhibits GnRH production, but the validity of this model in the human must remain in doubt. What is clear is that lowering prolactin levels, either by use of dopamine agonists or by surgical removal of a prolactin-secreting tumour, restores normal

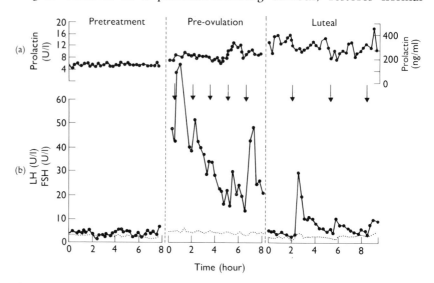

**Fig. 8.1.** Serum (a) prolactin, and (b) gonadotrophin (● LH, ---- FSH) concentrations measured at 15 min intervals for 8 h in a patient with hyperprolactinaemic amenorrhoea before and during treatment with pulsatile GnRH. The arrows indicate pulses of GnRH. Note the disordered pattern of pulsatile LH and FSH secretion before treatment and the response during the preovulatory and luteal phases of an ovulatory cycle. Ovulation occurred despite a further increase in serum prolactin.

gonadotrophin secretion and fertility (Thorner & Besser, 1977; Franks & Jacobs, 1983).

### Other pituitary endocrinopathies

Menstrual disorders are common in women of reproductive age who have acromegaly (Franks *et al.*, 1976; Nabarro, 1982). There are various possible causes of anovulation in this condition including concurrent hyperprolactinaemia (in *c.* 20% of such subjects) (Franks *et al.*, 1976), gonadotrophin deficiency (if the tumour is large) and associated poly-cystic ovaries.

Pituitary dependent Cushing's disease is also associated with an-ovulation; the mechanism may be linked to the development of poly-cystic ovaries possibly arising as a result of hypersecretion of adrenal androgens (Nabarro, 1982; Franks, 1989b).

### Non-functioning tumours of the hypothalamus and pituitary

Any destructive lesion of the hypothalamus or pituitary (e.g. cranio-pharyngioma or other 'non-functioning' tumours) can result in gon-adotrophin deficiency and therefore anovulation. It is worth nothing that such lesions may also cause hyperprolactinaemia by interfering with the secretion or transport of dopamine, the principle prolactin-inhibiting factor (Franks & Jacobs, 1983).

### Kallmann's syndrome and its variants

These are congenital disorders characterized by deficiency of GnRH which usually occurs in isolation but may sometimes be associated with deficiency of growth hormone releasing hormone (Franks, 1987). Classical Kallmanns's syndrome includes anosmia as well as other congenital abnormalities (Kallmann *et al.*, 1944; Rogol *et al.*, 1982), but the spectrum of presentation of isolated deficiency of GnRH is wide and the mildest forms of this disorder may present simply with primary amenorrhoea (or very occasionally secondary amenorrhoea) in a woman who has completed normal pubertal development.

### Functional disorders of gonadotrophin regulation

In these cases the disorder of gonadotrophin secretion resulting in anovulation occurs as a manifestation of an underlying disorder, the most common of which is reduced body weight. It was F.H. Marshall who first postulated the importance of the external environment, including nutrition, on the neural control of reproduction (1942). It was his work primarily which inspired Harris (1971) to explore the nature of the hypothalamic control of gonadotrophin secretion. The relevance of the work of Marshall, Harris and their more recent successors (Matsuo et al., 1971; Marshall, 1989) in understanding the mechanism and treatment of women with 'hypothalamic amenorrhoea' is now clear.

### Weight-loss-related amenorrhoea

Marked weight loss (<66% of ideal body weight or Body Mass Index <16 kg/m$^2$) is associated with profound gonadotrophin deficiency (Nillius & Wide, 1977) in which GnRH secretion as defined by analysis of leuteinizing hormone (LH) and FSH pulses is severely inhibited and displays a prepubertal pattern (Boyar et al., 1974a). Such patients have small ovaries with few antral follicles. In milder degrees of weight loss (or in partially recovered weight-related amenorrhoea) basal LH concentrations and the response to exogenous GnRH are still impaired compared with normal, but are significantly greater than in severely underweight women (Nillius & Wide, 1977). This is consistent with studies from Boyar and colleagues demonstrating that the pattern of gonadotrophin secretion in such subjects was analogous to that observed during mid-puberty (1974).

With the advent of high resolution ultrasound scanning of the ovaries it has recently been demonstrated that mild, or partially-recovered, weight loss is characterized by a 'multi-follicular' ovary (Adams et al., 1985; Treasure et al., 1985; Mason et al., 1988) in which there are several follicles (compare Figs 8.2 and 8.3) but without the increase in stroma which is typical of PCOS (see below and Fig. 8.9). It is striking that this pattern of ovarian follicles is also observed during normal puberty (Stanhope et al., 1985) and, as in puberty, it represents a normal ovary receiving an abnormal — or, in the case of puberty, an immature — gonadotrophic signal. The abnormal gonadotrophin pulse pattern is typically that of reduced LH pulse-frequency despite normal amplitude and normal mean LH concentrations (Fig. 8.4).

In some women (c. 20%) with multi-follicular ovaries, however, the LH-pulse pattern is normal during the 8-h sampling period and it is only when looking at the 24-h profile of gonadotrophin secretion that an abnormality can be detected. Figure 8.5 shows high amplitude LH pulses during sleep without the characteristic pattern of nocturnal slowing of LH which is observed in the early follicular phase of ovulatory cycles. This 'abnormality' is a pattern which is virtually identical to that which occurs normally in late puberty as described by Boyar et al. (1972); again emphasizing the parallel between multi-follicular ovaries and pubertal ovarian development (Mason et al., 1988).

Similar patterns of gonadotrophin secretion and ovarian follicles have been observed in the now commonly observed syndrome of exercise-related amenorrhoea suggesting that the mechanism of hypothalamic disorder shows some common features with that of weight-

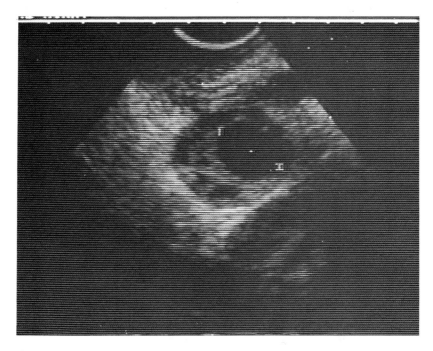

**Fig. 8.2.** Transvaginal ultrasonic image of a 'normal' ovary during the late follicular phase of the menstrual cycle. Note the single large preovulatory follicle, the major diameter of which is delineated by electronic calipers (centimetre scale). Photograph courtesy of Miss J.M. Adams.

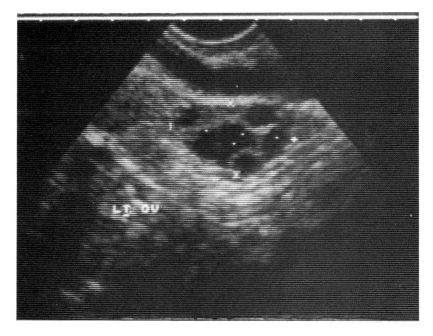

**Fig. 8.3.** Transvaginal ultrasonic image of a 'multicystic' ovary in a woman with weight-loss-related amenorrhoea. The two major diameters of the ovary are delineated by electronic calipers (centimetre scale). Note the presence of multiple follicles up to ~10 mm in diameter. Photograph courtesy of Miss J.M. Adams.

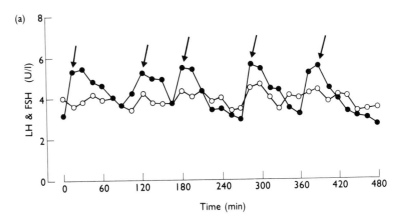

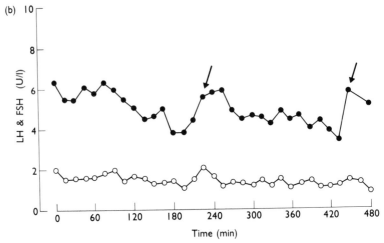

**Fig. 8.4.** Pulsatile gonadotrophin secretion (a) in a subject with normal ovaries in the mid-follicular phase, and (b) in an ovulatory woman with weight-loss-related amenorrhoea and multi-follicular ovaries (b). Note the reduced frequency of LH pulses in the woman with MFO. (●) LH, (○) FSH; arrow denotes the peak of a detectable pulse.

related amenorrhoea (Boyar *et al.*, 1974b). Interestingly, such women usually have a lower than normal proportion of body fat thus raising the possibility that the signal which determines the pattern of GnRH secretion may be related directly or indirectly to the function of adipose tissue (Boyar *et al.*, 1974b).

In weight- and exercise-related amenorrhoea, psychological factors may also be involved in the hypothalamic disorder but these are very difficult to distinguish from nutritional effects. It should be noted, however, that women who are underweight due to chronic illness (such as cystic fibrosis) have very similar patterns of gonadotrophin secretion and ovarian appearance to those in anorexia nervosa (Stead, 1987), suggesting that body weight (or body composition) is the more important factor in determining the hypothalamic abnormality.

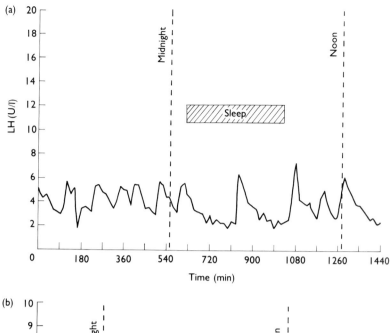

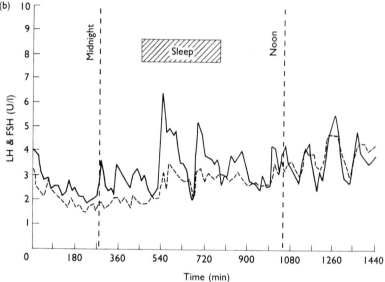

**Fig. 8.5.** Twenty-four hour pulse-pattern of LH (a) in a normal subject in the early follicular phase of the cycle, and (b) in a woman with weight-loss-related amenorrhoea and multifollicular ovaries following weight gain (b): (————) LH; (— — — —) FSH. The normal subject demonstrates sleep-related slowing of LH pulses whereas the pattern in the woman with MFO shows no nocturnal slowing and is reminiscent of that observed normally during late puberty (see text).

*Psychological causes*

The role of stress and other psychological disturbances in disorders of ovulation is far from clear. Many women report disorders of their menstrual cycle at 'stressful' times such as moving house or following divorce or bereavement. However, the endocrine features of such disorders have not been clearly defined. In more profound disturbances such as chronic depression, mania or schizophrenia the development of anovulation may, in part, be due to the use of psychotrophic drugs such as phenothiazines which can stimulate prolactin secretion (Franks & Jacobs, 1983).

*Idiopathic hypogonadotrophic hypogonadism*

This is an important, if somewhat heterogeneous, group of disorders of gonadotrophin secretion presenting with secondary amenorrhoea in which the underlying cause of the hypothalamic abnormality is unknown (Leyendecker *et al.*, 1980b; Coelingh-Benninck, 1983; Crowley *et al.*, 1985; Franks, 1987). Typically these women have marked abnormalities of gonadotrophin secretion characterized by reduced 8-h mean LH levels, low pulse-amplitude and diminished pulse-frequency (Crowley *et al.*, 1985; Adams, 1986). The ovaries are small and have few follicles (Adams, 1986).

## Polycystic ovary syndrome

Although PCOS is by far the most common cause of anovulation (Adams *et al.*, 1986; Hull, 1987) its pathogenesis remains unclear and little is known about the mechanism of anovulation (Table 8.4). It is a heterogeneous syndrome with more than one cause, but there is increasing evidence that the primary disorder has a familial basis, is ovarian in origin and may develop during, or even before, puberty (Leyendecker *et al.*, 1980b; Brook *et al.*, 1988; Hague *et al.*, 1988; Franks, 1989b). The syndrome is characterized by clinical and/or biochemical evidence of androgen excess which appears to be largely ovarian in origin (Kirschner *et al.*, 1976; Polson *et al.*, 1988a; Franks, 1989b). Another typical feature is elevated serum concentrations of LH (Nabarro, 1982; Franks, 1989b). Abnormalities of LH secretion appear to be due to abnormal feedback at hypothalamic or pituitary levels rather than because of a primary hypothalamic disorder (Franks, 1989b). Up to 20% of anovulatory women with PCOS have normal LH secretion and so although an elevated concentration of LH may contribute to the ovarian abnormality it is doubtful whether this is the primary mechanism of anovulation (Franks, 1989b).

**Table 8.4.** Anovulation in polycystic ovary syndrome

---

Possible mechanisms
  Inadequate circulating levels of FSH
  Decreased bioactivity of FSH
  Intrafollicular modulation of FSH action

---

Anovulation in PCOS is characterized by a failure of FSH-dependent follicle maturation (Franks *et al.*, 1988; Franks, 1989b). The normal intercycle rise in FSH is essential for follicle development (Hillier *et al.*, 1985) but serum FSH, at least as measured by radioimmunoassay, is normal in anovulatory women with PCOS and similar to levels in the early follicular phase of normal ovulatory cycles (Nabarro, 1982; Franks, 1989b). It is possible that the bioactivity of FSH is diminished in women with PCOS and with the recent development of sensitive bioassay methods for measurement of FSH in human serum it may soon be possible to address this issue. An alternative explanation to failure of follicle maturation despite normal immunoreactive levels of FSH is that its action may be modulated at the ovarian level by paracrine factors (Franks *et al.*, 1988) (Table 8.5). The role of such intra-ovarian paracrine factors in follicular development has been discussed in Chapter 3. It should be noted that in the context of anovulation, factors with negative regulatory effects would appear to be the most relevant.

Androgens enhance the action of FSH in stimulating oestradiol accumulation from rat granulosa cells (Hillier, 1981, 1985), but in the primate there is recent evidence that the oestrogen response of the granulosa cells to FSH is inhibited by androgen in large preovulatory follicles (Harlow *et al.*, 1988). Data from studies in clomiphene-induced cycles in women with PCOS provide some clinical evidence in support of the notion that intrafollicular androgen concentrations may be one important factor in determining the effect of FSH on follicular maturation in PCOS (Polson *et al.*, 1988b).

Polypeptide growth factors are also involved in modulation of the granulosa cells response to FSH. Both epidermal growth factor (EGF) (Hsueh *et al.*, 1981) and transforming growth factor α (TGFα) (Adashi & Resnick 1986) have potent inhibitory effects on granulosa cell oestrogen production (see Chapter 3) and recent data suggest that these effects may be important in the function of human follicles (Mason *et al.*, 1989).

It is likely that anovulation in PCOS is the result of a complex interaction between various factors including diminished biologically

**Table 8.5.** Paracrine modulators of FSH action

| | |
|---|---|
| Steroids | Oestrogens |
| | Androgens |
| Polypeptides | |
| Stimulatory | Insulin |
| | IGF I and II |
| | TGFβ |
| Inhibitory | TGFα |
| | EGF |
| | Inhibin? |

active FSH and intraovarian mechanisms (Fig. 8.6). Recent advances in our understanding of the ovarian paracrine system and its impact on folliculogenesis offer real hope of unravelling this complex problem.

## Diagnosis of anovulation

The basic approach to the differential diagnosis of anovulation is a simple one and depends on few biochemical tests. A careful history supplemented by information from examination will provide important guidelines to the diagnosis (Hull, 1981; Franks, 1987). The essential biochemical tests are measurements of serum FSH and prolactin and, in amenorrhoeic subjects, assessment of endogenous oestrogen production (Hull *et al.*, 1979b; Hull, 1981; Franks, 1987).

### Measurement of serum FSH

Measurement of FSH is a specific means of distinguishing between primary ovarian failure and other causes of anovulation. Serum LH levels will also of course be elevated in women with primary ovarian failure but may also be increased in patients with PCOS. The finding of a raised level of LH with normal serum FSH is suggestive of the diagnosis of PCOS but since 30–40% of women with anovulation due to polycystic ovaries may have normal (random) basal LH measurements (Franks, 1989b), direct measurement of LH is of limited use for diagnostic purposes. It is not, therefore, essential to perform LH measurements routinely.

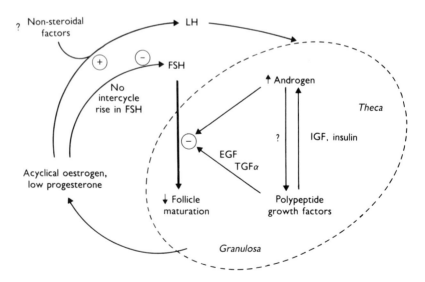

**Fig. 8.6.** Mechanism of anovulation in women with PCOS. It is suggested that the failure of FSH-dependent follicular maturation is the key abnormality. Hypersecretion of LH is a contributory but not an obligatory factor.

Measurement of FSH should not be confined to women with amenorrhoea since elevated FSH indicative of incipient ovarian failure may also be found in women with anovulatory menses.

## Prolactin

Measurement of serum prolactin will define hyperprolactinaemia. If this is confirmed further investigations are required, including measurement of thyroid function and radiology of the pituitary area (Franks & Jacobs, 1983).

## Assessment of oestrogen production

There is some debate as to the best method for assessment of endogenous oestrogen production. Measurement of serum oestradiol is of limited usefulness. Women with biological evidence of marked oestrogen deficiency (e.g. those with mild or partially recovered weight-loss-related amenorrhoea) may have serum oestradiol measurements which are within the normal range for the early to mid-follicular phase of ovulatory menstrual cycles (Treasure *et al.*, 1985). For this reason it is useful to perform an '*in vivo* bioassay' of oestrogen production by use of the progestagen withdrawal test (Hull *et al.*, 1979a,b; Hull, 1981). The conventional way to perform the test is to administer either natural progesterone (100 mg intramuscularly as a single injection) or, more conveniently, to give a synthetic, orally active, progestagen such as medroxyprogesterone acetate (5 mg daily for 5 days) (Hull *et al.*, 1979b). A positive test, that is menstrual bleeding following progesterone withdrawal, is good evidence of adequate follicular oestrogen production and furthermore (unlike serum oestradiol measurements) is a reliable index of a subsequent successful response to induction of ovulation with antioestrogens (Hull *et al.*, 1979a; Hull *et al.*, 1979b; Hull, 1981).

## Thyroid function tests

Measurement of serum thyroxine and thyroid-stimulating hormone (TSH) are often recommended in the diagnostic assessment of patients with anovulation (Hull, 1981). Unfortunately, it is very difficult to judge from the published literature whether thyroid disorders, either hypo- or hyperthyroidism, are an important cause of anovulation. Menstrual disorders have been reported in women with thyroid disease (Burrow, 1978; Franks, 1979) but there are no clear data regarding the prevalence of thyroid disorders amongst amenorrhoeic or oligomenorrhoeic patients. However, there is one condition in which measurement of thyroid function tests clearly has a place and that is in hyperprolactinaemia (Franks & Jacobs, 1983). Primary hypothyroidism can be associated with hyperprolactinaemic amenorrhoea, and it is important to identify this as a possible cause of hyperprolactinaemia because it has its own specific treatment, that is administration of thyroid hormone replacement which results in lower prolactin levels and resumption of ovulatory menstrual cycles (Semple *et al.*, 1983).

## Other diagnostic tests

### The GnRH test

Assessment of the LH and FSH response to a standard bolus (usually 100 μg) of natural-sequence GnRH has proved to be a useful research tool in understanding disorders of gonadotrophin regulation (Mortimer *et al.*, 1973; Nillius & Wide, 1977; Kandeel *et al.*, 1978). However, its use as a diagnostic test in individual subjects is limited by the fact that there is considerable overlap in gonadotrophin responsiveness to GnRH between groups of patients and, indeed, individual normal women (Franks, 1989a). This is illustrated by Fig. 8.7 which shows that although the mean LH response to 100 μg of GnRH is slightly lower in the group of subjects with a hypothalamic disorder of gonadotrophin regulation (all of whom presented with secondary amenorrhoea) the spectrum of responses is similar to that seen in normal subjects (Franks, 1989a).

### Analysis of pulsatile gonadotrophin secretion

This too is a useful means of delineating an underlying hypothalamic

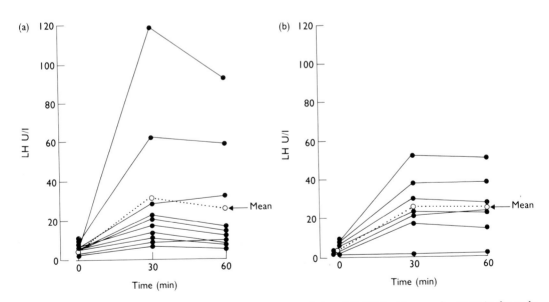

**Fig. 8.7.** The LH response to a 100 μg bolus of GnRH in (a) normal women in the early to mid-follicular phase, and (b) hypogonadotrophic hypo-oestrogenic subjects presenting with secondary amenorrhoea. Note the wide spectrum of responses in both groups with considerable overlap between them.

disturbance of gonadotrophin regulation (Crowley *et al.*, 1985) (Figs 8.1, 8.4, 8.5 and 8.8), but like the GnRH stimulation test it is of limited use in the management of anovulatory patients. In other words, if the preliminary assessment shows that serum levels of FSH are normal or low and there is evidence of oestrogen deficiency as determined by a negative response to progestagen withdrawal, no more information is required to make a diagnosis of deficiency of disordered regulation of gonadotrophins. If the serum prolactin measurement is added to the list of investigations, then patients with hyperprolactinaemia who require specific further investigation and treatment can be specifically identified within this group.

### Pelvic ultrasound

Modern imaging techniques, in particular high resolution ultrasound scanning of the pelvis, has provided a good deal of important information about normal follicular patterns and disorders of the ovary (Figs 8.2 and 8.3) and, particularly, in the identification of polycystic ovaries (Adams *et al.*, 1986; Franks, 1989b). The ovarian appearance in a subject with PCOS is shown in Fig. 8.9. In practice, however, an

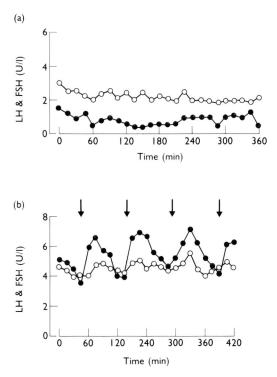

**Fig. 8.8.** Gonadotrophin concentrations (a) before, and (b) during treatment with pulsatile GnRH (arrows) in a hypogonadotrophic subject. (● LH, ○ FSH). Note very low pretreatment levels of LH with little evidence of pulsatile secretion and normalization of the gonadotrophin pattern during pulsatile GnRH therapy.

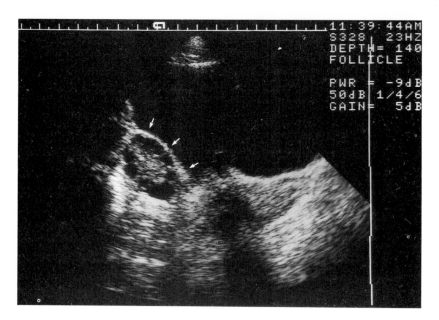

**Fig. 8.9** Transabdominal ultrasonic image of a 'polycystic' ovary (arrowed) in a patient with PCOS. Note the characteristically peripheral distribution of multiple immature follicles. Photograph courtesy of Miss D. Kiddy.

ultrasound scan of the ovaries is an essential diagnostic investigation in only a small proportion of patients with anovulation. Paradoxically, this situation arises because of the information provided by research into ovulatory disorders using pelvic ultrasound. Thus, it is clear that the majority of well-oestrogenized (progestagen-positive) subjects with normal levels of FSH have polycystic ovaries irrespective of the presence of hirsutism (Adams *et al.*, 1986; Hull, 1987; Franks, 1989b).

In hypogonadotrophic women the appearance of the ovaries provides useful but not essential information, but in women with primary ovarian failure it may be of prognostic importance to discover whether obvious antral follicles are present in the ovary.

Ultrasound is of considerable importance in assessing the response of the ovary during induction of ovulation, as discussed in more detail below.

## Treatment of anovulation — induction of ovulation

Perhaps the most important step in the management of anovulation is the selection of an appropriate form of treatment (Hull, 1981; Franks, 1987, 1988). This should be based on the results of investigations outlined in the previous section. The principle aims of treatment are either (1) to induce ovulation in infertile patients, or (2) to provide symptomatic treatment in women who do not wish to become pregnant. This includes correction of oestrogen-deficiency, management of menstrual disorders and treatment of associated problems such as hirsutism (Tan & Jacobs, 1985; Franks *et al.*, 1985a). This is, in itself, a large and important area of reproductive medicine but it is beyond the scope of this review to discuss this in detail. The emphasis will therefore be on induction of ovulation.

## Primary ovarian failure

There is no evidence that any form of treatment specifically influences the chance of ovulation in women with primary ovarian failure (Menon *et al.*, 1984). Attempts to induce 'rebound ovulation' after a period of gonadotrophin suppression by either contraceptive steroids (Starup *et al.*, 1978; Petsos, 1986) or GnRH-agonist analogues (Menon *et al.*, 1983) have enjoyed some popularity but without much scientific basis for their use. Certainly pregnancies have been reported in women treated in this way, but spontaneous ovulation and conception is known to occur without treatment in such cases (Shangold *et al.*, 1977; Wright & Jacobs, 1979; O'Herlihy *et al.*, 1980; Menon *et al.*, 1983, 1984) and there are no suitably designed controlled studies of the use of rebound ovulation or its variants in the literature. The successful use of donor eggs in the context of an *in vitro* fertilization (IVF) programme now offers some hope to childless couples with this problem (Lutjen *et al.*, 1984).

## Deficient or disordered regulation of gonadotrophins

### *With normal levels of oestrogen production*

The vast majority of women with normal FSH and normal oestrogen production have PCOS and management of this condition will be discussed specifically in the next section. This group also includes other causes of anovulation, for example women with anorexia who have recovered their weight but who have not yet started to menstruate regularly. The treatment of first choice is the antioestrogen, clomiphene.

### *With oestrogen deficiency*

These patients have a more profound disorder of gonadotrophin regulation or may have frankly lower levels of LH and FSH on random sampling. It is important to identify patients within this group with specific disorders such as hyperprolactinaemia.

### *Hyperprolactinaemic amenorrhoea*

Treatment is aimed at reducing circulating prolactin concentrations into the normal range. This leads to recovery of hypothalamic–

pituitary—gonadal function. The most convenient and effective means of treatment is medical therapy with long acting dopamine agonists (Thorner & Besser, 1977; Franks & Jacobs, 1983). Bromocriptine, a semisynthetic ergot derivative, will effectively and safely suppress prolactin secretion in the great majority of subjects irrespective of the height of the initial prolactin level (Thorner & Besser, 1977; Franks et al., 1977; Bergh et al., 1978). In other words, it will be effective in women with large prolactinomas as well as those with minimal elevation of prolactin and no obvious pituitary abnormality. The major debating point in recent years has been the advisability of the use of medical treatment to induce ovulation in patients with large prolactinomas who wish to become pregnant. This issue has been discussed widely in recent reviews (Franks & Jacobs, 1983; Nillius et al., 1985; Urdl et al., 1985; von Werder et al., 1985). Suffice it to say that the weight of evidence suggests that the risk of serious complications in pregnancy due to expansion of the pituitary (a phenomenon which also occurs in normal pregnancy) following primary treatment with bromocriptine has been shown to be small. This seems to be due partly to a direct effect of bromocriptine on the tumour, as it has been widely demonstrated that bromocriptine treatment results in shrinkage of the pituitary in c. 70% of cases (von Werder et al., 1985).

Pituitary surgery (usually by the trans-sphenoidal approach) is also effective treatment when necessary. However, it is best reserved for patients in whom dopamine agonists are poorly tolerated or ineffective: either in reducing prolactin levels to normal or in reducing the size of a large prolactinoma prior to attempting pregnancy (Franks & Jacobs, 1983; Nillius et al., 1985; von Werder et al., 1985b). Since the development of bromocriptine, a number of other long-acting dopamine agonists have become available, few of which have stood the test of time. However, recent trials of a non-ergot dopamine agonist (Rasmussen et al., 1988) with potentially fewer side-effects than bromocriptine offers some prospect of a wider choice of medication in the future.

### Weight-loss-related amenorrhoea

The treatment of choice is, of course, weight gain. This is specific and effective treatment although it may be rather a protracted process (Hull, 1981). It may be tempting to induce ovulation with exogenous gonadotrophins or pulsatile GnRH since these are rapidly effective (Adams et al., 1985; Homburg et al., 1989). However, there are at least two good reasons why this temptation should be resisted. The first is that women with a history of an eating disorder and who are still underweight may still require the support of psychotherapy to recover. Secondly, a woman who is underweight when she conceives runs a significantly higher risk of having an underweight baby than does a woman of normal weight (van der Spuy et al., 1988). However, there are some women who have returned to their pre-morbid weight but who have not regained ovulatory ovarian function and it is this group which merits consideration for induction of ovulation (Homburg *et al.*, 1989) (see below).

*Other disorders of gonadotrophin regulation including Kallman's syndrome and idiopathic hypogonadotrophic hypogonadism (IHH)*

These are ideally treated by pulsatile GnRH or human menopausal gonadotrophins (hMG).

*Pulsatile GnRH therapy.* The clinical application of the use of GnRH and its agonists has been one of the most exciting developments in reproductive endocrinology in the last decade. Early attempts to induce ovulation with GnRH using daily injections of the native decapeptide were frustrated by variable follicular responses and a poor rate of ovulation (Zarate *et al.*, 1976; Casas *et al.*, 1977). Following demonstration of the importance of pulsatile secretion of GnRH in obtaining a physiological pituitary response (Marshall, 1989), a number of groups were able successfully to induce ovulation using pulsed GnRH.

The early studies came from Leyendecker, Wildt and Hausmann (1980) who reported the use of intravenous treatment with GnRH delivered by an automatic pulsatile infusion pump. The efficacy of treatment was quickly confirmed by other groups (Skarin *et al.*, 1983; Mason *et al.*, 1984; Crowley *et al.*, 1985) and it has subsequently been demonstrated that in most cases subcutaneous delivery of GnRH pulses can be as effective as intravenous treatment (Mason *et al.*, 1984; Homburg *et al.*, 1989). The response of gonadotrophins to subcutaneous GnRH in a hypogonadotrophic patient is illustrated in Fig. 8.8.

Homburg *et al.* (1989) have recently reported a large series of women treated with pulsed GnRH, most of whom received subcutaneous therapy (Table 8.6). The ovulation and conception rates indicate that pulsatile GnRH therapy can be expected to restore normal fertility in women with hypothalamic amenorrhoea. Surprisingly, perhaps, it may also be effective in a substantial proportion of women with organic pituitary disease in whom primary gonadotrophic deficiency seems likely (Morris *et al.*, 1987; Homburg *et al.*, 1989). Clearly in many of these cases there is sufficient pituitary reserve to ensure a response to exogenous GnRH pulses.

Women with PCOS may also respond to treatment with pulsed GnRH (Burger *et al.*, 1980; Adams *et al.*, 1985; Bringer *et al.*, 1989; Homburg *et al.*, 1989) However LH concentrations, already high, are pushed even higher by exogenous GnRH and this may contribute to the poor rate of ovulation and conception observed in these women compared with hypogonadotrophic subjects and may also be associated with a very high rate of early pregnancy loss (Homburg *et al.*, 1989).

**Table 8.6.** Results of treatment with pulsatile GnRH

| | Disorders of gonadotrophin regulation | | Primary pituitary disease |
| | IHH | Weight-loss related | |
| --- | --- | --- | --- |
| Cases | 48 | 23 | 18 |
| Cycles | 129 | 60 | 52 |
| Ovulation | 112 | 55 | 38 |
| Conception | 38 | 21 | 11 |
| Miscarriages (EPL) | 6 (4) | 5 (0) | 5 (3) |
| CCR | 93% | 95% | 100% |

Data from Homburg *et al.*, 1989. IHH = idiopathic hypogonadotrophic hypogonadism. EPL = early pregnancy loss (≤6 weeks after ovulation). CCR = cumulative conception rate.

Because it allows the ovarian pituitary feedback mechanism to function normally, pulsatile GnRH therapy may be regarded as more 'physiological' than the use of exogenous gonadotrophins. However pulsed GnRH therapy may result in an increase in the rate of multiple pregnancy compared with pregnancy after spontaneous ovulation. Multiple pregnancies occur less commonly than after hMG treatment, but are still a feature of GnRH therapy (Coelingh-Bennink, 1983; Homburg *et al.*, 1989). Multiple pregnancies appear to occur predominantly as a result of conception in the first cycle of GnRH treatment. This is because multiple follicle development is more common than in subsequent cycles (Coelingh-Bennink, 1983). The explanation for this is not clear but may relate to the fact that the pituitary has not been recently exposed to the normal feedback effects of gonadal steroids. This in turn may affect the magnitude of the gonadotrophin response, or perhaps the bioactivity of the gonadotrophins released. From a practical viewpoint, the problem of multiple pregnancies can largely be overcome by careful ultrasound monitoring, particularly during the first cycle of treatment. Appropriate advice can then be offered to the couple if multiple follicles develop.

As elegantly demonstrated by Knobil *et al.* (1980) and Zeleznick and colleagues (Lunenfeld *et al.*, 1982; Hutchinson & Zeleznick, 1985) (see Chapter 6) pulsatile GnRH treatment can be used as a tool to investigate neuroendocrine control of the menstrual cycle and occasionally it is possible to perform such studies in women who do not wish to become pregnant. Various aspects of the gonadotrophic control of the ovarian cycle can be examined: from follicular growth in the early follicular phase, through ovulation to luteal function. As demonstrated in subjects with multi-follicular ovaries, reduced LH and FSH pulse-frequency is associated with disordered follicular growth (Mason *et al.*,

1988) and this situation can be reproduced experimentally by varying the interval between bolus injections of GnRH (Filicori *et al.*, 1988).

In the mid-luteal phase gonadotrophin concentrations are low, but appear to be necessary for support of the corpus luteum since inter-ruption of GnRH secretion in the luteal phase leads to a fall of pro-gesterone secretion and the onset of menses (Hutchinson & Zeleznik, 1984; Franks *et al.*, 1985b). It is however possible to 'rescue' the corpus luteum as originally demonstrated by Zeleznik and colleagues in the rhesus monkey (Hutchinson & Zeleznik, 1985) (see Chapter 6). In women, if the GnRH pump is restarted after 48 h, progesterone secre-tion resumes normally, showing that although progesterone synthesis ceases the corpus luteum remains functionally viable (Polson *et al.*, 1987b) (Fig. 8.10).

*hMG.* Exogenous gonadotrophins, usually of urinary origin, have been used for more than 30 years for induction of ovulation in hypogonado-trophic patients and with considerable success (Hull, 1981; Lunenfeld *et al.*, 1982) (Table 8.7). This form of treatment remains perfectly acceptable today, but the major disadvantage compared with GnRH is that the risk of multiple pregnancy is significantly higher. This problem can be resolved to a considerable degree by starting with a low dose of gonadotrophin and increasing the dose in a step-wise fashion ac-cording to the ovarian response (Brown, 1978; Hillier, 1981; Polson *et al.*, 1987a). We have applied this technique to the treatment of clomiphene-resistant patients with PCOS in whom multiple follicular growth is a particular problem (see below).

An intriguing development reported by Homburg and colleagues (Homburg *et al.*, 1988) is the use of short term low-dose growth hor-mone (GH) to improve ovarian responsiveness in hypogonadotrophic patients who prove resistant to hMG therapy. The addition of GH dramatically decreases the amount of gonadotrophin required to induce

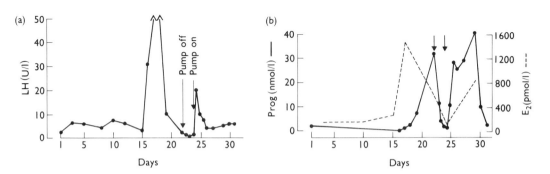

**Fig. 8.10.** LH, oestradiol and progesterone concentrations during a GnRH-induced ovulatory cycle in which the pulsatile infusion pump was stopped for 48 h from Day 22 of the cycle. Note the marked fall in progesterone but recovery of the normal luteal-phase pattern of secretion following reinstitution of GnRH therapy.

**Table 8.7.** Results of induction of ovulation with hMG in 279 women with amenorrhoea due to hypothalamic pituitary failure. (Data from Lunenfeld *et al.*, 1982)

| | Patient | Cycles | Pregnancies | Pregnancy (%) | Rate* (%) |
|---|---|---|---|---|---|
| Primary amenorrhoea | 91 | 354 | 77 | 84.6 | 81.23 |
| Primary amenorrhoea + galactorrhoea | 12 | 24 | 10 | 83.3 | 79.17 |
| Secondary amenorrhoea, oestrogen low | 106 | 293 | 67 | 63.2 | 87.6 |
| Secondary amenorrhoea, oestrogen low + galactorrhoea | 70 | 195 | 75 | – | 95.9 |

* Rate calculated by life-table analysis.

ovulation. The mechanism of action is not entirely clear but successful treatment is associated with a rise in circulating insulin-like growth factor I (IGF-I) concentrations, suggesting that hepatic response to growth hormone is the crucial factor.

## Polycystic ovary syndrome

As described above, this is the most common cause of anovulation and although the majority of ovulatory patients will respond to antioestrogen therapy, management of the 25% or so subjects who are clomiphene-resistant is one of the most challenging problems in infertility practice.

### Clomiphene citrate

This is the treatment of first choice in managing patients with PCOS or other subjects with a mild disorder of gonadotrophin regulation and/or action. In other words these are women who have no evidence of oestrogen deficiency associated with a hypothalamic disorder. The exact mechanism of action of clomiphene remains unclear (Adashi, 1984), but during treatment there is an increase in both LH and FSH concentrations in plasma within 2–5 days (Fig. 8.11). This may be regarded as mimicking the normal intercycle rise of FSH and results in further development of antral follicles from which the dominant follicle emerges and usually ovulates. This action of clomiphene is probably mediated by removal of the negative feedback effect of endogenous oestrogen but there is some evidence that clomiphene may have a direct stimulatory effect on pituitary gonadotrophin secretion (Adashi, 1984).

Interestingly, the prognosis for normal fertility following clomiphene appears to be better in women presenting with amenorrhoea than in those with anovulatory cycles (Hull, 1981, 1987). The reasons for this are far from clear. Some 60–90% of women with PCOS might be expected to ovulate after clomiphene, but the overall pregnancy rate is

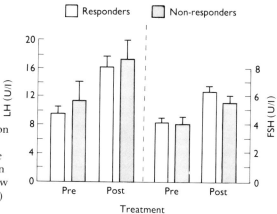

**Fig. 8.11.** Peak LH and FSH responses (occurring on Days 4–7) to treatment with clomiphene citrate (100 mg daily on Days 2–6 of the cycle). Note the similar magnitude of both LH and FSH responses in non-responders (i.e. those women who did not grow large follicles following treatment with clomiphene) and responders.

only 25–43% (MacGregor *et al.*, 1968; Thompson & Harson, 1970; Rust *et al.*, 1974; Genzell, 1977; Gorlitsky *et al.*, 1978; Tsapoulis *et al.*, 1978; Gysler *et al.*, 1982; Hammond, 1984; Table 8.8). These figures may be slightly misleading since a minority of the reports cited in the table included systematic measurement of progesterone concentrations; certainly none of the early studies had the benefit of ultrasound to assess the follicular response and to detect ovulation.

With the aid of ultrasound monitoring it is possible to assess carefully the ovarian response to treatment and a recent study has examined differences in hormone levels and ovarian ultrasound data between women with PCOS who ovulated after clomiphene and those who did not (Polson *et al.*, 1989a). Of the 40 cycles (in 27 women), 29 (73%) were ovulatory. Three of the 11 anovulatory cycles were characterized by development of a dominant follicle but without ovulation. All three of these cycles occurred in the same subject. In the remaining eight cycles, there was no evidence of follicular maturation (i.e. no follicles more than 10 mm) despite increases in FSH on days 3–5 after clomiphene which were similar to those occurring in the ovulators (Fig. 8.11). The failure of follicular growth does not therefore seem to depend on lack of an increase in FSH, at least as measured by radio-immunoassay. This phenomenon lends support to the hypothesis that

**Table 8.8.** Ovulation and conception rates following induction of ovulation with clomiphene citrate

| Reference | *n* | Ovulation | Pregnancies (%) |
|---|---|---|---|
| Kase *et al.* (1967) | 81 | 60 | 25 |
| MacGregor *et al.* (1968) | 4098 | 70 | 34 |
| Rust *et al.* (1974) | 105 | 91 | 38 |
| Gorlitsky *et al.* (1978) | 122 | 57 | 37 |
| Gysler *et al.* (1982) | 428 | 85 | 43 |
| Hammond *et al.* (1984) | 159 | 86 | 42 |

anovulation in women with PCOS may be related to either decreased bioactivity of FSH or interference with its action at ovarian level (Franks *et al.*, 1988).

From a practical point of view these results suggest that routine addition of hCG to treatment with clomiphene in patients who do not ovulate is not likely to be helpful and this process should be discouraged unless ultrasound monitoring demonstrates that a preovulatory follicle has developed.

Another important point is that women with PCOS who did not respond to clomiphene were significantly fatter than clomiphene-responders (Franks, 1989b; Polson *et al.*, 1989a). This emphasizes the importance of weight reduction in the management of anovulation in overweight subjects with PCOS.

### Low-dose gonadotrophin therapy for the treatment of PCOS

The choice of treatment for clomiphene-resistant women with PCOS remains a difficult one. There is an extensive literature on the use of gonadotrophin treatment (Buttram & Vaquero, 1975; Oeisner *et al.*, 1978; Gemzell & Wang, 1980; Adashi *et al.*, 1981; Lunde, 1982; Table 8.9), most of it relating to 'conventional' doses of hMG, that is starting at two ampoules/day and increasing rapidly until an ovarian response is obtained. The pregnancy rate varies from series to series but overall it is in the region of 30–40% (Table 8.9). However, conventional hMG treatment is associated with a high rate of multiple follicular growth, multiple pregnancy and miscarriage.

Recent availability of 'pure FSH' of urinary origin has encouraged trials of this gonadotrophin in women with PCOS (Yen, 1980; Kamrava *et al.*, 1982; Garcea *et al.*, 1985; Polson *et al.*, 1987a; Polson *et al.*, 1989b). Although this is effective in producing an ovarian response the problems of multiple follicular development remain. Initial studies using low doses of gonadotrophin, either hMG or FSH, have yielded more encouraging results with regard to a lower rate of multiple pregnancy.

We therefore embarked upon a study to investigate the effect of low-dose FSH using a regimen based on that suggested by Brown (1978), that is starting with a very low dose and gradually increasing the dose until the 'threshold' (Brown, 1978; Hillier, 1981) for the ovarian response was found. In initial studies, FSH was given by intermittent subcutaneous (i.e. pulsatile) injection in order to mimic endogenous FSH secretion (Polson *et al.*, 1987a). The results of the first 33 cycles of treatment in 10 women with clomiphene-resistant PCOS are summarized in Table 8.10. These results led us to further studies in which it was demonstrated that daily intramuscular administration of low-dose FSH was as effective as pulsatile subcutaneous treatment (Polson *et al.*, 1989b). More recently in a prospective comparative study it was shown that low-dose FSH had no particular advantage

**Table 8.9.** Summary of clinical results with hMG/hCG treatment in women with PCOS

| Reference | No. of patients | No. of treatment cycles | Ovulation rate (% patients) | Pregnancy rate (% patients) | Abortion rate | Multiple pregnancy rate | Complication rate (% cycles) |
|---|---|---|---|---|---|---|---|
| Thompson & Hansen (1970) | 212 | 546 | 162 (76%) | 50 (26%) | 21 (39%) | 8 (24.2%) | 6 (1.1%) |
| Gemzell* (1977) | 103 | 417 | | 47 (45.6%) | 27 (26.2%) | 14 (13.6%) | |
| Tsapoulis et al. (1978) | 40 | | 35 (87.5%) | | | | Mild 4.03% Severe 0.16% |
| Oeisner et al.** (1978) | 318 | | 68 (21.4%) | | | | |
| Gemzell & Wang (1980) | 41 | 77 | 39 (95.1%) | 27 (65.9%) | 7 (24.1%) | 8 (36.3%) | Mild 9.1% Severe 2.6% |

* Multiple pregnancy rate is calculated as the number of multiple pregnancies in relation to the total number of pregnancies less abortions.
** Includes all patients with endogenous oestrogen activity and anovulation.

**Table 8.10.** Outcome of 33 completed treatment cycles in women given low-dose pulsed FSH (Polson *et al.*, 1987a)

| | |
|---|---|
| Ovulatory cycles | 23 |
|    Single dominant follicles | 18 |
|    Two or three follicles | 5 |
| Anovulatory cycles | 10 |
|    No follicular growth | 4 |
|    Solitary cyst | 3 |
|    Four or more follicles | 3 |

All follicles referred to were ≥16 mm in diameter.

over hMG given at the same doses with respect to rates of ovulation, multiple follicular development (low for both treatments) and conception (Sagle *et al.*, 1989). The overall cumulative conception rate was 48% at 4 months of treatment (55% when corrected for ovulatory cycles) (Fig. 8.12).

A characteristic feature of low-dose gonadotrophin treatment is the high proportion of uni-ovulatory cycles (Polson *et al.*, 1987a; Polson *et al.*, 1989b). During these cycles the pattern of follicular growth on ultrasound, oestradiol production and luteal-phase progesterone secretion were very similar to those in spontaneous ovulatory cycles (Fig. 8.13). Interestingly there was a tendency for endogenous LH levels to fall from the high pretreatment levels to within the normal range in the late follicular phase (Fig. 8.14). This phenomenon was observed even when treatment with hMG was given (Sagle *et al.*, 1989). Furthermore, the incidence of a premature rise in LH (i.e. occurring

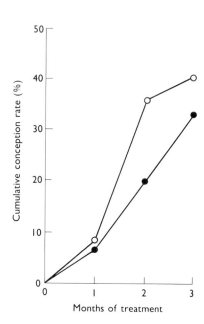

**Fig. 8.12.** Cumulative conception rate during treatment with hMG. (●) All patients; (○) excluding anovulatory cycles.

when the lead follicle was less than 16 mm in diameter) was very low (Polson *et al.*, 1987a; Sagle *et al.*, 1989), in contrast to the 25% incidence of premature luteinization observed during conventional hMG treatment (Fleming *et al.*, 1985).

### Use of GnRH-agonist analogues in treatment of PCOS

The rather low rate of pregnancy and the high incidence of premature luteinization following conventional hMG therapy prompted Fleming and colleagues to adopt a novel approach to induction of ovulation in women with PCOS (1985). They argued that if women with PCOS could be rendered 'hypogonadotrophic' then the chances of a good response of the ovary without risk of premature luteinization were much higher than with hMG alone. They therefore subjected patients to treatment with the long-acting GnRH analogue Buserelin which effectively led to pituitary–ovarian suppression. This was followed by administration of hMG. Their results have been most encouraging with

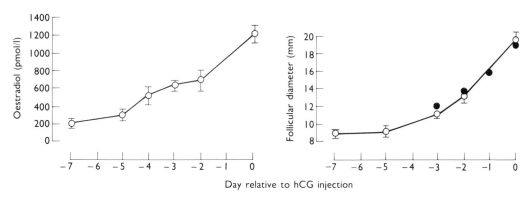

**Fig. 8.13.** Serum oestradiol concentrations (mean ±SEM) and diameter of the largest follicle measured by ultrasound in the follicular phase of ovulatory cycles, induced by low-dose FSH, in which a single dominant follicle developed. Mean follicular diameters in spontaneous cycles (in relation to the day of the LH surge) are indicated by the solid circles.

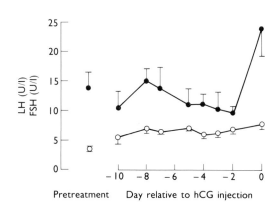

**Fig. 8.14.** Mean (±SEM) LH (●) and FSH (○) concentrations before treatment and during the follicular phase of ovulatory cycles induced by low-dose FSH.

reported pregnancy rates of c. 60% (Fleming et al., 1985; Coutts, 1989). Other groups have also had success with this approach although the results have not been quite as good as those of Fleming and colleagues (Fleming et al., 1985; Dodson et al., 1987; Coutts, 1989). It should, however, be noted that as yet there has been no randomized prospective study comparing hMG alone with the combined treatment.

Another obvious application of this combination of GnRH analogue and hMG is in the management of women with PCOS who are considered for IVF treatment (see Chapter 10).

### Ovarian wedge resection and its variants

Wedge resection of the ovaries has been used for many years as a way of inducing ovulation in women with PCOS. The reported ovulation rate is 30–90% but many of the studies are difficult to assess because the criteria for selection of patients are not always clear. To the author's knowledge, there has been no study comparing the effects of wedge resection with gonadotrophin therapy. Since wedge resection involves major surgery and the risk of adhesion formation is high, it would seem sensible to confine this treatment to that small subgroup of women with PCOS which fails to ovulate with gonadotrophin therapy.

A number of more recent and less traumatic modifications of wedge resections have been reported, again with encouragingly high rates of ovulation; (Table 8.11). Briefly these techniques range from laparoscopic biopsy to placing lesions in the surface of the ovary by electrocautery or laser under laparoscopic guidance. It is too early to assess the long-term results of such therapy but they carry the obvious advantage of less radical surgery than that associated with classic wedge resection.

## Conclusion

Differential diagnosis of disorders of ovulation is, in most cases, a single procedure which involves the minimum of biochemical tests. The basic investigation which includes measurement of serum FSH and prolactin

**Table 8.11.** Results of recent studies of effects of ovarian wedge resection on pregnancy rate. (Data from Cohen & Audebert, 1989)

| Reference | Year | No. of cases | Regular cycles (%) | Pregnancies (%) |
|---|---|---|---|---|
| Buttram | 1975 | 173 | 93.7 | 42.6 |
| Adashi et al. | 1981 | 90 | 91 | 47 |
| Lunde | 1982 | 92 | — | 40 |
| Tanaka | 1988 | 46 | 100* | 65.2 |

* Including patients treated subsequently with clomiphene or hMG.

and assessment of oestrogen production is, nevertheless, crucial to selecting the appropriate form of therapy for induction of ovulation. Well-oestrogenized anovulatory subjects (most of whom have PCOS) usually respond well to antioestrogens but treatment of clomiphene-resistant patients remains a challenging problem. In patients with hypothalamic disorders of gonadotrophin regulation, specific treatment of the underlying disorder should be instituted where possible, for example in women with weight-loss-related amenorrhoea or with hyperprolactinaemia. The remaining hypogonadotrophic patients with low oestrogen production can be effectively treated by pulsatile GnRH or exogenous gonadotrophins. Pelvic ultrasound scanning has proved to be an important development both in diagnosis of ovulatory disorders and, most importantly, in assessing their response to treatment.

# References

Adams, J. (1986) The use of ovarian ultrasound in the selection and monitoring of patients with hypothalamic amenorrhoea. In Bloom, S.R. & Jacobs, H.S. (eds) *Therapeutic Applications of LHRH*, pp. 77−87. Royal Society of Medicine Services, London.

Adams, J., Franks, S., Polson, D.W. *et al.* (1985) Multifollicular ovaries: clinical and endocrine features and response to pulsatile gonadotrophin releasing hormone. *Lancet*, **ii**, 1375−8.

Adams, J., Polson, D.W. & Franks S. (1986) Prevalence of polycystic ovaries in women with anovulation and idiopathic hirsutism. *Br. Med. J.*, **293**, 355−9.

Adashi, E.Y. (1984) Clomiphene citrate: mechanism(s) and site(s) of action − a hypothesis revisited. *Fertil. Steril.*, **42**, 331−4.

Adashi, E.Y. & Resnick, C.E. (1986) Antagonistic interactions of transforming growth factors in the regulation of granulosa cell differentiation. *Endocrinology*, **119**, 1879−81.

Adashi, E.Y., Rock, J.A., Guzick, D. *et al.* (1981) Fertility following bi-lateral ovarian wedge resection: a critical analysis of 90 consecutive cases of the polycystic ovary syndrome. *Fertil. Steril.*, **36**, 320−5.

Bergh, T., Nillius, S.J. & Wide, L. (1978) Clinical course and outcome of pregnancies in amenorrhoeic women with hyperprolactinaemia and pituitary tumours. *Br. Med. J.*, **2**, 875−80.

Bergh, T., Skarin, G., Nillius, S.J. *et al.* (1984) Pulsatile LRH administration to women with bromo-criptine-resistant hyperprolactinaemia. In Lamberts, S.W., Tilders, F.H.J., van der Veen, E.A. & Assies, J. (eds) *Trends in Diagnosis and Treatment of Pituitary Adenomas*, pp. 195−8. Free University Press, Amsterdam.

Board, J.A., Redwine, F.O., Moncure, C.W. *et al.* (1979) Identification of differing etiologies of clinically diagnosed premature menopause. *Am. J. Obstet. Gynecol.*, **134**, 936−44.

Bohnet, H.G., Dahlen, H.G., Wuttke, W. *et al.* (1976) Hyperprolactinaemic anovulatory syndrome. *J. Clin. Endocrinol. Metab.*, **42**, 132−43.

Boyar, R.M., Finkelstein, J., Roffwarg, H.P. *et al.* (1972) Synchronization of augmented luteinizing hormone secretion with sleep during puberty. *N. Engl. J. Med.*, **287**, 582−6.

Boyar, R.M., Katz, J., Finkelstein, J. *et al.* (1974) Immaturity of the 24-hour luteinizing hormone secretory pattern in anorexia nervosa. *N. Engl. J. Med.*, **291**, 861−5.

Bringer, J., Boulet, F. & Clouet, S. (1989) Induction de l'ovulation par l'administration de LHRH dans les infertilites avec ovaires polykystiques. In Audebert, A. (ed) *Dystrophies ovariennes*, pp. 157−166. Masson, Paris.

Brook, C.G.D., Jacobs, H.S. & Stanhope, R. (1988) Polycystic ovaries in childhood. (Editorial) *Br. Med. J.*, **296**, 878.

Brown, J.B. (1978) Pituitary control of ovarian function − concepts derived from gonadotrophin therapy. *Aust. NZ. J. Obstet. Gynaecol.*, **18**, 47−54.

Burger, C.W., Korsen, T.J.M., Hampes, P.G.A. *et al.* (1980) Ovulation induction with pulsatile luteinizing hormone-releasing hormone (LRH) in women with clomiphene resistant polycystic ovary-like disease: Clinical results. *Fertil. Steril.*, **46**, 1045−54.

Burrow, G.N. (1978) The thyroid gland and reproduction. In Yen, S.S.C. & Jaffe, R.B. (eds) *Reproductive Endocrinology*, pp. 373−87. W.B. Saunders, Philadelphia.

Burrow, G.N., Wortzman, G., Rewcastle, N.B. *et al.* (1981) Microadenomas of the pituitary and abnormal sellar tomograms in an unselected autopsy series. *N. Engl. J. Med.*, **304**, 156−8.

Buttram, V.C. Jr. & Vaquero, C. (1975) Post ovarian wedge resection adhesive disease. *Fertil. Steril.*, **26**, 874−9.

Casas, P.R.F., Miechi, H., Badano, A. *et al.* (1977)

Clinical and gonadotrophic response of amenorrheic patients treated with clomiphene and repeated injections of luteinizing hormone-releasing hormone. *Fertil. Steril.*, **28**, 293−4.

Coelingh-Bennink, H.J.T. (1983) Induction of ovulation by pulsatile intravenous administration of LHRH in polycystic ovarian disease. *Endocrinology, Suppl.* **112**, abstract 81.

Coutts, J.R.T. (1989) The use of LHRH analogues in ovulation induction and induction of multiple follicular growth for in vitro fertilisation. In Shaw R.W. & Marshall J.G. (eds) *LHRH and its Analogues*, pp. 198−213. Wright, London.

Crowley, W.F. Jr., Filicori, M., Spratt, D. *et al.* (1985) The physiology of gonadotrophin releasing hormone (GnRH) secretion in men and women. *Recent Prog. Horm. Res.*, **41**, 473−531.

Dodson, W.C., Hughes, C.L., Whitesides, D.B. *et al.* (1987) The effect of leuprolide acetate on ovulation induction with human menopausal gonadotrophins in polycystic ovary syndrome. *J. Clin. Endocrinol. Metab.*, **65**, 95−100.

Faglia, G., Beck-Peccoz, P., Travaglini, P. *et al.* (1977) Functional studies in hyperprolactinaemic states. In Crosignani, P.G. & Robyn, C. (eds) *Prolactin and Human Reproduction*, pp. 225−38. Academic Press, London.

Filicori, M., Ferrari, P. & Michelacci, L. (1988) The physiologic role of gonadotrophin-releasing hormone (GnRH) pulse frequency in the human menstrual cycle. *Endocrinology, Suppl.* **122** (Abstract 878).

Flemming, R., Haxton, M.J., Hamilton, M.P.R. *et al.* (1985) Successful treatment of infertile women with oligomenorrhoea using a combination of an LHRH agonist and exogenous gonadotrophins. *Br. J. Obstet. Gynaecol.*, **92**, 369−79.

Franks, S. (1979) Prolactin. In Gray, C.H. & James V.H.T. (eds) *Hormones in Blood*, pp. 279−331. Academic Press, London.

Franks, S. (1987) Primary and secondary amenorrhoea. *Br. Med. J.*, **294**, 815−19.

Franks, S. (1988) Treatment of anovulatory infertility. In Sheppard, M.C. (ed) *Advanced Medicine vol. 24*, pp. 22−30. Bailliére Tindall, London.

Franks, S. (1989a) Diagnostic uses of LHRH. In Shaw, R.W. & Marshall, J.C. (eds) *LHRH and its Analogues*, pp. 80−91. Wright, London.

Franks, S. (1989b) Polycystic ovary syndrome: a changing perspective. *Clin. Endocrinol. (Oxf.)* **31**, 87−120.

Franks, S., Adams, J., Mason, H.D. *et al.* (1985a) Ovulatory disorders in women with polycystic ovary syndrome. *Clin. Obstet. Gynaecol.*, **12**, 605−32.

Franks, S. & Jacobs, H.S. (1983) Hyperprolactinaemia. *Clin. Endocrinol. Metab.*, **12**, 641−68.

Franks, S., Jacobs, H.S., Hull, M.G.R. *et al.* (1977) Management of hyperprolactinaemic amenorrhoea. *Br. J. Obstet. Gynaecol.*, **84**, 241−53.

Franks, S., Jacobs, H.S. & Nabarro, J.D.N. (1976) Prolactin concentrations in patients with acromegaly: clinical significance and response to surgery. *Clin. Endocrinol. (Oxf.)*, **5**, 63−9.

Franks, S., Murray, M.A.F., Jequier, A.M. *et al.* (1975) Incidence and significance of hyperprolactinaemia in women with amenorrhoea. *Clin. Endocrinol. (Oxf.)*, **4**, 597−607.

Franks, S., Polson, D.W. & Reed, M.J. (1988) Physiopathology and diagnosis of polycystic ovary syndrome: the significance of 11β-hydroxy-androstenedione. In Genazzani, A.R., Petraglia, F., Volpe, A. & Facchinetti, F. (eds) *Advances in Gynaecological Endocrinology*, Vol 1 Parthenon, Carnforth, Lancs pp. 289.

Franks, S., van der Spuy, Z., Mason, W.P. *et al.* (1985b) Luteal function after ovulation induction by pulsatile luteinizing hormone releasing hormone. In Jeffcoate, S.L. (ed.) *The Luteal Phase*, pp. 89−100. John Wiley, London.

Fuxe, K., Anderson, L.F., Agnati, V. *et al.* (1981) Prolactin-lowering drugs. In Crosignani, P.G. & Rubin, B.L. (eds) *Endocrinology of Human Infertility: New Aspects*, pp. 93−128. Academic Press, London.

Garcea N., Campo S., Paretta, V. *et al.* (1985) Induction of ovulation with purified urinary follicle-stimulating hormone in patients with polycystic ovarian syndrome. *Am. J. Obstet. Gynecol.*, **151**, 635−40.

Gemzell, C.A. (1977) Induction of ovulation with human gonadotrophins. *J. Reprod. Med.*, **18**, 155−62.

Gemzell, C. & Wang, C.F. (1980) The use of human gonadotrophins for the induction of ovulation in women with polycystic ovarian disease. *Fertil. Steril.*, **33**, 479−86.

Glass, M.R., Shaw, R., Butt, W.R. *et al.* (1975) An abnormality of oestrogen feedback in amenorrhoea-galactorrhoea. *Br. Med. J.*, **iii**, 274−5.

Gorlitsky, G.A., Kase, N.G. & Speroff, L. (1978) Ovulation and pregnancy rates with clomiphene citrate. *Obstet. Gynaecol.*, **51**, 265−9.

Grossman, A., Moult, P.J.A., McIntyre, H. *et al.* (1982) Opiate mediation of amenorrhoea in hyperprolactinaemia and in weight-loss related amenorrhoea. *Clin. Endocrinol. (Oxf.)*, **17**, 379−88.

Gysler, M., March, C.M., Mishell, D.M. *et al.* (1982) A decade's experience with an individualized clomiphene citrate treatment regimen including its effect on the post-coital test. *Fertil. Steril.*, **37**, 161.

Hague, W.M., Tan, S.L., Adams, J. *et al.* (1987) Hypergonadotrophic amenorrhoea: aetiology and outcome in 93 young women. *Int. J. Obstet. Gynaecol.*, **25**, 121−5.

Hague, W., Adams, J., Reeders, S. *et al.* (1988) Familial polycystic ovaries: a genetic disease. *Clin. Endocrinol. (Oxf.)*, **29**, 593−606.

Hammond, M.G. (1984) Monitoring techniques for improved pregnancy rates during clomiphene citrate ovulation induction. *Fertil. Steril.*, **42**, 499−509.

Harlow, C.R., Shaw, H.J., Hillier, S.G. *et al.* (1988) Factors influencing follicle-stimulating hormone-responsive steroidogenesis in marmoset granulosa cells: effects of androgens and the stage of follicular maturity. *Endocrinology*, **122**, 2780−7.

Harris, G.W. (1971) Humours and hormones *J. Endocrinol.*, **53**, 2−23.

Hillier, S.G. (1981) Regulation of follicular oestrogen biosynthesis: a survey of current concepts. *J. Endocrinol., Suppl.* **89**, 3P−18P.

Hillier, S.G. (1985) Sex steroid metabolism and follicular development in the ovary. (Oxf.) *Rev. Reprod. Biol.*, **7**, 168−222.

Hillier, S.G., Afnan, A.M.M., Margara, R. *et al.* (1985) Superovulation strategy before in vitro fertilization. *Clin. Obstet. Gynaecol.*, **12**, 687−723.

Homburg, R., Eshel, A., Abdalla, H.I. *et al.* (1988) Growth hormone facilitates ovulation induction by gonadotrophins. *Clin. Endocrinol. (Oxf.)*, **29**, 113−17.

Homburg, R., Eshel, A., Armar, N.A. *et al.* (1989) One hundred pregnancies after treatment with pulsatile luteinising hormone releasing hormone to induce ovulation. *Br. Med. J.*, **298**, 809−12.

Hsueh, A.J.W., Welsh, T.H. Jr. & Jones, P.B.C. (1981) Inhibition of ovarian and testicular steroidogenesis by epidermal growth factor. *Endocrinology*, **108**, 2002−4.

Hull, M.G.R. (1981) Ovulation failure and induction. *Clin. Obstet. Gynaecol.*, **8**, 753−86.

Hull, M.G.R. (1987) Epidemiology of infertility and polycystic ovarian disease: endocrinological and demographic studies. *Gynecol. Endocrinol.*, **1**, 235−45.

Hull, M.G.R., Knuth, U.A., Murray, M.A.F. *et al.* (1979b) The practical value of the progestogen challenge test, serum oestradiol estimation or clinical examination in assessment of the oestrogen state and response to clomiphene in amenorrhoea. *Br. J. Obstet. Gynaecol.*, **86**, 799−805.

Hull, M.G.R., Savage, P.E. & Jacobs, H.S. (1979a) Investigations and treatment of amenorrhoea resulting in normal fertility. *Br. Med. J.*, **i**, 1257−61.

Hutchinson, J.S. & Zeleznik, A.J. (1984) The Rhesus monkey corpus luteum is dependent on pituitary gonadotrophin secretion throughout the luteal phase of the menstrual cycle. *Endocrinology*, **115**, 1780−6.

Hutchinson, J.S. & Zeleznik, A.J. (1985) The corpus luteum of the primate menstrual cycle is capable of recovering from a transient withdrawal of pituitary gonadotrophin support. *Endocrinology*, **117**, 1043−9.

Jacobs, H.S., Franks, S., Murray, M.A.F. *et al.* (1976) Clinical and endocrine features of hyperprolactinaemic amenorrhoea. *Clin. Endocrinol. (Oxf.)*, **5**, 439−54.

Jones, G.S. & De Moraes-Ruehsen, M. (1969) A new syndrome of amenorrhoea in association with hypergonadotropinism and apparently normal ovarian follicular apparatus. *Am. J. Obstet. Gynecol.*, **104**, 597−600.

Jung, R.T, White, M.C., Bowley, N.B. *et al.* (1982) CT abnormalities of the pituitary in hyperprolactinaemic women with normal or equivocal sellae radiologically. *Br. Med. J.*, **285**, 1078−81.

Kallman, F.J., Schoenfeld, W.A. & Barrera, S.E. (1944) The genetic aspects of primary eunuchoidism. *Am. J. Mental Deficiency*, **48**, 203−36.

Kamrava, M.M., Seibel, M.M., Berger, M.J. *et al.* (1982) Reversal of persistent anovulation in polycystic ovarian disease by administration of chronic low-dose follicle stimulating hormone. *Fertil. Steril.*, **37**, 520−3.

Kandeel, F.R., Butt, W.R., London, D.R. *et al.* (1978) Oestrogen amplication of the LH−RH response in the polycystic ovary syndrome and response to clomiphene. *Clin. Endocrinol. (Oxf.)*, **9**, 429−41.

Kase, N., Mroueh, A. & Olson, L.E. (1967) Clomid treatment for anovulatory infertility. *Am. J. Obstet. Gynecol.*, **98**, 1037−42.

Kirschner, M.A., Zucker, I.R. & Jespersen D. (1976) Idiopathic hirsutism − an ovarian abnormality. *N. Engl. J. Med.*, **294**, 637−40.

Knobil, E., Plant, T.M., Wildt, L. *et al.* (1980) Control of the Rhesus monkey menstrual cycle: permissive role of hypothalamic gonadotrophin releasing hormone. *Science*, **207**, 1371−3.

Lamberts, S.W.J., Timmers, J.M. & de Jong, F.H. (1981) The effect of long term naloxone infusion on the response of gonadotrophin to luteinising hormone releasing hormone and on plasma estradiol concentration in a patient with a prolactin secreting pituitary adenoma. *Fertil. Steril.*, **36**, 678−81.

Lancet editorial: Hyperprolactinaemia: Pituitary tumour or not? (1980) *Lancet*, **ii**, 517−19.

Leyendecker, G., Struve, T. & Plotz, E.J. (1980a) Induction of ovulation with chronic intermittent (pulsatile) administration of LHRH in women with hypothalamic and hyperprolactinaemic amenorrhoea. *Arch. Gynaecol.*, **229**, 172−90.

Leyendecker, G., Wildt, L. & Hausmann, M. (1980b) Pregnancies following chronic intermittent (pulsatile) administration of GnRH by means of a portable pump (Zyclomat) − a new approach to the treatment of infertility in hypothalamic amenorrhoea. *J. Clin. Endocrinol. Metab.*, **51**, 1214−16.

Lunde, O. (1982) Polycystic ovarian syndrome: a restrospective study of the therapeutic effect of ovarian wedge resection after unsuccessful treatment with Clomiphene citrate. *Gynecology*, **38**, 483−7.

Lunenfeld, B., Eshkol, A., Tikotzky, D. *et al.* (1982) Induction of ovulation: Human gonadotrophins. In Flamigni, C. & Givens, J.R. (eds) *The Gonadotrophins: Basic Science and Clinical Aspects in Females*, pp. 395−403. Academic Press, London.

Lutjen, P., Trounson, A., Leeton, J. *et al.* (1984) The establishment and maintenance of pregnancy using *in vitro* fertilization and embryo donation in a patient with primary ovarian failure. *Nature*, **307**, 174–5.

MacGregor, A.M., Johnson, J.E. & Burde, C.E. (1968) Further clinical experience with clomiphene citrate. *Fertil. Steril.*, **19**, 616.

McNatty, K.P. McNeilly, A.S. & Sawers, R.S. (1977) Prolactin and progesterone secretion by human granulosa cells *in vitro*. In Cosignani, P.G. & Robyn, C. (eds) *Prolactin and Human Reproduction*, pp. 109–17. Academic Press, London.

Marshall, F.H.A. (1942) Exteroceptive factors in sexual periodicity. *Biol. Rev.*, **17**, 68–90.

Marshall, J.C. (1989) Control of gonadotrophin secretion. In Shaw, R.W. & Marshall, J.C. (eds) *LHRH and its Analogues*, pp. 1–18. Wright Publishers, London.

Mason, H.D., Sagle, M., Polson, D.W. *et al.* (1988) Reduced frequency of luteinizing hormone pulses in women with weight loss-related amenorrhoea and multifollicular ovaries. *Clin. Endocrinol. (Oxf.)*, **28**, 611–18.

Mason, H.D., Margara, R., Winston, R.M.L. *et al.* (1989) Inhibition of estradiol production from human granulosa cells by epidermal growth factor (EGF): effects in normal and polycystic ovaries. *Proceedings of the 71st Annual Meeting of the Endocrine Society*, Seattle, USA (Abstr. 608).

Mason, P., Adams, J., Morris, D.V. *et al.* (1984) Induction of ovulation with pulsatile luteinizing hormone-releasing hormone. *Br. Med. J.*, **288**, 181–5.

Matsuo, H., Arimura A., Nair, R.M.G. *et al.* (1971) Synthesis of the porcine LH and FSH releasing hormone by the solid-phase method. *Biochem. Biophys. Res. Commun.*, **45**, 822–7.

Menon, V., Logan Edwards, R., Butt, W.R. *et al.* (1984) Review of 59 patients with hypergonadotrophic amenorrhoea. *Br. J. Obstet. Gynaecol.*, **91**, 63–6.

Menon, V., Logan Edwards, R., Lynch, S.S. *et al.* (1983) Luteinizing hormone releasing hormone analogue in treatment of hypergonadotrophic amenorrhoea. *Br. J. Obstet. Gynaecol.*, **90**, 539–42.

Morris, D.V., Abdulwahid, N., Armar, N.A. *et al.* (1987) Induction of fertility in patients with organic hypothalamic-pituitary disease: response to treatment with LHRH. *Fertil. Steril.*, **47**, 54–9.

Mortimer, C.H., Besser, G.M., McNeilly, A.S. *et al.* (1973) Luteinizing hormone and follicle stimulating hormone releasing hormone test in patients with hypothalamic–pituitary–gonadal dysfunction. *Br. Med. J.*, **iv**, 73–77.

Moult, P.J.A., Dacie, J.E., Rees, L.H. *et al.* (1981) Prolactin pulsatility in patients with gonadal dysfunction. *Clin. Endocrinol. (Oxf.)*, **14**, 387–94.

Nabarro, J.D.N. (1982) Pituitary prolactinomas. *Clin. Endocrinol. (Oxf.)*, **17**, 129–55.

Nillius, S.J., Rojanasakul, A. & Bergh, T. (1985) Management of prolactinomas in pregnancy. In Auer, L.M., Leb, G., Tscherne, G., Urdl, W. & Walter,

G.F. (eds) *Prolactinomas*, pp. 373–85. de Gruyter Publications.

Nillius, S.J. & Wide, L. (1977) The pituitary responsiveness to acute and chronic administration of gonadotrophin releasing hormone in acute and recovery stages of anorexia nervosa. In Vigersky, R.A. (ed). *Anorexia Nervosa*, pp. 225–41. Raven Press, New York.

Oeisner, G., Serr, D.M., Mashiach, S. *et al.* (1978) The study of induction of ovulation with menotropins: analysis of results of 1897 treatment cycles. *Fertil. Steril.*, **30**, 538.

O'Herlihy, C., Pepperell, R.J., Evans, J.H. (1980) The significance of FSH elevation in young women with disorders of ovulation. *Br. Med. J.*, **281**, 1447–50.

Pepperall, R.J. (1981) Prolactin and reproduction. *Fertil. Steril.*, **35**, 267–74.

Petsos, P., Buckler, H., Mamtora, H. *et al.* (1986) Ovulation after treatment with ethinyl-oestradiol and medroxyprogesterone acetate in a woman approaching premature menopause. Case report. *Br. J. Obstet. Gynaecol.*, **93**, 1155–60.

Polson, D.W., Kiddy, D.S., Mason, H.D. *et al.* (1989a) Induction of ovulation with clomiphene citrate in women with polycystic ovary syndrome: the difference between responders and nonresponders. *Fertil. Steril.*, **51**, 30–4.

Polson, D.W., Mason, H.D. & Kiddy, D.S. (1989b) Low-dose follicle-stimulating hormone in the treatment of polycystic ovary syndrome: a comparison of pulsatile subcutaneous with daily intramuscular therapy. *Br. J. Obstet. Gynaecol.*, **96**, 746–8.

Polson, D.W., Mason, H.D., Saldahna, M.B.Y. *et al.* (1987a) Ovulation of a single dominant follicle during treatment with low-dose pulsatile follicle stimulating hormone in women with polycystic ovary syndrome. *Clin. Endocrinol. (Oxf.)*, **26**, 205–12.

Polson, D.W., Reed, M.J., Franks, S. *et al.* (1988a) Serum 11-hydroxyandrostenedione as an indicator of the source of excess androgen production in women with polycystic ovaries. *J. Clin. Endocrinol. Metab.*, **66**, 946–50.

Polson, D.W., Reed, M.J., Scanlon, M.J. *et al.* (1988b) Androstenedione concentrations following dexamethasone suppression: correlation with clomiphene responsiveness in women with polycystic ovary syndrome. *Gynaecol. Endocrinol.*, **2**, 257–64.

Polson, D.W., Sagle, M., Mason, H.D. *et al.* (1986) Ovulation and normal luteal function during LHRH treatment of women with hyperprolactinaemic amenorrhoea. *Clin. Endocrinol. (Oxf.)*, **24**, 531–7.

Polson, D.W., Sagle, M., Mason, H.D. *et al.* (1987b) Recovery of luteal function after interruption of gonadotrophin secretion in the mid-luteal phase of the menstrual cycle. *Clin. Endocrinol. (Oxf.)*, **26**, 597–600.

Quigley, M.E., Sheehan, K.L., Casper, R.F. *et al.* (1980) Evidence for increased opioid inhibition of luteinizing hormone secretion in hyperprolactinaemic women with pituitary microadenomas. *J. Clin. Endocrinol. Metab.*, **50**, 427−30.

Rasmussen, C., Bergh, T., Wide, L. & Brownell, J. (1988) Long-term treatment with a new non-ergot long-acting dopamine agonist, CV 205−502, in women with hyperprolactinaemia. *Clin. Endocrinol. (Oxf.)*, **29**, 271−9.

Rogol, A.D., White, B.J., Lieblich, J.M. *et al.* (1982) The Kallman Syndrome: A clinical genetic and endocrine view of nine affected women. In Flamigni, C. & Givens, J.R. (eds) *The Gonadotrophins: Basic Science and Clinical Aspects in ·Females*, pp. 233−44. Academic Press, London.

Rust, L.A., Israel, R. & Mishell, D.R. (1974) *An individualised graduated therapeutic regimen for clomiphene citrate. Am. J. Obstet. Gynecol.*, **120**, 785−90.

Sagle, M., Kiddy, D.S. & Franks, S. (1989) A prospective comparative study of low-dose HMG and FSH in polycystic ovary syndrome (PCOS). *J. Endocrinol., Suppl.*, **121**, Abstract 307.

Semple, C.G., Beastall, G.H., Teasdale, G. *et al.* (1983) Hypothyroidism presenting with hyperprolactinaemia. *Br. Med. J.*, **286**, 1200−1.

Shangold, M., Turksoy, R.N., Bashford, R.A. *et al.* (1977) Pregnancy following the insensitive ovary syndrome. *Fertil. Steril.*, **28**, 1179−81.

Skarin, G., Nillius, S.J. & Wide, L. (1983) Pulsatile subcutaneous low-dose gonadotrophin-releasing hormone treatment of anovulatory infertility. *Fertil. Steril.*, **40**, 457−60.

Stanhope, R., Adams, J. & Jacobs, H.S. (1985) Ovarian ultrasound assessment in normal children, idiopathic precocious puberty and during low dose pulsatile gonadotrophin releasing hormone treatment of hypogonadotrophic hypogonadism. *Arch. Dis. Child.*, **60**, 116−19.

Starup, J., Philip, J. & Sele, V. (1978) Oestrogen treatment and subsequent pregnancy in two patients with severe hypergonadotrophic ovarian failure. *Acta Endocrinol. Copenh.*, **89**, 149−57.

Stead, R.J., Hodson, M.E., Batten, J.C. *et al.* (1987) Amenorrhoea in cystic fibrosis. *Clin. Endocrinol. (Oxf.)*, **26**, 187−95.

Tan, S.L. & Jacobs, H.S. (1985) Recent advances in the management of patients with amenorrhoea. *Clin. Obstet. Gynaecol.*, **12**, 725−47.

Tanaka, T., Oikawa, M., Sakuraji, N. *et al.* (1988) May wedge resection still be useful in patients with polycystic ovarian disease refractory to Clomiphene citrate? *Proceedings of the XIIth World Congress of Gynecology and Obstetrics,*, Rio de Janeiro.

Thompson, C.R. & Hanson, L.M. (1970) Pergonal (menotropins): a summary of clinical experience in the induction of ovulation and pregnancy. *Fertil. Steril.*, **21**, 844.

Thorner, M.O. & Besser, G.M. (1977) Hyperprolactinaemia and gonadal function: results of bromocriptine treatment. In Cosignani, P.G. & Robyn, C. (eds) *Prolactin and Human Reproduction*, pp. 285−302. Academic Press, London.

Treasure, J.L., Gordon, P.A.L., King, E.A. *et al.* (1985) Cystic ovaries: a phase of anorexia nervosa. *Lancet*, **ii**, 1379−81.

Tsapoulis, A.D., Zourlas, P.A. & Comninos, A.C. (1978) Observations on 320 infertile patients treated with human gonadotrophins (human menopausal gonadotrophin/human chorionic gonadotrophin). *Fertil. Steril.*, **29**, 492−5.

Urdl, W., Tscherne, G., Auer, L.M. *et al.* (1985) Pregnancies after treatment of prolactinomas: course and complications. In Auer, L.M., Leb, G., Tscherne, G., Urdl, W. & Walter, G.F. (eds). *Prolactinomas*, pp. 417−23. de Gruyter Publications.

Van Campenhout, J., Vauclair, R. & Maraghi, K. (1972) Gonadotropin resistant ovaries in primary amenorrhoea. *Obstet. Gynecol.*, **40**, 6−12.

van der Spuy, Z., Steer, P.J., McCusker, M. *et al.* (1988) Pregnancy outcome in underweight women following spontaneous and induced ovulation. *Br. Med. J.*, **296**, 962−5.

van Look, P.F.A., McNeilly, A.S., Hunter, W.M. *et al.* (1977) The role of prolactin in secondary amenorrhea. In Crosignani, P.G. & Robyn, C. (eds) *Prolactin and Human Reproduction*, pp. 217−24. Academic Press, London.

von Werder, K., Eversmann, T., Landgraf, R. *et al.* (1985) New aspects of medical treatment of prolactinomas. In Auer, L.M., Leb, G., Tscherne, G., Urdl, W. & Walter, G.F. (eds) *Prolactinomas*, pp. 309−18. de Gruyter Publications.

Wright, C.S.W. & Jacobs, H.S. (1979) Spontaneous pregnancy in a patient with hypergonadotrophic ovarian failure. *Br. J. Obstet. Gynaecol.*, **86**, 389−92.

Yen, S.S.C. (1980) The polycystic ovary syndrome. *Clin. Endocrinol. (Oxf.)*, **12**, 177−207.

Zarate, A., Canales, E.S., Soria, J. *et al.* (1976) Therapeutic use of ponado Liberin (follicle-stimulating hormone/luteinizing hormone-releasing hormone) in women. *Fertil. Steril.*, **27**, 1233−9.

# 9 Diagnosis and Treatment of Luteal Dysfunction

K.J. DOODY & B.R. CARR

## Introduction

### History

The first detailed description of the corpus luteum was published in 1672 by Regnier de Graaf (Short, 1977). The term 'corpus luteum' was introduced by Malpighi who noted the presence of a 'yellow body' in the cow ovary. This structure was demonstrated to be essential to the maintenance of early pregnancy as early as 1903 (Short, 1977). An extract of the corpus luteum 'progestin' was purified in 1933 and was demonstrated to possess this pregnancy maintaining capability (Allen & Wintersteiner, 1934).

Defective function of the corpus luteum was first postulated as a cause of reproductive failure by Jones (1949). It is known in the human that the corpus luteum is indispensible for the maintenance of pregnancy until after the seventh week of gestation (Fig. 9.1) (Csapo et al., 1972). Progesterone production is considered to be the primary function of the corpus luteum. However a multitude of substances are now known to be produced by the corpus luteum. Relaxin, for example, a product of the primate corpus luteum has been hypothesized to act

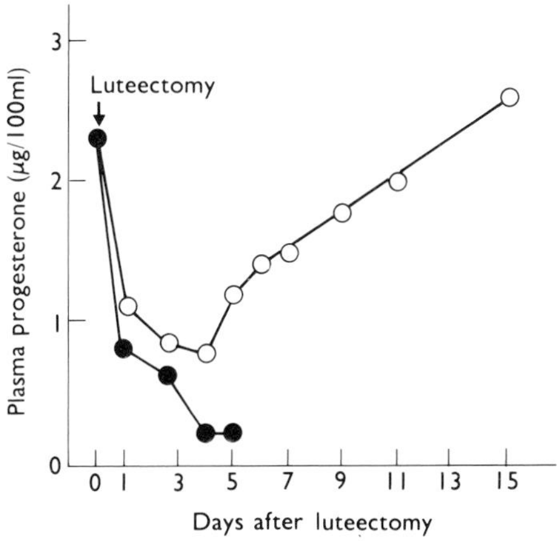

**Fig. 9.1.** The effect of removal of the corpus luteum (luteectomy) on pregnancy outcome. Arrow (time of luteectomy); before 7 weeks gestation, spontaneous abortion (●); after 8 weeks gestation, continuation of pregnancy (○). Adapted in part with permission from C.V. Mosby Co., Csapo *et al.* (1972) *Am. J. Obstet. Gynecol,* **112**, 106.

synergistically with oestrogen and progesterone to prepare the endometrium for implantation and development of the blood supply to the conceptus. Corpus luteum dysfunction has been proposed not only as a cause for recurrent pregnancy loss, but also for infertility (Jones, 1949; Hernandez Horta *et al.*, 1977).

## Definition

Luteal-phase dysfunction or deficiency is defined as the production of progesterone and/or oestrogen in a quantity or for a duration inadequate to result in initiation or maintenance of pregnancy. A broader definition of luteal dysfunction might include all aberrations of corpus luteum function which result in significant impairment of reproductive capacity. Additionally, some definitions have included defects of uterine origin which result in impairment of the interaction between the corpus luteum and the endometrium. Actions of gonadal steroids on the fallopian tube, cervix or directly with the gametes or embryo might also influence reproductive outcome, however, these interactions are not generally considered when discussing luteal dysfunction (Cline *et al.*, 1977; Margalioth *et al.*, 1988).

## Incidence

The reported incidence of luteal deficiency varies tremendously. The frequency of diagnosis is dependent on a multitude of factors including the nature of the patient population studied and the methods used to establish a diagnosis. When diagnosed by repeated endometrial biopsy, an incidence of 3.5% was reported by Jones (1976). It is generally reported that the incidence in unselected infertility patients is 3–10%, however, some investigators have reported luteal deficiency in up to 20% of infertile patients (Table 9.1) (Balasch & Vanrell, 1987). Patients

**Table 9.1.** Incidence of luteal-phase deficiency (LPD) in infertility

| Year | Authors | Patients (*n*) | LPD (%) |
|------|---------|----------------|---------|
| 1955 | Gillam | 123 | 10.7 |
| 1958 | Foss *et al.* | 856 | 15.7 |
| 1959 | Grant *et al.* | 165 | 20.0 |
| 1962 | Jones & Pourmand | 555 | 3.7 |
| 1962 | Botella-Llusia | 2000 | 6.0 |
| 1970 | Murthy *et al.* | 335 | 11.5 |
| 1974 | Sillo-Seidl & Dallenbach-Hellweg | 1915 | 20.0 |
| 1980 | Wentz | 149 | 19.0 |
| 1980 | Rosenberg *et al.* | 396 | 8.1 |
| 1982 | Nash | ? | 20.0 |
| 1983 | Downs & Gibson | 366 | 12.7 |
| 1983 | Pittaway *et al.* | 143 | 7.0 |
| 1986 | Balasch *et al.* | 355 | 12.9 |

Reproduced by permission from Balasch, J. & Vanrell, J.A. (1987) *Hum. Reprod.*, **2**, 557–67.

with a history of recurrent miscarriage, endometriosis or who are undergoing therapy with ovulation induction agents are apparently much more likely to demonstrate luteal inadequacy (25–35% or more) (Table 9.2) (Balasch & Vanrell, 1987).

Luteinized unruptured follicle syndrome (LUFS) — an apparently distinct type of luteal dysfunction — appears to occur statistically more frequently in women with unexplained infertility than in the fertile population (Moghissi & Wallach, 1983). The incidence of LUFS cycles in women with regular menses has been reported to be 4.9% (Kerin *et al.*, 1983). The reported incidence of LUFS in infertile patients varies considerably. This syndrome has been diagnosed in up to 5–79% of patients previously described as having unexplained infertility (Table 9.3) (Kerin *et al.*, 1983; Daly *et al.*, 1985; Petsos *et al.*, 1985; Ying *et al.*, 1987; Katz, 1988). Moreover, LUFS is seen much more frequently in women with luteal phase dysfunction (15%) and in patients with

**Table 9.2.** Incidence of luteal-phase deficiency (LPD) among patients with repeated abortion

| Year | Authors | Patients (*n*) | LPD (%) |
|------|---------|----------------|---------|
| 1951 | Jones & Delfs | 73 | 37.0 |
| 1959 | Grant *et al.* | 170 | 60.0 |
| 1962 | Botella-Llusia | 50 | 38.0 |
| 1977 | Yip | 10 | 30.0 |
| 1979 | Tho *et al.* | 100 | 23.0 |
| 1980 | Wentz | 8 | 37.5 |
| 1986 | Balasch *et al.* | 60 | 31.7 |

Adapted in part from Balasch, J. & Vanrell, J.A. (1987) *Hum. Reprod.*, **2**, 557–67.

**Table 9.3.** Incidence of luteinized unruptured follicle syndrome (LUFS) in fertile and infertile patients

| Author | Infertile | | | Fertile | | |
|---|---|---|---|---|---|---|
| | No. | LUFS | % | No. | LUFS | % |
| Schneller *et al.* | 47 | 26 | 55 | 18 | 9 | 50 |
| Dhont *et al.* | 21 | 7 | 33 | 45 | 25 | 56 |

Reproduced with permission from the American Fertility Society, Katz, E. (1988) *Fertil. Steril.*, **50**, 839.

corrected luteal phase dysfunction who do not conceive (38%) (Ying *et al.*, 1987).

## Classification

Several categories of luteal dysfunction have been described. Generally, these classifications are based on a description of the manifestations of the disease process rather than on the aetiology of the disorder.

### The short luteal phase

The occurrence of short luteal phases as a distinct clinical entity and the associated possible pathologic significance was recognized first by Strott *et al.* (1970). The short luteal phase was originally defined as a luteal phase of 8 days or less in duration in otherwise healthy women. Other investigators have defined the syndrome of short luteal phase as a duration less than 10 or even 11 days (Sherman *et al.*, 1974a; Quagliarello & Weiss, 1979; Lenton *et al.*, 1984). The incidence of short luteal phase in infertile females has been reported to be 3−11%. While follicular phase length may vary considerably between normal fertile women, duration of the luteal phase is remarkably constant (Vande Wiele *et al.*, 1970). A review of 327 cycles using a two-normal model observed a mean luteal phase duration in normal cycles to be 14.13 days with 95% confidence limits of 11.3 and 17.0 days (Lenton *et al.*, 1984). The incidence of short luteal phases which were considered to be abnormal was found to be 5.2%. In another study, short luteal phases have been demonstrated in seven of 26 apparently normally cyclic women (Strott *et al.*, 1970).

Although the association between short luteal phase and infertility has been suggested by several investigators, this remains controversial. Smith *et al.* (1984) found the incidence of short luteal phase in infertile women (9%) was not significantly different than that of a control population (8%). Jones has suggested that if pregnancy occurs, human chorionic gonadotrophin (hCG) can be detected within 7 or 8 days of the ovulatory luteinizing hormone (LH) surge and if the corpus luteum can be rescued by hCG, a corpus luteum that functions for 7 or 8 days should be sufficient to allow for pregnancy (Jones, 1976). On the other hand, a very high incidence of unsuspected subclinical pregnancies resulted in spontaneous abortion in patients with isolated short luteal phases (with in-phase endometrium) (Cline, 1979).

The pathogenesis of short luteal phase is unclear. In one study of patients with very short luteal phases as determined by basal body temperature, five of six patients demonstrated severe lags in endometrial maturation (Downs & Gibson, 1983a). This would imply that premature luteolysis of a normally functioning corpus luteum is not responsible for the short luteal duration in the majority of cases. The onset of menstruation does not always correlate with circulating levels of oestrogen or progesterone (Godfrey *et al.*, 1981). Menstruation has been reported to occur in the presence of higher levels of oestradiol and progesterone during cycles with short luteal phases as compared with normal cycles (Smith *et al.*, 1985). This would suggest that uterine factors rather than corpus luteum function might play a role in the pathogenesis of the short luteal phase in some women.

An association between short luteal phases and abnormal hormonal patterns has also been reported. Strott *et al.* (1970) demonstrated that short luteal phases were generally but not always associated with low luteal plasma progesterone levels. They also reported significantly lower follicle-stimulating hormone (FSH) levels and FSH:LH ratios in the follicular phase of cycles with short luteal phases (Fig. 9.2). Sherman and Korenman (1974a) confirmed lower follicular-phase FSH levels

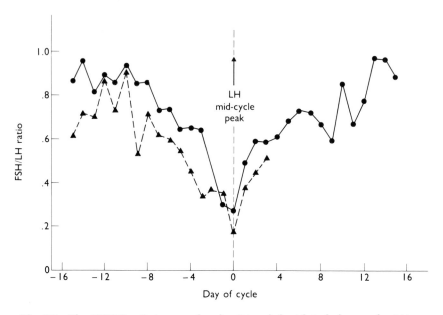

**Fig. 9.2.** The FSH:LH ratio in normal cycles (●) and short luteal-phase cycles (▲). Reproduced with permission by the Endocrine Society© from Strott *et al.* (1970) *J. Clin. Endocrinol. Metab.*, **30**, 246.

and luteal progesterone levels in cycles with short luteal phases. Additionally, they demonstrated that these cycles were also characterized by low mid-cycle and luteal oestradiol levels (Sherman & Korenman, 1974b). An association has been demonstrated between the length of the luteal phase and the mean luteal serum LH (Vandekerckhove & Dhont, 1972). A study of three women with recurrent short luteal phases revealed significantly elevated prolactin levels and absence of FSH surges (Aksel, 1980). Fredricsson *et al.* (1981) found higher prolactin levels and lower progesterone levels in 36 women with infertility and short luteal phase. It has been suggested that decreased FSH stimulation may result in a decrease in the number of LH receptors in these women. Examination of the hormonal profile of a single patient with sporadic short luteal phase revealed only an increased FSH:LH ratio throughout that cycle.

A short luteal phase has been demonstrated with high frequency in women undergoing superovulation with human menopausal gonadotrophins (hMG) (Kemeter *et al.*, 1977; Olson *et al.*, 1983; Laatikainen *et al.*, 1988) (Fig. 9.3). These cycles appear to be associated with certain hormonal patterns including very high or very low peak preovulatory oestradiol levels, low luteal progesterone levels and relatively decreased hCG levels at 24 h after hCG administration (Olson *et al.*, 1983).

All of these studies raise questions with regard to the significance of the short luteal phase as a cause of infertility in cases where luteal hormonal profiles appear normal.

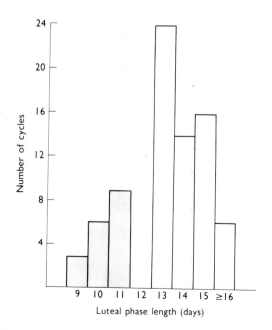

**Fig. 9.3.** Luteal-phase length in 78 ovulatory cycles of women treated with hMG and hCG. Sixty cycles had luteal-phase length ≥ 13 days (open bars), while 18 cycles had short luteal phases ≤ 11 days (shaded bars). Reproduced by permission of the American Fertility Society from Olson *et al.* (1983) *Fertil. Steril.*, **39**, 284.

## Aberrations of gonadal steroid production

It is well recognized that many cycles characterized by normal duration of the luteal phase are nevertheless marked by diminished production of gonadal steroids (Jones, 1976). Goldstein *et al.* (1982) identified three distinct hormonal profiles that can be associated with infertility and deficiency of endometrial maturation. Some patients were observed to have normal oestradiol levels and low progesterone values while others had low oestradiol and normal progesterone concentrations. A larger group of patients demonstrated a deficiency of both hormones.

Traditionally, a much greater emphasis has been placed on deficient progesterone levels than other hormonal patterns that may be associated with luteal dysfunction. Israel *et al.* (1972) reported that a progesterone concentration of 3 ng/ml (*c.* 10 nmol/l) or greater was indicative of ovulation. This value, however, appears useless as a criterion for the diagnosis of aberrant luteal steroid hormone production. A number of methods have been employed for this purpose including endometrial biopsy and serial blood sampling. These are discussed more extensively in the section on diagnosis (see later).

## Luteinized unruptured follicle syndrome

Recently, a syndrome of follicular/luteal dysfunction has been described in which the observed defect is a failure of rupture of the follicle in response to the LH surge (Marik & Hulka, 1978). This syndrome has been reported to occur spontaneously in fertile and infertile women (Dmowski *et al.*, 1980; Portuondo *et al.*, 1981; Kerin *et al.*, 1983). Additionally, this condition can be caused by preovulatory treatment with inhibitors of prostaglandin synthesis (Killick & Elstein, 1987). The aetiology of the defect observed in spontaneous cycles remains unknown. In a population of normal women LUFS tends to occur sporadically whereas patients with unexplained infertility may experience LUFS repeatedly in multiple cycles (Kerin *et al.*, 1983; Liukkonen *et al.*, 1984; Petsos *et al.*, 1985). An association of endometriosis and LUFS has been reported, however, no cause−effect relationship has been proven (Koninckx *et al.*, 1980).

Follicle growth does not appear to be altered in patients with LUFS, however, after the LH peak, LUF follicles, instead of rupturing, demonstrate a typical accelerated growth pattern (Hamilton *et al.*, 1985). Both the mid-cycle LH peak and the mid-luteal progesterone level appear to be significantly reduced in LUF cycles (Hamilton *et al.*, 1985). It appears that cycles characterized by LUFS may additionally demonstrate some degree of luteal inadequacy as manifested by decreased luteal plasma progesterone levels. Initially, LUFS was diagnosed at laparoscopy after presumed ovulation when ovulatory stigmas were observed to be absent (Table 9.4) (Katz, 1988). This technique has the obvious dis-

**Table 9.4.** Incidence of laparoscopic diagnosis of luteinized unruptured follicle syndrome (LUFS) in infertile women

| Author | No. of patients | LUFS | % |
|---|---|---|---|
| Marik & Hulka | 102 | 62 | 61 |
| Schneller *et al.* | 18 | 9 | 50 |
| Dhont *et al.* | 45 | 25 | 63 |
| Melega *et al.* | 12 | 10 | 83 |
| Temmerman *et al.* | 220 | 26 | 12 |
| Lemaire *et al.* | 3 | 14 | 40 |
| | 6 | 0 | 0 |
| | 13 | 7 | 54 |
| Brosens *et al.* | 16 | 1 | 6 |
| | 29 | 23 | 79 |

Reproduced with permission from the American Fertility Society, Katz E. (1988) *Fertil. Steril.*, **50**, 839.

advantages that surgery is required and that this surgery must be precisely timed. Additionally, rapid reperitonealization of the stigma may lead to an overestimation of this diagnosis by as much as 50% using this method (Portuondo *et al.*, 1981). More recently investigators have advocated the use of sonography (Coulam *et al.*, 1982; Daly *et al.*, 1985; Hamilton *et al.*, 1985; Ying *et al.*, 1987; Katz, 1988) (Table 9.5). Others have utilized determination of peritoneal fluid steroid levels for diagnosis of LUFS (Lesorgen *et al.*, 1984).

## Aetiology

A number of aetiologies for the development of luteal-phase dysfunction have been proposed (Table 9.6) (McNeely & Soules, 1988). A detailed knowledge of the function and interaction of the hypothalamus, pituitary, ovary and genital tract is essential to an understanding of the pathogenesis of luteal inadequacy. An understanding of the pathophysiology is in turn necessary for the initiation of appropriate diagnostic and therapeutic modalities.

Formation of a functionally normal corpus luteum is dependent on the luteinization of a mature, differentiated follicle. Primate studies have confirmed abnormal folliculogenesis and deficient FSH levels as a frequent cause of luteal dysfunction (Fig. 9.4) (DiZerega & Hodgen, 1981). Follicular development and the hormonal stimulus for luteinization are in turn dependent on a complex series of interactions involving several organs and numerous cell types. The initial stimulus for follicular growth is unknown. Paracrine interactions within the ovary have been hypothesized to result in the activation or 'recruitment' of cohorts of primordial follicles. Recruitment results in the induction of a capacity to respond to FSH. From these cohorts, under FSH stimulation, a dominant follicle emerges — a process often referred to as 'selection'.

**Table 9.5.** Incidence of luteinized unruptured follicle syndrome (LUFS) in infertile women on ultrasonography

| Author | No. of patients | LUFS | % |
|---|---|---|---|
| Daly | 33 | 3 | 9 |
| Gibbons et al. | 153 | 14 | 9 |
| Petsos et al. | 45 cycles | 8 cycles | 18 |
| Kerin et al. | 183 cycles (66 pts) | 9 cycles | 4 |
| Liukkonnen | 37 | 20 | 54 |
| Hamilton | 270 | 27 | 10 |

Reproduced with permission from the American Fertility Society, Katz E. (1988) *Fertil. Steril.*, **50**, 839.

**Table 9.6.** Postulated and proven causes of luteal-phase deficiency

Neuroendocrine
  Increased LH-pulse frequency
  Follicular-phase FSH deficiency
  Inadequate LH surge
  Abnormal follicular-phase LH:FSH ratio
  Mild hyperprolactinaemia
  Deficient luteal-LH levels

Ovarian
  Reduced numbers of primordial follicles
  Accelerated luteolysis

Uterine
  Inadequate endometrial progesterone receptors
  Endometritis

Other
  Physiological (postpartum, postmenarchal, premenopausal)
  Chronic hypoxia
  Drugs (e.g. clomiphene citrate; hMG)
  Chronic systemic disease (e.g. renal or liver failure)
  Exercise
  Psychosocial stress

Adapted with permission from the American Fertility Society, McNeely, M.J. & Soules, M.R. (1988) *Fertil Steril.*, **50**, 1–15.

This follicle continues on a path of maturation characterized by cell replication and expression of genes encoding steroidogenic enzymes. The preovulatory follicle can secrete up to 400 μg of oestradiol per day (Baird & Fraser, 1974), but perhaps the most important aspect of the differentiation of the cells which comprise the follicle is the induction of LH receptors (Lee *et al.*, 1973) (see Chapter 3).

The mid-cycle LH surge starts at or around the time that the pre-ovulatory follicle achieves a maximal rate of oestradiol secretion (Hoff *et al.*, 1983). LH, working via the second-messenger cyclic adenosine monophosphate (cAMP), has two fundamental actions: (1) the initiation of follicular rupture and ovum release, and (2) the induction of genes whose products are required for the synthesis of the hormones charac-

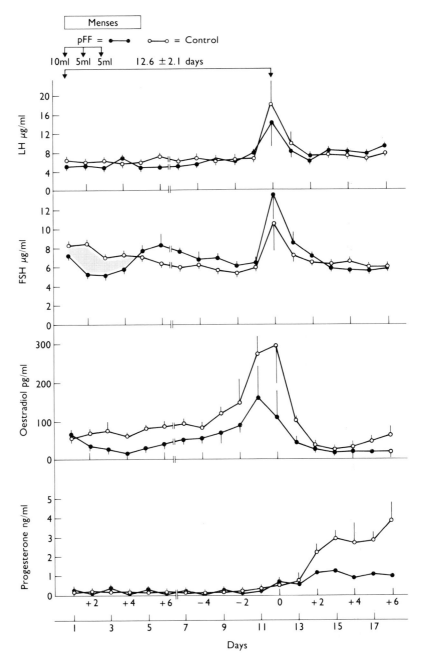

**Fig. 9.4.** Composite patterns of peripheral serum LH, FSH, oestradiol, and progesterone in cyclic monkeys treated with porcine follicular fluid (pff, $n=5$) or not (control). Note transient decrease in FSH levels during early follicular-phase treatment with pff (shaded area) and subsequent luteal phase dysfunction. Reproduced with permission of the American Fertility Society from DiZerega & Hogen (1981) *Fertil Steril.*, **35**, 489.

teristic of the luteal phase. Progesterone rises simultaneously with the LH surge. As progesterone levels begin to escalate, there is a sudden transient decline in plasma oestradiol levels which occurs prior to follicle rupture. This may reflect a decrease in the availability of the precursor, androstenedione, rather than an actual decrease in aromatase activity (Leung & Armstrong, 1980).

The preovulatory follicle undergoes a histamine-induced hyperaemia which is terminated by prostaglandin $F_{2\alpha}$ leading to damage and weakening of the follicular wall and ovulation (Murdoch & Myers, 1983; Murdoch & Cavender, 1989). After follicular rupture, vascularization of the granulosa cells occurs. The precise events mediating luteal angiogenesis in the human corpus luteum remain to be elucidated, but the major effect is the increase in availability of low-density lipoprotein (LDL)-cholesterol which can serve to supply cholesterol to granulosa cells (Fig. 9.5) (Carr *et al.*, 1982). LDL-cholesterol is the primary substrate for progesterone in the human corpus luteum (Fig. 9.6) (Carr *et al.*, 1981). In the absence of lipoprotein, corpus luteum cells secrete reduced amounts of progesterone. Uptake of LDL-cholesterol by corpus luteum tissues is a receptor-mediated event which can be stimulated by gonadotrophin (Carr *et al.*, 1981). Continued exposure of the human corpus luteum to gonadotrophic stimulation appears to be a prerequisite for normal luteal hormone production (Vande Wiele *et al.*, 1970) (see also Chapter 6).

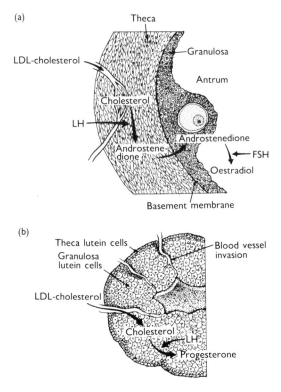

**Fig. 9.5.** Proposed model for the regulation of progesterone secretion by the human ovary. (a) Follicular phase; (b) luteal phase. Reproduced with permission of the American Fertility Society from Carr *et al.* (1982) *Fertil. Steril.*, **38**, 303.

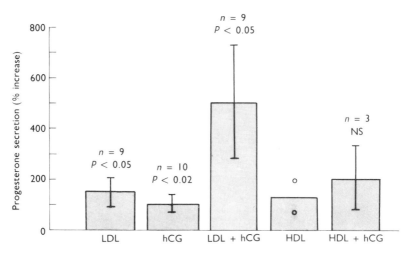

**Fig. 9.6.** Effects of low-density lipoprotein (LDL) and hCG on progesterone secretion by human luteal tissue. Tissue fragments were maintained in culture in medium containing lipoprotein-deficient serum (10%) and, where indicated, LDL (500 μg LDL-protein/ml), HDL (500 μg HDL-protein/ml), and hCG (1 IU/ml). The medium was changed daily and analysed for progesterone content by radioimmunoassay. Progesterone secretion rates on the third day of culture are shown. The tissues used were obtained from ovaries at various stages of the luteal phase of the ovarian cycle. Because of the variation in the rate of progesterone secretion from experiment to experiment, results are expressed as the percentage increase over control values obtained for progesterone secretion by tissue maintained in lipoprotein-deficient serum alone. Each bar represents the mean (± SE) result from the number of experiments indicated. The probability ($P$) values presented are for comparisons of progesterone secretion under each of the conditions indicated with progesterone secretion in the presence of lipoprotein-deficient serum, as determined using the unpaired Student's $t$-test. Reproduced with permission of the Endocrine Society© from Carr *et al.* (1981) *J. Clin. Endocrinol. Metab.*, **52**, 875.

Finally, the trophoblast of the early embryo is essential to the maintenance of the corpus luteum in early pregnancy. hCG secreted by the trophoblasts acts classically as a luteotrophin binding to LH/hCG receptors hence prolonging the steroidogenic lifespan of the corpus luteum. Impaired activity of the corpus luteum as evidenced by low serum concentrations of progesterone and oestradiol is also observed in patients with impending miscarriage or ectopic pregnancy. This is commonly believed to be the result of decreased production of hCG by the trophoblast. It has been demonstrated, however, in the case of ectopic pregnancy that the lower serum steroid levels cannot be completely explained by altered hCG bioactivity (Norman *et al.*, 1988). Primary defects of the corpus luteum or absence of other embryonic stimulators of ovarian steroid biosynthesis have been postulated.

Many substances other than steroid hormones (such as relaxin and inhibin) have been demonstrated to be produced by the corpus luteum and thus implicated in normal reproduction. However, implantation of donated embryos with subsequent normal fetal development to term has been demonstrated in women with gonadal failure and in castrate women who are administered exogenous oestrogen and progesterone

(Lutjen *et al.*, 1984; Rosenwaks, 1987). This would suggest that these two substances, produced by the corpus luteum, are not necessarily essential for implantation and maintenance of early pregnancy.

Progesterone and oestrogen are believed to mediate their effects on reproduction predominantly via their action on the endometrial lining of the uterus. Additionally, effects of these hormones on the oviduct and embryo have been suggested (Verhage *et al.*, 1979; Soules *et al.*, 1984a). The actions of these hormones on the endometrium have been investigated extensively. Oestradiol, secreted in large quantities by the granulosa cells during the follicular phase causes proliferation of the glandular epithelial cells and, perhaps more importantly, appears to induce receptors for oestradiol and for progesterone. Progesterone, together with oestrogen in the luteal phase is responsible for the differentiation of the endometrial cells which follows their proliferation. Gland secretion is very prominent during the luteal phase in women and is felt necessary for attachment of the blastocyst. Differentiation of the endometrial stroma including the proliferation of the stromal blood vessels and differentiation of fibroblasts into large decidual cells appears necessary for subsequent blastocyst invasion. These events are dependent on the levels of progesterone and oestradiol. It has been reported in monkeys that a specified absolute level of progesterone and oestradiol as well as a specified progesterone/oestradiol ratio is required for development of normal secretory endometrium (Good & Moyer, 1968).

Transient luteal deficiency has been demonstrated to occur in the cycles following menarche, abortion, postpartum and after cessation of birth control pills (see Table 9.6) (McNeely & Soules, 1988). Similarly, it is likely that normal women may experience occasional cycles which demonstrate characteristics of luteal inadequacy. Luteal dysfunction noted in association with these conditions is self-limiting, requires no treatment and does not cause significant long-term impairment of reproductive capacity.

Chronic or recurrent luteal dysfunction, does however, diminish reproductive capacity and an understanding of the aetiology of the disorder is essential to the diagnosis and therapy of patients thus affected. It appears that chronic or recurrent luteal deficiency, like chronic anovulation, is not a single specific disorder, but rather a syndrome which can be brought about by defects at any point in the hypothalamo–pituitary–gonadal–endometrial axis (see Table 9.6).

**Hypothalamus and pituitary**

Normal follicular and luteal function depends upon hypothalamic regulation of pituitary production of gonadotrophins. Hypothalamic secretion of appropriate amounts of gonadotrophin-releasing hormone (GnRH) in a precisely timed pulsatile fashion is required for adequate pituitary secretion of FSH. Luteal dysfunction has been induced in women treated with a GnRH agonist for 3 days in the early follicular phase (Fig. 9.7) (Sheehan *et al.*, 1982). Decreased pulse amplitude and frequency of GnRH secretion results in deficient FSH production by the pituitary. Decreased FSH production in turn leads to impaired follicular development with subsequent luteal dysfunction (Strott *et al.*, 1970; Sherman & Korenman, 1974a; Stouffer & Hodgen, 1980; DiZerega *et al.*, 1981). Increases in the pulse amplitude and frequency of GnRH secretion may lead to downregulation of the GnRH receptors and again gonadotrophin production is affected (usually an increased LH:FSH ratio). Soules *et al.* (1984) have demonstrated increased pulse frequency of LH in women with luteal deficiency. Immature follicles produced due to dysfunctional gonadotrophic secretion may yield abnormal responses to the LH surge and thus abnormal luteal function. The most widely accepted explanation for poor follicular response to the LH surge is lack of induction of LH receptors (Lee, 1987). Adequate FSH stimulation is necessary for induction of both the LH and FSH receptors.

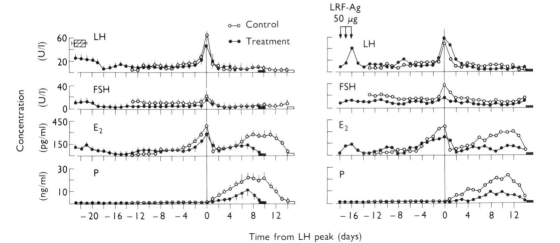

**Fig. 9.7.** Induction of luteal deficiency by treatment with a GnRH agonist. (*Left panel*) Time-course and quantitative changes in circulating concentrations (mean ± SE) of LH, FSH, oestradiol ($E_2$) and progesterone (P) during the menstrual cycle of four normal women treated with a GnRH-agonist (hatched box, top left) on the 3 days after onset of menstruation, and during the preceding control cycles. Data are centred around the mid-cycle gonadotrophin peak (Day 0). Onset of menstrual flow occurred on Day 9 in the treated cycles (solid boxes) and Day 14 after the mid-cycle surge in the control cycles (open boxes). (*Right panel*) Pattern of circulating concentrations of LH, FSH, $E_2$ and progesterone (P) during the control and GnRH-agonist (LRF-Ag) treated cycles in one subject. Treatment of this subject caused a prolonged follicular phase (19 days as opposed to 14 days) associated with reduced FSH concentrations. Concentrations of FSH and $E_2$ were suppressed at mid-cycle. A normal-length luteal phase ensued but concentrations of $E_2$ and progesterone were reduced throughout the entire luteal phase. Data are centred around the mid-cycle gonadotrophin surge (Day 0). (Solid boxes indicate the period of menstruation.) Reproduced with permission of the American Association for the Advancement of Science from Sheehan *et al.* (1982) *Science,* **215**, 170.

Increased LH secretion during the follicular phase has also been suggested to impair follicular development — presumably via increases in ovarian thecal androgen production which may have direct effects on the developing follicle. Serving not only as a substrate for FSH-induced aromatization, androgens in low concentrations may enhance aromatase activity. At higher levels, androstenedione is preferentially converted to potent 5α-reduced androgens which may in fact inhibit both aromatase activity and the FSH induction of LH receptors on granulosa cells (Hillier et al., 1980; Jia et al., 1985). Alternatively, the hypothalamic signals, together with the rising levels of oestradiol, may provoke a blunted LH surge. This, again, may be responsible for deficient luteinization of the preovulatory follicle.

A study of hypophysectomized rhesus monkeys has suggested that the corpus luteum might function independently of gonadotrophin secretion (Asch et al., 1982). In another study of rhesus monkeys, luteal-phase administration of a GnRH antagonist resulted in suppression of postovulatory gonadotrophin levels without affecting luteal function (Balmaceda et al., 1983). However, several other studies in various primates including humans have clearly demonstrated the importance of continuous LH stimulation during the luteal phase for maintenance of the corpus luteum throughout its functional life (Vande Wiele et al., 1970; Vandekerckhove & Dhont, 1972; Wardlaw et al., 1975; Groff et al., 1984; Mais et al., 1986). Interruption of LH secretion in the early, mid-, or late luteal phase causes progesterone levels to drop rapidly resulting in initiation of menses within 2—5 days. Reinstitution of gonadotrophic support after a hiatus of 3 days causes revival of luteal function in the early and mid-luteal phase but not in the late luteal phase. Surprisingly, the length of the luteal phase was not affected following a 3-day hiatus in LH stimulation (Hutchison & Zeleznik, 1985) (see Fig. 6.7). The dependence of the corpus luteum on LH for the maintenance of steroidogenesis reflects actions of the gonadotrophin which promote the transcription of the genes involved in sexmhormone biosynthesis. The hypothesis that inadequate luteal LH production may lead to decreased steroidogenesis and hence luteal dysfunction is the primary rationale for the use of hCG as a treatment modality.

Aberrant progesterone secretion may itself affect the gonadotrophic support of the corpus luteum. In women, it has been proposed that progesterone from the corpus luteum turn modulates GnRH secretion, and hence LH, thereby affecting its own production (Soules et al., 1984a). This hypothesis is supported by the observation that progesterone receptor blockade during the luteal phase may frequently lead to luteolysis (Fig. 9.8) (Garzol et al., 1988; Li et al., 1988a).

Hyperprolactinaemia has been a frequent finding in clinical investigations of infertile patients with ovulatory disturbances including luteal dysfunction (Seppala et al., 1976; Pozo et al., 1979; Michel &

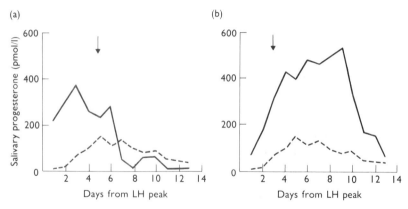

**Fig. 9.8.** The effects of a single, variable dose (5—200 mg) of RU486 on daily salivary progesterone profile. Arrow indicates the day of administration of RU486. The continuous line represents the profile of women who had received a dose of RU486. The dotted line represents the 5th percentile of a normal population of women and hence the lower limit of the normal range. (a) An example demonstrating how, in some cases, a significant fall of salivary progesterone concentration (i.e. luteolysis) occurred after the administration of RU486. (b) An example demonstrating that in other cases no apparent fall in salivary progesterone concentration was observed after the administration of RU486. Reproduced with permission by the American Fertility Society from Li *et al.* (1988) *Fertil. Steril.*, **50**, 732.

DiZerega, 1983). Additionally, metoclopromide induced hyperprolactinaemia has been demonstrated to impair ovarian follicular maturation and luteal function (Kauppila *et al.*, 1982). Several mechanisms have been proposed to account for this observed relationship. The presence of specific receptors for prolactin in human ovaries as well as the corpus luteum of various animals and *in vitro* studies suggest that prolactin may directly regulate ovarian function (Fig. 9.9) (Behrman *et al.*, 1978; McNeilly *et al.*, 1980; Demura *et al.*, 1982; Alila *et al.*, 1987). Additionally, central effects are also possible. Prolactin interferes with the hypothalamic dopaminergic tone and opioid tone, thus possibly affecting the pattern of the pulsatile secretion of GnRH (Bression *et al.*, 1980; Quigley *et al.*, 1980; Sauder *et al.*, 1984). Although an association has been observed, hyperprolactinaemia has not been definitively demonstrated to directly cause luteal deficiency and the exact relationship between the two conditions remains to be defined. The issue has been even more complicated by reports which dispute the association between hyperprolactinaemia and luteal dysfunction (Sarris *et al.*, 1978).

Luteal deficiency has also been associated with exercise and decreases in body weight (see Table 9.6) (Shangold *et al.*, 1979; Vanrell & Balasch, 1983; Bullen *et al.*, 1985; Minakami *et al.*, 1985). Although the mechanisms are still not understood, this disturbance is suspected to be largely secondary to effects at the level of the hypothalamus and pituitary. Decreases in pulsatile secretion of GnRH by the hypothalamus with concomitant decreases in pituitary secretion of

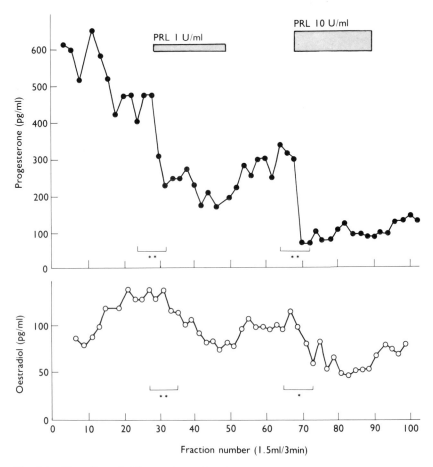

**Fig. 9.9.** The effect of different doses of prolactin on secretion of progesterone and oestrogen by *in vitro* perfused human ovaries. Reproduced by permission of the Endocrine Society©, from Demura *et al.* (1982) *J. Clin. Endocrinol. Metab.*, **54**, 1246.

gonadotrophins has been invoked as a possible mechanism of the ovulatory disturbances that have been noted to accompany high levels of exercise, as have increases of pituitary secretion of prolactin and cortisol. Increased baseline levels of endorphins have also been noted in athletes with ovulatory disorders and this may prove to play an important role in the pathophysiology of the disorder (Laatikainen *et al.*, 1986; Hohtari *et al.*, 1988). Schweiger and co-workers (1988) demonstrated that competitive athletes with cyclic menses demonstrated lower levels of luteal progesterone and oestradiol than non-athletic controls. This was evident despite similar levels of oestradiol seen in both groups during the follicular phase. In these patients, calorific intake correlated positively and subjective 'stress' correlated negatively with luteal progesterone levels.

Weight loss associated with calorific restriction has been associated with luteal deficiency in the absence of high levels of exercise. Some authors have attributed the diet-induced ovulatory disturbances to the resultant weight deficit, with its decreased contribution of adipose cells to oestrogen synthesis (Bates, 1985). Other data indicate that intermittent dieting with alternating losses and gains of c. 5% of body weight might be able to induce luteal disturbances without leading to weight deficit (Schweiger et al., 1987). Although it is difficult to separate the effects of long-term increases in calorific intake from the associated increases in body weight, this combination is undoubtedly the treatment of choice for luteal dysfunction secondary to low body weight. Low body weight women with infertility demonstrated a 62% incidence of short luteal phases prior to weight gain and an 8% incidence of short luteal phases after weight gain (Bates et al., 1982).

Obesity is also associated with a twofold increase in the incidence of infertility associated with ovulatory dysfunction (Green et al., 1988). This quoted incidence includes anovulation as well as more subtle ovulatory disorders. The association of obesity with luteal dysfunction specifically has not been thoroughly investigated, therefore, little is known with regard to the specific characteristics of this entity. One study of obese, oligomenorrhoeic, infertile women has demonstrated inadequate luteal progesterone secretion which was associated with low preovulatory FSH levels (Sherman & Korenman, 1974).

**Ovary**

As indicated previously, inadequate follicular stimulation by gonadotrophin has been suggested as a cause for luteal dysfunction. The basis for this inadequate stimulation may be inadequate blood levels of gonadotrophin or decreased ovarian responsiveness. Intrinsic deficiencies of gonadotrophin receptors within the ovary are probably rare causes of ovulatory dysfunction. The induction of these receptors is, however, dependent on hypothalamo/pituitary function, as previously discussed. Diminished ovarian responsiveness to gonadotrophins, may be seen in women with impending premature ovarian failure or age-related gonadal failure. This may result in ovulatory cycles with luteal insufficiency prior to cessation of menses (Sherman et al., 1976; Rosenberg et al., 1982).

Gonadotrophin receptors are linked to adenylyl cyclase by a guanine nucleotide binding protein (G protein). Membrane-associated G proteins are responsible for activating adenylyl cyclase to produce the second-messenger for gonadotrophin function — cAMP (see Fig. 3.2). Congenital deficiencies in these G proteins have been reported to result in anovulation despite normal gonadotrophin levels (Levine et al., 1983). The possibility that more minor deficiencies in G protein concentrations or defects in function may result in luteal dysfunction is a topic for speculation.

Numerous events in the ovary occur as a result of gonadotrophic stimulation. Oestradiol and progesterone produced as a consequence of such stimulation act at the hypothalamo/pituitary level to regulate follicular and luteal function. Deficient oestradiol and progesterone is usually considered a manifestation of follicular and luteal dysfunction rather than as a cause. Certain defects in steroid biosynthesis, however, are more appropriately considered as causal. Deficiency in production of LDL-cholesterol (as seen in the rare condition — abetalipoprotein- aemia) results in decreased availability and uptake of cholesterol by the corpus luteum and thus diminished substrate for steroidogenesis. The very low levels of progesterone in the luteal phase and during pregnancy associated with this condition, are however, compatible with implan- tation and normal fetal development (Figs 9.10 and 9.11) (Illingworth *et al.*, 1982; Parker *et al.*, 1986). This surprising finding supports the concept that luteal steroid levels typically associated with luteal-phase deficiency are merely a single manifestation of follicular and luteal function and that the associated subfertility may in fact be related to other important manifestations such as impaired ovum maturation. An alternative, but unproven explanation, would be that the low levels of oestradiol during pregnancy in this patient might have resulted in a progesterone to oestradiol ratio compatable with implantation.

In recent years, evidence has accumulated regarding a role for

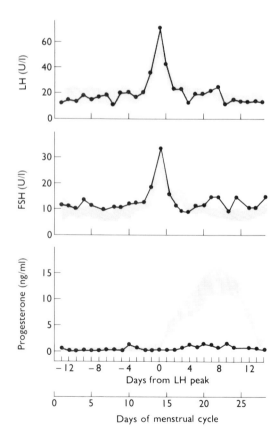

**Fig. 9.10.** Daily plasma levels of LH, FSH, and progesterone during the menstrual cycle of normally ovulating women (shaded area) and a woman with abetalipoproteinaemia (●). The data are expressed in relation to day of the LH peak and day of the menstrual cycle. (Modified from Carr *et al.*, 1982 Illingworth *et al.*, 1984 and Thorneycroft *et al.*, 1971. Reproduced with permission of the American Fertility Society from Carr *et al.* (1982) *Fertil. Steril.*, **38**, 303.

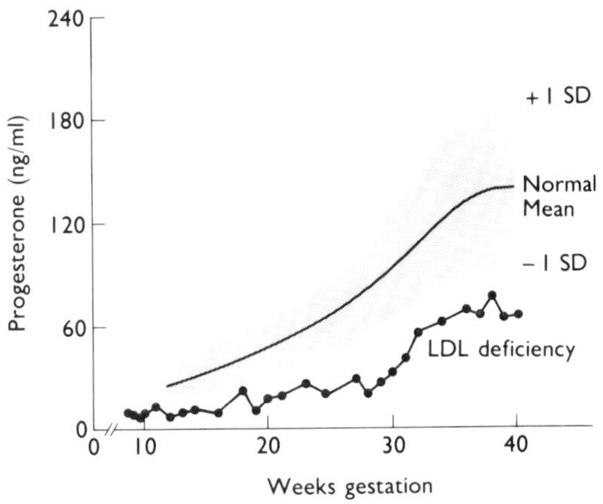

**Fig. 9.11.** Serum levels of progesterone throughout pregnancy in a woman with abetalipoprotenaemia. Values for the patient are indicated by the solid circles. Values for normal women during gestation (shaded area) are means ± SD. Adapted with permission from Parker *et al.* (1986) from *N. Engl. J. Med.*, **314**, 557.

prostaglandins in several functional processes in the ovary. Prostaglandin $F_{2\alpha}$ is essential for luteolysis in certain animal species (Horton & Poyser, 1976). There is accumulating evidence that prostaglandin $F_{2\alpha}$ is also important for regression of the corpus luteum in humans (Korda *et al.*, 1975; Patwardhan & Lanthier, 1984). Prostaglandin $E_2$ has been demonstrated to have luteotrophic effects on the human corpus luteum (Hahlin *et al.*, 1988). Both prostaglandins $F_{2\alpha}$ and $E_2$ are synthesized in the human corpus luteum (Challis *et al.*, 1976). Although the mechanism by which these substances affect luteal function is poorly understood, it is likely that processes which alter prostaglandin function in the ovary will in turn affect the corpus luteum.

### Endometrium (uterus)

Endometrial causes of luteal dysfunction have been infrequently cited. The uterus or endometrium in humans does not appear to directly affect the function of the corpus luteum (Doyle *et al.*, 1971). However, abnormal endometrial stromal development in women with normal luteal progesterone levels has been described (Keller *et al.*, 1979; Laatikainen *et al.*, 1983). This finding appears to result from a decrease in progesterone receptors. Attempts to quantify steroid receptor concentrations in the endometrium of patients with luteal inadequacy have led to conflicting findings. Some have reported decreased progesterone and oestrogen receptors in women with biopsy-diagnosed luteal phase deficiency (Levy *et al.*, 1980; Gautray *et al.*, 1981; Spirtos *et al.*, 1985). Others have failed to find significant alterations in endometrial progesterone receptor concentration in women with luteal phase defects (Table 9.7) (McRae *et al.*, 1984). One other study of endometrial steroid receptors in women with biopsy-confirmed luteal insufficiency revealed significantly increased progesterone receptor concentrations (Saracoglu *et al.*, 1985). This increase was postulated to

**Table 9.7.** Normal and inadequate luteal-phase blood levels of progesterone (P), receptors, and oestrogen receptors

|  | Normal luteal phase | Inadequate luteal phase |
|---|---|---|
| Blood P (ng/ml) | $25.88 \pm 8.63$ (19–23) | $14.44 \pm 3.98$ ($P = 0.018$) |
| P receptors (fmol/mg DNA) | $3808 \pm 2107$ | $2905 \pm 1764$ ($P = 0.174$) |
| Oestrogen receptors (fmol/mg DNA) | $463 \pm 357$ | $468 \pm 515$ ($P = 0.7$) |

Reproduced by permission of the American Fertility Society, McRae, M., Blasco, L. & Lyttle, C. (1984) *Fertil. Steril.*, **42**, 58–63.

represent an appropriate endometrial response to low serum progesterone levels. As previous studies have shown, progesterone will decrease its own receptor along with the oestrogen receptor (Bayard *et al.*, 1978).

The septate uterus has also been associated with luteal inadequacy. It has been suggested that the response of the endometrium overlying a uterine septum is analogous to that of the lower uterine segment where vascularity is less and the endometrial development lags behind that of the fundus. Medical treatment of the septate uterus with progesterone suppositories without surgical therapy resulted in term pregnancies in 60% of patients (Jones & Wheeless, 1969).

## Association with ovulation induction

The recent availability of a number of medications capable of inducing ovulation has led to profound improvement in the management of infertility secondary to chronic anovulation. Unfortunately, ovulation induction generally yields pregnancy rates which are much lower than the corresponding ovulation rates. Aberrant luteal steroidogenesis has frequently been put forward as an explanation for this observed discrepancy. However, a more plausible explanation is that undertreatment of anovulatory cycles or incomplete correction of amenorrhoea results in luteal phase deficiency. Women with transient luteal phase defects which may occur during extensive exercising or anorexia develop luteal dysfunction prior to developing anovulatory cycles or total amenorrhoea. With weight gain or decreased exercise these women begin to experience ovulatory cycles (Fig. 9.12).

### Clomiphene citrate

Since Greenblatt (1961) first reported the use of the non-steroidal compound clomiphene citrate, it has been established as the drug of choice in ovulation induction. Clomiphene citrate is most commonly

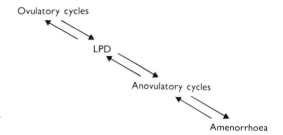

**Fig. 9.12.** Luteal-phase dysfunction (LPD). The development and transition of ovulatory cycles, LPD, anovulatory cycles and amenorrhoea in women.

employed to induce ovulation in patients with the diagnosis of polycystic ovarian syndrome (PCOS). Working as a competitive inhibitor of oestrogen action in the hypothalamus, clomiphene citrate serves to increase GnRH secretion which in turn leads to enhanced FSH secretion by the pituitary gland. Ovulation rates in properly selected patients often exceed 80%, whereas pregnancy rates are frequently less than 50% (Greenblatt, 1961; Kistner, 1965; MacLeod *et al.*, 1970; Garcia *et al.*, 1977). Spontaneous abortion rates following ovulation induction with clomiphene citrate may also be increased (MacLeod *et al.*, 1970).

Several mechanisms have been proposed to account for the low pregnancy rates observed with clomiphene therapy. Antioestrogenic effects on cervical mucus have been suggested as a cause of reduced pregnancy rates, as has luteinization of unruptured follicles (Lamb & Guderian, 1966; Garcia *et al.*, 1977). Van Hall and Mastboom reported a 65% incidence of short luteal phase (determined by basal body temperature) in clomiphene-treated patients (1969). Jones *et al.* (1970) reported on 70 women who responded to clomiphene with clinical evidence of ovulation. Thirty-two of these women had cycles with evidence of luteal dysfunction by endometrial biopsy. Most of these women had severe problems which occurred in repeated cycles and were not correctable by increasing the clomiphene dosage or the duration of the therapy. In these 32 women, 179 cycles led to three pregnancies all of which resulted in spontaneous miscarriage. In the 38 women with apparently normal luteal function, 130 treatment cycles led to 25 pregnancies of which 17 were carried to term. Garcia *et al.* (1977) observed delayed luteal endometrial maturation in one-half of 86 patients undergoing treatment with clomiphene citrate. On the other hand, Lamb *et al.* (1972) did not find an increased incidence of luteal-phase deficiency in anovulatory patients treated with clomiphene citrate. Luteal progesterone levels were normal or increased in patients who ovulated with clomiphene therapy (Wu, 1977).

Abnormal luteal steroidogenesis during clomiphene therapy might be a consequence either of incomplete correction of the underlying ovulatory defect (see Fig. 9.12), as discussed earlier, or may result from direct antioestrogenic effects on the ovary. Additionally, androgen secretion by the ovary may be increased with clomiphene therapy and this may impair follicular maturation and, consequently, lead to luteal dysfunction (Wu, 1977).

Investigations in rodents and non-human primates have shown synergism between FSH and oestrogen in the stimulation of follicular maturation (Ireland & Richards, 1978; DiZerega et al., 1981). In a study using relatively high-dose clomiphene to treat normally cyclic rhesus and cynamolgus monkeys, oestradiol levels were consistently reduced despite concurrent elevations in pituitary gonadotrophins (Marut & Hodgen, 1982). Direct effects of clomiphene on the ovary resulting in impaired folliculogenesis is suggested but unproven in humans.

Balasch et al. (1983) found a defective endometrial secretory pattern in 42.3% of patients after ovulation induction with clomiphene citrate and hCG, despite higher than normal luteal progesterone levels than fertile control subjects. This investigation would imply that clomiphene acts directly on the endometrium to impair responsiveness to gonadal steroids. Although direct antioestrogenic and progestational actions of clomiphene on endometrium has been suggested from in vivo studies, in vitro investigations suggest that clomiphene may actually exert an oestrogenic action on the endometrium (Ronnberg et al., 1985; Markiewicz et al., 1988).

Cook et al. (1984) found a 50% incidence of luteal-phase deficiency after clomiphene treatment of 10 ovulatory women. In a more recent study, administration of clomiphene citrate to 20 normally cyclic women with no prior evidence of luteal deficiency resulted in delayed endometrial histology in only one patient (Hecht et al., 1989). This would seem to imply that the most likely mechanism for the high incidence of luteal dysfunction seen during treatment of anovulation with clomiphene is an incomplete correction of the underlying ovulatory defect rather than effects of clomiphene on the endometrium or ovary.

### GnRH

The discovery of GnRH in 1971 led to its use in the treatment of infertility secondary to anovulation of hypothalamic origin. Initial attempts at using GnRH to induce ovulation were unsuccessful until the discovery that gonadotrophin secretion and hence follicular development was highly dependent on both the amplitude and frequency of administration. Administration of GnRH at too low or too high a pulse-frequency can lead to altered release of gonadotrophin, impaired ovarian stimulation and inadequate follicular maturation (Soules et al., 1987). Additionally, changes in frequency and amplitude of LH pulses have been observed throughout the human menstrual cycle (Reame et al., 1984; Soules et al., 1984). These changes, believed to result from steroid-induced changes in GnRH secretion in the hypothalamus, are likely to be important in the maintenance of normal luteal function (Soules et al., 1984).

Effects of GnRH administration on luteal function are therefore of concern when used to treat anovulatory infertility. Cessation of pulsatile GnRH administration after ovulation is followed by a defective luteal phase (Casas *et al.*, 1975; Nillius & Wide, 1975; Weinstein *et al.*, 1984). Many clinical protocols have been devised, attempting to achieve normal luteal function after induction of ovulation with GnRH. These include continuation of GnRH in a pulsatile fashion, administration of hCG every 3 to 4 days, or administration of exogenous progesterone (Berger & Zacur, 1985; Molloy *et al.*, 1985).

### Gonadotrophins

Since the induction of ovulation with exogenous human pituitary gonadotrophins was first achieved in 1958, the use of (hMG) together with hCG has become a successful form of ovulation induction therapy in anovulatory infertile women (Gemzell *et al.*, 1958). As with clomiphene citrate, treatment with hMG in women with anovulatory infertility usually results in a pregnancy rate which is much lower than the ovulation rate (Bergquist *et al.*, 1983). Additionally, fetal loss appears higher in gonadotrophin-induced pregnancies than in subsequent spontaneous pregnancies in the same patients (Lam *et al.*, 1989). Several studies have shown that the luteal phase of cycles stimulated with hMG can be shorter compared with spontaneous cycles (Townsent *et al.*, 1966; Olson *et al.*, 1983). Abnormal luteal function reflected in abnormal levels of circulating steroids during hMG/hCG cycles has been well described (Jones *et al.*, 1969; Cooke *et al.*, 1977). Investigation using a primate model has suggested that the type and length of gonadotrophin treatment employed for follicular stimulation greatly influences the property of the corpus luteum after ovulation (Stouffer *et al.*, 1986).

Although the exact mechanism responsible for luteal inadequacy in gonadotrophin-stimulated cycles remains to be defined, hyperprolactinaemia has been suggested as a possible aetiologic factor. Transient hyperprolactinaemia often occurs in patients undergoing ovarian superovulation with gonadotrophic hormones (Healy & Burger, 1983). This increase in prolactin production is believed to be secondary to increases in serum concentrations of oestrogens. Treatment with bromocriptine resulted in decreased prolactin levels in clomiphene-plus-FSH superovulated women. However, luteal serum progesterone concentrations were, unexpectedly, significantly reduced (Kauppila *et al.*, 1988). Adverse effects of the hyperprolactinaemia associated with gonadotrophic stimulation continues to remain a matter for speculation.

Interestingly, in unstimulated cycles the short luteal phase is usually associated with low levels of progesterone. In contrast, in hMG-stimulated cycles, progesterone secretion during the early luteal phase appears to be normal or exaggerated, typically followed by an unexpectedly rapid decline in the mid-luteal phase. High levels of oestradiol in the early luteal phase have also been noted in gonado-trophin stimulated cycles. This has been proposed to result in premature luteolysis (Laatikainen *et al.*, 1988). Some information is available which tends to support this hypothesis. Oestradiol administration has been demonstrated to be luteolytic *in vivo* (Johansson & Gemzell, 1971; Stouffer *et al.*, 1977). Additionally, oestradiol has been found to inhibit gonadotrophin-stimulated synthesis of progesterone in the corpus luteum *in vitro* (Thibier *et al.*, 1980). On the other hand, inhibition of luteal oestrogen formation by the administration of an aromatase in-hibitor did not alter luteal duration or mid-luteal phase progesterone production in spontaneously cyclic rhesus monkeys (Ellinwood & Resko, 1983).

## In vitro *fertilization/embryo transfer*

The establishment of successful pregnancies in women following the transfer of freeze-thawed embryos during the luteal phase of a normal non-stimulated cycle, where pregnancy previously failed to occur using multiple fresh embryos in a stimulated cycle, highlights the importance of recipient factors in achieving pregnancy through the use of *in vitro* fertilization (IVF) and embryo transfer (ET) (Trounson & Mohr, 1983). Corpus luteum dysfunction has been suggested as an explanation for the relatively low success rate seen with IVF/ET. Since IVF requires pharmacological hyperstimulation of the ovaries for optimal results, the aforementioned effects of clomiphene and/or hMG on luteal func-tion have been suggested as the cause of the luteal dysfunction. In addition, luteal function may be adversely affected by mechanical dis-ruption of the preovulatory follicle and loss of granulosa cells (future granulosa−lutein cells) during oocyte collection (Garcia *et al.*, 1981). This appears to be related to the vigorousness and number of aspir-ations. However, Kerin *et al.* (1981) noted normal luteal-phase hor-mone levels and no shortening of the luteal phase following follicular aspiration during unstimulated spontaneous cycles. Some have reported lower luteal progesterone levels in clomiphene-treated patients after follicular aspiration compared with stimulated patients not undergoing follicular aspiration (Vargyas *et al.*, 1986). The levels of progesterone in these women, however, remained significantly higher than in non-stimulated controls. Stress-induced hyperprolactinaemia or hyperpro-lactinaemia associated with general anaesthesia may also cause luteal dysfunction (Soules *et al.*, 1980). Transient hyperprolactinaemia is well documented in patients undergoing IVF/ET, as it is in gonadotrophin-stimulated cycles not connected with IVF. Current investigations do not, however, reveal any correlation of this finding with pregnancy-outcome (Denis *et al.*, 1989).

The hormonal aberrations observed in the luteal phase of stimulated cycles in patients undergoing IVF/ET are still a topic of some debate. Short luteal phases of 11 days or less were seen in 18 of 70 clomiphene/hMG/hCG-treated patients undergoing IVF (Laatikainen et al., 1988). Short cycle length has been associated with markedly reduced pregnancy rates in IVF cycles (Pampiglione et al., 1988). Huang et al. (1986) found no progesterone deficiency in patients treated with hMG/hCG for the purpose of IVF. The high oestradiol levels observed following oocyte recovery in stimulated cycles have been associated with a significant decrease in the pregnancy rate (Forman et al., 1987). The elevated levels of oestrogen have been hypothesized to inhibit implantation of the embryo. Premature luteolysis has also been suggested as a possible mechanism. Sterzik et al. (1988) examined luteal phase endometrial histology in 58 patients receiving superovulation therapy with either clomiphene/hCG, clomiphene/hMG/hCG, or hMG/hCG for IVF. The study group consisted of women who were not candidates for ET and endometrial histology was normal in only 30% of cases. The design of this study can be criticized, since it is likely that a majority of these women had received less than optimal ovarian stimulation.

Experiments in rodents indicate that implantation can be inhibited by relatively high serum oestradiol concentrations and that this effect can be overcome by concomitant administration of progesterone (Gidley-Baird et al., 1986). This hypothesis is supported by the data of Lejeune et al. (1986) who suggest that a high serum ratio of progesterone to oestradiol might have a favourable influence on the implantation process in human IVF.

## Association with endometriosis

Endometriosis is a condition in which functioning endometrium is found at sites outside the uterus. This is the most common diagnosis made in infertile women over the age of 25. It is clear that severe endometriosis can significantly alter tubal and ovarian anatomy and function, particularly if associated adhesions cause mechanical obstruction, fixation and diminished tubal motility. In the majority of cases of endometriosis, however, the degree of anatomical distortion fails to explain the associated infertility. Several studies have reported a higher than normal number of abortions in patients with endometriosis (Naples et al., 1981; Rock et al., 1981). Ovulatory disturbances and/or luteal deficiency have been postulated as mechanisms of infertility and recurrent pregnancy loss (Brosens et al., 1978; Naples et al., 1981; Balasch & Vanrell, 1987) in women with endometriosis.

Grant reported a 45% incidence of luteal-phase deficiency in infertile women with endometriosis (Grant, 1966). However, this investigation has been criticized for its use of basal body temperature for assessment of the date of ovulation used to interpret the endometrial biopsies. Kistner noted a high incidence of luteal dysfunction in patients following conservative surgery for endometriosis (1975). The mechanism by which endometriosis might bring about luteal dysfunction is not defined. Doody *et al.* (1988) found abnormal patterns of follicular growth in infertile women with endometriosis. Using linear-regression analysis of ultrasound findings, the authors detected slower and longer rates of follicular growth. Investigation by Tummon *et al.* (1988) demonstrated smaller follicles at LH surge, lower preovulatory oestradiol, and lower oestradiol at LH surge in infertile women with endometriosis. Another study detected lower follicular and luteal concentrations of LH receptors in women with endometriosis. However, the majority of studies were unable to detect a significant association of endometriosis and luteal dysfunction (Radwanska & Dmowski, 1981; Pittaway *et al.*, 1983; Balasch & Vanrell, 1985).

The use of danazol (a synthetic androgen) to treat endometriosis has become widespread since first described by Greenblatt *et al.* in 1971. Actions of danazol on the endometrium have been suggested to persist after discontinuation of the drug, thereby impairing normal response to gonadal steroid stimulation. Dmowski and Cohen (1978) reported increased fetal wastage in patients who conceived within 3 months after discontinuation of danazol. This, however, was not confirmed in a subsequent investigation (Daniell & Christianson, 1981). Additionally, a study by Balasch *et al.* (1986) of endometrial histology in 20 patients after discontinuation of therapy with danazol for endometriosis revealed abnormal secretory patterns in only three cases. This was the same incidence as that seen in the same patients prior to institution of danazol therapy.

## Diagnosis

Although luteal-phase deficiency is generally accepted to be a common cause of reproductive failure, the diagnosis of this disorder continues to be a source of great controversy. There appear to be no signs or symptoms which can be considered pathognomonic of luteal phase inadequacy. The mean age of patients with a defective corpus luteum does not differ significantly from the mean age of unselected infertility patients. Intermenstrual interval and the mean duration of menstruation falls within the normal range. Although some investigators have suggested that premenstrual spotting is a sign of luteal-phase inadequacy, this has not been confirmed by others (Jones, 1976; Tauber, 1978; Wentz, 1980). A number of methods have been employed in an attempt to identify abnormal luteal function and are described below. Each method has its own rationale and serves to identify overlapping, yet distinct ovulatory disorders.

## Basal body temperature

The correlation between changes in basal body temperature and events in the menstrual cycle was first recognized in 1904 (Table 9.8) Rubenstein in 1940 correlated ovulation with increase in basal body temperature. The dependence of the higher level of temperature in the later part of the menstrual cycle on progesterone secretion by the corpus luteum was demonstrated in 1948. Various authors have demonstrated that the rise in temperature coincides with the appearance of secretory changes in the endometrium. Buxton and Engle (1950) attempted to further define the temporal relationship between rise in basal body temperature and the age of the corpus luteum. They operated on 18 patients on the day of their temperature rise and found a large variation in the stage of maturity of the corpora lutea. Six patients had no definite evidence of ovulation, two corpora lutea appeared to be less than 12 h postovulatory, four appeared c. 24 h old, and two c. 36 h beyond ovulation. Two of the corpora lutea appeared to be 48 h old and the remaining two appeared to be 72 h old.

A study of basal body temperature graphs in 1134 menstrual cycles by Marshall (1963) demonstrated a biphasic response in 1088 with a mean of 13 days between temperature rise and initiation of menses. Other studies have suggested that a significant rise in basal body temperature occurs when the circulating level of progesterone surpasses 2.5 to 4 ng/ml (7.6−12.7 nmol/l) (Ross *et al.*, 1970; Moghissi *et al.*, 1972). Monophasic basal body temperature has, however, been identified in patients with normal luteal plasma progesterone and urinary oestrogen levels (Johansson *et al.*, 1972). Interestingly, up to 20% or more of ovulatory cycles may demonstrate no biphasic temperature

**Table 9.8.** Historical development of the relationship of basal body temperature (BBT) and ovulation

| Author | Year | Observations |
|---|---|---|
| Van de Velde | 1904 | Cyclic change in BBT during menstrual cycle |
| Van de Velde | 1930 | Temperature rise in function of corpus luteum |
| Rubenstein | 1940 | Correlation of ovulation with shift of BBT |
| Palmer | 1942 | Lack of cyclicity in BBT in non-ovulatory females |
| Davis & Fugo | 1948 | Demonstrated thermogenic property of progesterone |
| Palmer | 1949 | Correlation of high temperature phase and presence of secretory endometrium |
| Israel & Schneller | 1950 | Demonstration of thermogenic property of progesterone and correlation of temperature rise and ovulation with endometrial biopsy |
| Zuspan & Rao | 1974 | Progesterone-induced release of norepinephrine as the basic mechanism for the thermogenesis |

Adapted with permission from the American Fertility Society, Rosenfeld, D.L. & Garcia, C.R. (1976) *Fertil. Steril.*, **27**, 1256.

pattern (Moghissi, 1976; Bauman, 1981). Moreover, the mere presence of a biphasic basal body temperature does not establish normal luteal function. Ross *et al.* (1970) reported a rise in the basal body temperature with progesterone levels of 2.5 ng/ml (7.6 nmol/l) but concluded that 5 ng/ml (15.9 nmol/l) represented the lower limits of normal in the mid-luteal phase. Additionally, despite widespread use of basal body temperature charts to evaluate luteal-phase duration this test appears to be too insensitive to accurately determine the day of ovulation (Downs & Gibson, 1983).

Notwithstanding these reservations, both the apparent length of the luteal phase according to the basal body temperature and a slow rate of rise in the basal body temperature following ovulation (the so-called 'staircase effect') have been suggested as criteria for the diagnosis of luteal-phase deficiency (Andrews, 1979; Downs & Gibson, 1983). Jones suggested that a temperature rise of less than 0.8°F or an elevation lasting less than 10 days was indicative of luteal deficiency (Jones, 1949). Basal body temperature charts were indicative of luteal-phase defects in 13 of 16 (81%) patients documented to have luteal deficiency on the basis of two late luteal phase endometrial biopsies (Soules, 1977).

In summary, the basal body temperature graph is of limited use in making or confirming the diagnosis of luteal phase deficiency. The main value of the basal body temperature graph in patients suspected of having luteal dysfunction is to confirm the diagnosis of a short luteal phase, as discussed earlier.

## Endometrial biopsy

The endometrial biopsy has been hailed as the most reliable and practical means for the evaluation of luteal defects. Cyclic changes in the endometrium were observed through histologic examination as early as 1908 (Hitschmann & Adler, 1908). The differentiation and function of the endometrium were soon recognized to be very closely dependent on the production of gonadal steroids. Endometrial maturation occurs in such a manner that biopsies can be staged using only routine staining and light microscopy (Rock & Bartlett, 1937).

In a publication based upon the examination of *c.* 8000 endometrial biopsies, Noyes and Hertig (1950) presented a detailed description of the morphological features of human endometrium during the normal menstrual cycle and described a scheme for classifying the endometrium relative to an ideal 28-day cycle (Table 9.9 and Fig. 9.13) (see also Shangold *et al.*, 1983). These histological dating criteria have been employed clinically for more than 35 years. According to this method, ovulation occurs on cycle-day 14. On cycle-day 16, glycogen begins to accumulate in the basal portion of the glandular epithelium, and some of the nuclei appear to be displaced into the mid-portion of the cells,

**Table 9.9.** Criteria for dating the endometrium

| Day | Criteria |
|-----|----------|
| 15 | Vacuoles occasional (interval) |
| 16 | Vacuoles irregular |
| 17 | Vacuoles in picket-fence formation |
| 18 | Vacuoles above and below nuclei |
| 19 | Secretion (minimal) |
| 20 | Secretion (marked) |
| 21 | Oedema (minimal) |
| 22 | Oedema (marked) |
| 23 | Condensation around vessels (minimal) |
| 24 | Condensation around vessels (marked) |
| 25 | Decidua subcapsular |
| 26 | Decidua diffuse |
| 27 | Infiltration of leukocytes |
| 28 | Infiltration, clumping, and necrosis |

Reproduced by permission of the American Fertility Society, Shangold, M. *et al.* (1983) *Fertil. Steril.*, **40**, 627–30.

resulting in a pseudostratified configuration. In formalin-fixed material, the glycogen is solubilized, leaving large vacuoles in the base of the cells. This widespread subnuclear vacuolation of the glandular epithelium is taken as evidence that a functional, progesterone-producing corpus luteum has been formed. On Day 17 the glands become more tortuous and dilated. By Day 18, the vacuoles in the epithelium are smaller and are often located beside the nuclei. At this time the glycogen is present in the apex of the cells. On Day 19 intraluminal secretion is apparent and pseudostratification and vacuolation have nearly disappeared. On cycle-days 21 and 22, the endometrial stroma becomes oedematous. On Day 23, stromal cells surrounding the spiral arterioles begin to enlarge. Stromal mitoses become apparent. Day 24 is characterized by the appearance of predecidual cells around the spiral arterioles and numerous stromal mitoses. By Day 25, predecidua begins to differentiate under the surface epithelium. By Day 27, the upper portion of the endometrial stroma appears as a solid sheet of well-developed decidual-like cells. Differentiation of the decidua is accompanied by a marked increase in lymphocytic infiltration. Menstruation occurs on day 28.

More recently, Li *et al.* (1988) have used morphometric analysis in conjunction with multiple regression analysis to carry out histological dating of the endometrium. This method has been proposed to be more accurate than the traditional criteria set forth by Noyes and Hertig (1950).

Although the best criteria for dating the endometrium are topics for debate, in theory, the evaluation of endometrial histology in a patient with luteal insufficiency should serve as a bioassay — reflecting the quantity and duration of gonadal steroid production as well as the

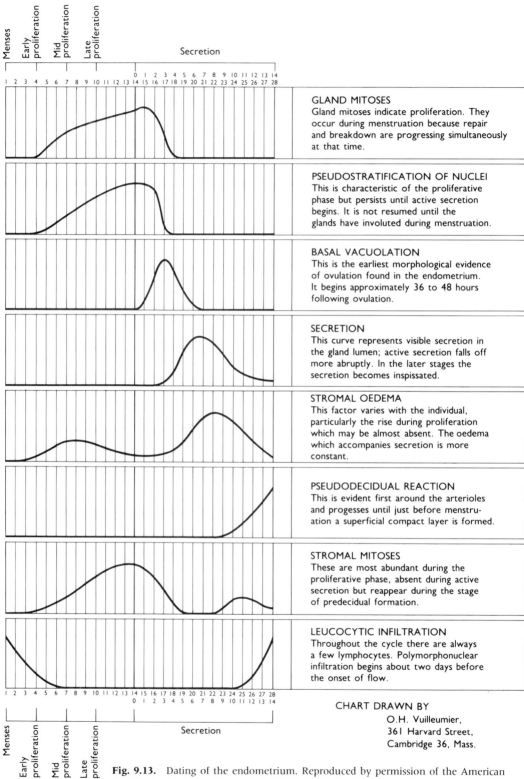

**Fig. 9.13.** Dating of the endometrium. Reproduced by permission of the American Fertility Society from Noyes *et al.* (1950) *Fertil. Steril.*, **1**, 3.

responsiveness of the endometrium to these hormones. Patients with luteal dysfunction will demonstrate delayed endometrial maturation. The optimum time to take the endometrial biopsy is debated. Some have proposed that the endometrium should be sampled at the time of expected implantation or c. 7 days after ovulation (Gautray et al., 1981). This is also the time of expected maximal luteal activity. Others have advocated biopsy immediately before the expected start of menstruation. The latter argue that this timing allows a more sensitive measure of cumulative stimulation of the endometrium by progesterone. It has also been claimed that dating of the endometrium is more accurate if performed later in the luteal phase. However, there is evidence that intraobserver variation at this time is no less than at any other point in the luteal phase (Scott et al., 1988).

The endometrial biopsy should be taken from two different locations high in the uterine fundus and should represent the full thickness of the endometrium. Endometrium from the lower uterine segment does not predictably respond to hormonal stimulation. It has been proposed that the histological dating of the specimen should reflect the most 'advanced' portion or feature rather than the average feature (Noyes & Hertig, 1950). Gillam has proposed that if 80% or more of the endometrium appears immature, this should be considered abnormal regardless of the normality of the remaining glands and stroma (1955).

Gillam (1955) and Witten and Martin (1985) emphasized that there were two distinct endometrial histology patterns associated with luteal deficiency and suggested that each should be treated differently. Most other investigators have suspected a luteal phase defect only if a biopsy demonstrates a lag in endometrial development of greater than 2 days relative to the time elapsed since ovulation. Typically, the time postovulation is calculated from the date of onset of the subsequent menstrual period (Jones, 1976). Iatrogenically shortened cycles have been suggested to be a consequence of postbiopsy bleeding although these have not been seen by all investigators (Noyes & Hertig, 1950; Noyes & Haman, 1953; Rosenfeld & Garcia, 1976). For this and other theoretical reasons, several investigators have proposed measurement of LH peak or shift in basal body temperature as a point of reference (Tredway et al., 1973; Koninckx et al., 1977; Johannisson et al., 1987). A significant rise in serum LH precedes the day of ovulation by c. 1 day (Tredway et al., 1973; Yussman & Taymor, 1973). Ultrasound assessment of the day of ovulation has been suggested to provide the most accurate correlation with endometrial dating (Shoupe et al., 1989).

The diagnosis of luteal dysfunction should not be made based on a single out-of-phase biopsy. For the luteal-phase endometrial defect to be a significant finding in the investigation of patients with impaired reproductive capacity, it must be made repeatedly. Thus, the diagnosis must be confirmed by a similarly timed biopsy in a subsequent cycle.

Despite its widespread acceptance, numerous criticisms have been put forth of endometrial biopsy as a means of evaluating suspected luteal defect. Results of an investigation in which 240 women underwent two, and 60 women three, endometrial biopsies revealed a highly significant tendency for change in the initial result (normal or abnormal) when two or more biopsies were performed (Balasch *et al.*, 1985). A number of patients with the histological finding of endometrial inadequacy become pregnant and eventually carried to term without treatment (Murthy *et al.*, 1970; Shepard & Senturia, 1977; Driessen *et al.*, 1980; Balasch *et al.*, 1986). These data suggest that endometrial defects are often sporadic. It has therefore been recommended that a third biopsy be performed in patients for whom divergent findings are made on two endometrial specimens, but this increases the cost and discomfort to the patient. Disagreement by different observers in dating the same biopsy further calls into question the accuracy of endometrial dating. Of 1007 biopsies dated by both Noyes and Hamon (1953), the two investigators agreed exactly on the dating in only 29%; dating was more than 2 days discordant in 19% of the biopsies. Scott *et al.* (1988) demonstrated that intraobserver variation would cause a change in diagnosis and management in 39% of all patients when the biopsy was analysed by a second pathologist.

Data put forth by Davis *et al.* (1989) raise further questions about the value of endometrial biopsy. They detected luteal phase deficiency (greater than a 2-day lag in endometrial histology) in 31.4% of biopsies done on fertile women. Recurrent endometrial lags were noted in two of 30 (7%) sequential pairs of biopsies performed in these same women. This information would suggest that the finding of histological endometrial immaturity, even in paired biopsies, may be a normal biological variant rather than a disease entity. Whether there are, in reality, two subpopulations of infertile patients, one with out-of-phase endometrium in every cycle and one with sporadic out-of-phase endometrium, remains to be determined. Tredway *et al.* (1973) have suggested that qualitative morphological differences between the glands and the stroma are more indicative of an inadequate luteal phase than the use of the standard criteria of a greater than 2-day lag in endometrial maturation.

Notwithstanding the diagnostic value of endometrial biopsy, some authors have objected to its use solely on the basis of the possible complications of this procedure. Early pregnancy can be inadvertently interrupted by the performance of endometrial biopsy attempting to diagnose the cause of infertility (Table 9.10) (Karow *et al.*, 1971). This appears, however, to be a rare complication of the procedure. However various authors have reported fetal wastage rates of up to 67% after biopsies taken in a conception cycle. More recent investigation by Sulewski *et al.* (1980) demonstrated that the incidence of abortion among 18 women who had undergone biopsy during a conception

**Table 9.10.** Summary of the literature of outcome of endometrial biopsy in the cycle of conception

| Author | No. of Cases | Term delivery | Premature | Abortion | Ectopic | % Fetal wastage | Still pregnant | Lost to follow-up |
|---|---|---|---|---|---|---|---|---|
| Mischell | 3 | 1 | | | 2 | 67 | | |
| Sturgis | 10 | 7 | | 1 | 2 | 33 | | |
| Simons | 31 | 31 | | | | 0 | | |
| Jackson | 29 | 17 | 1 | 3 | | 10 | 8 | |
| Hamblen | 10 | 9 | | 1 | | 11 | | |
| Hartman | 5 | 4 | | | | 0 | | 1 |
| Wilson | 14 | 11 | | | | 0 | 2 | 1 |
| Buxton | 22 | 20 | | 2 | | 9 | | |
| Karow | 28 | 22 | 3 | 2 | 1 | 11 | | |
| Arronet | 23 | 13 | | 7 | | 30 | 1 | 2 |
| Wentz | 10 | 9 | | | 1 | 10 | | |
| Wentz | 54 | 40 | | 9 | 2 | 20 | | |
| Rosenfeld | 23 | 14 | | 7 | | 30 | | |
| Jackobson | 7 | 6 | | 1 | | 14 | | |
| Balasch | 22 | 14 | | 7 | | 32 | | |

Adapted in part from Karow (1971) *Fertil. Steril.*, **22**, 482–95.

cycle did not differ from the incidence of spontaneous abortion among infertile women who did not undergo biopsy during a conception cycle. In spite of a lack of evidence of a significant relationship between endometrial biopsy and pregnancy loss, many investigators have proposed that this theoretical complication can be avoided altogether by the use of barrier methods of contraception during the cycle of biopsy.

Other investigators have reported other possible complications associated with biopsy of the endometrium for evaluation of infertility. Davidson *et al.*, (1987) in a retrospective analysis of 774 endometrial biopsies, noted excessive vaginal bleeding (five patients), fever (four patients), excessive pain (two patients), vasovagal reaction (two patients), and uterine perforation (two patients). Uterine contractions sufficient to preclude patient acceptance of a second endometrial biopsy are frequently encountered. Thirty-one of 52 patients considered a second biopsy unacceptable when the standard Novak curette was used to perform the procedure. This complication was reduced markedly with the use of a smaller disposable plastic curette (Check *et al.*, 1989).

Biochemical evaluation of endometrial response has been suggested to offer advantages over morphologic evaluation of the endometrium (Daly *et al.*, 1981; Ying *et al.*, 1985). Antibodies have been generated to various components of endometrial epithelial cell surfaces as well as secretory products and these may ultimately prove valuable in diagnosing luteal insufficiency (Aplin & Self, 1987; Self *et al.*, 1989).

## Progesterone determination

The development of techniques for accurate quantitation of circulating progesterone concentrations has brought about numerous attempts to correlate blood progesterone levels with luteal function (Yoshimi & Lipsett, 1968; Johansson, 1969). Israel *et al.* (1972) suggested that progesterone levels above 3 ng/ml (*c.* 10 nmol/l) were always accompanied by a secretory endometrium and, thus, progesterone assay was as accurate as endometrial biopsy in the indication of ovulation. This work was quickly confirmed by other investigators utilizing different methods of progesterone quantitation (Nadji *et al.*, 1975). With the availability of radioimmunoassay for measurements of progesterone in serum, it has been found that the progesterone pattern in infertile but otherwise normally menstruating women is often altered (Radwanska & Swyer, 1974; Dodson *et al.*, 1975; Brosens *et al*; 1978; Lenton *et al.*, 1978). The results of endometrial biopsies correlate well with daily serum progesterone assays (Fig. 9.14) (Jones & Wentz, 1974; McNeely & Soules, 1988). Serial progesterone determinations throughout the luteal phase therefore provide an accurate assessment of luteal function, but expense and inconvenience restrict the utility of this method (Andrews, 1979).

Single mid-luteal progesterone determinations have been advocated for the assessment of luteal function (Radwanska *et al.*, 1981). Radwanska and Swyer (1974) demonstrated that mid-luteal progesterone levels that were <10 ng/ml (*c.* 32 nmol/l) were observed in 60% of women with otherwise unexplained infertility. Only 10% of patients identified to have a non-hormonal cause of infertility were found to have mid-luteal progesterone values below that level. They therefore inferred that progesterone at levels of less than 10 ng/ml would identify inadequate luteal function. Hensleigh and Fainstat (1979) also suggested that the more stringent single values of 10 ng/ml in the mid-luteal phase or 15 ng/ml (*c.* 48 nmol/l) in the first trimester might be useful

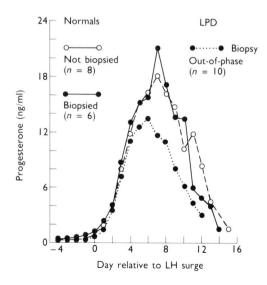

**Fig. 9.14.** Correlation of luteal-phase serum progesterone levels with histological assessment of endometrial development. Mean progesterone levels are illustrated for three groups of women: normal women (*n* = 8); normal women (*n* = 6) with in-phase endometrial biopsies; and infertile women (*n* = 10) with out-of-phase endometrial biopsies. The integrated progesterone concentration for the latter group was significantly decreased. Reproduced with permission of the American Fertility Society, McNeely & Soules (1988) *Fertil. Steril.*, **50**, 1.

in identifying luteal deficiency in a group of patients with recurrent abortion.

Plasma progesterone concentrations, however, reflect the episodic nature of steroid release from the corpus luteum (see Fig. 9.15) (Filicori *et al.*, 1984; Healy *et al.*, 1984; Veldhuis *et al.*, 1988). Large fluctuations (from 2.3 to 40.1 ng/ml; *c.* 6 to 128 nmol/l) have been reported in measurements obtained within a single day (Filicori *et al.*, 1984). This fact tends to diminish the value of a single progesterone determination. Several investigators have demonstrated a lack of correlation between endometrial development and single mid-luteal progesterone values in individual patients (Cooke *et al.*, 1972; Annos *et al.*, 1980; Rosenfeld *et al.*, 1980; Cumming *et al.*, 1985). Daya and co-workers (1988) demonstrated a lower mean luteal progesterone level in patients with recurrent abortion and luteal-phase deficiency diagnosed by endometrial histology (20 nmol/l) compared with controls (31 nmol/l). The range of values obtained, however, did not differ between the two groups (2–95 nmol/l). This group of investigators found 21 nmol/l to be the optimal discriminatory level of progesterone for the prediction of endometrial retardation. This cut-off level remains somewhat inaccurate

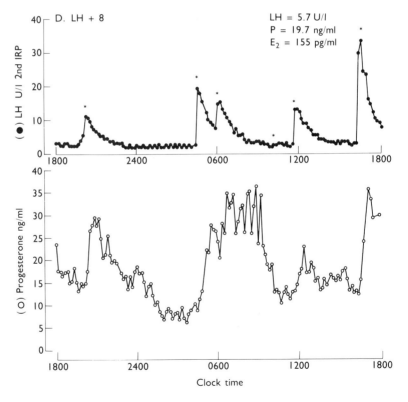

**Fig. 9.15.** The episodic secretion of LH (a) and progesterone (b) during the mid-luteal phase of a woman's menstrual cycle. Note the coincidence of peak progesterone values and pulses of LH(*). Reproduced with permission of the American Society for Clinical Investigation from Filicori *et al.* (1984) *J. Clin. Invest.*, **73**, 1638.

as a diagnostic test with a 70% sensitivity and a 71% specificity (Daya & Ward, 1988).

Abraham *et al.* (1974) reported that several patients with abnormal cycles had isolated luteal progesterone levels greater than 3 ng/ml (*c.* 10 nmol/l) and other 'normal' patients had isolated levels lower than 3 ng/ml. They advocated obtaining three blood samples from 4 to 11 days before the onset of menses. Using this method, they observed that in normal cycles, the sum of these three determinations was over 15 ng/ml (*c.* 48 nmol/l) whereas the total value in abnormal cycles fell below 15 ng/ml. Balasch *et al.* (1982b), however, studied 200 infertile women whose three progesterone estimations totalled over 15 ng/ml when taken from 4 to 11 days preceding menstruation. They found a 21.5% incidence of defective endometria following biopsies in two separate cycles. No difference was found when plasma progesterone concentrations in this group were compared with those of the remaining 157 infertile patients with normal endometrium.

Some investigators have suggested that the diagnosis of luteal phase dysfunction should be made by the simultaneous evaluation of an endometrial biopsy and a single mid-luteal progesterone level (Rosenfeld & Garcia, 1976). Shepard and Senturia (1977) observed a lack of correlation between progesterone level and endometrial histology. In this study, endometrial retardation had no prognostic significance for future fertility (six of eight patients conceived without therapy). These investigators concluded that progesterone was superior to histological evaluation of the endometrium for evaluation of luteal function. This study can be criticized, however, for the use of only a single biopsy in each patient to evaluate the presence or absence of possible luteal dysfunction.

More recently, Wu and Minassian (1987) have advocated the use of an integrated luteal progesterone in the assessment of luteal function. They observed that the typical pattern of daily luteal phase progesterone level is similar to a sine curve. They calculated the area under the curve of individual cycles based on the length of the luteal phase and a single luteal blood sample. This value was compared with findings of endometrial histology. The authors propose that this is a more meaningful test than a single progesterone level. More studies are needed to confirm the utility of this method of analysing luteal function.

Urinary progesterone and urinary pregnanediol (the major urinary metabolite of progesterone) have been advocated as a substitute for analysis of plasma progesterone in the evaluation of corpus luteum function (Chattoraj *et al.*, 1976; Chatterton *et al.*, 1982). In theory, urinary measurements could obviate some of the error inherent in the estimation of a single point in time of rapidly fluctuating blood levels. Unfortunately, there is considerable variation among individuals in the proportion of progesterone that is metabolized and excreted in the urine intact or as pregnanediol. Fifteen to 77% of progesterone entering the peripheral circulation is found in urine, and approximately one-half of this is in the form of pregnanediol conjugates. Urinary pregnanediol is also derived from precursors other than progesterone such as pregnenolone. For these reasons, urinary measurements of progesterone or pregnanediol are not appropriate for detailed clinical assessment of luteal function.

More recently, attempts have been made to correlate salivary progesterone measurements to normal luteal function (Walker et al., 1984; Zorn et al., 1984; Finn et al., 1988). The sensitivity and specificity of this method of analysis as a screening test for luteal dysfunction remains to be determined.

## Ultrasound

Because follicular dysfunction is held to be a common cause of luteal dysfunction, attempts have been made to identify abnormalities of follicular development. Ultrasound has been used to identify subtle abnormalities of follicular growth or to document premature ovulation in patients whose aetiology of infertility was otherwise not apparent (Lewinthal et al., 1986). More recently ultrasonography has been performed to evaluate the pattern of follicular growth in patients with short luteal phases or biopsy-proven luteal inadequacy (Ying et al., 1987). Three distinct patterns of follicular growth were seen in both treated and untreated patients. Untreated patients demonstrated normal sized follicles (46%), small follicles (39%) and luteinized unruptured follicles (15%). Ultrasonography has been suggested as a means of predicting response to treatment in women who have luteal dysfunction documented by other methods (blood progesterone or endometrial biopsy). It has been reported that treatment with clomiphene is more likely to benefit those patients who demonstrate poorly developed (smaller) follicles. Treatment with progesterone on the other hand may be the appropriate therapy for women who demonstrate luteal deficiency in the face of apparently normal follicular development as assessed by ultrasonography.

Additionally, in recent years, ultrasound has become the method of choice for the diagnosis of LUFS, as discussed previously. Initially, LUFS was diagnosed at laparoscopy after presumed ovulation when ovulatory stigmata were observed to be absent (Marik & Hulka, 1978). This technique has the obvious disadvantages that surgery is required and that it must be precisely timed (Dmowski et al., 1980). Additionally, rapid reperitonealization of the stigma may lead to an overestimation of LUFS by as much as 50% (Lesorgen et al., 1984). As with endometrial retardation, it appears that LUFS can be a sporadic phenomenon as well as a recurrent problem resulting in impaired reproductive capacity. The diagnosis of LUFS, therefore, should be made only if it is observed in a subsequent cycle (Daly et al., 1985).

# Therapy

Definitive diagnosis of luteal deficiency is an absolute prerequisite to initiation of therapy. The couple should be investigated thoroughly for the presence of other factors which might be responsible for subfertility or early pregnancy wastage. After the diagnosis of luteal deficiency is made, effort should be made to determine the cause of the dysfunction and to identify associated defects in follicular development. Response to any form of therapy should be evaluated objectively to assess its efficacy. If endometrial biopsy was used to make the initial diagnosis of luteal dysfunction, this should be repeated in a subsequent treatment cycle to prove that the endometrial histology has been corrected by treatment. Likewise, if a serum progesterone determination(s) was utilized to make the diagnosis, it should be repeated during a treatment cycle to confirm the correction of the luteal phase deficiency. LUFS may be observed in *c.* 38% of patients with 'corrected' luteal dysfunction who do not conceive and this possibility should be investigated in treatment failures. How to treat luteal-phase defect is highly controversial. Many treatments have been employed without the benefit of clinical trials demonstrating improvement in reproductive capacity over untreated control patients.

## Progesterone

Soon after its purification in 1933, progesterone became widely used in the treatment of a variety of gynaecological disorders. Its use in the treatment of luteal-phase dysfunction has been advocated by numerous investigators. This mode of therapy seems most appropriate for the treatment of luteal defects caused primarily by decreased progesterone biosynthesis. Progesterone therapy might also be considered in an attempt to overcome diminished endometrial responsiveness, however, this appears to be a rare cause of luteal dysfunction and the efficacy of progesterone supplementation in the treatment of this condition remains speculative. Although it is generally agreed that progesterone plays a central role in luteal-phase physiology, if the cause of the defect is suspected to involve hypothalamic or pituitary dysfunction or disorders of follicular maturation, initial treatment might be more appropriately directed elsewhere.

Supplementation of early pregnancy progesterone with synthetic progestins for the treatment of threatened abortion has been a common practice despite evidence that no benefits are gained (Johanssen, 1970). For the treatment of progesterone deficiency in patients demonstrating a defective luteal phase, some have advocated the use of natural progesterone instead of synthetic agents. Some synthetic progestins including norethisterone, norgestrel, chlormadinone acetate and medroxyprogesterone acetate have been shown to have luteolytic properties when administered during the luteal phase of the menstrual cycle (Johansson, 1971). Dehydrogesterone, an orally active, weak, non-thermogenic gestagen has been employed for treatment of luteal deficiency and has been reported not to provoke luteolysis (Balasch et al., 1982a). More experience is needed with this agent, however, before it can be used routinely to treat luteal dysfunction.

When initiating treatment for a deficiency in progesterone production, the aim should be to maintain physiological blood levels via exogenous administration of supplemental progesterone. It is possible that higher dosages of progesterone might be required if the defect is primarily one of endometrial insensitivity.

Progesterone is readily absorbed following vaginal, rectal, or intramuscular administration (Fig. 9.16a−c) (Nillius & Johansson, 1971). Administration of 100 mg progesterone vaginally or rectally results in peak serum levels in the range usually encountered in the mid-luteal phase, i.e. means of 13.5 and 22.5 ng/ml (44 and 72 nmol/l), respectively. Within 24 h, however, plasma levels of 2 ng/ml (c. 6 nmol/l) or lower are encountered. Intramuscular injection of progesterone results in higher peak levels (geometric mean 68 ng/ml or 213 nmol/l) and prolonged therapeutic blood levels (Nillius & Johansson, 1971). Severe myositis has been reported following the administration of progesterone intramuscularly in the thigh (Phipps et al., 1988). It has been suggested that this complication can be avoided if injections are administered into the gluteal muscles rather than the thigh or deltoid muscle. Progesterone suppositories are not commercially available (in the USA) and must be prepared by the pharmacist (Table 9.11). The base used to prepare the suppositories significantly affects the rate of steroid absorption (Fig. 9.17) (Price et al., 1983).

Pregnancy rates following progesterone therapy are difficult to interpret since patient populations, diagnostic procedures, routes and dosages of administration and duration of treatment vary considerably between studies. Additionally, controlled studies with untreated patients are lacking.

Jones and Pourmand (1962) reported an 80% pregnancy rate in 15 patients given 12.5 mg progesterone every day intramuscularly 10 days premenstrually to treat primary infertility due to luteal-phase defects. Rosenberg et al. (1980) treated 32 patients with luteal-phase defects diagnosed by endometrial biopsy with 25 mg vaginal suppositories twice daily. A 70% conception and 54% term pregnancy rate was obtained. Wentz et al. (1984) reported 23 pregnancies in 54 women treated with progesterone suppositories for delayed endometrial development. Soules et al. (1977) reported a 50% cumulative pregnancy rate after a mean of 5 months of therapy with twice daily progesterone suppositories (25 mg) in 16 patients with luteal deficiency documented by endometrial biopsy.

Daya and co-workers (1988) reported a 19% miscarriage rate in

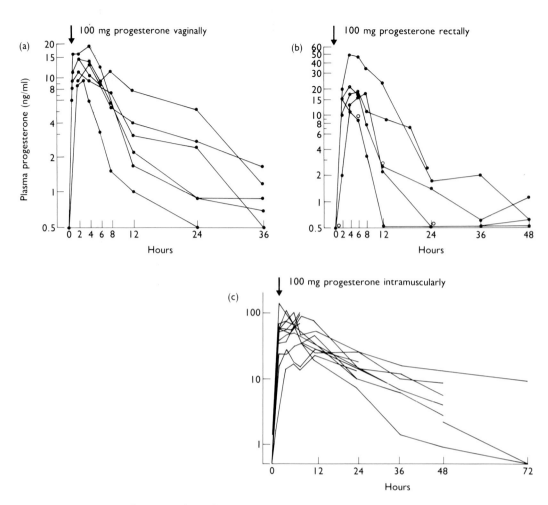

**Fig. 9.16.** Plasma levels of progesterone following 100 mg of progesterone given by (a) vaginal suppository; (b) rectal suppository or (c) by intramuscular injection. Adapted and reproduced by permission of the C.V. Mosby Co. from Nillius & Johansson (1971) *Am. J. Obstet. Gynecol.*, **110**, 470.

**Table 9.11.** Method for making progesterone suppositories

Progesterone suppositories for either vaginal or rectal administration can be made according to the following formula:

    progesterone powder (44 g);
    polyethylene glycol 400 (2096 g);
    polyethylene glycol 6000 (1392 g).

This gives a concentration of 25 mg in 1760 suppositories. Proportions must be altered according to mould size

Reproduced with permission from (Lippincott/Harper) Jones G.S. (1973) *Clin. Obstet. Gynecol.*, **16**, 255.

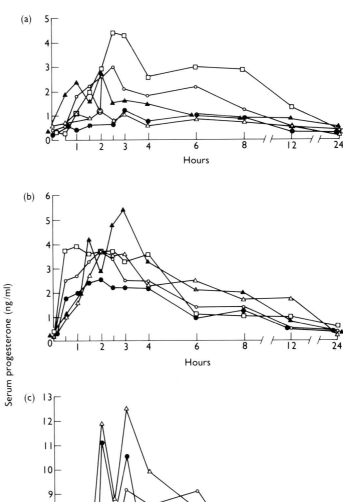

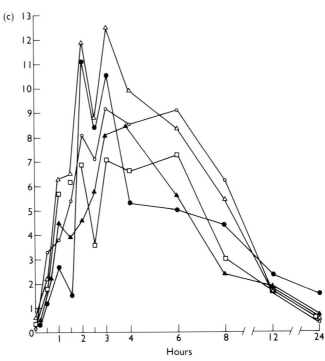

**Fig. 9.17.** Serum progesterone levels as a function of time following vaginal insertion of 25 mg of progesterone suppositories made with three different bases: (a) glycerinated gelation, (b) cocoa butter, and (c) polyethylene glycol. Reproduced with permission of the American Fertility Society from Price *et al.* (1983) *Fertil. Steril.,* **39**, 490 for (a).

patients with recurrent abortion and luteal-phase deficiency treated with 25 mg progesterone suppositories twice daily. Similarly, in a study by Tho *et al.* (1979) 91% of patients with luteal defect treated with progesterone carried pregnancies to term. Since all patients were treated in both of these studies, no data is available on the rate of spontaneous fetal loss that would have occurred in these same patients without treatment.

The possible teratogenicity of hormonal therapy for luteal deficiency has been a topic of much discussion. The US Food and Drug Administration (FDA) issued a warning advising of an increased risk of teratogenicity in infants born to women taking any progestational agents including natural progesterone itself, in the first trimester of pregnancy. Indications of adverse effects of hormone administration during pregnancy date back to the 1950s when androgens and synthetic progestins given therapeutically were reported to induce pseudohermaphroditism in female offspring. Subsequently, additional retrospective investigations reported increases in hypospadias, cardiovascular malformations and a syndrome manifested by multiple malformations including vertebral, anal, cardiac, tracheal, oesophageal, renal and limb defects (Nora & Nora, 1975; Heinonen *et al.*, 1977). A retrospective study of 40 children with dysmorphic anomalies revealed an antenatal exposure to sex steroids in nine (23%) cases (Lorber *et al.*, 1979). These studies included synthetic oestrogens and progestins as well as exposure to progesterone and conjugated oestrogens. Four of 16 patients with chromosomal anomalies also had histories of exogenous sex steroid exposure. More recently, retrospective and prospective studies indicate that the risk of fetal malformations is not increased with the use of natural progesterone or 17-hydroxyprogesterone (Matsunaga & Shiota, 1979; Ferencz *et al.*, 1980; Varma & Morsman, 1982; Michaelis *et al.*, 1983; Katz *et al.*, 1985; McDonough, 1985; Resseguie *et al.*, 1985; Rock *et al.*, 1985; Check *et al.*, 1986). Until the safety of the compound is established unequivocally, it is wise to clearly define for each woman the indication for treatment with progesterone and its potential risk (McDonough, 1985).

As previously suggested, although the aetiology of most cases of luteal dysfunction cannot be determined, it is likely that primary disorders of progesterone biosynthesis without associated defective function of the hypothalamus, pituitary or follicle is an uncommon cause of luteal dysfunction (Lenton *et al.*, 1984). Other authors have reported that luteal dysfunction characterized by endometrial inadequacy in spite of normal mid-luteal progesterone levels is far more frequent (86%) than luteal dysfunction associated with hormonal inadequacy (14%) (Balasch *et al.*, 1986a; Vanrell & Balasch, 1986). This may reflect the insensitivity of a serum progesterone level as a measure of hormonal function or a lack of specificity of endometrial biopsy as a test for luteal dysfunction. Alternatively, this might suggest end-organ insensitivity to normal levels of hormone production. Additionally, it is likely that the underlying cause of many of the cases in which hormonal inadequacy is a demonstrable finding, is aberrant folliculogenesis. In view of this, therapy aimed at maintaining physiological levels of blood progesterone may not be entirely appropriate. A more rational approach to treating luteal dysfunction must take into account possible causes of the apparent defect. If the diagnostic work-up is able to reveal an underlying cause, treatment is designed accordingly. If no cause can be demonstrated, empirical therapy might still be given. Unfortunately, published studies of treatment of luteal dysfunction, though frequently recognizing the heterogeneous nature of the disorder have infrequently sought to define the aetiology of the defect prior to initiation of therapy. The level of progesterone needed to initiate and maintain pregnancy is unclear, as discussed previously, since a woman with abetalipoproteinaemia is known to have had an uneventful pregnancy and a live-born infant in the presence of significantly reduced progesterone levels (see Fig. 9.11) (Parker *et al.*, 1986).

## Bromocriptine

As discussed previously, there appears to be an association between luteal deficiency and hyperprolactinaemia. Many investigators have reported correction of luteal dysfunction in women with hyperprolactinaemia treated with bromocriptine, 2.5 mg twice daily. However, oversuppression of prolactin to less than 5 ng/ml may be associated with luteal insufficiency. Del Pozo *et al.* (1979) reported improvement in luteal phase progesterone production and conception in five of eight women with luteal phase deficiencies and hyperprolactinaemia treated with bromocriptine. Andersen *et al.* (1979) described 12 hyperprolactinaemic, infertile patients with luteal deficiency in which treatment with bromocriptine resulted in normalization of prolactin secretion, increased progesterone levels and one pregnancy.

Check and Wu (1987) investigated the relative benefit of progesterone vs. bromocriptine for the treatment of infertility in hyperprolactinaemic women with luteal deficiency. All patients underwent assessment of patterns of follicular growth by ultrasound during spontaneous cycles. Two types of defects were observed: (1) luteal dysfunction associated with immature follicles, and (2) luteal dysfunction associated with mature follicles. Patients were randomized to progesterone vaginal suppositories or bromocriptine at dosages which corrected endometrial histology and follicular growth patterns. In the first group (women who demonstrated impaired follicular development), pregnancies were achieved in 15% of women treated with progesterone suppositories and 70% of women treated with bromocriptine. Patients who failed to conceive received the alternative therapy. Following this, 10 of 17 patients who failed progesterone therapy, conceived on bromocriptine while only one of six who failed bromocriptine therapy went on to conceive with progesterone. Results of treating the women in the second group (mature follicles) were markedly different. Seventy-seven per cent of women treated with progesterone conceived while only 17% treated with bromocriptine conceived. When conception failures were given the alternative treatment, only one of seven patients who failed progesterone therapy conceived with bromocriptine, while 20 of 25 women who failed bromocriptine conceived with progesterone. The value of bromocriptine for treatment of luteal deficiency in women with normal prolactin levels has not been demonstrated and, in fact, administration of bromocriptine to normally cyclic women results in diminished progesterone production in the luteal phase (Schulz et al., 1976; Saunders et al., 1979). Euprolactinaemic women with ovulatory disturbance and galactorrhoea have, however, been reported to respond to bromocriptine (Padilla et al., 1985) and this mode of therapy might be considered in this small subgroup of patients.

## Clomiphene citrate

First-line empirical therapy for luteal inadequacy in which the underlying defect is undefined has generally involved treatment with progesterone or clomiphene citrate. The rationale for the use of clomiphene citrate is the belief that luteal deficiency often results from aberrant follicular maturation. Clomiphene citrate acting at the level of the hypothalamus is capable of augmenting gonadotrophin release. It is used, therefore, as a pre-emptive measure designed to prevent the occurrence of luteal inadequacy through 'controlled hyperstimulation' of the early follicular phase (DiZerega & Hodgen, 1981). Hammond and Talbert (1982) reported 31 pregnancies in 69 patients treated with clomiphene for correction of infertility associated with low luteal progesterone levels. Quagliarello and Weiss (1979) reported correction of short luteal phase and pregnancy in seven of eight patients treated with clomiphene. Downs and Gibson (1983) reported a conception rate of 79% in a group of patients with a histological delay of 5 days or more after treatment with clomiphene. When the histological lag was less severe, the conception rate with this therapy was much lower (8.9%).

Murray et al. (1989), in a retrospective investigation, compared clomiphene citrate with vaginal progesterone for the treatment of infertile patients with luteal inadequacy diagnosed by impaired endometrial development on at least two occasions. The mean duration of infertility was more than 3 years in each group. Clomiphene was administered to a group of 34 patients at a dose of 50 mg orally on Days 2−6 of the cycle. This was increased to 100 mg if post-treatment biopsy continued to demonstrate a maturational lag. Four patients were excluded from the study because of failure to correct endometrial histology at this dose. Progesterone was administered to a second group of 35 patients at a maximum dose of 25 mg twice a day beginning on the third day after ovulation as estimated by basal body temperature. Four patients in the progesterone treatment group and three in the clomiphene group were lost to follow-up before completion of 1 year of therapy. Of the 31 remaining patients in the progesterone treatment group, all (100%) were pregnant by 1 year. Of the 27 remaining clomiphene-treated patients, 23 (81%) had conceived within the year. These differences were not statistically significant. Huang (1986), in a similarly designed study, also demonstrated no significant difference between the two modes of therapy, however, pregnancy rates were much lower. Normal endometrial biopsies were achieved in only 26 of 51 patients (51%) using progesterone and 25 of 56 patients (45%) using clomiphene citrate. Only 17 progesterone-treated patients and 13 clomiphene-treated patients conceived. The cause of the marked discrepancy in overall pregnancy rates between these two studies is not readily apparent.

Check and co-workers (1987) compared treatment with clomiphene or hMG versus treatment with progesterone in patients with luteal dysfunction, in whom sonographic investigation of patterns of follicular growth were made. Two groups were identified: (1) women with normal follicular growth, and (2) women with luteal dysfunction associated with immature follicles. Patients in the first group were randomized to treatment with progesterone suppositories or treatment with clomiphene or hMG. In this group of patients, 22 of 25 treated with progesterone suppositories conceived within 6 months (one miscarriage) while only three of 27 conceived in the group treated with clomiphene or hMG (two miscarriages). Cross-over studies during the next 6 months demonstrated that 21 of 26 women with pure luteal dysfunction who failed to have a successful pregnancy on treatment with ovulation inducing agents conceived on treatment with progesterone suppositories, and only two aborted. Patients with abnormal follicular growth patterns were randomized into three treatment groups: (1) ovulation inducing drugs, where seven of 10 conceived but four aborted, (2) progesterone suppositories only, where three of 12 conceived and none aborted, or (3) a combination of ovulation inducing drugs and luteal progesterone, where 14 of 16 conceived and only one aborted. Thirteen of 16 patients who failed single-agent therapy conceived when treated with both ovulation drugs and progesterone. These data strongly suggest that studies of follicular maturation may help determine the optimal form of treatment for luteal dysfunction.

## hMG

hMG has been reported to be successful in the treatment of luteal dysfunction even after failure to respond to clomiphene citrate (Caspi & Hirsch, 1971; Shapiro, 1972). Similarly, it has been reported that 'pure' FSH might also be of benefit in selected cases. However, extensive data on the use of FSH to treat this disorder are not presently available (Huang *et al.*, 1984). Because of the need for intensive monitoring of these patients and the risk of multiple pregnancy, treatment with gonadotrophin should be reserved for those who respond poorly to more 'conventional' therapy. Moreover, as previously indicated, gonadotrophin therapy is itself associated with a relatively high incidence of luteal-phase dysfunction.

## GnRH

GnRH given intravenously in a pulsatile fashion throughout the menstrual cycle has also been suggested to be effective in the correction of luteal defects (Phansey *et al.*, 1985). Larger studies are needed to confirm this and identify the subset of patients which might benefit most from this form of therapy. This method would seem most appropriate for treating ovulatory dysfunction with an hypothalamic aetiology and may not be applicable to other causes of luteal deficiency. Additionally, the expense of this method seems to preclude its use as a first-line treatment.

## Superovulation and IVF/ET

The benefit of pharmacological luteal support in gonadotrophin-stimulated cycles remains a topic of debate. Blumenfeld and Nahhas (1988) reported a marked benefit in women treated with hCG every 3 days during the luteal phase. Women undergoing ovulation induction with clomiphene/hCG, hMG/hCG or clomiphene/hMG/hCG, demonstrated higher luteal-phase plasma concentrations of progesterone, increased luteal phase duration, increased pregnancies per cycle and reduced pregnancy wastage. Messinis *et al.* (1988) found significantly increased pregnancy rates in hypo-oestrogenic anovulatory women who received luteal-phase hCG support in hMG/hCG ovulation-induction cycles, however, they observed no improvement in similarly treated normo-oestrogenic women.

Treatments directed at correcting the abnormal hormonal milieu in IVF cycles have included both progesterone supplementation and luteal-phase hCG administration. Leeton *et al.* (1985) demonstrated no improvement in pregnancy rate in women treated with progesterone beginning on Day 7 after oocyte collection. Other investigators have also found that giving progesterone supplementation of the periovulatory period, and/or of the luteal phase does not modify pregnancy rate following ET (Yovich *et al.*, 1985).

One novel approach has been the administration of progesterone 4 h before the administration of hCG (Mahadevan *et al.*, 1988). This resulted in significantly increased LH levels compared with similar patients given progesterone at the time of hCG. Progesterone levels tended to be higher at the time of embryo transfer in all patients who received progesterone (4 h before, or at the time of hCG) as compared with untreated controls. There was also a 50% decrease in the oestrogen to progesterone ratio. Clinical pregnancy rates, however, were identical in both groups.

Randomized trials of support with hCG following IVF–ET have also been conducted. In a study reported by O'Neill *et al.* (1985), 60 patients with high luteal-phase serum oestradiol levels were assigned randomly to receive either no support or hCG support during the luteal phase. Of the 25 patients who received no luteal-phase support, none became pregnant, whereas 14 of the 35 patients given hCG during the luteal phase achieved pregnancy. Another randomized study of 17 patients undergoing 20 cycles of IVF/ET compared the administration of daily progesterone (25 mg intramuscularly) with hCG (1500 IU intramuscularly) on Days 4, 7, 10 and 13 after the ovulatory dose of hCG (Nader *et al.*, 1988). In this small series, hCG administration resulted in significantly higher serum levels of both progesterone and oestradiol. All three clinical pregnancies occurred in the hCG treatment group despite there being a significantly lower progesterone to oestradiol ratio in this group.

Other studies have not demonstrated increases in pregnancy rates with luteal hCG administration. Buvat *et al.* (1988) reported that hCG (1500 IU) administered three times at 2-day intervals following ET resulted in significantly increased progesterone levels, progesterone/oestradiol ratios and luteal phase length. Pregnancy rates in the hCG treated group (15%) were not significantly different than the rate in the untreated group (14.5%). Mahadevan *et al.* (1985) also reported increases in luteal-phase duration but no improvement in pregnancy rates with low-dose luteal hCG administration in IVF cycles.

## Summary

Luteal-phase dysfunction is a common cause of reproductive failure in women. However, it remains unclear as to the true incidence of this disorder because of the difficulty in making a diagnosis. It has multiple causes and therapy, if appropriate, should be directed accordingly.

## Acknowledgements

This work was supported in part by Training Grant No. NIH 5-T32-HDO7190.

# References

Abraham, G.E., Maroulis, G.B. & Marshall, J.R. (1974) Evaluation of ovulation and corpus luteum function using measurements of plasma progesterone. *Obstet. Gynecol.*, **44**, 522–5.

Aksel, S. (1980) Sporadic and recurrent luteal phase defects in cyclic women: comparison with normal cycles. *Fertil. Steril.*, **33**, 372–7.

Alila, H.W., Rogo, K.O & Gombe, S. (1987) Effects of prolactin on steroidogenesis by human luteal cells in culture. *Fertil. Steril.*, **47**, 947–55.

Allen, W.M. & Wintersteiner, O. (1934) Crystalline progestin. *Science*, **80**, 190–1.

Andersen, A.N., Larsen, J.F., Eskidsen, P.C., Knoth, M., Micic, S., Svenstrup, B. & Nielsen, J. (1979) Treatment of hyperprolactinemic luteal insufficiency with bromocriptine. *Acta Obstet. Gynecol. Scand.*, **58**, 379–83.

Andrews, W.C. (1979) Luteal phase defects. *Fertil. Steril.*, **32**, 501–9.

Annos, T., Thompson, I.E. & Taymor, M.L. (1980) Luteal phase deficiency and infertility: difficulties encountered in diagnosis and treatment. *Obstet. Gynecol.*, **55**, 705–10.

Aplin, J.D. & Self, M.W. (1987) A monoclonal antibody to a cell surface determinant in human endometrial epithelium: stage-specific expression in the menstrual cycle. *Am. J. Obstet. Gynecol.*, 250–3.

Asch, R.H., Abou-Samra, M., Braunstein, G.D. & Pauerstein, C.J. (1982) Luteal function in hypophysectomized rhesus monkeys. *J. Clin. Endocrinol. Metab.*, **55**, 154–61.

Baird, D.T. & Fraser, I.S. (1974) Blood production and ovarian secretion rates of estradiol-17β and estrone in women throughout the menstrual cycle. *J. Clin. Endocrinol. Metab.*, **38**, 1009–17.

Balasch, J., Creus, M., Marquez, M., Burzaco, I. & Vanrell, J.A. (1986a) The significance of luteal phase deficiency on fertility: a diagnostic and therapeutic approach. *Hum. Reprod.*, **1**, 145–7.

Balasch, J. & Vanrell, J.A. (1985) Mild endometriosis and luteal function. *Int. J. Fertil.*, **30**, 4–6.

Balasch, J. & Vanrell, J.A. (1987) Corpus luteum insufficiency and fertility: a matter of controversy. *Hum. Reprod.*, **2**, 557–67.

Balasch, J., Vanrell, J.A., Creus, M., Marquez, M. & Gonzalez-Merlo, J. (1985) The endometrial biopsy for diagnosis of luteal phase deficiency. *Fertil. Steril.*, **44**, 699–701.

Balasch, J., Vanrell, J.A., Creus, M., Marquez, M. & Gonzalez-Merlo, J. (1986b) Early luteal function following danazol therapy for endometriosis. *Hum. Reprod.*, **1**, 291–3.

Balasch, J., Vanrell, J.A., Duran, M. & Gonzalez-Merlo, J. (1983) Luteal phase evaluation after clomiphene-chorionic gonadotrophin-induced ovulation. *Int. J. Fertil.*, **28**, 104–6.

Balasch, J., Vanrell, J.A., Marquez, M., Burzaco, I &

Gonzalez-Merlo, J. (1982a) Dehydrogesterone versus vaginal progesterone in the treatment of the endometrial luteal phase deficiency. *Fertil. Steril.*, **37**, 751–4.

Balasch, J., Vanrell, J.A., Marquez, M., Rivera, F. & Gonzalez-Merlo, J. (1982b) Luteal phase in infertility: problems of evaluation. *Int. J. Fertil.*, **27**, 60–2.

Balmaceda, J.P., Borghi, M.R., Coy, D.H., Schally, A.V. & Asch, R.H. (1983) Suppression of postovulatory gonadotrophin levels does not affect corpus luteum function in Rhesus monkeys. *J. Clin. Endocrinol. Metab.*, **57**, 866–8.

Bates, G.W. (1985) Body weight control practice as a cause of infertility. *Clin. Obstet. Gynecol.*, **28**, 632–44.

Bates, G.W., Bates, S.R. & Whitworth, N.S. (1982) Reproductive failure in women who practice weight control. *Fertil. Steril.*, **37**, 373–8.

Bauman, J.E. (1981) Basal body temperature: unreliable method of ovulation detection. *Fertil. Steril.*, **36**, 729–33.

Bayard, F., Damilano, S., Robel, P. & Baulieu, E.E. (1978) Cytoplasmic and nuclear estradiol and progesterone receptors in human endometrium. *J. Clin. Endocrinol. Metab.*, **46**, 635–48.

Behrman, H.R., Grinwich, D.L., Hichens, M. & MacDonald, G.J. (1978) Effect of hypophysectomy, prolactin, and prostaglandin $F_{2\alpha}$ on gonadotrophin binding *in vivo* and *in vitro* in the corpus luteum. *Endocrinology*, **103**, 349–57.

Berger, N.G. & Zacur, H.A. (1985) Exogenous progesterone for luteal support following gonadotrophin-releasing hormone ovulation induction: case report. *Fertil. Steril.*, **44**, 133–5.

Bergquist, C., Nillius, S.J. & Wide, L. (1983) Human gonadotrophin therapy. I. Serum estradiol and progesterone patterns during conceptual cycles. *Fertil. Steril.*, **39**, 761–5.

Blumenfeld, Z. & Nahhas, F. (1988) Luteal dysfunction in ovulation induction: the role of repetitive human chorionic gonadotrophin supplementation during the luteal phase. *Fertil. Steril.*, **50**, 403–7.

Bression, D., Brandi, A.M., Martres, M.P., Nousbaum, A., Cesselin, F., Racadot, J. & Peillon, F. (1980) Dopaminergic receptors in human prolactin-secreting adenomas: a quantitative study. *J. Clin. Endocrinol. Metab.*, **51**, 1037–43.

Brosens, I.A., Koninckx, P.R. & Corveleyn, P.A. (1978) A study of plasma progesterone, oestradiol-17β, prolactin and LH levels, and of the luteal phase appearance of the ovaries in patients with endometriosis and infertility. *Br. J. Obstet. Gynaecol.*, **85**, 246–50.

Bullen, B.A., Skrinar, G.S., Beitns, Z., von Mering, G., Turnbull, B.A. & McArthur, J.W. (1985) Induction of menstrual disorders by strenuous exercise in untrained women. *N. Engl. J. Med.*, **312**, 1349–53.

Buvat, J., Marcolin, G., Herbaut, J.C., Dehaene, J.L., Verbecq, P. & Fourlinnie, J.C. (1988) A randomized trial of human chorionic gonadotrophin support following in vitro fertilization and embryo transfer. *Fertil. Steril.*, **49**, 458–61.

Buxton, C.L. & Engle, E.T. (1950) A correlation between basal temperature, the appearance of the endometrium, and the appearance of the ovary. *Am. J. Obstet. Gynecol.*, **60**, 539–51.

Carr, B.R., MacDonald, P.C., & Simpson, E.R. (1982) The role of lipoproteins in the regulation of progesterone secretion by the human corpus luteum. *Fertil. Steril.*, **38**, 303–11.

Carr, B.R., Sadler, R.K., Rochelle, D.B., Stalmach, M.A., MacDonald, P.C. & Simpson, E.R. (1981) Plasma lipoprotein regulation of progesterone biosynthesis by human corpus luteum tissue in organ culture. *J. Clin. Endocrinol. Metab.*, **52**, 875–81.

Casas, P.R.F., Badano, A.R., Aparicio, N., Lencioni, L.J., Berli, R.R., Badano, H., Biccoca, C. *et al.* (1975) Luteinizing hormone-releasing hormone in the treatment of anovulatory infertility. *Fertil. Steril.*, **26**, 549–53.

Caspi, E. & Hirsch, H. (1971) Therapy of ovulatory sterility and corpus luteum insufficiency with human menopausal and chorionic gonadotrophins. *Isr. J. Med. Sci.*, **7**, 1040–5.

Challis, J.R.G., Calder, A.A., Dilley, S., Forster, C.S., Hillier, K., Hunter, D.J.S., MacKenzie, I.Z. & Thorburn, G.D. (1976) Production of prostaglandins E and $F_\alpha$ by corpora lutea, corpora albicantes and stroma from the human ovary. *J. Endocrinol.*, **68**, 401–8.

Chatterton, R.T. Jr., Haan, J.N., Jenco, J.M. & Cheesman, K.L. (1982) Radioimmunoassay of pregnanediol concentrations in early morning urine specimens for assessment of luteal function in women. *Fertil. Steril.*, **37**, 361–6.

Chattoraj, S.C., Rankin, J.S., Turner, A.K. & Lowe, E.W. (1976) Urinary progesterone as an index of ovulation and corpus luteal function. *J. Clin. Endocrinol. Metab.*, **43**, 1402–5.

Check, J.H., Chase, J.A., Nowroozi, K., Wu, C.H. & Chern, R. (1989) Clinical evaluation of the pipelle endometrial suction curette for timed endometrial biopsies. *J. Reprod. Med.*, **34**, 219–20.

Check, J.H., Nowroozi, K. & Wu, C.H. (1987) Ovulation-inducing drugs versus progesterone therapy for infertility in patients with luteal phase defects. *43rd Annual Meeting of the American Fertility Society.* (Abstr. P-297).

Check, J.H., Rankin, A. & Teichman, M. (1986) The risk of fetal anomalies as a result of progesterone therapy during pregnancy. *Fertil. Steril.*, **45**, 575–7.

Check, J.H. & Wu, C.H. (1987) Bromocriptine versus progesterone therapy for infertility related luteal phase defects in hyperprolactinemic patients. *43rd Annual Meeting of the American Fertility Society, Reno, NV.* (Abstr. P-151).

Cline, D.L. (1979) Unsuspected subclinical pregnancies in patients with luteal phase defects. *Am. J. Obstet. Gynecol.*, **134**, 438–44.

Cline, E.M., Randall, P.A. & Oliphant, G. (1977) Hormone-mediated oviductal influence on mouse embryo development. *Fertil. Steril.*, **28**, 766–71.

Cook C.L., Schroeder, J.A. Yussman, M.A. & Sanfilippo, J.S. (1984) Induction of luteal phase defect with clomiphene citrate. *Am. J. Obstet. Gynecol.*, **149**, 613–16.

Cooke, I.D., Lenton, E.A., Adams, M., Pearce, M.A., Fahmy, D. & Evans, C.R. (1977) Some clinical aspects of pituitary–ovarian relationships in women with ovulatory infertility. *J. Reprod. Fertil.*, **51**, 203–13.

Cooke, I.D., Morgan, C.A. & Parry T.E. (1972) Correlation of endometrial biopsy and plasma progesterone levels in infertile women. *Br. J. Obstet. Gynecol.*, **79**, 647–50.

Coulam, C.B., Hill, L.M. & Breckle, R. (1982) Ultrasonic evidence for luteinization of unruptured preovulatory follicles. *Fertil. Steril.*, **37**, 524–9.

Csapo, A.I., Pulkkinen, M.O., Ruttner, B., Sauvage, J.P. & Wiest, W.G. (1972) The significance of the human corpus luteum in pregnancy maintenance. *Am. J. Obstet. Gynecol.*, **112**, 1061–7.

Cumming, D.C., Honore, L.H., Scott, J.Z. & Williams, K.P. (1985) The late luteal phase in infertile women: comparison of simultaneous endometrial biopsy and progesterone levels. *Fertil. Steril.*, **43**, 715–19.

Daniell, J.F. & Christianson, C. (1981) Combined laparoscopic surgery and danazol therapy for pelvic endometriosis. *Fertil. Steril.*, **35**, 521–5.

Daly, D.C., Maslar, I.A., Rosenbert, S.M., Tohan, N. & Riddick, D.H. (1981) Prolactin production by luteal phase defect endometrium. *Am. J. Obstet. Gynecol.*, **140**, 587–91.

Daly, D.C., Soto-Albors, C., Walters, C., Ving, Y. & Riddick, D.H. (1985) Ultrasonographic assessment of luteinized unruptured follicle syndrome in unexplained infertility. *Fertil. Steril.*, **43**, 62–5.

Davidson, B.J., Thrasher, T.V. & Seraj, I.M. (1987) An analysis of endometrial biopsies performed for infertility. *Fertil. Steril.*, **48**, 770–4.

Davis, O.K., Berkeley, A.S., Naus, G.J., Cholost, I.N. & Freedman, K.S. (1989) The incidence of luteal phase defect in normal, fertile women, determined by serial endometrial biopsies. *Fertil. Steril.*, **51**, 582–6.

Daya, S. & Ward, S. (1988) Diagnostic test properties of serum progesterone in the evaluation of luteal phase defects. *Fertil. Steril.*, **49**, 168–70.

Daya, A., Ward, S. & Burrows, E. (1988) Progesterone profiles in luteal phase defect cycles and outcome of progesterone treatment in patients with recurrent spontaneous abortion. *Am. J. Obstet. Gynecol.*, **158**, 225–32.

Del Pozo, E.D., Wyss, H., Tolis, G., Alcaniz, J., Campana, A. & Naftolin, F. (1979) Prolactin and deficient luteal function. *Obstet. Gynecol.*, **53**, 282–5.

Demura, R., Ono, M., Demura, H., Shizume, K. & Oouchi, H. (1982) Prolactin directly inhibits basal as well as gonadotropin-stimulated secretion of progesterone and 17β-estradiol in the human ovary. *J. Clin. Endocrinol. Metab.*, **54**, 1246–50.

Denis, A.L.C., Hofmann, G.E., Scott, R.T. & Muasher, S.J. (1989) The incidence of hyperprolactinemia during gonadotropin stimulation and its effect on outcome in in-vitro fertilization (IVF). *Society for Gynecologic Investigation. 36th annual meeting.* (Abstr. 398).

DiZerega, G.S. & Hodgen, G.D. (1981a) Luteal phase dysfunction infertility: a sequel to aberrant folliculogenesis. *Fertil. Steril.*, **35**, 489–99.

DiZerega, G.S., Turner, C.K., Stouffer, R.L., Anderson, L.D., Channing, C.P. & Hodgen, G.D. (1981b) Suppression of follicle-stimulating hormone-dependent folliculogenesis during the primate ovarian cycle. *J. Clin. Endocrinol. Metab.*, **52**, 451–6.

Dmowski, W.P. & Cohen, M.R. (1978) Antigonadotropin (danazol) in the treatment of endometriosis. *Am. J. Obstet. Gynecol.*, **130**, 41–8.

Dmowski, W.P., Rao, R. & Scommegna, A. (1980) The luteinized unruptured follicle syndrome and endometriosis. *Fertil. Steril.*, **33**, 30–4.

Dodson, K.S., Macnaughton, M.C. & Coutts, J.R.T. (1975) Infertility in women with apparently ovulatory cycles. *Br. J. Obstet. Gynaecol.*, **82**, 615–24.

Doody, M.C., Gibbons, W.E. & Buttram, V.C. Jr. (1988) Linear regression analysis of ultrasound follicular growth series: evidence for an abnormality of follicular growth in endometriosis patients. *Fertil. Steril.*, **49**, 47–51.

Downs, K.A. & Gibson, M. (1983a) Basal body temperature graph and the luteal phase defect. *Fertil. Steril.*, **40**, 466–8.

Downs, K.A. & Gibson, M. (1983) Clomiphene citrate therapy for luteal phase defect. *Fertil. Steril.*, **39**, 34–8.

Doyle, L.L., Barclay, D.L., Dungan, G.W. & Kirton, K.T. (1971) Human luteal function following hysterectomy as assessed by plasma progestin. *Am. J. Obstet. Gynecol.*, **110**, 92–7.

Driessen, F., Holwerda, P.J., Putte, S.C.J.v.d. & Kremer, J. (1980) The significance of dating an endometrial biopsy for the prognosis of the infertile couple. *Int. J. Fertil.*, **25**, 112–16.

Ellinwood, W.E. & Resko, J.A. (1983) Effect of inhibition of estrogen synthesis during the luteal phase on function of the corpus luteum in rhesus monkeys. *Biol. Reprod.*, **28**, 636–44.

Ferencz, C., Matanoski, G.M., Wilson, P.D., Rubin, J.D., Neill, C.A. & Gutberlet, R. (1980) Maternal hormone therapy and congenital heart disease. *Teratology*, **21**, 225–39.

Filicori, M., Butler, J.P. & Crowley, W.F. Jr. (1984) Neuroendocrine regulation of the corpus luteum in the human. *J. Clin. Invest.*, **73**, 1638–47.

Finn, M.M., Gosling, J.P., Tallon, D.F., Madden, A.T.S., Meehan, F.P. & Fottrell, P.F. (1988) Normal salivary progesterone levels throughout the ovarian cycle as determined by a direct enzyme immunoassay. *Fertil. Steril.*, **50**, 882–7.

Forman, R., Fries, N., Blacker, C., Hazout, A., Allart, J.B., Testart, J. & Frydman, R. (1987) Evidence for an adverse effect of elevated serum estradiol on embryo implantation following IVF. *Fifth World Congress on In Vitro Fertilization and Embryo Transfer, Norfolk, VA* (Abstr. 118).

Fredricsson, B., Carlstrom, K., Bjork, G. & Messinis, I. (1981) Effects of prolactin and bromocriptine on the luteal phase in infertile women. *Eur. J. Obstet. Gynecol. Reprod. Biol.*, **11**, 319–33.

Garcia, J., Jones, G.S., Acosta, A.A. & Wright, G.L. Jr. (1981) Corpus luteum function after follicle aspiration for oocyte retrieval. *Fertil. Steril.*, **36**, 565–72.

Garcia, J., Jones, G.S. & Wentz, A.C. (1977a) The use of clomiphene citrate. *Fertil. Steril.*, **28**, 707–17.

Garrett, J.E., Geisert, R.D., Zavy, M.T. & Morgan, G.L. (1988) Evidence for maternal regulation of early conceptus growth and development in beef cattle. *J. Reprod. Fertil.*, **84**, 437–46.

Garzol, V.G., Liu, J., Ulmann, A., Baulieu, E. & Yen, S.S.C. (1988) Effects of an antiprogesterone (RU486) on the hypothalamic-hypophyseal-ovarian-endometrial axis during the luteal phase of the menstrual cycle. *J. Clin. Endocrinol. Metab.*, **66**, 508–17.

Gautray, J.P., De Brux, J., Tajchner, G., Robel, P. & Mouren, M. (1981) Clinical investigation of the menstrual cycle. III. Clinical, endometrial, and endocrine aspects of luteal defect. *Fertil. Steril.*, **35**, 296–303.

Gemzell, C.A., Diczfalusy, E. & Tillinger, G. (1958) Clinical effect of human pituitary follicle-stimulating hormone (FSH) *J. Clin. Endocrinol. Metab.*, **18**, 1333–48.

Gidley-Baird, A.A., O'Neill, C., Sinosich, M.J., Porter, R.N., Pike, I.L. & Saunders, D.M. (1986) Failure of implantation in human *in vitro* fertilization and embryo transfer patients: the effects of altered progesterone/estrogen ratios in humans and mice. *Fertil. Steril.*, **45**, 69–74.

Gillam, J.S. (1955) Study of the inadequate secretion phase endometrium. *Fertil. Steril.*, **6**, 18–36.

Godfrey, K.A., Aspillaga, M.O., Taylor, A. & Lind, T. (1981) The relation of circulating progesterone and oestradiol concentrations to the onset of menstruation. *Br. J. Obstet. Gynaecol.*, **88**, 899–903.

Goldstein, D., Zuckerman, H., Harpaz, S., Barkai, J., Geva, A., Gordon, S., Shalev, E. *et al.* (1982) Correlation between estradiol and progesterone in cycles with luteal phase deficiency. *Fertil. Steril.*, **37**, 348−54.

Good R.G. & Moyer, D.L. (1968) Estrogen−progesterone relationship in the development of secretory endometrium. *Fertil. Steril.*, **19**, 37−49.

Grant, A. (1966) Additional sterility factors in endometriosis. *Fertil. Steril.*, **17**, 514−19.

Green, B.B., Weiss, N.S. & Daling, J.R. (1988) Risk of ovulatory infertility in relation to body weight. *Fertil. Steril.*, **50**, 721−6.

Greenblatt, R.B., Barfield, W.E., Jungck, E.C. & Ray, A.W. (1961) Induction of ovulation with MRL/41. *J. Am. Med. Assoc.*, **178**, 101−30.

Greenblatt, R.B., Dmowski, W.P., Manesh, V.B. & Scholer, H.F.L. (1971) Clinical studies with an antigonadotrophin-Danazol. *Fertil. Steril.*, **22**, 102−12.

Groff, T.R., Raj, H.G.M., Talbert, L.M. & Willis, D.L. (1984) Effects of neutralization of luteinizing hormone on corpus luteum function and cyclicity in *Macaca fascicularis*. *J. Clin. Endocrinol. Metab.*, **59**, 1054−7.

Hahlin, M., Dennefors, B., Johanson, C. & Hamberger, L. (1988) Luteotropic effects of prostaglandin E$_2$ on the human corpus luteum of the menstrual cycle and early pregnancy. *J. Clin. Endocrinol. Metab.*, **66**, 909−14.

Hamilton, C.J.C.M., Wetzels, L.C., Evers, J.L.H., Hoogland, H.J., Muijtjens, A. & de Haan, J. (1985) Follicle growth curves and hormonal patterns in patients with the luteinized unruptured follicle syndrome. *Fertil. Steril.*, **43**, 541−8.

Hammond, M.G. & Talbert, L.M. (1982) Clomiphene citrate therapy of infertile women with low luteal phase progesterone levels. *Obstet. Gynecol.*, **59**, 275−9.

Healy, D.L. & Burger, H.G. (1983) Serum follicle-stimulating hormone, luteinizing hormone, and prolactin during the induction of ovulation with exogenous gonadotrophin. *J. Clin. Endocrinol. Metab.*, **56**, 474−8.

Healy, D.L., Schenken, R.S., Lynch, A., Williams, R.F. & Hodgen, G.D. (1984) Pulsatile progesterone secretion: its relevance to clinical evaluation of corpus luteum function. *Fertil. Steril.*, **41**, 114−21.

Hecht, B.R., Bardawil, W.A., Khan-Dawood, F.S. & Dawood, M.Y. (1989) Luteal insufficiency: correlation between endometrial dating and integrated progesterone output in clomiphene citrate induced cycles. *36th Annual Meeting of the Society for Gynecologic Investigation*. (Abstr. 577).

Heinonen, O.P., Slone, D., Monson, R.R., Hook, E.B. & Shapiro, S. (1977) Cardiovascular birth defects and antenatal exposure to female sex hormones. *N. Engl. J. Med.*, **296**, 67−70.

Hensleigh, P.A. & Fainstat, T. (1979) Corpus luteum dysfunction: serum progesterone levels in diagnosis and assessment of therapy for recurrent and threatened abortion. *Fertil. Steril.*, **32**, 396−400.

Hernandez Horta, J.L., Gordillo Fernandez, J., Soto de Leon, B. & Cortex-Gallegos, V. (1977) Direct evidence of luteal insufficiency in women with habitual abortion. *Obstet. Gynecol.*, **49**, 705−8.

Hillier, S.G., van den Boogard, A.M.J., Reichert, L.E. Jr. & Van Hall, E.V. (1980) Intraovarian sex steroid hormone interactions and the regulation of follicular maturation: aromatization of androgens by human granulosa cells *in vitro*. *J. Clin. Endocrinol. Metab.*, **50**, 640−7.

Hitschmann, F. & Adler, L. (1908) Der Bau der Uterus-schleimhaut des geschlectsreifen Weibes mit besonderer Berrucksichtigung der Menstruation. *Monatschr. Geburtsch. Gynakl.*, **27**, 1.

Hoff, J.D., Quigley, M.E. & Yen, S.S.C. (1983) Hormonal dynamics at midcycle: a reevaluation. *J. Clin. Endocrinol. Metab.*, **57**, 792−6.

Hohtari, H., Elovainio, R., Salminen, K. & Laatikainen, T. (1988) Plasma corticotropin-releasing hormone, corticotropin, and endorphins at rest and during exercise in eumenorrheic and amenorrheic athletes. *Fertil. Steril.*, **50**, 233−8.

Horton, E.W. & Poyser, N.L. (1976) Uterine luteolytic hormone: a physiological role for prostaglandin F$_{2\alpha}$. *Physiol. Rev.*, **56**, 595−651.

Huang, K. (1986) The primary treatment of luteal phase inadequacy: progesterone versus clomiphene citrate. *Am. J. Obstet. Gynecol.*, **155**, 824−8.

Huang, K., Muechler, E.K. & Bonfiglio, T.A. (1984) Follicular phase treatment of luteal phase defect with follicle-stimulating hormone in infertile women. *Obstet. Gynecol.*, **64**, 32−6.

Huang, K.E., Muechler, E., Schwarz, K.R., Goggin, M. & Graham, M.C. (1986) Serum progesterone levels in women treated with human menopausal gonadotropin and human chorionic gonadotropin for *in vitro* fertilization. *Fertil. Steril.*, **46**, 903−6.

Hutchison, J.S. & Zeleznik, A.J. (1985) The corpus luteum of the primate menstrual cycle is capable of recovering from a transient withdrawal of pituitary gonadotropin support. *Endocrinology*, **117**, 1043−9.

Illingworth, D.R., Corbin, D.K., Kemp, E.D. & Keenan, E.J. (1982) Hormone changes during the menstrual cycle in abetalipoproteinemia: reduced luteal phase progesterone in a patient with homozygous hypobetalipoproteinemia. *Proc. Natl. Acad. Sci. USA*, **70**, 6685−9.

Ireland, J.J. & Richards, J.S. (1978) Acute effects of estradiol and follicle-stimulating hormone on specific binding of human [$^{125}$I]Iodo-follicle-stimulating hormone to rat ovarian granulosa cells *in vivo* and *in vitro*. *Endocrinology*, **102**, 876−83.

Israel, R., Mishell, D.R., Stone, S.G., Thorneycroft, I.H. & Moyer, D.L. (1972) Single luteal phase serum progesterone assay as an indicator of ovulation. *Am. J. Obstet. Gynecol.*, **112**, 1043−6.

Jia, X.C., Kessel, B., Welsh, T.H. & Hsueh, A.J. (1985) Androgen inhibition of follicle-stimulating hormone-stimulated luteinizing hormone receptor formation in cultured rat granulosa cells. *Endocrinology*, **117**, 13—22.

Johannisson, E., Landgren, B.M., Rohr, H.P. & Diczfalusy, E. (1987) Endometrial morphology and peripheral hormone levels in women with regular menstrual cycles. *Fertil. Steril.*, **48**, 401—8.

Johannsen, A. (1970) The prognosis of threatened abortion. *Acta Obstet. Gynecol. Scand.*, **49**, 89—93.

Johansson, E.D.B. (1969) Progesterone levels in peripheral plasma during the luteal phase of the normal human menstrual cycle measured by a rapid competitive protein binding technique. *Acta Endocrinol. Copenh.*, **69**, 592—606.

Johansson, E.D.B. (1971) Depression of the progesterone levels in women treated with synthetic gestagens after ovulation. *Acta Endocrinol. Copenh.*, **68**, 779—92.

Johansson, E.D.B. & Gemzell, C. (1971) Plasma levels of progesterone during the luteal phase in normal women treated with synthetic oestrogens (RS 2874, F 6103 and ethinyloestradiol) *Acta. Endocrinol. Copenh.*, **68**, 551—60.

Johansson, E.D.B., Larsson-Cohn, U. & Gemzell, G. (1972) Monophasic basal body temperature in ovulatory menstrual cycles. *Am. J. Obstet. Gynecol.*, **113**, 933—7.

Jones, F.S., Ruehsen, M.D.M., Johanson, A.J., Ratti, S. & Blizzard, R.M. (1969b) Elucidation of normal ovarian physiology by exogenous gonadotropin stimulation following steroid pituitary suppression. *Fertil. Steril.*, **20**, 14—34.

Jones, G.E.S. (1949) Some newer aspects of the management of infertility. *J. Am. Med. Assoc.*, 1123—9.

Jones, G.S. (1976) The luteal phase defect. *Fertil. Steril.*, **27**, 351—6.

Jones, G.S., Maffezzoli, R.D., Strott, C.A., Ross, G.T. & Kaplan, G. (1970) Pathophysiology of reproductive failure after clomiphene-induced ovulation. *Am. J. Obstet. Gynecol.*, **108**, 847—67.

Jones, G.S. & Pourmand, K. (1962) An evaluation of etiologic factors and therapy in 555 private patients with primary infertility. *Fertil. Steril.*, **13**, 398—410.

Jones, G.S. & Wentz, A.C. (1974) Serum progesterone values in the luteal phase defects. *Obstet. Gynecol.*, **44**, 26—34.

Jones, Jr., H.W. & Wheeless, C.R. (1969a) Salvage of the reproductive potential of women with anomalous development of the Mullerian ducts. *Am. J. Obstet. Gynecol.*, **104**, 348—64.

Karow, W.G., Gentry, W.C., Skeels, R.F. & Payne, S.A. (1971) Endometrial biopsy in the luteal phase of the cycle of conception. *Fertil. Steril.*, **22**, 482—95.

Katz E. (1988) The luteinized unruptured follicle and other ovulatory dysfunctions. *Fertil. Steril.*, **50**, 839—50.

Katz, Z., Lancet, M., Skornik, J., Chemke, J., Mogilner, B.M. & Klinberg, M. (1985) Teratogenicity of progestogens given during the first trimester of pregnancy. *Obstet. Gynecol.*, **65**, 775—80.

Kauppila, A., Keinonen, P., Vihko, R. & Ylostalo, P. (1982) Metoclopramide-induced hyperprolactinemia impairs ovarian follicle maturation and corpus luteum function in women. *J. Clin. Endocrinol. Metab.*, **54**, 955—60.

Kauppila, A., Martikainen, H., Puistola, U., Reinila, M. & Ronnbert, L. (1988) Hypoprolactinemia and ovarian function. *Fertil. Steril.*, **49**, 437—41.

Keller, W., Wiest, W.G., Askin, F.B., Johnson, L.W. & Strickler, R.C. (1979) Pseudocorpus luteum insufficiency: a local defect of progesterone action on endometrial stroma. *J. Clin. Endocrinol. Metab.*, **48**, 127—32.

Kemeter, P., Breitenecker, G., Salzer, H., Friedrich, F. & Husslein, H. (1977) Gonadotrophin-induced ovulation and pregnancy in hypergonadotropic amenorrhea. *Fertil. Steril.*, **28**, 373.

Kerin, J.F., Broom, T.J., Ralph, M.M., Edmonds, D.K., Warnes, G.M., Jeffrey, R. & Crocker, J.M. *et al.* (1981) Human luteal phase function following oocyte aspiration from the immediately preovular graafian follicle of spontaneous ovular cycles. *Br. J. Obstet. Gynaecol.*, **88**, 1021—8.

Kerin, J.F., Kirby, C., Morris, D., McEvoy, M., Ward, B. & Cox, L.W. (1983) Incidence of the luteinized unruptured follicle phenomenon in cycling women. *Fertil. Steril.*, **40**, 620—6.

Killick, S. & Elstein, M. (1987) Pharmacologic production of luteinized unruptured follicles by prostaglandin synthetase inhibitors. *Fertil. Steril.*, **47**, 773—7.

Kistner, R.W. (1965) Induction of ovulation with clomiphene citrate (Clomid) *Obstet. Gynecol. Surv.*, **20**, 873—900.

Kistner, R.W. (1975) Management of endometriosis in the infertile patient. *Fertil. Steril.*, **26**, 1151—66.

Koninckx, P.R., Goddeeris, P.G., Lauweryns, J.M., De Hertogh, R.C. & Brosens, I.A. (1977) Accuracy of endometrial biopsy dating in relation to the midcycle luteinizing hormone peak. *Fertil. Steril.*, **28**, 443—5.

Koninckx, P.R., Ide, P., Vandenbrouck, W. & Brosens, I.A. (1980) New aspects of the pathophysiology of endometriosis and associated infertility. *J. Reprod. Med.*, **24**, 257—60.

Korda, A.R., Shutt, D.A., Smith, I.D., Shearman, R.P. & Lyneham, R.C. (1975) Assessment of possible luteolytic effect of intra-ovarian injection of prostaglandin $F_{2\alpha}$ in the human. *Prostaglandins*, **9**, 443—9.

Laatikainen, T., Andersson, B., Karkkainen, J. & Wahlstrom T. (1983) Progestin receptor levels in endometria with delayed or incomplete secretory changes. *Obstet. Gynecol.*, **62**, 592—5.

Laatikainen, T., Kurunmaki, H. & Koskimies, A. (1988) A short luteal phase in cycles stimulated with clomiphene and human menopausal gonadotropin for *in vitro* fertilization. *J. In Vitro Fertil.*

*Embryo Transfer.*, **5**, 14−17.

Laatikainen, T., Virtanen, T. & Apter, D. (1986) Plasma immunoreactive β-endorphin in exercise-associated amenorrhea. *Am. J. Obstet. Gynecol.*, **154**, 94−7.

Lam, S.Y., Baker, H.W.G., Evans, J.H. & Pepperell, R.J. (1989) Factors affecting fetal loss in induction of ovulation with gonadotropins: increased abortion rates related to hormonal profiles in conceptual cycles. *Am. J. Obstet. Gynecol.*, **160**, 621−8.

Lamb, E.J., Colliflower, W.W. & Williams, J.W. (1972) Endometrial histology and conception rates after clomiphene citrate. *Obstet. Gynecol.*, **39**, 389−96.

Lamb, E.J. & Guderian, A.M. (1966) Clinical effects of clomiphene in anovulation. *Obstet. Gynecol.*, **28**, 505−12.

Lee, C.S. (1987) Luteal phase defects. *Obstet. Gynecol. Surv.*, **42**, 267−74.

Lee, C.Y., Coulam, C.B., Jiang, N.S. & Ryan R.J. (1973) Receptors for human luteinizing hormone in human corpora luteal tissue. *J. Clin. Endocrinol. Metab.*, **36**, 148−52.

Lejeune, B., Camus, M., Deschart, J. & LeRoy, F. (1986) Differences in the luteal phases after failed or successful *in vitro* fertilization and embryo replacement. *J. In Vitro Fert. Embryo Transfer.*, **3**, 358−65.

Lenton, E.A., Adams, M. & Cooke, I.D. (1978) Plasma steroid and gonadotrophin profiles in ovulatory but infertile women. *Clin. Endocrinol.*, **8**, 241−55.

Lenton, E.A., Landgren, B.M. & Sexton, L. (1984) Normal variation in the length of the luteal phase of the menstrual cycle: identification of the short luteal phase. *Br. J. Obstet. Gynaecol.*, **91**, 685−9.

Lesorgen, P.R., Wu, C.H., Green, P.J., Gocial, B. & Lerner, L.J. (1984) Peritoneal fluid and serum steroids in infertility patients. *Fertil. Steril.*, **42**, 237−42.

Leeton, J., Trounson, A. & Jessup, D. (1985) Support of the luteal phase in *in vitro* fertilization programs: results of a controlled trial with intramuscular proluton. *J. In Vitro Fert. Embryo Transfer.*, **2**, 166−9.

Leung, P.C.K. & Armstrong, D.T. (1980) Interactions of steroids and gonadotropins in the control of steroidogenesis in the ovarian follicle. *Annu. Rev. Physiol.*, **42**, 71−82.

Levine, M.A., Downs, R.W. Jr., Moses, A.M., Breslau, N.A., Marx, S.J., Lasker, R.D., Rizzoli, R.E. *et al.* (1983) Resistance to multiple hormones in patients with pseudohypoparathyroidism. *Am. J. Med.*, **74**, 545−56.

Levy, C., Robel, P., Gautray, J.P., De Brux, J., Verma, U. & Baulieu, E.E. (1980) Estradiol and progesterone receptors in human endometrium: normal and abnormal menstrual cycles and early pregnancy. *Am. J. Obstet. Gynecol.*, **136**, 646−51.

Lewinthal, D., Furman, A., Blankstein, J., Corenblum, B., Shalev, J. & Lunenfeld, B. (1986) Subtle abnormalities in follicular development and hormonal profile in women with unexplained infertility. *Fertil. Steril.*, **46**, 833−9.

Li, T.C., Dockery, P., Thomas, P., Rogers, A.W., Lenton, E.A. & Cooke, I.D. (1988a) The effects of progesterone receptor blockade in the luteal phase of normal fertile women. *Fertil. Steril.*, **50**, 732−42.

Li, T.C., Rogers, A.W., Dockery, P., Lenton, E.A. & Cooke, I.D. (1988b) A new method of histologic dating of human endometrium in the luteal phase. *Fertil. Steril.*, **50**, 52−60.

Liukkonen, S., Koskimies, A.I., Tenhunen, A. & Ylostalo, P. (1984) Diagnosis of luteinized unruptured follicle (LUF) syndrome by ultrasound. *Fertil. Steril.*, **41**, 26−30.

Lorber, C.A., Cassidy, S.B. & Engel, E. (1979) Is there an embryo-fetal exogenous sex steroid exposure syndrome (EFESSES)? *Fertil. Steril.*, **31**, 2124.

Lutjen, P., Trounson, A., Leeton, J., Findlay, J., Wood, C. & Renou, P. (1984) The establishment and maintenance of pregnancy using *in vitro* fertilization and embryo donation in a patient with primary ovarian failure. *Nature*, **307**, 174−5.

McDonough, P.G. (1985) Progesterone therapy: benefit versus risk. *Fertil. Steril.*, **44**, 13−16.

MacLeod, S.C., Mitton, D.M., Parker, A.S. & Tupper, W.R.C. (1970) Experience with induction of ovulation. *Am. J. Obstet. Gynecol.*, **108**, 814−24.

McNeely, M.J., & Soules, M.R. (1988) The diagnosis of luteal phase deficiency: a critical review. *Fertil. Steril.*, **50**, 1−5.

McNeilly, A.S., Kerin, J., Swanston, I.A., Bramley, T.A. & Baird D.T. (1980) Changes in the binding of human chorionic gonadotrophin/luteinizing hormone, follicle-stimulating hormone and prolactin to human corpora lutea during the menstrual cycle and pregnancy. *J. Endocrinol*, **87**, 315−25.

McRae, M.A., Blasco, L. & Lyttle, C.R. (1984) Serum hormones and their receptors in women with normal and inadequate corpus luteum function. *Fertil. Steril.*, **42**, 58−63.

Mahadevan, M.M., Fleetham, J. & Taylor P.J. (1988) Effects of progesterone on luteinizing hormone release and estradiol/progesterone ratio in the luteal phase of women superovulated for *in vitro* fertilization and embryo transfer. *Fertil. Steril.*, **50**, 935−7.

Mahadevan, M.M., Leader, A. and Taylor P.J. (1985) Effects of low-dose human chorionic gonadotropin on corpus luteum function after embryo transfer. *J. In Vitro Fert. Embryo Transfer*, **2**, 190−4.

Mais, V., Kazar, R.R., Cetel, N.S., Rivier, J., Vale, W. & Yen S.S.C. (1986) The dependency of folliculogenesis and corpus luteum function on pulsatile gonadotropin secretion in cycling women using a gonadotropin-releasing hormone antagonist as a probe. *J. Clin. Endocrinol. Metab.*, **62**, 1250−5.

Margalioth, E.J., Bronson, R.A., Cooper, G.W. & Rosenfeld, D.L. (1988) Luteal phase sera and progesterone enhance sperm penetration in the hamster egg assay. *Fertil. Steril.*, **50**, 117−22.

Marik, J. & Hulka, J. (1978) Luteinized unruptured follicle syndrome: a subtle cause of infertility. *Fertil. Steril.*, **29**, 270−4.

Markiewicz, L., Laufer, N. & Gurpide, E. (1988) *In vitro* effects of clomiphene citrate on human endometrium. *Fertil. Steril.*, **50**, 772−6.

Marshall, J. (1963) Thermal changes in the normal menstrual cycle. *Br. Med. J.*, **1**, 102−4.

Marut, E.L. & Hodgen, G.D. (1982) Antiestrogenic action of high-dose clomiphene in primates: pituitary augmentation but with ovarian attenuation. *Fertil. Steril.*, **38**, 100−4.

Matsunaga, E. & Shiota, K. (1979) Threatened abortion, hormone therapy and malformed embryos. *Teratology*, **20**, 469−80.

Messinis, I.E., Bergh, T. & Wide, L. (1988) The importance of human chorionic gonadotropin support of the corpus luteum during human gonadotropin therapy in women with anovulatory infertility. *Fertil. Steril.*, **50**, 31−5.

Michaelis, J., Michaelis, H., Gluck, E. & Koller, S. (1983) Prospective study of suspected associations between certain drugs administered during early pregnancy and congenital malformations. *Teratology*, **27**, 57−64.

Michel, P.S. & Dizerega, G.S. (1983) Hyperprolactinemia and luteal phase dysfunction infertility. *Obstet. Gynecol. Surv.*, **38**, 248−54.

Minakami, H., Kimura, K. & Tamada, T. (1985) Low serum levels of FSH, LH and prolactin in luteal phase inadequacy. *Endocrinol. Jpn.*, **32**, 265−70.

Moghissi, K.S. (1976) Accuracy of basal body temperature for ovulation detection. *Fertil. Steril.*, **27**, 1415−21.

Moghissi, K.S., Syner, F.N. & Evans, T.N. (1972) A composite picture of the menstrual cycle. *Am. J. Obstet. Gynecol.*, **114**, 405−18.

Moghissi, K.S. & Wallach, E.E. (1983) Unexplained infertility. *Fertil. Steril.*, **39**, 5−21.

Molloy, B.G., Hancock, K.W. & Glass, M.R. (1985) Ovulation induction in clomiphene non-responsive patients: the place of pulsatile gonadotropin-releasing hormone in clinical practice. *Fertil. Steril.*, **43**, 26−33.

Murdoch, W.J. & Cavender, J.L. (1989) Effect of indomethacin on the vascular architecture of pre-ovulatory ovine follicles: possible implication in the luteinized unruptured follicle syndrome. *Fertil. Steril.*, **51**, 153−5.

Murdoch, W.J. & Myers, D.A. (1983) Effect of treatment of estrous ewes with indomethacin on the distribution of ovarian blood to the periovulatory follicle. *Biol. Reprod.*, **29**, 1229−32.

Murray, D.L., Reich, L. & Adashi, E.Y. (1989) Oral clomiphene citrate and vaginal progesterone suppositories in the treatment of luteal phase dysfunction: a comparative study. *Fertil. Steril.*, **51**, 35−41.

Murthy, Y.S., Arronet, G.H. & Parekh, M.C. (1970) Luteal phase inadequacy. *Obstet. Gynecol.*, **36**, 758−61.

Nader, S., Berkowitz, A.S., Ochs, D., Held, B. & Winkel C.A. (1988) Luteal-phase support in stimulated cycles in an in vitro fertilization/embryo transfer program: progesterone versus human chorionic gonadotropin. *J. In Vitro Fert. Embryo Transfer.*, **5**, 81−4.

Nadji, P., Reyniak, V., Sedlis, A., Szarowski, D. & Bartosid, D. (1975) Endometrial dating correlated with progesterone levels. *Obstet. Gynecol.*, **45**, 193−4.

Naples, J.D., Batt, R.E. & Sadigh, H. (1981) Spontaneous abortion rate in patients with endometriosis. *Obstet. Gynecol.*, **57**, 509−12.

Nillius, S.J. & Johansson, E.D.B. (1971) Plasma levels of progesterone after vaginal, rectal, or intramuscular administration of progesterone. *Am. J. Obstet. Gynecol.*, **110**, 470−7.

Nillius, S.J., & Wide, L. (1975) Gonadotrophin-releasing hormone treatment for induction of follicular maturation and ovulation in amenorrhoeic women with anorexia nervosa. *Br. Med. J.*, **3**, 405−8.

Nora, A.H. & Nora, J.J. (1975) A syndrome of multiple congenital anomalies associated with teratogenic exposure. *Arch. Environ. Health*, **30**, 17−21.

Norman, R.J., Buck, R.H., Kemp, M.A. & Joubert S.M. (1988) Impaired corpus luteum function in ectopic pregnancy cannot be explained by altered human chorionic gonadotropin. *J. Clin. Endocrinol. Metab.*, **66**, 1166−70.

Noyes, R.W. & Haman, J.O. (1953) Accuracy of endometrial dating. *Fertil. Steril.*, **4**, 504−17.

Noyes, R.W. & Hertig, A.T. (1950) Dating the endometrial biopsy. *Fertil. Steril.*, **1**, 3−25.

Olson, J.L., Rebar, R.W., Schreiber, J.R. & Vaitukaitis, J.L. (1983) Shortened luteal phase after ovulation induction with human menopausal gonadotropin and human chorionic gonadotropin. *Fertil. Steril.*, **39**, 284−91.

O'Neill, C., Ferrier, A.J., Vaughan, J., Sinosich, M.J. & Saunders, D.M. (1985) Causes of implantation failure after *in vitro* fertilisation and embryo transfer. *Lancet*, **ii**, 615.

Padilla, S.L., Person, G.K., McDonough, P.G. & Reindollar, R.H. (1985) The efficacy of bromocriptine in patients with ovulatory dysfunction and normoprolactinemic galactorrhea. *Fertil. Steril.*, **44**, 695−8.

Pampiglione, J.S., Sharma, V., Riddle, A.F., Mason, B.A. & Campbell, S. (1988) The effect of cycle length on the outcome of *in vitro* fertilization. *Fertil. Steril.*, **50**, 603−6.

Parker, C.R. Jr., Illingworth, D.R., Bissonnette, J. & Carr, B.R. (1986) Endocrinology of pregnancy in abetalipoproteinemia: studies in a patient with homozygous familial hypobetalipoproteinemia. *N.*

Engl. J. Med., **314**, 557–60.

Patwardhan, V.V. & Lanthier, A. (1984) Effect of prostaglandin F$_{2\alpha}$ on the hCG-stimulated progesterone production by human corpora lutea. *Prostaglandins*, **27**, 465–73.

Petsos, P., Chandler, C., Oak, M., Ratcliffe, W.A., Wood, R. & Anderson D.C. (1985) The assessment of ovulation by a combination of ultrasound and detailed serial hormone profiles in 35 women with long-standing unexplained infertility. *Clin. Endocrinol. (Oxf.)*, **22**, 739–51.

Phansey, S.A., Toffle, R., Curtin, J., Nagel, T.C., Tagatz, G.E., Barnes, M.A. & Nair, R. (1985) Alternative indications for pulsatile gonadotropin-releasing hormone therapy in infertile women. *Fertil. Steril.*, **44**, 589–94.

Phipps, W.R., Benson, C.B. & McShane, P.M. Severe thigh myositis following intramuscular progesterone injections in an *in vitro* fertilization patient. *Fertil. Steril.*, **49**, 536–7.

Pittaway, D.E., Maxson, W., Daniell, J., Herbert, C. & Wentz, A.C. (1983) Luteal phase defects in infertility patients with endometriosis. *Fertil. Steril.*, **39**, 712–3.

Portuondo, J.A., Agustin, A., Herran, C. & Echanojauregui, A.B. (1981) The corpus luteum in infertile patients found during laparoscopy. *Fertil. Steril.*, **36**, 37–40.

Price, J.H., Ismail, H., Gorwill, R.H. & Sarda, I.R. (1983) Effect of the suppository base on progesterone delivery from the vagina. *Fertil. Steril.*, **39**, 490–3.

Quagliarello, J. & Weiss, G. (1979) Clomiphene citrate in the management of infertility associated with shortened luteal phases. *Fertil. Steril.*, **31**, 373–7.

Quigley, M.E., Sheehan, K.L., Casper, R.F. & Yen, S.S.C. (1980) Evidence for an increased opioid inhibition of luteinizing hormone secretion in hyperprolactinemic patients with pituitary microadenoma. *J. Clin Endocrinol. Metab.*, **50**, 427–30.

Radwanska, E. & Dmowski, W.P. (1981) Luteal function in infertile women with endometriosis. *Infertility*, **4**, 269–78.

Radwanska, E., Hammond, J. & Smith, P. (1981) Single midluteal progesterone assay in the management of ovulatory infertility. *J. Reprod. Med.*, **26**, 85–9.

Radwanska, E. & Swyer, G.I.M. (1974) Plasma progesterone estimation in infertile women and in women under treatment with clomiphene and chorionic gonadotrophin. *Br. J. Obstet. Gynecol.*, **81**, 107–12.

Reame, N., Sauder, S.E., Kelch, R.P. & Marshall, J.C. (1984) Pulsatile gonadotropin secretion during the human menstrual cycle: evidence for altered frequency of gonadotropin-releasing hormone secretion. *J. Clin. Endocrinol. Metab.*, **59**, 328–37.

Resseguie, L.J., Hick, J.F., Bruen, J.A., Noller, K.L., O'Fallon, W.M. & Kurland, L.T. (1985) Congenital malformations among offspring exposed *in utero* to progestins, Olmsted County, Minnesota, 1936–1974. *Fertil. Steril.*, **43**, 514–9.

Rock, J. & Bartlett, M.K. (1937) Biopsy studies of human endometrium. *J. Am. Med. Assoc.*, **108**, 2022–8.

Rock, J.A., Guzick, D.S., Sengos, C., Schweditsch, M., Sapp, K.C. & Jones, H.W. Jr. (1981) The conservative surgical treatment of endometriosos: evaluation of pregnancy success with respect to the extent of disease as categorized using contemporary classification systems. *Fertil. Steril.*, **35**, 131–7.

Rock, J.A., Wentz, A.C., Cole, K.A., Kimbal, A.W. Jr., Zacur, H.A., Early, S.A. & Jones, G.S. (1985) Fetal malformations following progesterone therapy during pregnancy: a preliminary report. *Fertil. Steril.*, **44**, 17–19.

Ronnberg, L., Isotalo, H., Kauppila, A., Martikainen, H. & Vihko, R. (1985) Clomiphene-induced changes in endometrial receptor kinetics on the day of ovum collection after ovarian stimulation: a study on cytosol and nuclear estrogen and progestin receptors and 17β-hydroxysteroid dehydrogenase. *Ann. NY Acad. Sci.*, **442**, 408–15.

Rosenfeld, D.L., Chudow, S. & Bronson, R.A., (1980) Diagnosis of luteal phase inadequacy. *Obstet. Gynecol.*, **56**, 193–6.

Rosenfeld, D.L. & Garcia, C.R. (1976) A comparison of endometrial histology with simultaneous plasma progesterone determinations in infertile women. *Fertil. Steril.*, **27**, 1256–66.

Rosenberg, S.M., Johnson, M. & Riddick, D.H. (1982) Luteal phase defect as a marker of imminent ovarian failure. *Obstet. Gynecol.*, **59**, 895–915.

Rosenberg, S.M., Luciano, A.A. & Riddick, D.H. (1980) The luteal phase defect: the relative frequency of, and encouraging response to, treatment with vaginal progesterone. *Fertil. Steril.*, **34**, 17–20.

Rosenwaks, Z. (1987) Donor eggs: their application in modern reproductive technologies. *Fertil. Steril.*, **47**, 895–909.

Ross, G.T., Cargille, C.M., Lipsett, M.B., Rayford, P.L., Marshall, J.R., Strott, C.A. & Rodbard, D. (1970) Pituitary and gonadal hormones in women during spontaneous and induced ovulatory cycles. *Recent Prog. Horm. Res.*, **26**, 1–62.

Saracoglu, O.F., Aksel, S., Yeoman, R.R. & Wiebe, R.H. (1985) Endometrial estradiol and progesterone receptors in patients with luteal phase defects and endometriosis. *Fertil. Steril.*, **43**, 851–5.

Sarris, S., Swyer, G.I.M., McGarrigle, H.H.G., Lawrence, D.M., Little, V. & Lachelin, G.C.L. (1978) Prolactin and luteal insufficiency. *Clin. Endocrinol. (Oxf.)*, **9**, 543–7.

Sauder, S.E., Frager, M., Case, G.D., Kelch, R.P. & Marshall, J.C. (1984) Abnormal patterns of pulsatile luteinizing hormone secretion in women with hyperprolactinemia and amenorrhea: responses to bromocriptine. *J. Clin. Endocrinol. Metab.*, **59**, 941−8.

Saunders, D.M., Hunter, J.C., Haase H.R. & Wilson, G.R. (1979) Treatment of luteal phase inadequacy with bromocriptine. *Obstet. Gynecol.*, **53**, 287−9.

Schulz, K.D., Geiger, W., Pozo, E.D., Lose, K.H., Kunzig, H.J. & Lancranjan, I. (1976) The influence of the prolactin-inhibitor bromocriptin (CB 154) on human luteal function *in vivo. Arch. Gynak.*, **221**, 93−6.

Schweiger, U., Laessle, R., Pfister, H., Hoehl, C., Schwingenschloegel, M., Schweiger, M. & Pirke, K.M. (1987) Diet-induced menstrual irregularities: effects of age and weight loss. *Fertil. Steril.*, **48**, 746−51.

Schweiger, U., Laessle, R., Schweiger, M., Herrmann, F., Riedel, W. & Pirke, K.M. (1988) Caloric intake, stress, and menstrual function in athletes. *Fertil. Steril.*, **49**, 447−50.

Scott, R.T., Snyder, R.R., Strickland, D.M., Tyburski, C.C., Bagnall, J.A., Reed, K.R., Adair, C.A., *et al.* (1988b) The effect of interobserver variation in dating endometrial histology on the diagnosis of luteal phase defects. *Fertil. Steril.*, **50**, 888−92.

Self, M.W., Aplin, J.D., Foden, L.J. & Tindall, V.R. (1989) A novel approach for monitoring the endometrial cycle and detecting ovulation. *Am. J. Obstet. Gynecol.*, **160**, 357−62.

Seppala, M., Hirvonen, E. & Ranta, T. (1976) Hyperprolactinemia and luteal insufficiency. *Lancet*, **i**, 229−30.

Shangold, M., Berkeley, A. & Gray, J. (1983) Both midluteal serum progesterone levels and late luteal endometrial histology should be assessed in all infertile women. *Fertil. Steril.*, **40**, 627−30.

Shangold, M., Freeman, R., Thysen, B. & Gatz, M. (1979) The relationship between long-distance running, plasma progesterone, and luteal phase length. *Fertil. Steril.*, **31**, 130−3.

Shapiro, A.G. (1972) New treatment for the inadequate luteal phase. *Obstet. Gynecol.*, **40**, 826−8.

Sheehan, K.L., Casper, R.F. & Yen, S.S.C. (1982) Luteal phase defects induced by an agonist of luteinizing hormone-releasing factor: a model for fertility control. *Science*, **215**, 170−2.

Shepard, M.K. & Senturia, Y.D. (1977) Comparison of serum progesterone and endometrial biopsy for confirmation of ovulation and evaluation of luteal function. *Fertil. Steril.*, **28**, 541−8.

Sherman, B.M. & Korenman, S.G. (1974a) Measurement of plasma LH, FSH, estradiol and progesterone in disorders of the human menstrual cycle: the short luteal phase. *J. Clin. Endocrinol. Metab.*, **38**, 89−93.

Sherman, B.M. & Korenman, S.G. (1974b) Measurement of serum LH, FSH, estradiol and progesterone in disorders of the human menstrual cycle: the inadequate luteal phase. *J. Clin. Endocrinol. Metab.*, **39**, 145−9.

Sherman, B.M., West, J.H. & Korenman, S.G. (1976) The menopausal transition: analysis of LH, FSH, estradiol, and progesterone concentrations during menstrual cycles of older women. *J. Clin. Endocrinol. Metab.*, **42**, 629−36.

Short, R.V. (1977) The discovery of the ovaries. In S. Zuckerman & Weir B.J. (eds) *The Ovary*, pp. 1−39, 2nd ed., Academic Press, New York.

Shoupe, D., Mishell, D.R., Jr., Lacarra, M., Lobo, R.A., Horenstein, J., d'Ablaing, G. & Moyer, D. (1989) Correlation of endometrial maturation with four methods of estimating day of ovulation. *Obstet. Gynecol.*, **73**, 88−92.

Smith, S.K., Lenton, E.A. & Cooke, I.D. (1985) Plasma gonadotrophin and ovarian steroid concentrations in women with menstrual cycles with a short luteal phase. *J. Reprod. Fertil.*, **75**, 363−8.

Smith, S.K., Lenton, E.A., Landgren, B.M. & Cooke, I.D. (1984) The short luteal phase and infertility. *Br. J. Obstet. Gynaecol.*, **91**, 1120−2.

Soules, M.R., Clifton, D.K., Bremner, W.J. & Steiner, R.A. (1987) Corpus luteum insufficiency induced by a rapid gonadotropin-releasing hormone-induced gonadotropin secretion pattern in the follicular phase. *J. Clin. Endocrinol. Metab.*, **65**, 457−64.

Soules, M.R., Steiner, R.A., Clifton, D.K. & Bremner, W.J. (1984b) Abnormal patterns of pulsatile luteinizing hormone in women with luteal phase deficiency. *Obstet. Gynecol.*, **63**, 626−9.

Soules, M.R., Steiner, R.A., Clifton, D.K., Cohen, N.L., Aksel, S. & Bremner, W.J. (1984a) Progesterone modulation of pulsatile luteinizing hormone secretion in normal women. *J. Clin. Endocrinol. Metab.*, **58**, 378−83.

Soules, M.R., Sutton, G.P., Hammond, C.B. & Haney, A.F. (1980) Endocrine changes at operation under general anesthesia: reproductive hormone fluctuations in young women. *Fertil. Steril.*, **33**, 364−71.

Soules, M.R., Wiebe, R.H., Aksel, S. & Hammond, C.B. (1977) The diagnosis and therapy of luteal phase deficiency. *Fertil. Steril.*, **28**, 1033−7.

Spirtos, N.J., Yurewicz, E.C., Moghissi, K.S., Magyar, D.M., Sundareson, A.S. & Bottoms, S.F. (1985) Pseudocorpus luteum insufficiency: a study of cytosol progesterone receptors in human endometrium. *Obstet. Gynecol.*, **65**, 535−40.

Sterzik, K., Dallenbach, C., Schneider, V., Sasse, V. & Dallenbach-Hellweg, G. (1988) In vitro fertilization: the degree of endometrial insufficiency varies with the type of ovarian stimulation. *Fertil. Steril.*, **50**, 457−62.

Stouffer, R.L. & Hodgen G.D. (1980) Induction of luteal phase defects in rhesus monkeys by follicular fluid administration at the onset of the menstrual cycle. *J. Clin. Endocrinol. Metab.*, **51**, 669−71.

Stouffer, R.L., Hodgen, G.D., Graves, P.E., Danforth, D.R., Eyster, K.M. & Ottobre, J.S. (1986) Characterization of corpora lutea in monkeys after superovulation with human menopausal gonadotropin or follicle-stimulating hormone. *J. Clin. Endocrinol. Metab.*, **62**, 833–9.

Stouffer, R.L., Nixon, W.E. & Hodgen, G.D. (1977) Estrogen inhibition of basal and gonadotropin-stimulated progesterone production by rhesus monkey. *Endocrinology*, **101**, 1157–63.

Strott, C.A., Cargille, C.M., Ross, G.T. & Lipsett M.B. (1970) The short luteal phase. *J. Clin. Endocrinol. Metab.*, **30**, 246–51.

Sulewski, J.M., Ward, S.P. & McGaffic, W. (1980) Endometrial biopsy during a cycle of conception. *Fertil. Steril.*, **34**, 548–51.

Tauber, H. (1978) Luteal phase insufficiency. *Contrib. Gynecol. Obstet.*, **4**, 78–113.

Thibier, M., El-Hassan, N., Clark, M.R., LeMaire, W.J. & Marsh, J.M. (1980) Inhibition by estradiol of human chorionic gonadotropin-induced progesterone accumulation in isolated human luteal cells: lack of mediation by prostaglandin F. *J. Clin. Endocrinol. Metab.*, **50**, 590–2.

Tho, P.T., Byrd, J.R. & McDonough, P.G. (1979) Etiologies and subsequent reproductive performance of 100 couples with recurrent abortion. *Fertil. Steril.*, **32**, 389–95.

Townsent, S.L., Brown, J.B., Johnston, J.W., Adey, F.D., Evans, J.H. & Taft, H.P. (1966) Induction of ovulation. *Br. J. Obstet. Gynecol.*, **73**, 529–43.

Tredway, D.R., Mishell, D.R. Jr. & Moyer, D.L. (1973) Correlation of endometrial dating with luteinizing hormone peak. *Am. J. Obstet. Gynecol.*, **117**, 1030–3.

Trounson, A. & Mohr, L. (1983) Human pregnancy following cryopreservation, thawing and transfer of an eight-cell embryo. *Nature*, **305**, 707–9.

Tummon, I.S., Maclin, V.M., Radwanska, E., Binor, Z. & Dmowski, W.P. (1988) Occult ovulatory dysfunction in women with minimal endometriosis or unexplained infertility. *Fertil. Steril.*, **50**, 716–20.

Vandekerckhove, D. & Dhont, M. (1972) The relationship between serum LH levels, as determined by radioimmunoassay, and the life span of the corpus luteum. *Ann. Endocrinol. (Paris)*, **33**, 205–10.

Vande Wiele, R.L., Bogumil, J., Dyrenfurth, I., Ferin, M., Jewelewicz, R., Warren, M., Rizkallah, T. & Mikhail, G. (1970) Mechanisms regulating the menstrual cycle in women. *Recent Prog. Horm. Res.*, **26**, 63–103.

Van Hall, E.V. & Mastbroom, J.L. (1969) Luteal phase insufficiency in patients treated with clomiphene. *Am. J. Obstet. Gynecol.*, **103**, 165–71.

Vanrell, J.A. & Balasch, J. (1983) Prolactin in the evaluation of luteal phase in infertility. *Fertil. Steril.*, **39**, 30–3.

Vanrell, J.A. & Balasch, J. (1986) Luteal phase defects in repeated abortion. *Int. J. Gynaecol. Obstet.*, **24**, 111–15.

Vargyas, J., Kletzky, O. & Marrs, R.P. (1986) The effect of laparoscopic follicular aspiration on ovarian steroidogenesis during the early preimplantation period. *Fertil. Steril.*, **45**, 221–5.

Varma, T.R. & Morsman, J. (1982) Evaluation of the use of proluton-depot (hydroxyprogesterone hexanoate) in early pregnancy. *Int. J. Gynaecol. Obstet.*, **20**, 13–17.

Veldhuis, J.D., Christiansen, E., Evans, W.S., Kolp, L.A., Rogol, A.D. & Johnson, M.L. (1988) Physiological profiles of episodic progesterone release during the midluteal phase of the human menstrual cycle: analysis of circadian and ultradian rhythms, discrete pulse properties, and correlations with simultaneous luteinizing hormone release. *J. Clin. Endocrinol. Metab.*, **66**, 414–21.

Verhage, H.G., Bareither, M.L., Jaffe, R.C. & Akbar, M. (1979) Cyclic changes in ciliation, secretion and cell height of the oviductal epithelium in women. *Am. J. Anat.*, **156**, 505–22.

Walker, S.M., Walker, R.F. & Riad-Fahmy, D. (1984) Longitudinal studies of luteal function by salivary progesterone determinations. *Horm. Res.*, **20**, 231–40.

Wardlaw, S., Lauersen, N.H. & Saxena, B.B. (1975) The LH-hCG receptor of human ovary at various stages of the menstrual cycle. *Acta Endocrinol. Copenh.*, **79**, 568–76.

Weinstein, F.G., Seibel, M.M. & Taymor, M.L. (1984) Ovulation induction with subcutaneous pulsatile gonadotropin-releasing hormone: the role of supplemental human chorionic gonadotropin in the luteal phase. *Fertil. Steril.*, **41**, 546–50.

Wentz, A.C. (1980) Premenstrual spotting: its association with endometriosis but not luteal phase inadequacy. *Fertil. Steril.*, **33**, 605–7.

Wentz, A.C., Herbert, C.M., Maxson, W.S. & Garner, C.H. (1984) Outcome of progesterone treatment of luteal phase inadequacy. *Fertil. Steril.*, **41**, 856–62.

Witten, B.I. & Martin, S.A. (1985) The endometrial biopsy as a guide to the management of luteal phase defect. *Fertil. Steril.*, **44**, 460–5.

Wu, C.H. (1977) Plasma hormones in clomiphene citrate therapy. *Obstet. Gynecol.*, **49**, 443–8.

Wu, C.H. & Minassian, S.S. (1987) The integrated luteal progesterone: an assessment of luteal function. *Fertil. Steril.*, **48**, 937–40.

Ying, Y.K., Daly, D.C., Randolph, J.F., Soto-Albors, C.E., Maier, D.B., Schmidt, C.L. & Riddick, D.H. (1987) Ultrasonographic monitoring of follicular growth for luteal phase defects. *Fertil. Steril.*, **48**, 433–6.

Ying, Y.K., Walters, C.A., Kuslis, S., Lin, J.T., Daly, D.C. & Riddick, D.H. (1985) Prolactin production by explants of normal, luteal phase defective, and corrected luteal phase defective late secretory endometrium. *Am. J. Obstet. Gynecol.*, **151**, 801–4.

Yoshimi T. & Lipsett, M.B. (1968) The measurement of plasma progesterone. *Steroids*, **11**, 527–40.

Yovich, J.L., McColm, S.C., Yovich, J.M. & Matson, P.L. (1985) Early luteal serum progesterone concentrations are higher in pregnancy cycles. *Fertil. Steril.*, **44**, 185−9.

Yussman, M.A. & Taymor, M.L. (1973) Serum levels of follicle stimulating hormone and luteinizing hormone and of plasma progesterone related to ovulation by corpus luteum biopsy. *J. Clin. Endocrinol. Metab.*, **30**, 396−9.

Zorn, J.R., McDonough, P.G., Nessman, C., Janssens, Y. & Cedard L. (1984) Salivary progesterone as an index of the luteal function. *Fertil. Steril.*, **41**, 248−53.

# 10 Manipulation of Normal Ovarian Function

D.W. POLSON & D.L. HEALY

## Introduction

Controlled manipulation (augmentation or suppression) of normal ovarian function is an important strategy in contemporary reproductive medicine. The main reason for wanting to stimulate the ovaries is to increase the number of mature eggs which become available to treat infertility by *in vitro* fertilization/embryo transfer (IVF/ET), gamete-intrafallopian transfer (GIFT) or related assisted-conception techniques. Suppression of cyclic ovarian endocrine function is important as a prelude to certain forms of ovarian stimulation therapy or as a contraceptive strategy and can also afford a non-surgical means for treating various gynaecological conditions exacerbated by ovarian steroids, for example uterine fibroids and oestrogen-dependent tumours.

In recent years, endocrinological and pharmacological methods for manipulating ovarian function have been refined and developed hand-in-hand with rapid increases in our understanding of fundamental aspects of ovarian endocrinology. Earlier chapters in this book have emphasized the endocrine and paracrine mechanisms which regulate spontaneous follicular development, ovulation and luteinization in normal menstrual cycles. The aim of this final chapter is to critically assess the clinical protocols in current use for manipulating ovarian function, stressing their physiological basis and highlighting some of the practical benefits and disadvantages associated with their use.

# Treatment regimens for manipulating ovarian function

The principal reason for aiming to stimulate ovarian function is to improve fertility. With the discovery of antioestrogenic drugs and the purification of gonadotrophins from postmenopausal urine during the 1960s, it became possible to use these agents to stimulate the ovaries to yield multiple mature oocytes within a single cycle of treatment. Although the primary indication has usually been treatment of anovulation (see Chapter 8), augmentation of ovarian function has also been used to treat couples with male-related infertility (Melis *et al.*, 1987; Fioretti *et al.*, 1989) or idiopathic (unexplained) infertility (Welner *et al.*, 1988; Fisch *et al.*, 1989), and to treat endometriosis. Variable success has been reported using this strategy to increase the likelihood of a conception occurring *in vivo*.

It was IVF, and the realization that multiple follicular development led to improved rates of success (Trounson *et al.*, 1981) which provided the stimulus for improving and refining techniques of ovarian stimulation. The historic arrival of the first 'test-tube' baby in 1978 not only provided hope to countless infertile women, but also opened the door to dramatic advances in ovarian manipulation for other purposes. This first successful IVF pregnancy was conceived in a natural cycle, following recovery and fertilization of a single egg. However, IVF failed to achieve world-wide success until it was recognized that the likelihood of starting a pregnancy using this approach was directly related to the number of embryos transferred to the uterus (see Fig. 10.1) (Trounson *et al.*, 1981; Wood *et al.*, 1985; Hughes *et al.*, 1989). Following the initial report of this effect by Trounson and colleagues, the use of ovarian

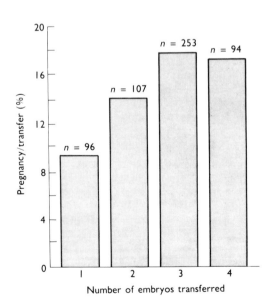

**Fig. 10.1.** The effect of the number of embryos transferred on the pregnancy rate after IVF (from Hughes *et al.*, 1989, with permission).

stimulation has facilitated the growth of IVF as an assisted-conception strategy. Furthermore, by providing clinical endocrinologists with an opportunity to manipulate normal ovaries, knowledge of folliculogenesis, intraovarian regulatory mechanisms and the control of ovulation has also been improved.

To achieve 'superovulation' a number of different therapeutic regimens have been described:

1 Antioestrogen therapy, for example clomiphene citrate, tamoxifen.
2 Treatment with exogenous gonadotrophins.
3 Combination-therapy with antioestrogens and exogenous gonadotrophins.
4 Combination-therapy with gonadotrophin-releasing hormone (GnRH) agonists and exogenous gonadotrophins.
5 Treatment with 'pure' follicle-stimulating hormone (FSH).

In the following sections we review the clinical success of the different treatment protocols and discuss various recent developments in reproductive medicine which have been facilitated by their use.


## Antioestrogens

During the 1950s a number of scientists discovered the potential benefits of drugs with oestrogenic and antioestrogenic activity. Various non-steroidal substances were synthesized which were noted to have syn- and antioestrogenic effects at different sites within the body. Among these clomiphene citrate and tamoxifen have been the two compounds most widely used to stimulate ovarian function. Despite the latter having the purer antioestrogenic activity, most clinical experience has been gained with clomiphene citrate. Its mode of action has been comprehensively reviewed (Adashi, 1984). In essence, clomiphene produces its effect by binding to oestradiol receptors in the hypothalamus, anterior pituitary and ovaries. The drug has been shown to have both syn- and antioestrogenic actions at various target sites. This property is related to the presence in most pharmaceutical preparations of two steroisomers: the *zu* congener which is predominantly antioestrogenic (Van Campenhout *et al.*, 1973) and the *en* congener which is oestrogenic (Ross *et al.*, 1973; Glasier *et al.*, 1989). The drug appears to work primarily through the antioestrogenic action of *zu* clomiphene (Glasier *et al.*, 1989) which blocks the negative feedback action of endogenous oestrogen at the level of the adenohypophysis (Ross *et al.*, 1970; Vaitukaitis *et al.*, 1971) and increases the frequency of pulsatile GnRH release by the hypothalamus (Miyake *et al.*, 1980). The attendant rise in serum concentration of endogenous luteinizing hormone (LH) and FSH leads to augmentation of spontaneous ovarian activity and increased folliculogenesis.

Clomiphene citrate has been used extensively for the induction of ovulation in anovulatory women and is particularly successful in women with polycystic ovaries, who comprise the largest group of anovulatory women (Adams et al., 1985) (see Chapter 8). Such patients usually have normal serum oestradiol concentrations (Polson et al., 1987) and normal oestradiol receptor numbers in hypothalamic and pituitary target-cells. Women with hypothalamic amenorrhoea and hypo-oestrogenism may have reduced oestrogen receptor numbers and therefore be less responsive to antioestrogenic drugs.

Among women with polycystic ovaries, 75–85% will develop regular ovulatory cycles when prescribed antioestrogens (Garcia et al., 1977; Gysler et al., 1982). A recent study suggests that the reason some fail to respond is ovarian refractoriness to what would otherwise be appropriate increases in serum gonadotrophin concentrations (Polson et al., 1989). This may be secondary to an ovarian abnormality, for example reduced gonadotrophin receptors or aberrant paracrine control. Alternatively, their endogenous FSH may be biologically inactive (Reichert, 1986).

Such deficiencies in responsiveness to gonadotrophin should not, however, apply to women with normal ovarian function. Administering clomiphene citrate to women with cyclic ovarian activity provokes an acute release of gonadotrophin which enhances follicular recruitment and development similar to that usually seen in anovulatory women. Clomiphene citrate has therefore been used as an adjunct to treat many forms of infertility (e.g. donor insemination, artificial insemination with the partner's semen, endometriosis and idiopathic infertility) on the assumption that increasing the number of follicles ovulated will increase the pregnancy rate. However, there have been few controlled trials and little evidence to suggest that treatment with clomiphene citrate does actually increase the pregnancy rate in ovulatory women with these forms of infertility.

Administration of clomiphene citrate alone has also been used to induce multiple follicular development in IVF patients (Wood et al., 1981; Trounson & Leeton, 1982; Fishel et al., 1984). However, the average number of follicles which develops is usually much lower than when therapy is given with exogenous gonadotrophins or when the clomiphene is given in combination with exogenous gonadotrophins (see later). Treatment with clomiphene citrate alone is, therefore, not widely used for this purpose.

Principal advantages of antioestrogen therapy are its simple (oral) administration, its low cost, and the fact that relatively few side-effects are associated with its use. The relatively low number of suitably mature oocytes which its use affords is its main disadvantage. There is also the concern that the antioestrogenic action of clomiphene citrate may interfere with endometrial development conducive to embryo implantation (Kokko et al., 1981).

To conclude, treatment with clomiphene citrate stimulates ovarian function in both ovulatory and anovulatory women. For women with normal ovarian function it increases the number of follicles which develop but does not appear to improve the *in vivo* pregnancy rate; its application to IVF is restricted by the relatively low numbers of oocytes yielded as compared with other treatments which are available (see below). The principal indication for antioestrogen therapy remains in the management of anovulatory infertility.

## Gonadotrophins

Use of exogenous gonadotrophin therapy to stimulate folliculogenesis became widespread with the extraction of biologically active gonadotrophins from menopausal urine. The pharmaceutical preparation in most common use contains approximately equal amounts (*c.* 75 IU/ ampoule) of FSH and LH bioactivity and is known generically as human menopausal gonadotrophin (hMG). Until the advent of IVF, therapy with hMG was mainly confined to the treatment of patients with ovulatory disorders due to polycystic ovaries, hypothalamic amenorrhoea and (prior to the introduction of bromocriptine) hyperprolactinaemia (see Chapter 8).

Exogenous gonadotrophins act directly at the ovarian level to stimulate follicular growth. One of the initial problems encountered in anovulatory women treated with hMG was the tendency towards multiple follicular development — particularly in women with polycystic ovaries (Oelsner *et al.*, 1978). Women with hypothalamic amenorrhoea had a more conservative and predictable response, but multiple pregnancy remained a problem (Schwartz *et al.*, 1980). It soon became clear that careful monitoring of ovarian response was essential to the safe and successful use of hMG. Initially physical parameters (e.g. changes in cervical mucus and ovarian volume) were monitored. Later on measurement of urinary oestrogen or serum oestradiol was incorporated, and in recent years ovarian ultrasonography to monitor ovarian responses directly has entered into widespread use.

There are numerous reviews of exogenous gonadotrophin usage in anovulatory women (e.g. Oelsner *et al.*, 1978; Wang & Gemzell, 1980), but few studies have been performed in women with normal ovarian function due to the close monitoring that is required (Weiner *et al.*, 1988). We have treated with hMG 39 women from couples with idiopathic infertility of at least 3 years' duration (Wade *et al.*, 1988). Each woman received 150 IU hMG from Day 3 of the cycle and the response was monitored by serial (daily) measurement of serum oestrogen concentrations and pelvic ultrasound. There were two pregnancies in 82 control cycles compared with 18 of 96 cycles with ovarian stimulation ($\bar{x} = 7.66$; $P < 0.01$). This significant improvement may have been due to the correction of subtle ovulatory defects which have been reported in these couples (Marik & Hulka, 1978; Dmowski *et al.*, 1981) or to increasing the number of oocytes which were released from the ovaries and passed into the fallopian tube. Further larger studies are needed to confirm the value of this form of treatment for idiopathic infertility.

Due to its obvious potential for stimulating multiple follicular development, hMG has been used extensively in IVF clinics (Jones *et al.*, 1982; Laufer *et al.*, 1983). Numerous studies have presented data on the efficacy of hMG-stimulation regimens in terms of number/ quality of oocytes and embryos which result and pregnancy outcome. Jones *et al.* (1982) advocate administration of four ampoules of hMG (i.e. *c.* 300 IU each of FSH and LH) on day 3 of the treatment cycle followed by three ampoules (*c.* 225 IU) on each of the following 3 days; thereafter the daily dose of hMG is titrated to the serum oestradiol concentration.

Our experience with use of hMG alone for this purpose has not met with the expected level of success. In a recent study we compared the use of hMG alone with the use of hMG in combination with a GnRH-agonist (see below). Fifteen of the 56 cycles (27%) using hMG alone were abandoned — 13 due to a premature LH rise and two due to poor follicular development. The pregnancy rate was also disappointing. Only three of 26 IVF/ET cycles resulted in a clinical pregnancy and none of 10 GIFT cycles. This was significantly lower than the 17% clinical pregnancy rate obtained in the GnRH-agonist/hMG group. The poor rate of success in GIFT patients receiving hMG alone may reflect oocyte immaturity, as has previously been reported in hMG-treated IVF patients (Laufer *et al.*, 1984). Similarly disappointing results from using hMG alone have been reported in other studies (Sathanadan *et al.*, 1989). A discharge rate of 27% is obviously unsatisfactory for an IVF programme and we therefore no longer use this stimulation regimen.

In summary, treatment with exogenous gonadotrophins can be used to stimulate ovarian function and results in multiple follicular development. Where conception *in vivo* is the objective, use of hMG with careful monitoring of ovarian function by oestrogen assays and ovarian ultrasound can improve pregnancy rates in couples with idiopathic infertility. The potential value of using hMG to augment ovarian function before artificial insemination or to treat endometriosis requires further evaluation. In our experience, the use of hMG alone for IVF is limited by the high incidence of abandoned cycles and low pregnancy rates.

## Antioestrogens with gonadotrophins

Numerous studies have suggested this form of combination-therapy to be the most successful for stimulation of multiple follicular development in IVF or GIFT treatment cycles (e.g. Hillier *et al.*, 1985; Healy *et al.*, 1987). Daily administration of clomiphene citrate (usually for 5 days at a dose of 50–100 mg/day) from Days 2 to 3 of the cycle elicits an increase in endogenous gonadotrophin levels which recruits a cohort of developing antral follicles at the beginning of the follicular phase of the treatment cycle. Simultaneous or sequential (i.e. starting on the day when clomiphene therapy is stopped) treatment with exogenous gonadotrophins (usually two or three ampoules of hMG/day) allows supranormal circulating gonadotrophin concentrations to be maintained such that multiple ovarian follicles enter oestrogen-secretory, pre-ovulatory stages of development. Supplementation of clomiphene citrate with exogenous gonadotrophins thereby overrides the physiological mechanism which would otherwise lead to the development of a single ovulatory follicle. Gonadotrophins are given daily until oestrogen levels and follicular development based on ovarian ultrasonography are consistent with the presence of multiple preovulatory follicles, whereupon ovulation is usually induced with hCG (see below).

A recent review of our experience with this form of combination-therapy confirmed successful induction of multiple folliculogenesis in 80–85% of treatment cycles. For women undergoing oocyte recovery the median number of oocytes obtained was six with a range of 1–26. The fertilization rate was 62%, and 70% of women starting treatment had an embryo transferred. The success as defined by clinical pregnancy per embryo transfer was 15% (unpublished data). Comparable success has been reported in other studies.

A retrospective analysis of endocrine changes during the stimulation phase of these cycles confirmed the existence of subtle differences between those cycles in which there were satisfactory follicular responses (peak serum oestradiol concentrations >3600 pmol/l) and those in which there were lesser ovarian responses (peak serum oestradiol concentrations <3600 pmol/l). In a series of 203 consecutive clomiphene/hMG treatment cycles, 166 were judged satisfactory and 37 unsatisfactory according to these criteria. All patients received the same stimulation regimen of clomiphene citrate (100 mg/day on Days 3–7) and hMG (150 IU/day from Day 4 onwards). From Day 8 on-wards the daily dose of hMG was adjusted according to the individual response as judged by serum oestradiol concentration and ovarian ultrasound. Figure 10.2 shows mean daily serum oestradiol levels for the satisfactory and poor responders. The difference between the two groups is highly significant after only 2 days of hMG therapy. Daily fluctuations in the mean serum FSH concentrations for the two groups are shown in Fig. 10.3. The pre-treatment FSH concentrations were similar, but significantly higher serum FSH concentrations were present in poor responders only 72 h after commencing clomiphene citrate and after only two injections of hMG. During this time, the dose of hMG given was similar in both groups so the higher FSH concentration in the poor responders presumably reflects higher endogenous release of FSH. This may be because less oestradiol and inhibin were produced by the ovaries of the

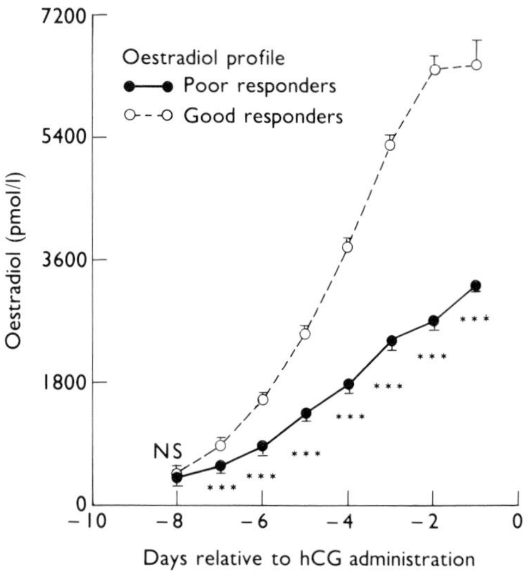

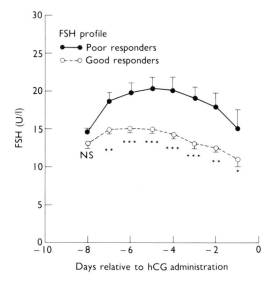

**Fig. 10.2.** Comparison of mean (±SE) serum oestradiol concentrations during the follicular phase on treatment with clomiphene citrate and hMG in 166 women with a satisfactory response (o − − − −o) and 37 women with an unsatisfactory response (o——o) (*** P<0.001).

**Fig. 10.3.** Comparison of mean (±SE) serum FSH concentrations during the follicular phase on treatment with clomiphene citrate and hMG in 166 women with a satisfactory response (o − − − −o) and 37 women with an unsatisfactory response (o——o) (* P <0.05; ** P <0.01; *** P <0.001).

poor responders (McLachlan, Robertson, Healy, deKretser & Burger, 1986). Women with a poor follicular response were then given higher doses of hMG which could account for the subsequent sustained elevation of their serum FSH concentrations. The serum LH concentration was similar in both groups. Comparing the outcome between these two groups confirmed a lower number of oocytes obtained, lower number of embryos transferred and lower overall pregnancy rate in those patients with a poor ovarian response and elevated serum FSH concentrations. The FSH concentration early in the stimulation phase may therefore prove to be a useful predictor of satisfactory folliculogenesis.

Previous work has established the importance of serum oestradiol measurements during stimulation with clomiphene citrate/hMG for timing of oocyte recovery (Jones *et al.*, 1984; Quigley *et al.*, 1984). Using data from 102 singleton conception cycles, the 5th, 50th and 95th centile values have been calculated for the oestradiol concentration on each day of the treatment cycle relative to the day of hCG administration (Okamoto *et al.*, 1986). These data provide a guide to an appropriate response, but fail to delineate the optimal response for conception to occur. We have recently reviewed the oestradiol profiles in 562 cycles receiving clomiphene citrate/hMG to determine the relationship between the serum oestradiol concentration and conception. These cycles were divided into six groups according to their serum oestradiol concentration: being less than the 5th centile; 5th to the 25th; 25th to the 50th; 50th to the 75th; 75th to the 95th; and greater than 95th centile. Within each group the number of oocytes obtained, the fertilization rate, number of embryos transferred and pregnancy rates were compared. As may be expected, there was a positive correlation between the serum oestradiol concentration and the number of oocytes obtained. Fertilization rates were similar and a similar median number of embryos was transferred in all groups. Pregnancy was significantly more likely to occur in IVF cycles in which women had a serum oestradiol concentration between 5500 and 9000 pmol/l, whereas in GIFT cycles the pregnancy rate (20%) was independent of serum oestrogen concentration (unpublished data). Thus for IVF, serum oestradiol concentration seems to influence pregnancy outcome. However, it is clear that the endogenous steroidal milieu during and following superovulation may not promote a degree of endometrial development optimal for implantation to occur (Dehou *et al.*, 1987). Only 66% of women undergoing endometrial biopsy at the time of embryo transfer following clomiphene/hMG therapy were noted to have histological changes consistent with the day of their cycle (Abate *et al.*, 1987). This asynchrony may be related to supraphysiological oestrogen concentrations and inappropriately high oestradiol:progesterone ratios. Our own experience would appear to confirm that while moderately elevated oestradiol concentrations are associated with higher pregnancy rates, excessive ovarian stimulation is undesirable for IVF cycles.

Another study assessing the endometrial response to alternative stimulation regimens has suggested that clomiphene citrate itself may have a detrimental effect on endometrial development (Sterzik *et al.*, 1988). Only four of 19 endometrial biopsies taken 2 days after oocyte collection from women receiving clomiphene citrate/hMG had a histological appearance consistent with the second day postovulation compared with an 'in-phase' biopsy rate of 50% in women who had been treated with hMG alone. This apparent negative influence of clomiphene citrate on the endometrium may be explained by its antioestrogenic properties (see earlier). However, the true impact of

327 MANIPULATION OF OVARIAN FUNCTION

clomiphene citrate on endometrial development remains to be established.

The combination of clomiphene citrate and hMG remains the most widely used superovulation regimen for IVF/GIFT and will elicit satisfactory multiple follicular development in 80–85% of cycles (McBain & Trounson, 1984; Rogers *et al.*, 1986). For the remainder, we have found the most common reason for abandoning treatment to be a failure of follicular development. In a review of 255 consecutive abandoned IVF treatment cycles, 46% patients were discharged due to a poor oestradiol response. The two other major indications were an elevated serum LH or progesterone concentration, in 9 and 11% of cases respectively (Oliver *et al.*, 1988). To determine whether this group of women had endocrinologically normal ovulatory cycles, weekly blood hormone tests were done from Day 1 of a spontaneous cycle. This confirmed that only 94 had a normal pattern of gonadotrophin, oestradiol and progesterone release. The most common abnormalities were (1) an inadequate luteal phase (peak progesterone concentration <20 nmol/1); (2) premature follicular luteinization (progesterone concentration 15 nmol/1 on Day 15); or (3) occult ovarian failure (serum LH and FSH levels above the 90th centile during the follicular phase of the cycle) (Cameron *et al.*, 1988). Following their initial failure, 33 of these women had a repeat cycle of IVF treatment using the same stimulation regimen. In 70%, the second cycle was also abandoned for the same reason. Six of nine women with seemingly normal endocrinology failed to have a satisfactory ovarian response to the repeat stimulation.

Thus it is clear that a group of patients exist who require an alternative stimulation protocol. The reason for their lack of follicular responsiveness is uncertain. One suggestion is that high follicular-phase levels of LH lead to increased ovarian androgen levels. This may be associated with both an inhibition of follicular development and an increased rate of follicular atresia (Louvet *et al.*, 1975) (see also Chapter 3). A second possibility is that subtle defects exist in the intraovarian control of follicular growth preventing multiple folliculogenesis. It should also be recalled that an LH surge is the appropriate physiological response to a rise in serum oestradiol concentration above a threshold level of *c.* 500 pmol/1 (see Chapter 1). When multiple follicular growth is induced, an inappropriately early LH surge often occurs when supraphysiological oestrogen levels are produced due to the presence of multiple small follicles containing immature oocytes. Such an artefactual response is obviously inappropriate for IVF or GIFT where the aim is to collect multiple mature oocytes from follicles which have undergone normal preovulatory development, including timely exposure to an ovulation-inducing surge of LH or human chorionic gonadotrophin (hCG). Therefore, in recent years considerable work to circumvent this problem has addressed the potential benefit of using treatment with GnRH-agonists to inhibit pituitary gonadotrophin release, thereby blocking inappropriate increases in levels of endogenous LH, whilst simultaneously administering exogenous gonadotrophins to stimulate the ovaries, as discussed below.

## GnRH-agonists with gonadotrophins

Use of exogenous gonadotrophins to produce multiple follicular development in normally cyclic women is often associated with abnormal ovarian changes and discordant pituitary responses to circulating ovarian hormones. Both of these problems may be overcome by suppressing endogenous gonadotrophin release whilst simultaneously treating with exogenous gonadotrophins. Selective inhibition of pituitary gonadotrophin release can be achieved by therapy with GnRH-agonists (Dericks-Tan et al., 1977; McLachlan, Healy & Burger, 1986). Administration either by subcutaneous injection or nasal insufflation of various synthetic GnRH-agonists has been shown to result in an initial stimulatory phase with increased pituitary release of gonadotrophins. However sustained administration of the GnRH-agonist depletes the pituitary gland of gonadotrophins and desensitizes it to the trophic actions of endogenous GnRH. Serum levels of FSH and LH therefore fall, follicular development is suppressed and ovarian secretion of oestrogen ceases. Early reports of pituitary−ovarian suppression using GnRH-agonist therapy to improve follicular development in response to exogenous gonadotrophins were encouraging (Porter et al., 1984; Fleming et al., 1985). Since then numerous confirmatory publications have followed.

In this study GnRH-agonist/gonadotrophin combination-therapy was initially given to 29 consecutive women in whom conventional combination-therapy with clomiphene citrate and hMG had failed to stimulate an adequate follicular response. The GnRH agonist Buserelin (Hoechst) was administered by intranasal insufflation (100 mg six times daily at regular intervals). Treatment with Buserelin was begun in the luteal phase of the cycle and maintained until serum oestradiol concentrations had fallen below 180 pmol/l for 2 consecutive days. Daily treatment with hMG (225 IU) was then initiated while treatment with Buserelin was continued. Both drugs were given until the time of hCG administration. If the serum oestradiol concentration did not increase after 3 days of therapy with hMG the daily dose of hMG was raised by 150 IU every 3 days to a maximum of 13 ampoules (c. 975 IU gonadotrophin/day). When adequate folliculogenesis was obtained as judged by blood oestradiol levels, and ovarian ultrasound examination confirmed the presence of at least three follicles >17 mm diameter, 10 000 IU hCG were administered to complete oocyte maturation and stimulate ovulation. Transvaginal ultrasound-guided oocyte recovery was performed 36 h later. The response to treatment was compared with that obtained in a similar group of 15 women undergoing repeat combination-therapy with clomiphene citrate and hMG women after a previously abandoned cycle. Nine of the 15 receiving a repeat cycle of clomiphene citrate and hMG failed to achieve follicular development suitable for oocyte recovery, compared with only five of 29 women receiving Buserelin and hMG. The median duration and dose of treatment with hMG was significantly higher when Buserelin was used, and resulted in a higher median number of oocytes being collected (see Table 10.1 and Fig. 10.4). Oocyte quality — as suggested by fertilization rates — was similar in both groups but there was a significantly higher percentage of triple-embryo transfers in the Buserelin-treated group. Three pregnancies occurred in this group and none in the clomiphene citrate/hMG group.

This study demonstrated a significant improvement in folliculogenesis in women receiving Buserelin. By suppressing endogenous gonadotrophin release, the tendency towards premature follicular selection with an early rise in serum LH or progesterone concentration was overcome. The initial phase of ovarian suppression may also have helped to promote the existence of a cohort of developmentally similar follicles which were able to begin preovulatory development more synchronously in response to the treatment with exogenous gonadotrophin than would otherwise occur using stimulation with clomiphene citrate/hMG in the presence of endogenous gonadotrophic activity (Hillier *et al.*, 1985).

It is clear from this and other studies that prior treatment with a GnRH-agonist may improve multiple follicular development and prevent cancellation of treatment cycles in women with a previously

**Table 10.1.** Comparison of responses of women with a previously abandoned clomiphene citrate (CC)/hMG cycle, to either a repeat CC/hMG cycle ($n = 15$) or treatment with Buserelin/hMG ($n = 29$). Figures given are median (range)

|  | Repeat CC/hMG cycle | Buserelin/hMG cycle |
|---|---|---|
| % of abandoned cycles | 53% | 14%* |
| Days of hMG therapy | 7 (4−9) | 12** (6−24) |
| Ampoules of hMG used | 12 (6−24) | 59** (15−194) |
| No. of oocytes collected | 0 (0−5) | 4* (0−19) |
| >3 oocytes retrieved | 20% | 62%* |
| Fertilization rate | 76.5% | 75.8% |
| Three-embryo transfer | 13% | 54%* |
| Pregnancy rate | 0% | 16% |

  * $P<0.01$; chi-squared.
** $P<0.001$; Wilcoxon Rank Sum.

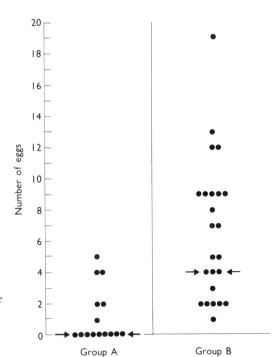

**Fig. 10.4.** Number of oocytes collected in 15 women receiving stimulation with clomiphene citrate and hMG (Group A) compared with 29 women receiving stimulation with Buserelin and hMG (Group B). Arrows indicate median number of oocytes collected.

unsatisfactory response to clomiphene citrate/hMG. To establish whether similar benefits might apply to women who respond normally to a standard clomiphene citrate/hMG superovulation protocol, we have recently completed a large study using two different doses of Buserelin (600 and 1200 μg/day) with hMG. Women who had previously shown an adequate follicular response to clomiphene citrate/hMG were randomized to receive either hMG alone, Buserelin (600 μg/day) plus hMG, or Buserelin (1200 μg/day) plus hMG. We hoped to establish if an individual's previous response to clomiphene citrate/hMG cycle could be improved by alternative treatment with Buserelin/hMG cycle and to determine whether there were any differences between the two doses of Buserelin. The results from this randomized study were also compared with a similar group of women concurrently receiving a second or subsequent cycle of therapy with clomiphene citrate/hMG stimulation. Table 10.2 summarizes the number of completed cycles in each group and the indication for abandoning treatment. Women receiving hMG alone were significantly more likely to be discharged — usually due to a premature LH surge. Only seven of the 120 (6%) Buserelin cycles were abandoned and none were due to an LH surge. Four of the abandonments were because of inadequate follicular development, two had elevated serum progesterone concentrations, and one woman stopped sniffing for social reasons. It was of interest that for these women who had shown a previously normal response to clomiphene citrate/hMG, the 6% discharge-rate from cycles of treatment with Buserelin was not

**Table 10.2.** Details of IVF/GIFT treatment groups randomized to receive ovarian stimulation with Buserelin (600 μg/day) plus hMG, Buserelin (1200 μg/day) plus hMG, hMG alone or (in a separate but concurrent study) clomiphene citrate plus hMG

| | Randomized study | | | |
| --- | --- | --- | --- | --- |
| | Bus. 600+hMG | Bus. 1200+hMG | hMG alone | CC/hMG |
| No. of women | 51 | 56 | 50 | 176 |
| No. of cycles | 56 | 64 | 56 | 176 |
| No. of abandoned cycles | 4 | 3 | 15* | 18 |
| Serum oestradiol <1600 pmol/l | 1 | 3 | 2 | 11 |
| Premature LH surge | — | — | 13 | 4 |
| Serum progesterone >7 nmol/l | 2 | — | — | 1 |
| Serum LH >30 IU/l | — | — | — | 2 |
| Self discharge | 1 | — | — | — |

* $P<0.01$ vs. Bus. 600, Bus. 1200 and CC/hMG (Fisher's test)
Bus. 600 = Buserelin 600 μg/day.
Bus. 1200 = Buserelin 1200 μg/day.
CC = clomiphene citrate.

significantly lower than the 10% discharge-rate seen in women undergoing a repeat cycle of stimulation with clomiphene citrate/hMG.

Both doses of Buserelin produced ovarian suppression within a similar period of time (see Fig. 10.5) and in both groups there was a significant increase in the dose and duration of hMG therapy given compared with hMG alone or clomiphene citrate/hMG. Despite this need for more hMG, a similar median number of follicles was aspirated in each group and a similar median number of oocytes was obtained. There was no significant difference in fertilization rates between any of the groups. Therefore, in this randomized study, Buserelin did not improve the number of oocytes obtained compared with hMG alone, nor were the fertilization rates increased, suggesting that oocyte quality was not improved. For individual women, comparison of the Buserelin cycle with the previous clomiphene citrate/hMG cycle revealed no significant differences in terms of the number of follicles aspirated, number of oocytes recovered or fertilization rate.

Comparing the clinical pregnancy rate per cycle started, treatment with Buserelin/hMG and clomiphene citrate/hMG achieved significantly higher pregnancy rates than treatment with hMG alone (see Table 10.3). This appeared to be due to a reduction in the number of abandoned cycles rather than an improvement in folliculogenesis *per se*. There was no difference in the pregnancy rates between the Buserelin-600 μg and Buserelin-1200 μg groups, and neither group had a higher pregnancy rate than women receiving concurrent clomiphene citrate/hMG combination-therapy. Therefore, in this group of women who respond satisfactorily to clomiphene citrate/hMG stimulation, Buserelin confers no advantage and repeat treatment with clomiphene citrate/

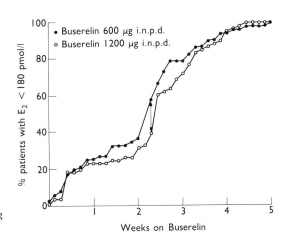

**Fig. 10.5.** Comparison of time taken to achieve suppression of oestradiol levels in women receiving Buserelin 600 μg/day and Buserelin 1200 μg/day.

**Table 10.3.** Clinical pregnancy rates in IVF and GIFT patients who were randomized to receive ovarian stimulation with Buserelin (600 μg/day) plus hMG, Buserelin (1200 μg/day) plus hMG, hMG alone or (in a separate but concurrent study) clomiphene citrate plus hMG

| | Randomized study | | | |
|---|---|---|---|---|
| Treatment | Bus. 600+hMG | Bus. 1200+hMG | hMG alone | CC/hMG |
| **IVF** | | | | |
| 1−2 Embryos transferred | 0/8 | 1/8 | 1/11 | 4/43 |
| 3−4 Embryos transferred | 6/24 | 4/29 | 2/15 | 10/66 |
| Total | 6/32 | 5/37 | 3/26 | 14/109 |
| | (18.8%) | (13.5%) | (11.5%) | (12.8%) |
| **GIFT** | | | | |
| 1−3 oocytes | 0/2 | 0/0 | 0/2 | 3/10 |
| 4−6 oocytes | 3/8 | 6/14 | 0/8 | 12/22 |
| Total | 3/10 | 6/14 | 0/10* | 15/32 |
| | (30%) | (42.8%) | (0%) | (46.8%) |
| **IVF and GIFT** | | | | |
| Clinical pregnancy rate/transfer | 9/42 | 11/51 | 3/36 | 29/141 |
| | (21.4%) | (21.6%) | (8.3%) | (20.6%) |
| Clinical pregnancy/cycle started | 9/56 | 11/64 | 3/56* | 29/176 |
| | (16.1%) | (17.2%) | (5.4%) | (16.5%) |

\* $P<0.05$ vs. Bus. 1200 and CC/hMG (Fisher's test)
Bus. 600 = Buserelin (600 μg/day)
Bus. 1200 = Buserelin (1200 μg/day)
CC = clomiphene citrate

hMG is to be recommended. On the other hand, for women in whom there is inadequate folliculogenesis or a premature LH surge in response to clomiphene citrate/hMG therapy, alternative GnRH-agonist/hMG therapy will significantly improve both the number who reach oocyte-recovery and the pregnancy rate achieved. Our study confirms that Buserelin 600 μg/day is effective for this purpose and we would therefore recommend that this dose be used.

Another group for whom we would recommend the use of GnRH-agonist therapy is women aged over 37 years. A recent retrospective review of prognostic features of couples undergoing IVF treatment has confirmed that there is a significant reduction in pregnancy rates in women over 37 years (Hughes *et al.*, 1989). With increasing age there is a tendency towards higher serum gonadotrophin concentrations, indicative of increasing ovarian resistance. Thus the ability of older women to evince multiple follicular development is reduced. Also their higher baseline-LH concentrations may increase their tendency to elicit an inappropriate LH surge early on in the follicular phase of the ovarian cycle (Droesch *et al.*, 1988).

To determine whether treatment with Buserelin might improve folliculogenesis and reduce the number of abandoned cycles in older IVF patents, we randomized a group of women aged over 37 years in whom there was a previously satisfactory response to clomiphene citrate/hMG, to receive either a second cycle of clomiphene citrate/hMG, or to receive Buserelin (1200 µg/day) followed by hMG when pituitary downregulation was confirmed. Nine of the 41 women (22%) allocated to receive clomiphene citrate/hMG were discharged from treatment compared with only one of the 36 women (3%) treated with Buserelin/hMG ($P<0.001$). The number of oocytes obtained, fertilization rates and number of eggs (GIFT) or embryos available for transfer were similar in both groups. The clinical pregnancy rate per ET and per cycle started were both significantly higher in women receiving Buserelin than clomiphene citrate/hMG (29 vs. 6.7%; and 25 vs. 4.9%, respectively). In this study, Buserelin not only significantly reduced the likelihood of being discharged from the treatment cycle, but it also increased the pregnancy rate. This may have been due to better embryo quality or improved endometrial receptivity. Whatever the reason, it seems clear that GnRH-agonist therapy should be recommended for women aged over 37 years.

As mentioned earlier, drawbacks of GnRH-agonist therapy are the increased duration and dose of hMG required to elicit an appropriate follicular response. The reason for this is unclear, but could be due to the absence of endogenous FSH or a reduction in circulating growth hormone (GH) concentrations. There is increasing evidence from both *in vitro* and *in vivo* studies that GH facilitates FSH action at the granulosa cell level (Jiu *et al.*, 1986; Homburg *et al.*, 1988) which has general implications for the use of GH as an adjunct in superovulation therapy (see below). It is possible that Buserelin may suppress GH production by the anterior pituitary gland such that higher levels of FSH are required to overcome a GnRH-agonist induced state of relative GH-deficiency. The need for higher doses and longer duration of hMG therapy when used in combination with GnRH-agonist unfortunately increases the cost per treatment cycle. Therefore, to prove cost-effective there will have to be an improvement in the pregnancy rates currently obtainable using combination-therapy with GnRH-agonist and hMG.

Towards this end, it may be possible to exploit the ability of GnRH-agonists acutely to stimulate gonadotrophin release as well as to produce longer-term pituitary downregulation. The short-term response to administration of a GnRH-agonist is an acutely increased release of both FSH and LH such that if exogenous gonadotrophins are administered the following day, folliculogenesis is enhanced (see Figs 10.6 and 10.7). Advantage has been taken of this 'flare-up' response to produce multiple follicular development in IVF/GIFT treatment cycles. We prefer the term 'BOOST' to describe this endogenous gonadotrophic supplement to treatment with exogenous hMG. Continued administration of the GnRH-agonist will produce pituitary downregulation within 7−10 days and in most women there will not be a LH surge. Timing of oocyte recovery can therefore be improved and fewer cycles cancelled. Most studies have confirmed that this 'short' treatment protocol for Buserelin with hMG reduces the total dosage of hMG required compared with the 'long' treatment protocol which requires that pituitary downregulation be fully established before any treatment with hMG is started (Sathanadan et al., 1989). There have been studies in which treatment has been randomized to either clomiphene citrate/hMG or GnRH-agonist/hMG using the short protocol. Some confirm a lower number of abandoned cycles in the Buserelin group, whereas others claim no difference (MacNamee et al., 1989). Overall, there seems to be little convincing evidence of any improvement in the clinical pregnancy rate using this protocol, but further studies are needed as most of the

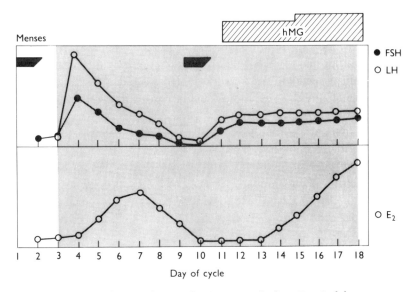

**Fig. 10.6.** Schema indicating the use of a GnRH-agonist from Day 3 of the treatment cycle (shaded area) to induce pituitary downregulation and ovarian suppression. Treatment with hMG is then commenced (hatched area) to stimulate folliculogenesis.

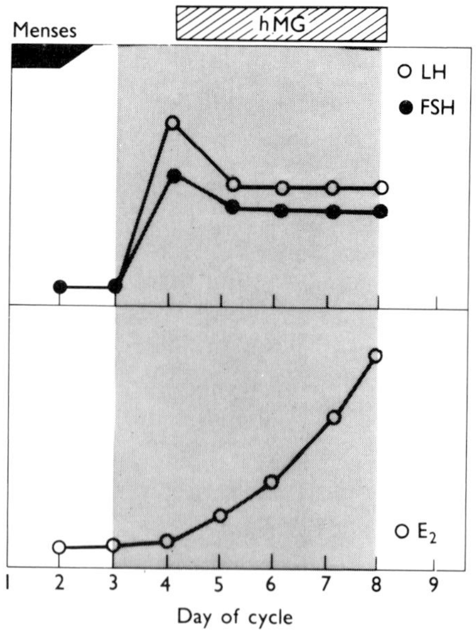

**Fig. 10.7.** Schema indicating the use of a GnRH-agonist in a 'BOOST' mode to promote folliculogenesis before IVF. The agonist is taken daily from Day 3 (shaded area) and induces a rise in serum FSH and LH. The next day, hMG therapy is commenced (hatched area) to augment this endogenous gonadotrophin release and maintain multiple folliculogenesis.

earlier work has been non-randomized and without suitable control groups.

In summary, GnRH-agonists play a major role in the manipulation of normal ovarian function. Their use removes the influence of endogenous gonadotrophins on the ovary, and prevents the ovulatory LH surge. Thereby exogenous gonadotrophin can be used to control folliculogenesis and allow accurate timing of ovulation following hCG administration. Used in conjunction with IVF, Buserelin/hMG therapy significantly improves the overall pregnancy rate in women who have previously failed to respond appropriately to clomiphene citrate/hMG and in women who are more than 37 years of age. However, combination treatment with GnRH-agonist and hMG appears to offer little advantage to women who show normal ovarian responsiveness to clomiphene citrate/hMG.

## 'Pure' FSH

There have been reports that high serum LH concentrations during the follicular phase of IVF stimulation cycles may be detrimental to oocyte maturation (Howles *et al.*, 1986; Stanger & Yovich, 1985). Recent evidence from ovulation-induction programmes also suggests an association between elevated blood LH levels and spontaneous miscarriage (Homburg *et al.*, 1988a; Sagle *et al.*, 1988). This may reflect the deleterious influence of premature exposure of immature oocytes to LH. It has therefore been suggested that an LH-free gonadotrophin preparation may be preferable to hMG for augmenting ovarian function before IVF.

'Pure' FSH, an extract of menopausal urine containing *c*. 75 IU FSH and <1 IU of LH, has been available as 'Metrodin' (Ares-Serono) for some years. It is used both for ovulation-induction in anovulatory women (see Chapter 8) and for superovulation in conjunction with IVF and GIFT (Kamrava *et al.*, 1982; Polson, Mason, Saldahana & Franks, 1987). Protocols are extremely variable between different clinics, but one non-randomized study comparing pure FSH with hMG for ovulation-induction in clomiphene-resistant women with polycystic ovaries failed to show any improvement in pregnancy rate with pure FSH and no reduction in the likelihood of a miscarriage occurring (Sagle *et al.*, 1989).

To determine the contribution of follicular-phase blood LH levels to the outcome of ovarian-stimulation therapy, we established a reference range of LH values from measurements made during 102 consecutive clomiphene citrate/hMG IVF conception-cycles (Thomas *et al.*, 1989). We then examined rates of oocyte recovery, fertilization and pregnancy in 596 consecutive IVF/GIFT patients according to their plasma LH concentrations. The number of oocytes retrieved was not related to LH concentration, nor was there any difference in the fertilization or pregnancy rates. This study did not therefore suggest that serum LH levels were predictive of IVF success. Also there was no evidence that high LH concentrations were detrimental to follicular development or the ability of oocytes to be fertilized and establish a pregnancy. Unfortunately, this study did not ascertain if high LH levels were associated with an increased incidence of early pregnancy loss. It did, however, suggest that LH levels are of little clinical value in predicting clinical response. It is therefore questionable if an LH-free gonadotrophin preparation is currently necessary for ovarian stimulation in association with IVF.

## Induction and timing of ovulation with hCG

In the normal menstrual cycle, the ovulatory LH surge is initiated in response to oestradiol secreted by the preovulatory follicle. With rising serum oestradiol levels in the late follicular phase of the cycle GnRH release by the hypothalamus is modified (Schuilling & Lappohn, 1985) as reflected in increased frequency and amplitude of pulsatile LH secretion by the pituitary, resulting in an increase in the peripheral serum LH concentration (Kapen *et al.*, 1973; Hoff *et al.*, 1977). Increased stimulation of the preovulatory follicle by LH not only drives follicular oestrogen secretion but also gradually· initiates changes in steroid metabolism associated with luteinization and increased secretion of progesterone (Laborde *et al.*, 1976) (see also Chapter 3). Rising serum progesterone levels may provide the final cue for onset of the oestrogen-induced LH surge which triggers the final stages of oocyte maturation and follicular rupture (Edwards, 1980).

Oocyte recovery for IVF or GIFT can conveniently be timed to an ovulatory dose of hCG. The aim should be to give the hCG injection as close as possible to the time of spontaneous LH surge onset. If it is given before the preovulatory phase of follicle and oocyte maturation is complete, the eggs obtained may be immature or of reduced developmental potential (Laufer et al., 1984). Since normal oocyte maturation is influenced by the intrafollicular environment, fertilization of human oocytes matured in vitro is relatively unsuccessful (Veeck, 1988).

In patients not receiving GnRH-agonist therapy to suppress pituitary gonadotrophin release, the aim should be to give an ovulation inducing injection of hCG (usually 5000 or 10 000 IU) not more than 24 h before onset of the endogenous LH surge. Inevitably, this means that a proportion of patients will have started their surge by the time that hCG is given. Unless this is detected, spontaneous follicular rupture may occur before the egg collection can be carried out. If the time of surge onset is known (blood or urinary LH assays) the egg collection can be brought forward accordingly. However, reliance on an endogenous LH surge to time oocyte recovery is associated with recovery of a higher proportion of immature oocytes (Droesch et al., 1988), probably due to difficulty in determining precisely when an LH surge begins.

Use of hCG to time oocyte-recovery before IVF or GIFT therefore confers a number of advantages, however, the decision when to give hCG is critical. Most centres use a combination of follicular number and size with serum oestradiol concentrations to determine when hCG should be given. In the Infertility Medical Centre, Victoria, we have used the serum oestradiol levels in the follicular phases of 102 clomiphene citrate/hMG stimulated cycles which resulted in a singleton IVF pregnancy to determine optimal values of oestradiol for each day of ovarian stimulation, as a guide to a satisfactory response (Okamato et al., 1986). This has proved useful for recognizing abnormal responses and in our programme women with oestradiol levels less than the 5th centile are discharged due to unsatisfactory folliculogenesis.

Further data has provided a guide to the timing of hCG administration and would suggest that serum oestradiol levels between 5500 and 9000 pmol/l are optimal for IVF success. Levels less than this were associated with fewer oocytes being collected and a lower pregnancy rate. Higher levels also had a lower pregnancy rate, possibly due to the detrimental influence of elevated serum oestradiol concentrations on endometrial development, as a high oestrogen:progesterone ratio early in the luteal phase has been associated with reduced pregnancy rates (Gidley-Baird et al., 1986).

## Physiological effects of suppressing ovarian activity

Since gonadotrophins stimulate ovarian activity, inhibition of their release by the pituitary gland causes a reversible suppression of ovarian function. Recognition of the physiological negative feedback role of ovarian oestradiol at the putuitary level prompted work in the 1950s to manufacture a synthetic oestrogen for use as a contraceptive pill. It soon became clear that progesterone was needed to afford cycle control, but that oestrogens given alone could effectively inhibit folliculogenesis by reducing peripheral serum gonadotrophin concentrations. This pointed the way to medical suppression of folliculogenesis as a clinical strategy in the management of certain oestrogen-responsive gynaeco-logical conditions such as fibroids and endometriosis. For obvious reasons, exogenous oestrogen cannot be used as a medication in the treatment of such conditions. However, long-acting GnRH-agonists which inhibit gonadotrophin release and suppress the ovaries (see above) are finding widespread application for this purpose.

## GnRH-agonist therapy and endometriosis

Pelvic endometriosis is a variable clinical entity, being an unexpected finding in some asymptomatic women and, in others, a debilitating and aggressive disease. Medical therapy is usually first-time management, particularly among the infertile, with a progestogen or Danazol being the usual treatment offered. Both of these are not without unpleasant side-effects including weight-gain, nausea, abdominal distension with progestogens, and more serious virilizing effects with Danazol such as facial hair growth, acne, and deepening of the voice (Buttram *et al.*, 1985). Cure rates depend on a subjective pelvic reassessment with reports of 60–80% success for both types of treatment. Suppression of ovarian steroid biosynthesis with a GnRH-agonist has been shown in many studies to improve clinical symptoms and pelvic evidence of endometriosis (Meldrum *et al.*, 1985). Unfortunately, one of the effects of this 'medical castration' is a reduction in bone-density secondary to prolonged hypo-oestrogenism. This has been observed after only 6 months of treatment (Matta *et al.*, 1987).

The precise role for GnRH-agonists in the clinical management of endometriosis therefore remains uncertain. Short-term GnRH-agonist therapy only is to be recommended in view of the bone demineralization effects, and there is always the possibility of a recurrence. The large ovarian endometriomas are probably better dealt with surgically, but pretreatment with a GnRH-agonist or similar suppressive agent is sen-sible. However, recent evidence suggests that for women with mild pelvic endometriosis, laser-ablative therapy at the time of diagnostic laparoscopy produces a clinical cure and correction of subfertility (Gast *et al.*, 1988). It is therefore possible that if the development of this surgical approach continues, medical therapy for endometriosis will play a less important role in the future.

**GnRH-agonists and fibroids**

Leiomyomata, or uterine fibroids are oestrogen-dependent tumours, occurring in 20–25% of women over the age of 30 years. Oestrogen is thought to play a role in the formation of these tumours as increased numbers of oestrogen receptors have been found in fibroid muscle compared with adjacent normal myometrium.

Uterine fibroids have been shown to reduce in size with relief of clinical symptoms following suppression of ovarian function with GnRH-agonists. In our own experience (75 patients aged between 17 and 52 years) a 4-month course of GnRH-agonist treatment typically results in fibroid regression from a pretreatment volume of $257\pm42$ cm$^3$ (mean$\pm$SE) to $131\pm41$ cm$^3$. The most significant decrease in fibroid size occurs within the first 12 weeks of treatment. A strong correlation has been found between initial fibroid size and the subsequent degree of regression with larger tumours responding most markedly to oestrogen deprivation induced by GnRH-agonist treatment (unpublished data). Reduction in fibroid size is seen as early as 3 weeks after initiating treatment in the mid-luteal phase of the menstrual cycle. The time of commencement of GnRH-agonist treatment is critical when used to manipulate ovarian function in patients with endometriosis and leimyomata. Commencement in the mid-luteal phase, in the presence of circulating progesterone concentrations indicative of recent ovulation, leads to more rapid suppression of pituitary FSH and LH secretion, and hence of ovarian oestradiol production.

Unlike its application to endometriosis, GnRH-agonist therapy for uterine fibroids represents the first medical treatment which has become available to improve the clinical symptoms and reduce the size of these tumours. In clinical practice, GnRH-agonists might be used in selected patients with uterine fibroids as an alternative to surgery, or used in combination with a surgical approach using the GnRH-agonist preoperatively. Of significance in this regard is the use of GnRH-agonist therapy before undertaking hysteroscopic resection of submucous leiomyomata. We recently used this approach to treat a 17-year-old woman who was so sick that she had originally presented with a haemoglobin of 2.8 gm/dl. By combining GnRH-agonist therapy and hysteroscopic resection she was able to retain her uterus.

# Physiological effects of stimulating ovarian activity

During ovarian stimulation with antioestrogenic drugs and exogenous gonadotrophins, blood oestradiol levels rise in parallel with the follicular response. Elevated oestradiol levels are a useful indication of satisfactory folliculogenesis, but they also have unwanted sequelea. The endometrium is oestrogen-responsive and histological changes take place as oestradiol levels rise. One suggested cause of low IVF success-rates (in 1988, 75% of our patients reached ET but only 15% of these conceived) is reduced endometrial receptivity or asynchronous endometrial−ovum development (Abate *et al.*, 1987). In a normal ovulatory cycle, endometrial maturity is regulated by oestradiol secreted by the preovulatory follicle and is synchronized with oocyte-release and corpus luteum formation. Luteal progesterone then causes secretory changes in the endometrium which are conducive to embryo-implantation 5−7 days after ovulation. During IVF treatment cycles, follicular-phase oestradiol levels become supraphysiologically elevated and although luteal-phase progesterone concentrations also become elevated, the oestradiol:progesterone ratio early-on in the luteal phase may not be adequate to provide a suitably receptive (i.e. 'in-phase') endometrium. Evidence to support this is provided by reports of improved pregnancy rates in cycles with relatively high progesterone concentrations early in the luteal phase (Jones *et al.*, 1984; Taylor *et al.*, 1986). Furthermore, one-third of the endometrial biopsies taken from IVF patients at the time of ET 2 or 3 days after oocyte-recovery were 'out of phase' (Abate *et al.*, 1987).

Progesterone supplementation has been used in many centres to try to improve endometrial receptivity and overcome the consequences of elevated serum oestradiol concentrations (see also Chapter 9). However, there is little evidence that pregnancy rates have improved (Leeton *et al.*, 1985; Howles *et al.*, 1987; Van Steirteghem *et al.*, 1988). It is clear that luteal support with hCG is essential following ovarian stimulation using GnRH-agonist/gonadotrophin combination-therapy (Smith *et al.*, 1989), and that treatment with hCG is better than systemic progesterone. There is evidence from both animal and human studies of an ovarian−uterine counter-current system of blood flow (Riesen *et al.*, 1970; Ginther *et al.*, 1974), and it seems possible that high local concentrations of progesterone are important for endometrial maturation. Evidence from our donor-oocyte programme (for women with premature menopause receiving hormonal replacement therapy to mimic the follicular-luteal phasic steroid pattern of a normal cycle) also suggests that local administration of progesterone may be preferable to systemic steroid therapy. In a series of 14 ETs over a 12-month period, five pregnancies were achieved from seven transfers when a combination of intravaginal progesterone pessaries plus systemic progesterone (Proluton, 50 mg intramuscularly daily) was administered throughout the luteal phase, compared with no pregnancies from the other seven transfers when Proluton alone was used (Leeton *et al.*, 1989). It remains to be determined whether luteal-phase support with progesterone pessaries improves IVF pregnancy rates.

Clearly, the manipulation of normal ovarian function is not without its drawbacks, and the physiological changes produced by superovulation can result in bodily changes that may be detrimental to achieving and maintaining a pregnancy. Furthermore, a percentage of women will either fail to respond to the drugs used to stimulate multiple follicular development, or will have an undesirable response with a premature elevation of the serum LH or progesterone concentration. In the retrospective analysis of 255 consecutive abandoned cycles in our IVF programme mentioned earlier (Oliver *et al.*, 1988), 45% of the abandonments were due to a failure of adequate folliculogenesis and up to 15% had occult ovarian failure (i.e. supranormal FSH and LH levels). When these women were subsequently given Buserelin/hMG combination-therapy, folliculogenesis was significantly improved in those who had normal FSH plasma LH levels with 19 of 21 women obtaining oocytes and three of these achieving a pregnancy. In contrast, in women with occult ovarian failure there was a disappointing response with only four of eight reaching oocyte recovery and no pregnancies (see Fig. 10.8) (Cameron *et al.*, 1988).

Thus in poor responders, an IVF pregnancy rate similar to that seen following routine clomiphene citrate/hMG therapy can be produced by using a Buserelin/hMG stimulation regimen. Results from other centres support these data. However, for women with occult ovarian failure, it seems unlikely that ovarian stimulation with exogenous gonadotrophins will improve their ovarian response, and this group of women should be redirected to a donor oocyte programme (Cameron *et al.*, 1989).

From our experience with clomiphene citrate/hMG combination-therapy and IVF, 9% of abandoned cycles are due to an inappropriate LH surge and 11% to a premature rise in serum progesterone concentration (Oliver *et al.*, 1988). The gonadotrophin surge is usually physiologically appropriate in relation to the serum oestradiol level, but inappropriate in terms of follicle number and maturity. Similarly a rise in the serum progesterone concentration in the late follicular phase, secondary to premature luteinization, is associated with poor IVF outcome (Kerin & Warnes, 1986). Both events can be circumvented by combining pituitary suppression using a GnRH-agonist with hMG. In 90 of our patients who previously showed this type of abnormal response

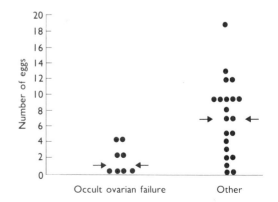

**Fig. 10.8.** Number of oocytes collected following therapy with Buserelin and hMG in eight women with occult ovarian failure compared with 21 other women with normal serum FSH concentrations.

to clomiphene citrate/hMG, subsequent treatment with Buserelin/hMG led to a cycle cancellation rate of only 6% and an IVF pregnancy rate per ET of 17% (unpublished data). Therefore this group of women show a much better response than those who simply display a quantitatively inadequate follicular response. This points to a primary intra-ovarian defect in women with poor follicular responsiveness to clomiphene citrate/hMG, as opposed to aberrances within the hypothalamo–pituitary axis.

Another potential problem for women receiving gonadotrophin therapy is ovarian hyperstimulation. This has been recognized for many years and in severe cases may result in excessive ovarian enlargement, ascites, pleural oedema and renal failure (Schenker & Weinstein, 1978). One death has been reported (Moses et al., 1965). It is clear that the likelihood of developing the hyperstimulation syndrome is increased by the administration of hCG (Hancock, 1970). In ovulation-induction programmes, hCG can be withheld if necessary and the multiple developing follicles which are present will usually undergo spontaneous regression and atresia. For women undergoing IVF, however, the intention is to collect a large number of oocytes and it is essential to administer hCG when multiple mature follicles are present. The potential for developing full-blown clinical hyperstimulation is reduced by aspirating all accessible antral follicles within the ovary, as removal of the granulosa cells will diminish the potential for the excessive degree of ovarian steroid production associated with hyperstimulation (Hodgen, 1982). In women for whom luteal support has been suggested, or is necessary (i.e. GnRH-agonist/hMG cycles), further doses of hCG are usually administered after the collection of oocytes. If more than 10 oocytes are obtained and multiple follicles are present, it may be preferable to support the luteal phase with systemic progesterone or vaginal progesterone pessaries rather than to stimulate the ovaries further with repeated doses of hCG and increase the risk of hyperstimulation (MacNamee et al., 1989). As most women will show a similar response to ovarian stimulation therapy in a subsequent cycle, the dose of hMG used in the next cycle should be reduced following a treatment cycle resulting in hyperstimulation.

## Future directions

Current work in this area indicates that optimal ovarian stimulation before IVF or GIFT is associated with the collection of five to seven mature oocytes (Hughes et al., 1989) and that for in the majority of patients this can be achieved using antioestrogen/gonadotrophin combination-therapy. For those who do not respond adequately, and in whom the diagnosis of occult ovarian failure has been excluded, success comparable with that otherwise expected of clomiphene citrate/hMG combination-therapy can usually be achieved by combined treatment with a GnRH-agonist and hMG. There remains, however, a small group of women who repeatedly undergo unsuccessful attempts at ovarian stimulation. They may have regular ovulatory cycles with apparently normal serum gonadotrophin, oestradiol and progesterone levels. However, their ovaries consistently fail to develop multiple preovulatory follicles in response to treatment with exogenous gonadotrophins, with or without GnRH-agonist pretreatment.

There is evidence that for this group of women treatment with exogenous GH may provide a useful adjunct to gonadotrophin therapy. Experiments have shown that treatment with GH *in vivo* or *in vitro* augments the action of FSH on granulosa cell function. The action of GH may be direct at the granulosa cell level (Jiu *et al.*, 1986), or indirect through increased hepatic production of insulin-like growth factors (IGF-I) (Davoren & Hsueh, 1986). Other experimental work has established that IGF-I of hepatic origin or produced within the ovary is able to augment the trophic action of FSH on granulosa cells (see Chapter 3). Moreover, there is evidence from clinical studies that GH/hMG combination-therapy in anovulatory women undergoing ovulation-induction significantly improves the response otherwise seen with hMG alone (Homburg *et al.*, 1988b).

Properly controlled, randomized studies are now underway in a number of clinical centres to evaluate the potential benefits of GH as an adjunct to the use of hMG to stimulate multiple follicular development before IVF or GIFT. Use of GH in combination with GnRH-agonists (or possibly in the future, GnRH antagonists: see, e.g. Fraser & Baird, 1987) and exogenous gonadotrophins may allow satisfactory ovarian responses to be achieved in those 10−15% of patients who fail to respond adequately to conventional therapy with clomiphene citrate and hMG.

Trials are also needed to evaluate the 'BOOST' response elicited by treatment with GnRH-agonist as an adjunct to exogenous gonadotrophin therapy (see above). This form of combination-therapy holds out a means of achieving satisfactory ovarian responses to exogenous gonadotrophins without causing inappropriate or untimely increases in endogenous LH release, such that the overall number of abandoned treatment cycles should fall. A further benefit is that uterine receptivity and implantation rates may be improved once clomiphene citrate is deleted from the treatment regimen.

Meanwhile, contemporary techniques for manipulating normal ovarian function usually allow multiple oocytes to be collected for use in programmes of assisted conception such as IVF and GIFT. There are few side-effects or problems associated with the use of current treatment regimens if ovarian responses are monitored properly with a combination of blood or urinary oestrogen assays and pelvic ultrasonography.

In conclusion, we confidently predict that continuing advances in basic and applied research in the field of ovarian endocrinology will come together over the next few years to allow further improvements in ovarian manipulation therapy. Prominent among such developments are likely to be (1) an improved understanding of the paracrine control mechanisms which subserve gonadotrophin action on the ovaries, and (2) an increase in the availability of molecularly pure, genetically engineered forms of FSH, LH and other hormones and growth factors which can be used to selectively manipulate the ovarian paracrine system. Thus in the future, more women receiving therapy aimed at ovarian augmentation or suppression can expect to have a satisfactory outcome.

# References

Abate, V., deCorato, R., Cali, A. & Stinchi, A. (1987) Endometrial biopsy at the time of embryo transfer: correlation of histological diagnosis with therapy and pregnancy rate. *J. In Vitro Fertil. Embryo Transfer*, **4**, 173−6.

Adams, J., Polson, D.W. & Franks, S. (1985) Prevalence of polycystic ovaries in women with anovulation and idiopathic hirsutism. *Br. Med. J.*, **297**, 1024−6.

Adashi, E.Y. (1984) Clomiphene citrate: mechanisms and sites of action − a hypothesis revisited. *Fertil. Steril.*, **42**, 331−44.

Buttram, V.C. Jr, Reiter, R.C. & Ward, S. (1985) Treatment of endometriosis with danazol: report of a 6 year prospective study. *Fertil. Steril.*, **43**, 353−60.

Cameron, I.T., O'Shea, F.C., Rolland, J.M., Hughes, E.G., deKretser, D.M. & Healy, D.L. (1988) Occult ovarian failure: a syndrome of infertility, regular menses and elevated follicle-stimulating hormone concentrations. *J. Clin. Endocrinol. Metab.*, **67**, 1190−4.

Cameron, I.T., Rogers, P.A.W., Caro, C., Harman, J., Healy, D.L. & Leeton, J.L. (1989) Oocyte donation: a review. *Br. J. Obstet. Gynaecol.*, **96**, 893−9.

Davoren, B. & Hsueh, A.J.W. (1986) Growth hormone increases ovarian levels of immunoreactive somatomedin-c/insulin-like growth factor-1 *in vivo*. *Endocrinology*, **118**, 888−90.

Dehou, M.F., Lejeune, B., Arijs, C. & Leroy, F. (1987) Endometrial morphology in stimulated *in vitro* fertilization cycles and after steroid replacement therapy in cases of primary ovarian failure. *Fertil. Steril.*, **48**, 995−1000.

Dericks-Tan, J.S., Hammer, E. & Taubert, H.D. (1977) The effect of D-Ser (TBU)$^6$-LH-RH-EA$^{10}$ upon gonadotropin release in normally cyclic women. *J. Clin. Endocrinol. Metab.*, **45**, 597−600.

Dmowski, W.P., Rezai, P., Anletta, F.J. & Scommegna, A. (1981) Abnormal follicle-stimulating hormone and luteinizing hormone patterns contrasting with normal estradiol and progesterone secretion in women with long standing unexplained infertility. *J. Clin. Endocrinol. Metab.*, **52**, 1218.

Droesch, K., Muasher, S.J., Kreimer, D., Seeger Jones, G., Acosta, A.A. & Rosenwaks, Z. (1988) Timing of oocyte retrieval in cycles with a spontaneous luteinizing hormone surge in a large *in vitro* fertilization program. *Fertil. Steril.*, **50**, 451−6.

Edwards, R.G. (1980) *Conception in the Human Female*, pp. 316−44. London, Academic Press.

Fioretti, P., Paoletti, A.M., Strigini, F., Mais, V., Olivieri, L. & Melis, G.B. (1989) Induction of multiple follicular development as a therapy for unexplained or male-related infertility. *Gynecol. Endocrinol.*, **3**, 45−53.

Fisch, P., Casper, R.F., Brown, S.E., Wrixon, W., Collins, J.A., Reid, R. L. & Simpson, C. (1989) Unexplained infertility: evaluation of treatment with clomiphene citrate and human chorionic gonadotrophin. *Fertil. Steril.*, **51**, 828−33.

Fishel, S.B., Edwards, R.G. & Purdy, J.M. (1984) Analysis of infertile patients treated consecutively by *in vitro* fertilization at Bourne Hall. *Fertil. Steril.*, **42**, 191−3.

Fleming, R., Haxton, M.J., Hamilton, W.P.R. *et al.* (1983) Successful treatment of infertile women with oligomenorrhoea using a combination of an LHRH agonist and exogenous gonadotropins. *Br. J. Obstet. Gynaecol.*, **92**, 369−72.

Fraser, H.M. & Baird, D.T. (1987) Clinical applications of LHRH analogues. *Baillierés Clin. Endocrinol. Metab.*, **1**, 43−70.

Garcia, J.E., Jones, G.S. & Wentz, A.C. (1977) The use of clomiphene citrate. *Fertil. Steril.*, **28**, 708−13.

Gast, M.J., Tobler, R., Strickler, R.C., Odem, R. & Pineda, J. (1988) Laser vaporization of endometriosis in an infertile population: the role of complicating infertility factors. *Fertil. Steril.*, **49**, 32−6.

Gidley-Baird, A.A., O'Neill, C., Sinosich, M.J., Porter, R.N., Pike, L. & Saunders, D.M. (1986) Failure of implantation in human *in vitro* fertilization and embryo transfer: the effects of altered progesterone/estrogen ratios in humans and mice. *Fertil. Steril.*, **45**, 69–74.

Ginther, O.J., Dierschke, D.J., Walsh, S.W. & del Campo, O.H. (1974) Anatomy of arteries and veins of uterus and ovaries in rhesus monkeys. *Biol. Reprod.*, **11**, 205–19.

Glasier, A.F., Irvine, D.S., Wickings, E.J., Hillier, S.G. & Baird, D.T. (1989) A comparison of the effects on follicular development between clomiphene citrate, its two isomers and spontaneous cycles. *Hum. Reprod.*, **4**, 252–6.

Gysler, M., Marsh, C.M., Mishell, D.R. & Bailey, E.J. (1982) A decade's experience with an individualised clomiphene treatment regimen including its effect on the postcoital test. *Fertil. Steril.*, **37**, 161–7.

Hancock, K.W., Stitch, S.R., Oakey, R.E., Scott, J.S., Levell, M.J. & Ellis, F.R. (1970) Ovarian stimulation; problems of prediction of response to gonadotrophins. *Lancet*, **ii**, 482–5.

Healy, D.L., Morrow, L., Jones, M. *et al.* (1987) Contribution of *in vitro* fertilization to the knowledge of the reproductive endocrinology of the menstrual cycle. *Clin. Endocrinol. Metab.*, **1**, 133–52.

Hillier, S.G., Afnan, A.M.M., Margara, R.A. & Winston, R.M.L. (1985) Superovulation strategy before *in vitro* fertilization. *Baillierés Clin. Obstet. Gynaecol.*, **12**, 687–723.

Hodgen, G.D. (1982) The dominant ovarian follicle. *Fertil. Steril.*, **38**, 281.

Hoff, J.D., Lasley, A.L., Wang, C.F. & Yen, S.S.C. (1977) The two pools of gonadotrophin: regulation during the menstrual cycle. *J. Clin. Endocrinol. Metab.*, **44**, 302–12.

Homburg, R., Armar, N.A., Eshel, A., Adams, J. & Jacobs, H.S. (1988a) Influence of serum luteinizing hormone concentrations on ovulation, conception, and early pregnancy loss in polycystic ovary syndrome. *Br. Med. J.*, **297**, 1024–6.

Homburg, R., Eshel, A., Abdalla, H.I. & Jacobs, H.S. (1988b) Growth hormone facilitates ovulation induction by gonadotrophins. *Clin. Endocrinol. (Oxf.)*, **29**, 113–17.

Howles, C.M., MacNamee, M.C., Edwards, R.G., Goswamy, R. & Steptoe, P.C. (1986) Effects of high tonic levels of luteinizing hormone on outcome of *in vitro* fertilization. *Lancet*, **ii**, 521–3.

Howles, C.M., MacNamee, M.L. & Edwards, R.G. (1987) The effect of progesterone supplementation prior to the induction of ovulation in women treated for *in vitro* fertilization. *Hum. Reprod.*, **2**, 91–4.

Hughes, E.G., King, C. & Wood, C. (1989) A prospective study of prognostic factors in *in vitro* fertilization and embryo transfer. *Fertil. Steril.*, **51**, 838–44.

Jiu, X.-C., Kalniju, J. & Hseuh, M.R.W. (1986) Growth hormone enhances follicle stimulating hormone-induced differentiation of cultured rat granulosa cells. *Endocrinology*, **118**, 1401–9.

Jones, H.W. Jr, Jones, G.S., Andrews, M.C. *et al.* (1982) The program for *in vitro* fertilization at Norfolk. *Fertil. Steril.*, **38**, 14–21.

Jones, H.W. Jr, Andrews, M.C., Acosta, A.A. *et al.* (1984) Three years of *in vitro* fertilization at Norfolk. *Fertil. Steril.*, **42**, 826–33.

Kamrava, M.M., Seibel, M.M., Berger, M.J., Thompson, I. & Taymor, M.L. (1982) Reversal of persistent anovulation in polycystic ovarian disease by administration of chronic low dose follicle stimulating hormone. *Fertil. Steril.*, **37**, 520–3.

Kapen, S., Boyar, R., Hellman, L. & Weitzman, E.D. (1973) Episodic release of luteinizing hormone at mid-menstrual cycle in normal adult women. *J. Clin. Endocrinol. Metab.*, **36**, 724–9.

Kerin, J.F. & Warnes, G.M. (1986) Monitoring of ovarian response to stimulation in *in vitro* fertilization cycles. *Clin. Obstet. Gynaecol.*, **29**, 158–70.

Kokko, E., Janne, O., Kanppila, A. & Vikko, R. (1981) Cyclic clomiphene citrate treatment lowers cytosol estrogen and progestin receptor concentrations in the endometrium of post-menopausal women on estrogen replacement therapy. *J. Clin. Endocrinol. Metab.*, **52**, 345–9.

Laborde, N., Carril, M., Cheviakoff, S., Croxatto, H.D., Pedroza, E. & Rosner, J.M. (1976) The secretion of progesterone during the periovulatory period in women with certified ovulation. *J. Clin. Endocrinol. Metab.*, **43**, 1157–63.

Laufer, N., DeCherney, A.H., Haseltine, F.P. *et al.* (1983) The use of high-dose human menopausal gonadotropin in an *in vitro* fertilization program. *Fertil. Steril.*, **40**, 734–7.

Laufer, N., Tarlatzis, B.C., DeCherney, A.H. *et al.* (1984) Asynchrony between human cumulus–corona cell complex and oocyte maturation after human menopausal gonadotrophin treatment for *in vitro* fertilization. *Fertil. Steril.*, **42**, 366–72.

Leeton, J., Trounson, A. & Jessup, D. (1985) Support of the luteal phase in *in vitro* fertilization programmes; results of a controlled trial with intramuscular proluton. *J. In Vitro Fertil. Embryo Transfer*, **2**, 166–74.

Leeton, J., Rogers, P.A.W., Cameron, I.T., Caro, C. & Healy, D.L. (1989) Pregnancy results following embryo transfer in women receiving low dose variable length estrogen replacement therapy for premature ovarian failure. *J. In Vitro Fertil. Embryo Transfer* **6**, 232–5.

Louvet, J.P., Harman, J.M., Schreiber, J.R. & Ross, G.T. (1975) Evidence for role of androgens in follicular maturation. *Endocrinology*, **97**, 366–72.

MacNamee, M.C., Howles, C.M., Taylor, P.J., Elder, K.T. & Edwards, R.G. (1989) Short-term luteinizing hormone-releasing hormone agonist treatment: prospective trial of a novel ovarian stimulation regimen for *in vitro* fertilization. *Fertil. Steril.*, **52**, 264–9.

Marik, J. & Hulka, J. (1978) Luteinized unruptured follicle syndrome; a subtle cause of infertility. *Fertil.*

Steril., **29**, 270.

Matta, W.H., Shaw, R.W., Hesp, R. & Katz, D. (1987) Hypogonadism induced by luteinizing hormone-releasing hormone analogues: effects on bone density in premenopausal women. *Br. Med. J.*, **294**, 1523—4.

McBain, J.C. & Trounson, A.O. (1984) Patient management—treatment cycle. In Wood, C. & Trounson, A. (eds) *Clinical In Vitro Fertilization*, pp. 49—65. Springer-Verlag, Berlin.

McLachlan, R.I., Healy, D.L. & Burger, H.G. (1986) Clinical aspects of LHRH analogues in gynaecology: a review. *Br. J. Obstet. Gynaecol.*, **93**, 411—54.

McLachlan, R.I., Robertson, D.M., Healy, D.L., deKretser, D.M., Burger, H.G. (1986) Plasma inhibin levels during gonadotrophin-induced ovarian hyperstimulation for IVF: a new index of follicular function? *Lancet*, **i**, 1233—4.

Meldrum, D.R. (1985) Clinical management of endometriosis with luteinizing hormone releasing hormone analogues. *Semin. Reprod. Endocrinol.*, **3**, 371—80.

Melis, G.B., Paoletti, A.M., Strigini, F., Menchini, Fabris, F., Canale, D. & Fioretti, P. (1987) Pharmacological induction of multiple follicular development improves the success rate of artificial insemination with husband's semen in couples with male-related or unexplained infertility. *Fertil. Steril.*, **47**, 441—5.

Miyake, A., Aone, T., Minagawa, J., Kawamura, Y. & Kurachi, K. (1980) Changes in plasma luteinizing hormone releasing hormone during clomiphene induced ovulatory cycles. *Fertil. Steril.*, **34**, 172—4.

Moses, M., Bogokowsky, H., Antebi, E., Lunenfeld, B., Raban, E., Serr, D.M. & Salonj, D.A. (1965) Thrombo-embolic phenomenon after ovarian stimulation with human gonadotrophins. *Lancet*, **ii**, 1213—15.

Oelsner, G., Serr, D.M., Mashiach, S., Blackstein, J., Snyder, M. & Lunenfeld, B. (1978) The study of induction of ovulation with menotropins: analysis of results of 1897 treatment cycles. *Fertil. Steril.*, **30**, 538.

Okamoto, S., Healy, D.L., Howlett, D.T. *et al.* (1986) An analysis of plasma estradiol concentrations using clomiphene citrate (cc)-human menopausal gonadotropin (HMG) stimulation in an in vitro fertilization-embryo transfer (IVF-ET) program. *J. Clin. Endocrinol. Metab.*, **63**, 736—40.

Oliver, E., Krapez, J., MacLachlan, V., Thomas, A. & Healy, D.L. (1988) Natural history of unsatisfactory superovulation responses in IVF. *Proc. Soc. Fertil.* (Abstr. 16).

Polson, D.W., Franks, S., Reed, M.J., Cheng, R.W., Adams, J. & James, V.H.T. (1987) The distribution of oestradiol in plasma in relation to uterine cross-sectional area in women with polycystic or multifollicular ovaries. *Clin. Endocrinol. (Oxf.)*, **26**, 581—8.

Polson, D.W., Mason, H.D., Saldahana, M.B.Y. & Franks, S. (1987) Ovulation of a single dominant follicle during treatment with low dose pulsatile follicle stimulating hormone in women with polycystic ovary syndrome. *Clin. Endocrinol. (Oxf.)*, **26**, 205—10.

Polson, D.W., Kiddy, D.S., Mason, H.D. & Franks, S. (1989) Induction of ovulation with clomiphene citrate in women with polycystic ovary syndrome: the difference between responders and nonresponders. *Fertil. Steril.*, **51**, 30—4.

Porter, R.N., Smith, W., Craft, I.L., Abdulwahid, N.A. & Jacobs, H.S. (1984) Induction of ovulation for *in vitro* fertilization using Buserelin and gonadotropins. *Lancet*, **ii**, 1284—5.

Quigley, M., Berkowitz, A.S., Gilbert, S.A. & Wolf, D.P. (1984) Clomiphene citrate in an *in vitro* fertilization program: hormonal comparisons between 50 and 150 mg daily dosage. *Fertil. Steril.*, **41**, 809—16.

Reichert, L.E. (1986) Factors affecting follitropin stimulation of target tissue. *J. Endocrinol. Suppl.* **108** (Abstr. 28).

Riesen, J.W., Koering, M.J., Meyer, R.K. & Wolf, R.C. (1970) Origin of ovarian venous progesterone in the rhesus monkey. *Endocrinology*, **86**, 1212—14.

Rogers, P., Molloy, D., Healy, D.L. *et al.* (1986) Crossover trial of superovulation protocols from two major *in vitro* fertilization centres. *Fertil. Steril.*, **46**, 424—31.

Ross, G.T., Cargille, C.M., Lipsett, M.B., Rayford, P.L., Marshall, J.R., Strott, C.A. & Rodbard, D. (1970) Pituitary and gonadal hormones in women during spontaneous and induced ovulatory cycles. *Recent Prog. Horm. Res.*, **26**, 1—62.

Ross, J.W., Paup, D.C., Brant-Zawadzki, M., Marshall, J.R. & Gorski, R.A. (1973) The effects of cis and trans-clomiphene in the induction of sexual behaviour. *Endocrinology*, **93**, 681—5.

Sagle, M., Bishop, K., Ridley, N. *et al.* (1988) Recurrent early miscarriage and polycystic ovaries. *Br. Med. J.*, **297**, 1027—8.

Sagle, M., Kiddy, D.S. & Franks, S. (1989) A prospective comparative study of low-dose HMG and FSH in polycystic ovary syndrome. *J. Endocrinol. Suppl.* **119** (Abst. 307).

Sathanadan, M., Warnes, G.M., Kirby, C.A., Petrucco, D.M. & Matthews, C.D. (1989) Adjuvant leuprolide in normal, abnormal and poor responders to controlled ovarian hyperstimulation for IVF/GIFT. *J. Clin. Endocrinol. Metab.*, **51**, 988—1006.

Schenker, J.G. & Weinstein, D. (1978) Ovarian hyperstimulation syndrome; a current survey. *Fertil. Steril.*, **30**, 255—68.

Schuilling, G.A. & Lappohn, R.E. (1985) Secretion of LH and FSH: modulation by GnRH and estrogen — basic and clinical aspects. In Coelingh Bennink, H.J.T., Dogterom, A.A., Lappohn, R.E., Rolland, R. & Schoemaker, J. (eds) *Pulsatile GnRH 1985.*

pp. 29–42. Ferring Publications, Haarlem.

Schwartz, M., Jewelewicz, R., Dyrenfurth, I., Tropper, P. & Vande Wiele, R.L. (1980) The use of human menopausal and chorionic gonadotrophin for induction of ovulation. *Am. J. Obstet. Gynecol.*, **138**, 801–7.

Smith, E.M., Anthony, F.W., Gadd, S.G. & Masson, G.M. (1989) Trial of support treatment with buserelin and human and menopausal gonadotrophin in women taking part in an *in vitro* fertilization programme. *Br. Med. J.*, **298**, 1483–6.

Stanger, J.D. & Yovitch, J.L. (1985) Reduced *in vitro* fertilization of human oocytes from patients with raised basal luteinizing hormone levels during the follicular phase. *Br. J. Obstet. Gynaecol.*, **92**, 385–90.

Sterzik, K., Dallenbach, C., Schneider, V., Sasse, V. & Dallenbach-Hellweg, C. (1988) *In vitro* fertilization: the degree of endometrial insufficiency varies with the type of ovarian stimulation. *Fertil. Steril.*, **50**, 457–62.

Taylor, P.J., Trounson, A., Besanko, M., Burger, H.G. & Stockdale, J. (1986) Plasma progesterone and prolactin changes in superovulated women before, during and immediately after laparoscopy for *in vitro* fertilization and their relation to pregnancy. *Fertil. Steril.*, **45**, 680–6.

Thomas, A., Okamoto, S., O'Shea, F., MacLachlan, V., Besanko, M. & Healy, D.L. (1989) Do raised serum luteinizing hormone levels during IVF stimulation really predict fertilization rates and clinical outcome? *Br. J. Obstet. Gynaecol.* **96**, 1328–32.

Trounson, A.O. & Leeton, J.F. (1982) The endocrinology of clomiphene stimulation. In Edwards, R.G. & Purdy, J.M. (eds) *Human Conception In Vitro*, p. 51. Academic Press, New York.

Trounson, A.O., Leeton, J.F., Wood, C., Webb, J. & Wood, J. (1981) Pregnancies in humans by fertilization *in vitro* and embryos in the control of ovulatory cycles. *Science*, **212**, 681–4.

Vaitukaitis, J.L., Bermudez, J.A., Cargille, C.M., Lipsett, M.B. & Ross, G.T. (1971) New evidence for an anti-estrogenic action of clomiphene citrate in women. *J. Clin. Endocrinol. Metab.*, **32**, 503–8.

Van Campenhout, J.C., Borreman, E.T., Wyman, H. & Antaki, I. (1973) Induction of ovulation with cis clomiphene. *Am. J. Obstet. Gynecol.*, **115**, 321.

Van Steirteghem, A.C., Smitz, J., Camus, M. *et al.* (1988) The luteal phase after *in vitro* fertilization and related procedures. *Hum. Reprod.*, **3**, 161–4.

Veeck, L.L. (1988) Oocyte assessment and biological performance. *Ann. NY Acad. Sci.*, **541**, 259–74.

Wade, H., O'Shea, F., Phillips, S., MacLachlan, V., Leahy, F. & Healy, D.L. (1988) Improving pregnancy rates using ovarian stimulation in women with idiopathic infertility. *Proc. Fertil. Soc. Aust.*, p. 18.

Wang, C.F. & Gemzell, C. (1980) The use of human gonadotropins for the induction of ovulation in women with polycystic ovary disease. *Fertil. Steril.*, **33**, 479–86.

Welner, S., DeCherney, A.H. & Polan, M.L. (1988) Human menopausal gonadotropins — a justifiable therapy in ovulatory women with long standing idiopathic infertility. *Am. J. Obstet. Gynecol.*, **158**, 111.

Wood, C., Trounson, A., Leeton, J.F. *et al.* (1981) A clinical assessment of nine pregnancies obtained by *in vitro* fertilization and embryo transfer. *Fertil. Steril.*, **35**, 502–7.

Wood, C., McMaster, R., Rennie, G., Trounson, A.O. & Leeton, J.F. (1985) Factors influencing pregnancy rates following in vitro fertilization and embryo transfer. *Fertil. Steril.*, **43**, 245–50.

# Index